Advanced Thyroid and Parathyroid Ultrasound

Mira Milas • Susan J. Mandel
Jill E. Langer
Editors

Advanced Thyroid and Parathyroid Ultrasound

Springer

Editors
Mira Milas
Department of Surgery and the Endocrinology & Metabolism Institute
University of Arizona College of Medicine - Phoenix
Banner - University Medical Center Phoenix
Phoenix, AZ, USA

Susan J. Mandel
Department of Endocrinology, Diabetes and Metabolism
Perelman School of Medicine
University of Pennsylvania
Philadelphia, PA, USA

Jill E. Langer
Department of Radiology
The Perelman School of Medicine at the University of Pennsylvania
Philadelphia, PA, USA

Videos can also be accessed at
http://link.springer.com/book/10.1007/978-3-319-44100-9

ISBN 978-3-319-44098-9 ISBN 978-3-319-44100-9 (eBook)
DOI 10.1007/978-3-319-44100-9

Library of Congress Control Number: 2017932093

Printed on acid-free paper

This Springer imprint is published by Springer Nature
The registered company is Springer International Publishing AG
The registered company address is: Gewerbestrasse 11, 6330 Cham, Switzerland

Foreword

Ultrasound for the past two or more decades has been the optimal and recommended modality for the evaluation of thyroid and parathyroid gland diseases. Basic textbooks of ultrasound relating to thyroid and parathyroid have been developed. The authors of this new textbook *Advanced Thyroid and Parathyroid Ultrasound* have compiled a large imaging atlas and resource to delineate all of the findings to date that have been associated with various features of benign and malignant nodules and disorders of the thyroid and parathyroid glands.

The important concepts are both the imaging and the advanced components. Over and above basic ultrasonography of the thyroid and parathyroid, this textbook utilizes a large amount of imagery so the latest references and characteristics related to benign and malignant characteristics can be detailed for nodular thyroid disease.

This represents an important step forward as a very useful textbook for those who are active in fields of endocrine neck ultrasound including endocrinologists, radiologists, surgeons, other clinicians, and also for teaching residents and fellows. This book serves as a practical guide and reference source for understanding the rationale of how all thyroid nodules are assessed relative to the risk of their imaged findings. It is rich with cine clips and practical illustrations of parathyroid disease findings, needle aspiration.

It promises to be a stand-alone, new book highly desirable for acquisition and utilization. Since it is based on primarily imagery, it represents an important addition to the endocrine neck literature and practical elements of endocrine patient care. The three highly experienced and respected editors are authorities, practitioners, and teachers of ultrasound with endocrine surgery, endocrinology, and radiology backgrounds. They represent the multidisciplinary spirit and content of this textbook, and this editorial collaboration emphasizes the broad applicability of this text to all clinical fields using ultrasound for endocrine diseases of the neck.

Daniel S. Duick, M.D., M.A.C.E.

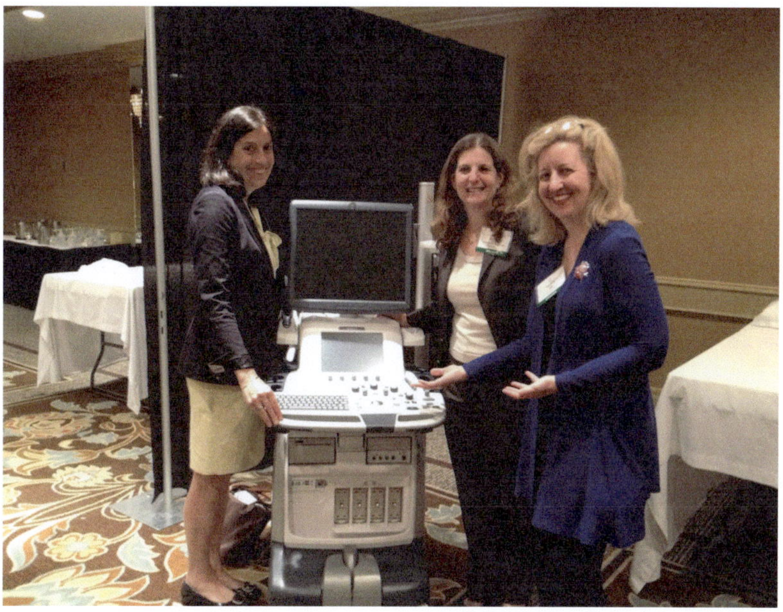

With heartfelt gratitude and appreciation to our families, colleagues, students, and patients for the gift of an inspiring life in medicine

Preface

Ultrasound is the single most essential companion to the medical care of patients with thyroid and parathyroid disease. Ultrasound is both the imaging modality of choice and the means of guiding interventions, literally for biopsies or ablations and figuratively for clinical and surgical decisions. This ultrasound book is a state-of-the-art atlas of contemporary knowledge and performance of neck ultrasound for endocrine disorders. It continues a tradition of excellence that Springer has established in the field of ultrasound education. It also establishes a new style of ultrasound education that, like the images themselves, is rich in real-time, dynamic content.

The inspiration for this ultrasound textbook came from the numerous invaluable teaching sessions that the authors and editors have engaged in via our professional societies over the years. Each author was specifically drawn from experts who as clinicians use ultrasound daily. Authors from all medical specialties relevant to thyroid and parathyroid ultrasound were purposefully represented. Comprehensive topics and all innovations that are currently in use were included so that the textbook can serve as an in-depth resource to novice and advanced sonographers. We wished to recreate the energy and eureka moments of appreciating ultrasound images that often occurred during didactic conferences. There, as those who have attended these conferences know, the interactions were case-based, practical, and infused with pearls from clinical experience. Often actual patient volunteers would give of their time and privacy to be ultrasound models. To them we are especially grateful and because of them ultrasound exists.

As editors we have learned tremendously from each other over the years. Converging on the topic of ultrasound has enhanced the way we bring diagnostic and therapeutic care to our patients and been a joyful dimension of our professional careers. We wished to pass this forward in a way that stimulates colleagues, residents, fellows, and students and all who encounter ultrasound to continue to learn new skills, refine interpretations, and innovate better ultrasound applications. A guiding philosophy is that the responsibility of working with ultrasound extends beyond the care of the patient to ongoing motivation and education of those who provide that care.

Internet Access to Video Clip: The owner of this text will be able to access these video clips through Springer with the following Internet link: http:// link.springer.com/book/10.1007/978-3-319-44100-9.

A unique and pioneering component is that the book is associated with a video library of ultrasound cine clips and case-based discussions. This allows the best aspect of ultrasound—the real-time viewing—to exist as an effective learning venue. A video icon in the chapters marks that additional material can be viewed in the online version of the book. The commentary accompanying the various themes hopes to enhance the understanding of ultrasound details and the fact that these details matter. As a visual discipline, ultrasound is inherently subject to interobserver variability and the truth of the proverbial expression, "the eyes cannot see what the mind does not know." We hope that the readers benefit from hearing the rationale behind the technical and medical parameters of ultrasound and broaden their knowledge and application of this technology.

The book is intended for all who care about patients with thyroid and parathyroid conditions, of all specialties. Communication, collegiality, and a multidisciplinary engagement have been the hallmark of our experience with ultrasound at its best. Although a novice sonographer will be able to understand all of the topics, they are presented from a vantage point of complex and nuanced decision-making encountered in real clinical scenarios. The sections are organized according to a logical structure covering benign and malignant thyroid conditions, parathyroid disease, and ultrasound technology, ultrasound-guided interventions, educational opportunities, and innovations. The style of the chapters is intended to communicate practical, actionable information with rich illustration. We also highlight how different specialists uniquely apply ultrasound in given clinical scenarios. Significantly, the book's publication was timed to coincide with all the most current guidelines for management of thyroid nodules, thyroid cancer, and hyperparathyroidism, both national and international. Therefore, a novel contribution is the emphasis on pattern recognition and risk stratification as the advised approach to and the new lexicon of ultrasound interpretation.

As surgeons, endocrinologists, and radiologists we appreciate the role ultrasound has played in our fields and the invaluable way in which it improves patient encounters. We are grateful to countless mentors, colleagues, and patients who enabled the creation of this book and dedicate it to those who will continue to advance ultrasound in modern medicine.

Phoenix, AZ, USA — Mira Milas, M.D.
Philadelphia, PA, USA — Susan J. Mandel, M.D., M.P.H.
Philadelphia, PA, USA — Jill E. Langer, M.D.

Contents

Contributors

Devaprabhu Abraham, M.D. Department of Medicine, University of Utah, Salt Lake City, UT, USA

Salmaan Ahmed, M.D. Department of Diagnostic Radiology, The University of Texas MD Anderson Cancer Center, Houston, TX, USA

Zubair W. Baloch, M.D., Ph.D. Department of Pathology and Laboratory Medicine, University of Pennsylvania Medical Center, Perelman School of Medicine, Philadelphia, PA, USA

Eren Berber, M.D. Department of Endocrine Surgery, The Cleveland Clinic, Cleveland, OH, USA

Denise Carneiro-Pla, M.D., F.A.C.S. Division of Oncologic and Endocrine Surgery, Department of Surgery, Medical University of South Carolina, Charleston, SC, USA

Yufei Chen, M.D. Department of Surgery, Massachusetts General Hospital, Harvard Medical School, Boston, MA, USA

Vijayaratna Chockalingham, M.D. Department of Endocrinology, Banner - University Medical Center Phoenix, University of Arizona College of Medicine – Phoenix, Phoenix, AZ, USA

Jean-François Cléroux, M.D., F.R.C.P.C. Jt Department of Medical Imaging, University Health Network – Mt Sinai Hospital – Women's College Hospital, University of Toronto, Toronto, ON, Canada

James M. Debnam, M.D. Section of Neuro Radiology, Department of Diagnostic Radiology, The University of Texas M. D. Anderson Cancer Center, Houston, TX, USA

Manish Dhyani, M.D. Department of Radiology, Massachusetts General Hospital, Harvard Medical School, Boston, MA, USA

Manjiri K. Dighe, M.D. Department of Radiology, University of Washington, Seattle, WA, USA

William S. Duke, M.D., F.A.C.S. Department of Otolaryngology—Head and Neck Surgery, Augusta University, Augusta, GA, USA

Renee K. Dversdal, M.D. Division of Hospital Medicine, Department of Medicine, Oregon Health and Science University, Portland, OR, USA

Beth S. Edeiken-Monroe, M.D., F.A.C.R. Department of Diagnostic Imaging, The University of Texas MD Anderson Cancer Center, Houston, TX, USA

Dina Elaraj, M.D., F.A.C.S. Section of Endocrine Surgery, Department of Surgery, Northwestern University Feinberg School of Medicine, Chicago, IL, USA

Andrea Frasoldati, M.D. Endocrine Unit, Arcispedale Santa Maria Nuova - Research Hospital (IRCCS) for Advanced Technologies and Clinical Pathways in Oncology, Reggio Emilia, Italy

Jeremy L. Freeman, M.D., F.R.C.S., F.A.C.S. Department of Otolaryngology—Head and Neck Surgery, Mount Sinai Hospital, University of Toronto, Toronto, ON, Canada

Sangeet Ghai, M.D., F.R.C.R. Jt. Department of Medical Imaging, University Health Network – Mt Sinai Hospital – Women's College Hospital, University of Toronto, Toronto, ON, Canada

Andrew G. Gianoukakis, M.D. Department of Medicine, Division of Endocrinology, Harbor-UCLA Medical Center and the David Geffen School of Medicine at UCLA, Torrance, CA, USA

Allan Golding, M.D., F.A.C.E., E.C.N.U. Department of Endocrine Surgery, Memorial Physician Group, Hollywood, FL, USA

Edward G. Grant, M.D. Department of Radiology, Keck Hospital of USC, University of Southern California, Los Angeles, CA, USA

Marlon A. Guerrero, M.D., F.A.C.S. Department of Surgery, Banner – University Medical Center, Tucson Campus, University of Arizona, Tucson, AZ, USA

Maria K. Gule-Monroe, M.D. The Department of Diagnostic Radiology, The University of Texas M. D. Anderson Cancer Center, Houston, TX, USA

Nicholas J. Hangiandreou, Ph. D. Department of Radiology, Mayo Clinic, Rochester, MN, USA

R. Mack Harrell, M.D., F.A.C.P., F.A.C.E., E.C.N.U. Department of Endocrine Surgery, Memorial Health Systems, Hollywood, FL, USA

P. Ryan Hungerford, M.D., F.A.C.E., E.C.N.U. Rogue Valley Physicians, Medford, OR, USA

John Interlandi, M.D., F.A.C.E., E.C.N.U. Department of Endocrinology, Advanced Health Partners, Hermitage, TN, USA

Jason Michael Johnson, M.D. The Department of Diagnostic Radiology, The University of Texas M. D. Anderson Cancer Center, Houston, TX, USA

Sathya Jyothinagaram, M.D., F.A.C.E. Diabetes and Endocrinology Institute, Banner - University Medical Center Phoenix, University of Arizona College of Medicine – Phoenix, Phoenix, AZ, USA

Colleen M. Kiernan, M.D., M.P.H. Department of General Surgery, Vanderbilt University, Nashville, TN, USA

Lawrence T. Kim, M.D., F.A.C.S. Division of Surgical Oncology, Department of Surgery, University of North Carolina, Chapel Hill, NC, USA

Vikram D. Krishnamurthy, M.D. Department of Endocrine Surgery, The Cleveland Clinic, Cleveland, OH, USA

Vinodh A. Kumar, M.D. Department of Diagnostic Radiology, The University of Texas M. D. Anderson Cancer Center, Houston, TX, USA

Michael Kwon, M.D., Ph.D. Department of Diagnostic Radiology, The University of Texas MD Anderson Cancer Center, Houston, TX, USA

Brian H. Lang, M.S., F.R.A.C.S., F.C.S.H.K., F.H.K.A.M. Division of Endocrine Surgery, Department of Surgery, Queen Mary Hospital, The University of Hong Kong, Pokfulam, Hong Kong, SAR, China

Jill E. Langer, M.D. Department of Radiology, The Perelman School of Medicine at the University of Pennsylvania, Philadelphia, PA, USA

Robert A. Levine, M.D., F.A.C.E., E.C.N.U. Thyroid Center of New Hampshire, St. Joseph Hospital Endocrinology, Geisel School of Medicine at Dartmouth College, Nashua, NH, USA

Changtian Li, M.D., Ph.D. Department of Ultrasound, Chinese PLA General Hospital, Beijing, China

Ilya Likhterov, M.D. Department of Otolaryngology Head and Neck Surgery, Mount Sinai Beth Israel, New York, NY, USA

Mark A. Lupo, M.D., F.A.C.E., E.C.N.U. Thyroid & Endocrine Center of Florida, Florida State University, College of Medicine, Sarasota, FL, USA

Harshawn Malhi, M.D. Department of Radiology, Keck Hospital of USC, University of Southern California, Los Angeles, CA, USA

Susan J. Mandel, M.D., M.P.H. Division of Endocrinology, Diabetes and Metabolism, Perelman School of Medicine, University of Pennsylvania, Philadelphia, PA, USA

Nicole A. Massol, M.D., F.A.S.C.P. Division of Cytopathology, University of Arkansas for Medical Sciences, Little Rock, AR, USA

Peter J. Mazzaglia, M.D. Rhode Island Hospital, The Warren Alpert School of Medicine, Brown University, University Surgical Associates, Providence, RI, USA

Caitlin P. McMullen, M.D. Department of Otolaryngology—Head and Neck Surgery, Mount Sinai Hospital, University of Toronto, Toronto, ON, Canada

William D. Middleton, M.D. Mallinckrodt Institute of Radiology, Washington University School of Medicine, Saint Louis, MO, USA

Mira Milas, M.D., F.A.C.S. Department of Surgery and the Endocrinology & Metabolism Institute, University of Arizona College of Medicine - Phoenix, Banner - University Medical Center Phoenix, Phoenix, AZ, USA

Zvonimir Luka Milas, M.D., F.A.C.S. Department of Surgery, Levine Cancer Center at the Carolinas Medical Center, University of North Carolina Chappell Hill, Charlotte, NC, USA

Barbra S. Miller Division of Endocrine Surgery, Section of General Surgery, University of Michigan, Ann Arbor, MI, USA

Liudmila Muraveika, M.D., P.H.D. Department of Surgery, Stanford University Medical Center, Palo Alto, CA, USA

Lisa A. Orloff, M.D. F.A.C.S., F.A.C.E. Director of Endocrine Head & Neck Surgery, Professor of Otolaryngology - Head & Neck Surgery, Thyroid & Parathyroid Surgery, Stanford University School of Medicine and Stanford Cancer Center, Stanford, CA, USA

Claudio Maurizio Pacella, M.D. Department of Diagnostic Imaging and Interventional Radiology, Regina Apostolorum Hospital, Rome, Italy

Enrico Papini Department of Endocrinology and Metabolism, Regina Apostolorum Hospital, Rome, Italy

Sareh Parangi, M.D. Department of Surgery, Massachusetts General Hospital, Harvard Medical School, Boston, MA, USA

Daniel Rocke, M.D., J.D. Division of Head and Neck Surgery & Communication Sciences, Department of Surgery, Duke University Medical Center, Durham, NC, USA

Anthony E. Samir Department of Radiology, Harvard Medical School, Massachusetts General Hospital, Boston, MA, USA

Dawid Schlingerhout, M.D. Section of Neuro Radiology, Department of Diagnostic Radiology, The University of Texas M. D. Anderson Cancer Center, Houston, TX, USA

Merry E. Sebelik, M.D., F.A.C.S. Department of Otolaryngology, Head & Neck Surgery, Veterans Affairs Medical Center-Atlanta, Emory University School of Medicine, Atlanta, GA, USA

Komal B. Shah, M.D. Department of Diagnostic Radiology, The University of Texas MD Anderson Cancer Center, Houston, TX, USA

Joyce J. Shin, M.D., F.A.C.S. Department of Endocrine Surgery, The Cleveland Clinic, Cleveland, OH, USA

Maisie L. Shindo Director of Thyroid & Parathyroid Center, Director of Head & Neck Endocrine Surgery, Department of Otolaryngology, Oregon Health & Science University, Portland, OR, USA

Allan E. Siperstein Endocrine Surgery Department, Cleveland Clinic, Cleveland, OH, USA

Jennifer A. Sipos, M.D. Division of Endocrinology, Diabetes and Metabolism, The Ohio State University Wexner Medical Center, Columbus, OH, USA

Amy Sisley, M.D. University of Arizona College of Medicine Phoenix, Banner – University Medical Center Phoenix, Phoenix, AZ, USA

John Woody Sistrunk, M.D., E.C.N.U. Jackson Thyroid & Endocrine Clinic, PLLC, Jackson, MS, USA

Robert A. Sofferman, M.D., F.A.C.S. Division of Otolaryngology—HNS, University of Vermont Medical Center, Burlington, VT, USA

Carmen C. Solórzano, M.D., F.A.C.S. Division of Surgical Oncology and Endocrine Surgery, Department of Surgery, Vanderbilt University Medical Center, Nashville, TN, USA

Antonia E. Stephen, M.D. Department of Surgery, Massachusetts General Hospital, Harvard Medical School, Boston, MA, USA

David Steward, M.D. University of Cincinnati, Cincinnati, OH, USA

Nicole L. Strissel, M.S., R.V.T., R.D.M.S. Department of Radiology, Mayo Clinic, Rochester, MN, USA

Cord Sturgeon, M.D., M.S., F.A.C.S. Department of Surgery, Northwestern University, Chicago, IL, USA

David J. Terris, M.D., F.A.C.S., F.A.C.E. Department of Otolaryngology—Head and Neck Surgery, Augusta University, Augusta, GA, USA

Dubravka Milas Tollison, M.D. Department of Family Medicine, Banner - University Medical Center Phoenix, University of Arizona College of Medicine – Phoenix, Phoenix, AZ, USA

Petros Tsamatropoulos, M.D. Endocrine Unit, Arcispedale Santa Maria Nuova - Research Hospital (IRCCS) for Advanced Technologies and Clinical Pathways in Oncology, Reggio Emilia, Italy

Mark L. Urken, M.D. Department of Otolaryngology Head and Neck Surgery, Mount Sinai Beth Israel, New York, NY, USA

Roberto Valcavi, M.D., F.A.C.E. Endocrine Unit, Centro Palmer, Reggio Emilia, Italy

Thinh Vu, M.D. Department of Diagnostic Radiology, The University of Texas MD Anderson Cancer Center, Houston, TX, USA

Emily Watters, M.D., M.P.H. Phoenix Integrated Surgery Residency, University of Arizona College of Medicine Phoenix, Banner – University Medical Center Phoenix, Phoenix, AZ, USA

Elizabeth O. Westfall, M.D. Department of Medical Imaging, Banner - University Medical Center Phoenix, Phoenix, AZ, USA

Teresa Wu, M.D. Center for Simulation & Innovation, University of Arizona, College of Medicine-Phoenix, Phoenix, AZ, USA

Department of Emergency Medicine, Banner - University Medical Center Phoenix, Phoenix, AZ, USA

Marcelle Yehuda, M.D. Department of Medicine, Division of Endocrinology, Harbor-UCLA Medical Center and the David Geffen School of Medicine at UCLA, Torrance, CA, USA

Part I

Ultrasound in Clinical Practice: Philosophy and Logistics

Thyroid and Parathyroid Ultrasound: Comprehensive and Problem-Focused Point-of-Care Utilization in Clinical Practice

1

Marelle Yehuda, Elizabeth O. Westfall, Mira Milas, and Andrew G. Gianoukakis

1.1 Introduction

The modern use of bedside ultrasonography has changed the practice of medical care. Ultrasonography's relative ease of use, low cost, and bedside availability have made it invaluable in many clinical settings including those in which patients with thyroid and parathyroid disease are evaluated.

This chapter provides an overview of comprehensive and point-of-care applications of ultrasound (US) in the medical and surgical evaluation of patients with thyroid or parathyroid pathology. We also address potential pitfalls in the use of point-of-care neck ultrasound: the interobserver variability, the limited sensitivity of ultrasound to detect various pathologies, and the need to employ other imaging methods when appropriate.

1.1.1 History of Sonography

The modern ultrasound arises from the concept of echolocation and the pulse echo principle. In the late eighteenth century, experimental biologist Lazzaro Spallanzani, demonstrated that bats use sound waves for hunting and navigation [1]. In the ensuing centuries, scientists continued to study the concept of sound and echolocation and eventually began utilizing knowledge of sound waves and principles of physics to measure distance underwater, known as Sound Navigation and Ranging or SONAR. As this technology became more refined during World War II, the medical profession attempted to employ ultrasound as a therapeutic treatment for various ailments, such as arthritis [2]. The first physician credited with producing clinical ultrasound images for diagnostic purposes was Karl Dussik, an Austrian neurologist at the University of Vienna who used ultrasound

M. Yehuda, M.D. • A.G. Gianoukakis, M.D. (✉)
Department of Medicine, Division of Endocrinology, Harbor-UCLA Medical Center and the David Geffen School of Medicine at UCLA, 1124 West Carson St. RB-1, Torrance, CA 90502, USA
e-mail: marelleyehuda@gmail.com; agianoukakis@mednet.ucla.edu

E.O. Westfall, M.D.
Department of Medical Imaging, Banner - University Medical Center Phoenix, 1111 E. McDowell Road, Phoenix, AZ 85006, USA
e-mail: Elizabeth.westfall@bannerhealth.com

M. Milas, M.D., F.A.C.S.
Department of Surgery and the Endocrinology & Metabolism Institute, University of Arizona College of Medicine - Phoenix, Banner - University Medical Center Phoenix, 1441 North 12th Street 2nd floor, Phoenix, AZ 85006, USA
e-mail: Mira.Milas@bannerhealth.com

M. Milas et al. (eds.), *Advanced Thyroid and Parathyroid Ultrasound*,
DOI 10.1007/978-3-319-44100-9_1

to image and measure the intracranial ventricles [2]. Around the same time, George Ludwig, a researcher at the Naval Medical Research Institute, began experimenting with A-mode ultrasound to detect gallstones in animal models [1]. In the 1960s and 1970s, researchers began using ultrasound to evaluate the thyroid gland. An early thyroid ultrasound apparatus is seen pictured in Fig. 1.1 [3]. Due to a lack of widespread ultrasound availability and expertise, thyroid ultrasonography was not routinely used in clinical practice for the next two decades [4]. By the early 2000s, more affordable equipment made the acquisition and use of ultrasound feasible for clinicians. Figure 1.2 shows the dramatic progress in ultrasound technology with regard to quality of imaging and design of ultra-compact sonographic machines over the past 15 years.

Today, ultrasound machines are found in almost every emergency room and are used for the rapid assessment of trauma patients and the bedside evaluation of a plethora of medical conditions. Ultrasonography has also been incorporated into medical care facilities at a distance from tertiary referral centers. Ultrasound probes remotely operated by technicians via robotics can be used to obtain diagnostic images in rural medical clinics or remote locations, such as the South Pole [5]. Even the International Space Station has an ultrasound machine in its Human Research

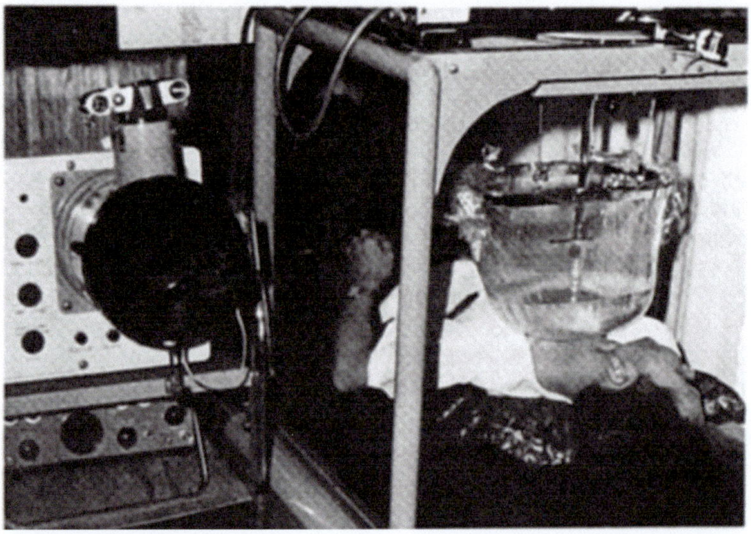

Fig. 1.1 A historical image circa 1967 of the beginning of thyroid ultrasound. Fujimoto Y, Oka A, Omoto R, Hirose M. Ultrasound scanning of the thyroid gland as a new diagnostic approach. Ultrasonics. 1967;5(3):177–80. With permission

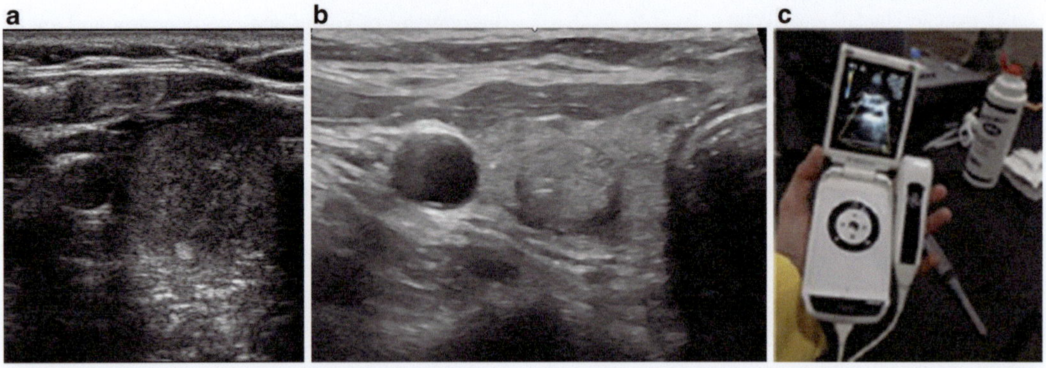

Fig. 1.2 Improvements in ultrasound image quality are evident when comparing a right thyroid nodule image from 2005 (**a**) to one obtained in 2015 (**b**). A handheld ultrasound is capable of detecting major thyroid abnormalities though models currently available still await high-frequency transducers to provide fine imaging details (**c**). Author's image

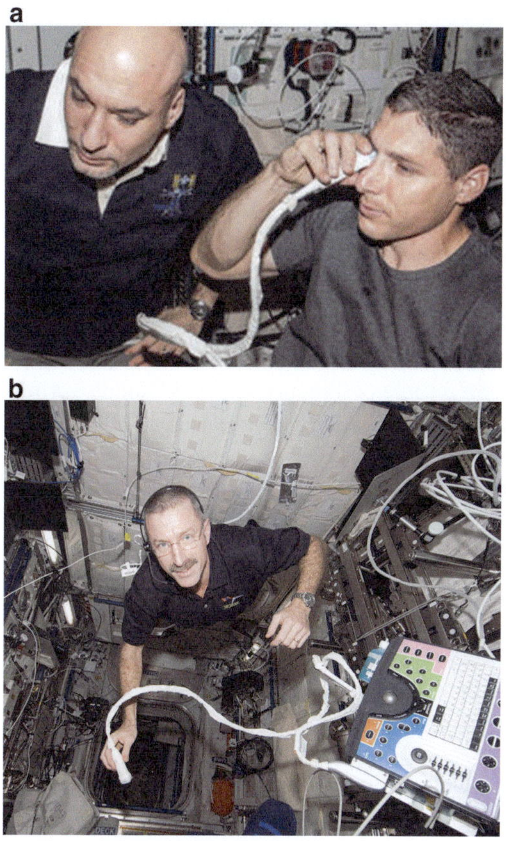

Fig. 1.3 (**a**, **b**) Human Research Facility Ultrasound on the International Space Station 2 [6, 7]

Facility, the Advanced Diagnostic Ultrasound in Microgravity (ADUM). The ADUM ultrasound is a commercial ultrasound that has been modified to allow astronaut crew members to perform their own ultrasound exams, guided by ground medical personnel [6, 7] (Fig. 1.3). The utility and scope of ultrasound are expanding, and providers in all fields of medicine, working in a variety of settings, are incorporating its use into their practice.

1.1.2 What Is Point-of-Care Ultrasound?

Point-of-care ultrasound, also called bedside, provider-performed, or focused ultrasound, can be defined as the utilization of sonography to answer a specific clinical question at the time of patient presentation and examination [8]. In a 2011 New England Journal of Medicine review article, Moore defined point-of-care ultrasonography as the use of "real-time dynamic images (rather than images recorded by a sonographer and interpreted later), which allow findings to be directly correlated with the patient's presenting signs and symptoms" [9]. The paradigm shift created by point-of-care ultrasound is that the clinician develops a clinical question and then performs and interprets the imaging test in real time, as opposed to the traditional practice of sending the patient for a sonogram and waiting for the results.

Point-of-care ultrasound was first utilized for trauma evaluation in Europe in the 1970s and became common in US trauma care by the mid-1980s. The first standardized point-of-care use of ultrasound was the Focused Assessment with Sonography for Trauma (FAST) exam. The FAST exam, adopted in the 1990s, includes a basic series of four views for the evaluation of free abdominal fluid and has replaced diagnostic peritoneal lavage for the evaluation of blunt abdominal trauma. FAST has now been expanded to include the evaluation for pneumothorax and fluid or blood in the thorax post trauma [10].

Today, point-of-care clinician-performed ultrasound is the standard of care in surgery, obstetrics and gynecology, emergency medicine, ophthalmology, as well as internal medicine and most of its subspecialties (cardiology, gastroenterology, endocrinology, and intensive care). The term comprehensive ultrasound, in a very traditional sense, refers to an ultrasound that is conducted in a radiology department, where the main goal is to communicate information to clinicians who themselves may not view or interpret the images and require a thorough description in order to make clinical decisions. Comprehensive ultrasound may also refer to the provision of diagnostic, interventional, and therapeutic ultrasonography for patient care, whether this occurs in a radiology department or a clinical office setting. Descriptions of point-of-care and comprehensive ultrasound contain complementary and overlapping concepts.

1.2 Point-of-Care Ultrasound of the Thyroid and Parathyroid Glands

In the late 1960s, researchers began experimenting with sonography to estimate the weight of the thyroid gland and to identify solid and cystic lesions. In 1970, the Journal of Clinical Endocrinology and Metabolism published its first paper describing thyroid ultrasound. Patients were scanned using two-dimensional B-mode and, if a lesion was detected, one-dimensional A-mode, to differentiate cystic from solid lesions. The images, which were transferred to film, were basic and of poor quality when compared to today's standards (Fig. 1.4) [11]. Despite these shortcomings, early thyroid ultrasonography was recognized for its utility to detect and measure lesions as well as to distinguish between solid and cystic thyroid lesions. Furthermore, even in those early days of thyroid ultrasonography, investigators hypothesized that ultrasound may have the potential to distinguish between benign and malignant thyroid lesions [11].

1.3 Why Perform Point-of-Care Neck Ultrasound

The point-of-care neck ultrasound can be used to evaluate suspected anatomical or functional thyroid and parathyroid disease (Table 1.1). Along with a history and physical exam, the point-of-care neck ultrasound can be used by the provider to assess the thyroid and generate a differential diagnosis and plan of care. Whether a patient presents complaining of a neck mass or the provider palpates a lesion on neck exam, the bedside ultrasound can be utilized to identify the presence of intrathyroidal lesions, extrathyroidal lesions, or diffuse enlargement of the thyroid. In cases in which the patient presents with signs or symptoms of hyperthyroidism, a bedside ultrasound can discover a solitary nodule, leading to suspicion for a hyperfunctioning "hot" nodule, or recognize a diffusely enlarged and vascular gland, characteristic of Graves' disease.

1.3.1 Nodules

Thyroid nodules are highly prevalent in the general population, and their incidence increases with age [12]. The superficial location of the thyroid gland permits the palpation and recognition of larger lesions, and the frequent use of imaging in medicine leads to the discovery of incidental small lesions. No matter the method of discovery of a thyroid nodule, bedside ultrasound can be used to evaluate and characterize the lesion. Ultrasound is used to assess a nodule's risk of malignancy based on US characteristics, and to guide further decision-making and management by facilitating and guiding fine-needle aspiration (FNA) [13]. Ultrasound also facilitates the evaluation of cervical lymph nodes in the context of

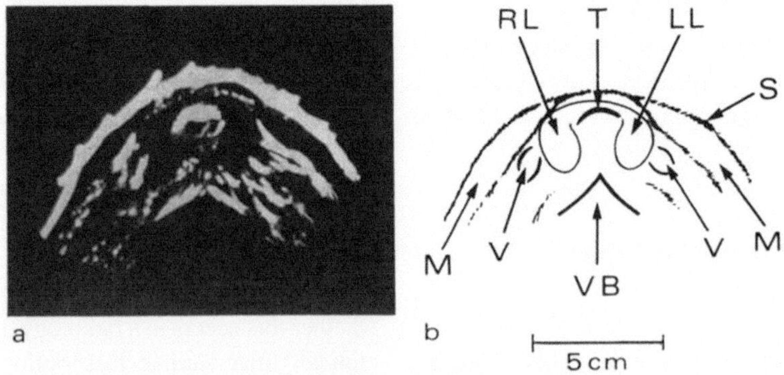

Fig. 1.4 Early ultrasound image of normal thyroid. (**a**) Ultrasonic tomogram (B-scan) at low sensitivity. (**b**) Schematic representation: RL, right thyroid lobe; LL, left thyroid lobe; T, anterior wall of the trachea; VB, vertebral body; V, vascular sheath; S, skin and transducer artifact; and M, sternomastoid muscle. From J Clin Endocrinol Metab. 1971; (32): 709. With permission

Table 1.1 Indications and information from point-of-care ultrasound

• Clarification of clinical exam findings
• Accurate diagnosis of thyroid and parathyroid disease
• Differentiation of cystic vs. solid masses
• Measurement of lesions
• Thyroid nodule ultrasonographic feature characterization and pattern recognition
• Malignancy risk assessment of thyroid nodules
• Lymph node screening with initial thyroid nodule detection
• Lymph node mapping with thyroid cancer
• Localization of abnormal parathyroid glands
• Visual guidance for interventions (biopsy, cyst drainage, alcohol ablation)
• Improvement of biopsy accuracy
• Monitoring of response to therapy
• Identification of recurrent/persistent cancer
• Evaluation of cervical lymphadenopathy or metastases
• Optimization of surgical incision placement
• Optimization of surgical planning based on details of findings (signs of local invasion, substernal goiter extension, tracheal deviation)
• Laryngeal ultrasound for vocal cord mobility
• Identification of coexisting pathology
• Intraoperative evaluation
• Education
• Communication of findings to multidisciplinary providers

thyroid or other neck masses and guides the need for FNA.

1.3.2 Parathyroid

Hyperparathyroidism can be due to a single adenoma, multiglandular disease, or, in rare cases, parathyroid cysts or carcinoma [14, 15]. The incidence of primary hyperparathyroidism is much higher in women than in men, and the prevalence increases with age [14]. The parathyroid glands can be imaged with a variety of modalities; CT, MRI, ultrasound, and scintigraphy. The various imaging modalities for the parathyroid glands provide complementary information for the diagnosis of parathyroid disease and for surgical preparation and planning [16]. Ultrasound's benefits are that it easily locates and defines anatomical features of superficial, enlarged, parathyroid glands as well as coexistent thyroid abnormalities. While it can be a useful tool, the practitioner must be aware of its limitations and pitfalls and be ready to utilize additional diagnostic testing to ensure the correct diagnosis and treatment. The ultrasound imaging characteristics of abnormal parathyroid glands are addressed in detail in Chap. 24 of this book.

1.4 Expanding the Traditional Use of Thyroid and Parathyroid Ultrasound: Perils and Pitfalls

Originally, in the domain of radiologists, ultrasound is now used by practitioners in almost all specialties. In the 1970s, trauma physicians became the first to employ non-radiologist-performed ultrasonography, and its application has expanded since then. Ultrasound is now utilized by a wide range of providers, from medical students to physician assistants, nurse practitioners, residents, fellows, and practicing clinicians.

Performing and interpreting ultrasound is a learned skill. As this imaging modality has moved to the bedside, a debate has ensued regarding who should be performing and interpreting point-of-care ultrasound, how these tests should be documented and billed, as well as how the accuracy and quality of the test can be assured [17, 18].

In point-of-care ultrasonography, the operator is both obtaining and interpreting images; thus, adequate operator training and experience are essential to its performance. In a prospective 2010 study by Kim et al., ultrasound diagnostic performance of radiology residents was compared to that of radiology faculty. Diagnostic performance was statistically significantly greater among faculty compared to junior and senior residents ($p=0.007$ and $p=0.003$, respectively) [19]. In another prospective study demonstrating the importance of sonographer experience, 52 post-thyroidectomy patients with high-risk thyroid cancer had ultrasounds performed by two different providers with different levels of experience. Neck ultrasounds performed by the less experienced provider found six proven cases of recurrent disease. In the same group of patients, an expert sonographer found 16 proven cases of recurrence, demonstrating that identification of disease recurrence is operator dependent [20]. Other studies have compared ultrasound interpretation between practitioners in different specialties. A retrospective analysis of surgeon- vs. radiologist-performed bedside ultrasounds at the University of Wisconsin found that when surgeons performed the preoperative ultrasound, they documented lymph node status more frequently (69 % vs. 20 %, $p<0.01$) compared to radiologists. In postsurgical follow-up, the patients scanned by the surgeons exhibited less neck RAI uptake at the time of ablation and had lower recurrence rates (12 % vs. 0 %, $p=0.01$) suggesting that surgeon-performed sonography allows for better preoperative planning and more extensive surgical resection when indicated [21]. This study which examined provider-specific point-of-care imaging vs. comprehensive ultrasonography reflects the importance of problem-focused use of ultrasound. Since the operative plan is dependent on preoperative radiologic evaluation, the surgeon is focused on gaining anatomic information that will guide surgery and minimize unexpected findings in the operating room. Radiologists face inherent limitations when presented with interpreting an ultrasound study ordered simply as a "thyroid ultrasound." Images saved by a sonographer following a routine thyroid protocol may not capture anatomic areas important to the surgeon such as the tracheoesophageal groove, the recurrent laryngeal nerve, and lateral neck lymph nodes. In conclusion, the diagnostic performance of ultrasound may be dependent on both operator experience, as well as the goals and role, of the sonographer.

1.5 Radiologic Studies Complementing Thyroid/Parathyroid US

While this textbook is devoted to ultrasound imaging, other radiologic modalities may be needed to complement, clarify, and expand upon the findings of ultrasound. These imaging methods include computed tomography scanning (CT), four-dimensional computed tomography (4DCT), magnetic resonance imaging (MRI), positron emission tomography (PET), nuclear medicine applications of radioiodine scanning, and Tc99m-sestamibi scanning. These additional imaging modalities can be of assistance in: (1) Evaluating the mediastinum including cases of goiter with substernal extension, (2) Evaluating retropharyngeal cervical metastases or invasion of thyroid cancer into surrounding anatomical structures such as the trachea or esophagus, (3) Discovering distant metastases, (4) Determining the etiology of and quantifying hyperthyroidism (5) Further characterizing and localizing abnormal parathyroid glands.

Innovations in radiology techniques have expanded the options for patient evaluation and treatment. A case in point is parathyroid imaging. As minimally invasive parathyroidectomy gained popularity over the traditional bilateral neck exploration, preoperative identification of autonomously functioning parathyroid glands became crucial. While ultrasound is a sensitive modality to identify superficial parathyroid adenomas, it has limitations in identifying supernumerary, substernal, or ectopic parathyroids. Therefore, ultrasonography and scintigraphy are often utilized as complementary imaging modalities. A 2005 meta-analysis by Ruda et al. [22] found that for the detection of single parathyroid adenomas, Tc99m-sestamibi was superior to ultrasound with a sensitivity of 88.4 % vs. 78.5 %. The sensitivity of both imaging modalities in this study decreased dramatically when multiglandular disease (MGD) or double adenomas (DA) were present (sestamibi 44.46 % vs. 34.86 % for ultrasound and 29.95 % vs. 16.20 %, respectively). Contemporary practice calls for combining neck ultrasound imaging with either 4DCT or Tc99m-sestamibi prior to parathyroid surgery in all cases [23]. It is important to recognize the limitations of technology, interobserver variability, and local expertise when selecting how to combine these imaging modalities.

1.6 The Rationale for a Multidisciplinary Ultrasound Textbook

In January 2016, guidelines for the management of thyroid nodules and thyroid cancer were published by the American Thyroid Association [13], and it is anticipated that the American Association of Endocrine Surgeons will publish guidelines for the management of primary hyperparathyroidism later in 2016. This textbook has been compiled shortly following these updated guidelines. The spirit and content of the new ultrasound-related recommendations of these guidelines are illustrated in this textbook. The emphasis is on practical implementation and improved interpretation of ultrasound, as well as illustration of specific features using cine-clips and high-resolution ultrasound images. The authors of this texbook, purposefully represent the key specialists utilizing thyroid and parathyroid ultrasound—endocrinologists, surgeons, and radiologists and increasingly pathologists, internists, and emergency medicine physicians.

The ultrasound themes are covered in a comprehensive manner: logistics, technology, sonographic features of disease, US features of thyroid, parathyroid and lymph node structures, pattern recognition, interventional ultrasound, educational resources, and novel applications. While incorporating advanced concepts and cutting edge information, the themes underscore the basics of ultrasound: *who* performs and interprets it, *how* it can be optimized and performed most effectively, *why* and *when* to use ultrasound and FNA, *where* in the clinical setting can point-of-care ultrasound be implemented, and *what* future opportunities exist for ultrasound. With the accompanying, web-accessible illustration supplement of cine-clips and images, readers will hopefully find the textbook to be a valuable resource as they incorporate ultrasound into routine clinical care and professional practice.

1.7 Summary

Sonography has evolved and proven to be a valuable imaging modality in a variety of clinical settings. Specifically, ultrasound of the neck is a useful imaging modality for thyroid and parathyroid disease that can be performed at the time of a patient encounter, in order to answer a specific clinical question or direct further care. Point-of-care ultrasound can be performed by the primary care practitioner, emergency room physician, endocrinologist or surgeon, to evaluate suspected neck disease, characterize the thyroid parenchyma or lesions, and evaluate parathyroid disease. Perioperatively, the surgeon can make use of ultrasound to direct surgery for thyroid malignancy or parathyroid disease. The main challenges in the utilization of bedside ultrasound include variable operator skill and interpretation of images, as well as standardization of reporting. It is also essential that providers recognize the limitations of point-of-care ultrasound and be knowledgeable regarding which complementary radiologic imaging modalities to employ when necessary, in-order to accurately and definitively diagnose thyroid and parathyroid conditions.

References

1. History of Ultrasound in Obstetrics and Gynecology, Part 1 [Internet]. [cited 2016 Jan 13]. Available from: http://www.ob-ultrasound.net/history1.html.
2. Edler I, Lindström K. The history of echocardiography. Ultrasound Med Biol. 2004;30(12):1565–644.
3. Fujimoto Y, Oka A, Omoto R, Hirose M. Ultrasound scanning of the thyroid gland as a new diagnostic approach. Ultrasonics. 1967;5(3):177–80.
4. Baskin HJ. Thyroid ultrasound—just do it. Thyroid. 2004;14(2):91.
5. Otto C, Shemenski R, Scott JM, Hartshorn J, Bishop S, Viegas S. Evaluation of tele-ultrasound as a tool in remote diagnosis and clinical management at the Amundsen-Scott South Pole Station and the McMurdo Research Station. Telemed J E Health. 2013;19(3): 186–91.
6. NASA - Human Research Facility Ultrasound on the International Space Station 2 [Internet]. [cited 2016 Jan 19]. Available from: http://www.nasa.gov/mission_pages/station/research/experiments/749.html#publications.
7. Garcia M. NASA Studies Link Genetics and Nutrition with Astronaut Vision Changes [Internet]. 2016. Available from: http://www.nasa.gov/feature/nasa-studies-link-genetics-and-nutrition-with-astronaut-vision-changes.
8. Levitov A, Dallas P, Slonim A. Bedside ultrasonography in clinical medicine. New York, NY: McGraw-Hill Education; 2010. p. 332.
9. Moore CL, Copel JA. Point-of-care ultrasonography. N Engl J Med. 2011;364(8):749–57.

10. Noble VE, Nelson BP. Manual of emergency and critical care ultrasound. Cambridge: Cambridge University Press; 2011.
11. Thijs LG, Stroes W. Diagnostic ultrasound in clinical thyroid investigation. J Clin Endocrinol Metab. 1971;32:709.
12. Guth S, Theune U, Aberle J, Galach A, Bamberger CM. Very high prevalence of thyroid nodules detected by high frequency (13 MHz) ultrasound examination. Eur J Clin Invest. 2009;39(8):699–706.
13. Haugen BR, Alexander EK, Bible KC, Doherty G, Mandel SJ, Nikiforov YE, et al. 2015 American thyroid association management guidelines for adult patients with thyroid nodules and differentiated thyroid cancer. Thyroid. 2015;26:1.
14. Ghasemi-Rad M, Lesha E, Abkhiz S, Mohammadi A. Primary hyperparathyroidism: comparing between solid and cystic adenomas and the efficacy of ultrasound and single-photon emission computed tomography in their diagnosis. Endocr Pract. 2015;21(11):1277–81.
15. Cappelli C, Rotondi M, Pirola I, De Martino E, Leporati P, Magri F, et al. Prevalence of parathyroid cysts by neck ultrasound scan in unselected patients. J Endocrinol Invest. 2009;32(4):357–9.
16. Tublin ME, Pryma DA, Yim JH, Ogilvie JB, Mountz JM, Bencherif B, et al. Localization of parathyroid adenomas by sonography and technetium tc 99m sestamibi single-photon emission computed tomography before minimally invasive parathyroidectomy: are both studies really needed? J Ultrasound Med. 2009;28(2):183–90.
17. Greenbaum LD. It is time for the sonoscope. J Ultrasound Med. 2003;22(4):321–2.
18. Hoffenberg SR, Tayal VS, Greenbaum LD, Filly RA. Time for the sonoscope? * Replies. J Ultrasound Med. 2003;22(7):753–7.
19. Kim SH, Park CS, Jung SL, Kang BJ, Kim JY, Choi JJ, et al. Observer variability and the performance between faculties and residents: US criteria for benign and malignant thyroid nodules. Korean J Radiol. 2010;11(2):149–55.
20. Rosario PW. Ultrasonography for the follow-up of patients with papillary thyroid carcinoma: how important is the operator? Thyroid. 2010;20(7):833–4.
21. Oltmann SC, Schneider DF, Chen H, Sippel RS. All thyroid ultrasound evaluations are not equal: sonographers specialized in thyroid cancer correctly label clinical N0 disease in well differentiated thyroid cancer. Ann Surg Oncol. 2015;22(2):422–8.
22. Ruda JM, Hollenbeak CS, Stack BC. A systematic review of the diagnosis and treatment of primary hyperparathyroidism from 1995 to 2003. Otolaryngol Head Neck Surg. 2005;132(3):359–72.
23. Solorzano CC, Carneiro-Pla D. Minimizing Cost and Maximizing Success in the Preoperative Localization Strategy for Primary Hyperparathyroidism. Surg Clin North Am. 2014;94(3):587–605.

Key Components of a Comprehensive Thyroid and Parathyroid Ultrasound Report

2

Ilya Likhterov and Mark L. Urken

2.1 Introduction

The diagnosis, the management, and the surveillance of thyroid and parathyroid pathology rely heavily on the information provided by high-resolution ultrasound (US) imaging of the neck. Ultrasonography is an established, safe, and accurate way of detection and characterization of thyroid nodules and cervical lymph nodes and localization of enlarged parathyroid glands in the workup and preparation for surgery [1]. The examination is being performed more and more commonly in an office setting by non-radiology physicians (e.g., endocrinologists, general practitioners, pathologists, and surgeons).

The report describing the findings of an US examination must be comprehensive and convey relevant information. The description of what was seen during the ultrasonographic evaluation must communicate the location and the level of clinical concern to the treating clinician. This actionable data must be accurate and consistent from patient to patient and from exam to exam. The challenge arises not only because the interpretation of US imaging findings is subjective but because the techniques for performing the examination are often varied among practitioners. The heterogeneity of the US reports that are generated often affects the clinical utility of a particular study, as well as the potential necessity to repeat that study, adding unnecessary costs to an already overburdened healthcare system. The need to subject a patient to a repeat examination in order to gain critical information is not uncommon. The clinicians should be cognizant of the variability of ultrasound reporting and be aware of how this heterogeneity influences their particular practice. Centers with a wide referral base and a larger number of US report sources will experience more variability than practices that rely on one source for their imaging needs.

Unfortunately, while a number of recommendations on what constitutes a complete US report have been published, no universal system is currently in use. In this chapter, we explore the features thought to be salient in the description of the thyroid and parathyroid pathology by professional organizations and by groups of experts focusing on this issue. In addition, we will describe a thyroid patient database that may help to track the comprehensiveness of the reports and the role it may play in the path toward standardization.

I. Likhterov, M.D. (✉) • M.L. Urken, M.D.
Department of Otolaryngology Head and Neck Surgery, Mount Sinai Beth Israel,
10 Union Square East 5B,
New York, NY 10003, USA
e-mail: ilikhterov@chpnet.org; murken@chpnet.org

M. Milas et al. (eds.), *Advanced Thyroid and Parathyroid Ultrasound*,
DOI 10.1007/978-3-319-44100-9_2

2.2 Recommendations for Thyroid Ultrasound Reporting

The evaluation of the thyroid gland may be performed for a variety of reasons. However, no matter what the indication, it is important to examine and report on all of the clinically significant areas of the neck. For patients with thyroid nodules, for whom thyroid cancer is one of the differential diagnoses, the evaluation of the gland alone is not sufficient. Papillary thyroid carcinoma has a high propensity to metastasize to the regional lymph nodes in the central and lateral cervical compartments [2]. These anatomic regions must be evaluated during the initial and surveillance ultrasound studies.

Tables 2.1, 2.2, and 2.3 highlight the recommendations on thyroid ultrasound reporting from a multidisciplinary group of experts [3] (Table 2.1), the American Thyroid Association (ATA) [4] (Table 2.2), and the American Association of Clinical Endocrinologists (AACE) [5] (Table 2.3).

All three groups recommend measuring the thyroid lobes in all three dimensions.

In addition, at least two of the three guidelines recommend including the description of the gland parenchyma (heterogeneous vs. homogeneous), the general thyroid echogenicity, the vascularity patterns, and the measurement of the isthmus.

In the description of the thyroid nodules, there is agreement that the following features should be reported: size of each nodule in three dimensions, the number of nodules in each lobe, the internal architecture, the echogenicity, the presence of calcifications, vascularity patterns, whether the nodule is taller or wide, and the location in the thyroid lobe in the cranial-caudal and in the anterior/posterior orientation. In addition, there were two other features included in two of the three guidelines: suspicion for extrathyroidal extension and the contour of the nodule.

The need for evaluation of the lymphatic compartments was highlighted in all three recommendations. However, the degree of detail of the description of the lymph nodes varied. Clinical

Table 2.1 Multidisciplinary consensus report [3]

Thyroid gland/general	Thyroid nodule	Lymph nodes
Thyroid parenchyma (homogeneous or heterogeneous)	Number of nodules in each lobe	Purpose of lymph node evaluation
Size in three dimensions	Clinical significance of each nodule	Size in three dimensions
Size of the isthmus	Size in three dimensions	Location
Echogenicity	Location in the gland (both in the superior/inferior and in the anterior/posterior orientation)	Internal architecture
Vascularity	Whether the nodule is taller than wider	Presence of hilum
Calcification patterns not associated with nodules	Contour	Shape
Pyramidal lobe	Suspicion for extrathyroidal extension	Calcifications
Mediastinal extension	Internal architecture	Vascularity
Tracheal deviation	Echogenicity	Suspicion of invasion of nearby structures/extranodal extension
Thyroglossal duct cyst	Non-suspicious echogenic foci Calcifications Vascularity	Overall impression (suspicion of metastasis)

Table 2.2 ATA recommendations [4]

Thyroid gland/general	Thyroid nodule	Lymph nodes
Thyroid parenchyma (homogeneous or heterogeneous)	Number of nodules in each lobe	Purpose of lymph node evaluation
Size in three dimensions	Clinical significance of each nodule	Size in three dimensions
Size of the isthmus	Size in three dimensions	Location
Echogenicity	Location in the gland (both in the superior/inferior and in the anterior/posterior orientation)	Internal architecture
Vascularity	Whether the nodule is taller than wider	Presence of hilum
Calcification patterns not associated with nodules	Contour	Shape
Pyramidal lobe	Suspicion for extrathyroidal extension/margins	Calcifications
Mediastinal extension	Internal architecture	Vascularity
Tracheal deviation	Echogenicity	Suspicion of invasion of nearby structures/extranodal extension
Thyroglossal duct cyst	Non-suspicious echogenic foci Calcifications Vascularity	Overall impression (suspicion of metastasis)

Table 2.3 AACE recommendations [5]

Thyroid gland	Thyroid nodule	Lymph nodes
Thyroid parenchyma (homogeneous or heterogeneous)	Number of nodules in each lobe	Purpose of lymph node evaluation
Size in three dimensions	Clinical significance of each nodule	Size in three dimensions
Size of the isthmus	Size in three dimensions	Location
Echogenicity	Location in the gland (both in the superior/inferior and in the anterior/posterior orientation)	Internal architecture
Vascularity	Whether the nodule is taller than wider	Presence of hilum
Calcification patterns not associated with nodules	Contour	Shape
Pyramidal lobe	Suspicion for extrathyroidal extension	Calcifications
Mediastinal extension	Internal architecture	Vascularity
Tracheal deviation	Echogenicity	Suspicion of invasion of nearby structures/extranodal extension
Thyroglossal duct cyst	Non-suspicious echogenic foci Calcifications Vascularity Presence of peripheral halo	Overall impression (suspicion of metastasis)

suspicion for metastatic disease in the lymph node is mentioned consistently. The high-risk features, such as size, internal architecture, the absence of a hilum, shape, calcifications, and vascular patterns of a lymph node, were not mentioned in the ATA or the AACE recommendations.

Attempts to combine the ultrasound features of each thyroid nodule and assign a measure of risk for malignancy have been made. The Thyroid Imaging Reporting and Data System (TIRADS) is modeled on the BI-RADS for breast imaging. A TIRADS category is assigned to each nodule based on how many of the following suspicious US features are identified: solidity, hypo-echogenicity or marked hypo-echogenicity, microlobulated or irregular margins, microcalcifications, and taller-than-wide shape [6]. The TIRADS classification incorporates some of the thyroid nodule features described in the recommendations above; however, it is not a comprehensive ultrasound reporting system since it does not incorporate the imaging characteristics of the thyroid gland itself, nor does it address the risk of lymphatic metastasis. This system has not been widely adopted in the United States. A committee representing the American College of Radiology (ACR) has published a list of recommended terminology and lexicon in an attempt to standardize the diagnostic approach to thyroid nodules and to develop the use of TIRADS in the United States [7].

One feature that is not mentioned in the above recommendations is real-time strain elastography. This measure of tissue stiffness has been evaluated as a tool in differentiating malignant from benign thyroid nodules [8]. Classification of nodule elastography includes the Rago [9] and the Asteria criteria [10]. Addition of elastography to the gray-scale US features appears to increase the negative predictive value of the exam [11, 12]. Technology needed to evaluate compression properties of a thyroid nodule is not routinely available; however, when elastography data is generated, it should be incorporated in the ultrasound report [13].

One of the most critical ultrasonographic findings in management of thyroid nodules is the change in size as tracked over time. A nodule that remains stable over a number of years can be monitored with repeat imaging. On the other hand, a significant change in any of the three dimensions must warrant a biopsy and possibly surgical excision. Given the inconsistencies inherent to ultrasonographic measurements, a certain margin of error must be accounted for in the clinical decision-making [14, 15]. One of the largest observational trials tracking differentiated thyroid cancers with repeat surveillance ultrasounds used a 3 mm increase in size as an indication of clinically significant growth [16]. The ATA guidelines define growth as a 20 % increase in the nodule diameter or a 50 % increase in the nodule volume [4]. The change in the size measurements of the nodule and changes in the dimensions of the lymph nodes should be reported and tracked. The rate at which these changes are occurring can be as valuable as the absolute size measurement.

Appearance of any new adverse ultrasonographic features, not noted on previous ultrasounds, must be included in the report. Development of microcalcifications, changes in the vascular patterns of a nodule, suspicion for invasion, disappearance of a lymph node hilum, and other interval changes may be indications to a change in the biology of the disease. Repeat biopsy may be warranted. Whenever possible, the repeat ultrasounds should be performed by the same practitioner to reduce the inter-rater variability.

Clinicians following patients with thyroid disease must employ a reliable system for recognizing changes on surveillance US exams. Tracking the size and the features of thyroid nodules and lymph nodes over time in a clear, easily reviewable format is imperative to initiating a timely intervention in cases of sudden change. The Thyroid Care Collaborative (TCC) is an example of a robust and user-friendly database that helps to facilitate these goals [17]. The three-dimensional location of each nodule and lymph node is tracked through schematic representation. The measurements of the size in three dimensions are reported for each nodule in a table format, which facilitates recognition of a potentially clinically significant change. Reporting change in this manner is especially helpful when following patients with multinodular disease and/or multiple lymph nodes. The program can further alert the clinician of any significant changes and make suggestions regarding additional workup by cross-referencing the ATA guidelines and its reported stratification of risk based on ultrasound features.

In addition, the TCC promotes consistency in ultrasound data recording by prompting clinicians to fill in the predetermined categories. A library of representative ultrasound images highlighting each of the key features in a user-friendly fashion is provided to assist less experienced clinicians to identify the appropriate diagnostic features. If a particular feature is not available in the ultrasound report, the clinician's awareness is raised. Additional steps can then be taken to obtain the missing data point, if considered significant. It is our hope that a standardized and complete data entry framework, such as the one available in the TCC, can be employed by all ultrasonographers in the future.

2.2.1 Recommendations for Ultrasound Reporting of Parathyroid Pathology

Ultrasound evaluation of the central neck is often the first step in the localization of parathyroid adenoma candidates in patients with hyperparathyroidism. The hypoechoic appearance of the enlarged gland(s) is a distinguishing feature of parathyroid adenomas. Localization of the candidate for an adenoma in the superior vs. inferior and intraglandular vs. extraglandular location should be reported. The degree of localization provided by the US of the central neck facilitates performing a directed, minimally invasive parathyroidectomy. Suspected ectopic location (e.g., carotid sheath) identified on an US can be invaluable at the time of surgery. In addition, US findings may suggest presence of coexisting thyroid pathology that warrants further diagnostic workup.

References

1. Yassa L, Cibas ES, Benson CB, Frates MC, Doubilet PM, Gawande AA, Moore Jr FD, Kim BW, Nosé V, Marqusee E, Larsen PR, Alexander EK. Long-term assessment of a multidisciplinary approach to thyroid nodule diagnostic evaluation. Cancer. 2007;111(6):508–16.
2. Wada N, et al. Lymph node metastasis from 259 papillary thyroid microcarcinomas: frequency, pattern of occurrence and recurrence, and optimal strategy for neck dissection. Ann Surg. 2003;237(3):399–407.
3. Su HK, Dos Reis LL, Lupo MA, Milas M, Orloff LA, Langer JE, Brett EM, Kazam E, Lee SL, Minkowitz G, Alpert EH, Dewey EH, Urken ML. Striving toward standardization of reporting of ultrasound features of thyroid nodules and lymph nodes: a multidisciplinary consensus statement. Thyroid. 2014;24(9):1341–9.
4. Haugen BR, Alexander EK, Bible KC, Doherty G, Mandel SJ, Nikiforov YE, Pacini F, Randolph G, Sawka A, Schlumberger M, Schuff KG, Sherman SI, Sosa JA, Steward D, Tuttle RM, Wartofsky L. 2015 American Thyroid Association Management Guidelines for adult patients with thyroid nodules and differentiated thyroid cancer. Thyroid. 2016;26:1.
5. Gharib H, Papini E, Paschke R, Duick DS, Valcavi R, Hegedüs L, Vitti P, AACE/AME/ETA Task Force on Thyroid Nodules. American Association of Clinical Endocrinologists, Associazione Medici Endocrinologi, and European Thyroid Association medical guidelines for clinical practice for the diagnosis and management of thyroid nodules: executive summary of recommendations. J Endocrinol Invest. 2010;33(5):287–91.
6. Kwak JY, Han KH, Yoon JH, Moon HJ, Son EJ, Park SH, Jung HK, Choi JS, Kim BM, Kim EK. Thyroid imaging reporting and data system for US features of nodules: a step in establishing better stratification of cancer risk. Radiology. 2011;260(3):892–9.
7. Grant EG, Tessler FN, Hoang JK, Langer JE, Beland MD, Berland LL, Cronan JJ, Desser TS, Frates MC, Hamper UM, Middleton WD, Reading CC, Scoutt LM, Stavros AT, Teefey SA. Thyroid ultrasound reporting lexicon: white paper of the ACR thyroid imaging, reporting and data system (TIRADS) committee. J Am Coll Radiol. 2015;12(12 Pt A):1272–9.
8. Razavi SA, Hadduck TA, Sadigh G, Dwamena BA. Comparative effectiveness of elastographic and B-mode ultrasound criteria for diagnostic discrimination of thyroid nodules: a meta-analysis. AJR Am J Roentgenol. 2013;200(6):1317–26.
9. Rago T, Santini F, Scutari M, Pinchera A, Vitti P. Elastography: new developments in ultrasound for predicting malignancy in thyroid nodules. J Clin Endocrinol Metab. 2007;92(8):2917–22.
10. Asteria C, Giovanardi A, Pizzocaro A, Cozzaglio L, Morabito A, Somalvico F, Zoppo A. US-elastography in the differential diagnosis of benign and malignant thyroid nodules. Thyroid. 2008;18(5):523–31.
11. Trimboli P, Guglielmi R, Monti S, Misischi I, Graziano F, Nasrollah N, Amendola S, Morgante SN, Deiana MG, Valabrega S, Toscano V, Papini E. Ultrasound sensitivity for thyroid malignancy is increased by real-time elastography: a prospective multicenter study. J Clin Endocrinol Metab. 2012;97(12):4524–30.

12. Moon HJ, Sung JM, Kim EK, Yoon JH, Youk JH, Kwak JY. Diagnostic performance of gray-scale US and elastography in solid thyroid nodules. Radiology. 2012;262(3):1002–13.
13. Park VY, Kim EK, Kwak JY, Yoon JH, Kim MJ, Moon HJ. Thyroid imaging reporting and data system and ultrasound elastography: diagnostic accuracy as a tool in recommending repeat fine-needle aspiration for solid thyroid nodules with non-diagnostic fine-needle aspiration cytology. Ultrasound Med Biol. 2016;42(2):399–406.
14. Wienke JR, Chong WK, Fielding JR, Zou KH, Mittelstaedt CA. Sonographic features of benign thyroid nodules: interobserver reliability and overlap with malignancy. J Ultrasound Med. 2003;22(10):1027–31.
15. Brauer VF, Eder P, Miehle K, Wiesner TD, Hasenclever H, Paschke R. Interobserver variation for ultrasound determination of thyroid nodule volumes. Thyroid. 2005;15(10):1169–75.
16. Ito Y, Miyauchi A, Inoue H, Fukushima M, Kihara M, Higashiyama T, Tomoda C, Takamura Y, Kobayashi K, Miya A. An observational trial for papillary thyroid microcarcinoma in Japanese patients. World J Surg. 2010;34(1):28–35.
17. Dos Reis LL, Tuttle RM, Alon E, Bergman DA, Bernet V, Brett EM, Cobin R, Doherty G, Harris JR, Klopper J, Lee SL, Lupo M, Milas M, Machac J, Mechanick JI, Orloff L, Randolph G, Ross DS, Smallridge RC, Terris DJ, Tufano RP, Mehra S, Scherl S, Clain JB, Urken ML. What is the gold standard for comprehensive interinstitutional communication of perioperative information for thyroid cancer patients? A comparison of existing electronic health records with the current American Thyroid Association recommendations. Thyroid. 2014;24(10):1466–72.

3 Pathways to Thyroid and Parathyroid Ultrasound Certification

P. Ryan Hungerford and John Woody Sistrunk

3.1 Introduction

As endocrinologist-performed neck ultrasound is now mainstream, formal certification and practice accreditation have become necessary as an affirmation of both quality and consistency to benefit patients and to satisfy insurance carrier requirements. Certification of endocrinologists and other specialty physicians, attesting their ability in thyroid/parathyroid ultrasound, is available through the American Association of Clinical Endocrinologist's Endocrine Certification in Neck Ultrasound (ECNU) program. Practice accreditation is available through the American Institute of Ultrasound in Medicine (AIUM).

3.2 Background

At present, community- and university-based hospital radiology departments commonly produce thyroid ultrasound reports that have variable quality. It is not uncommon for the target audience of these reports, the clinician, to be informed of multiple thyroid nodules without provision of key descriptive details. For examples, reports can be too brief, use the unhelpful term "indeterminate," or erroneously caution about "microcalcifications," a very significant finding commonly associated with papillary thyroid carcinoma and often incorrectly applied to almost invariably benign colloid nodules or cysts. Furthermore, a careful cervical lymph node evaluation, essential for a comprehensive evaluation of the nodular thyroid gland, is rarely performed or documented.

Real-time ultrasound in the hands of the endocrinologist produces a study highly influenced not only by the clinician's deep understanding of thyroid physiology and pathology but also by their awareness of the patient-specific context in which the study is being performed. The clinician is able to correlate sonographic features with laboratory findings, physical examination, and the patient's unique medical history. This allows for a detailed and clinically relevant ultrasound study and report. The same philosophy applies to other specialists who care for patients with thyroid and parathyroid diseases.

P.R. Hungerford, M.D., F.A.C.E., E.C.N.U. (✉)
Rogue Valley Physicians,
2900 Doctor's Park Drive, Medford, OR 97504, USA
e-mail: hungerfordr@rvpdocs.com

J.W. Sistrunk, M.D., E.C.N.U.
Jackson Thyroid & Endocrine Clinic, PLLC,
971 Lakeland Drive, Suite 353, Jackson, MS 39216, USA
e-mail: woodysistrunk@gmail.com

M. Milas et al. (eds.), *Advanced Thyroid and Parathyroid Ultrasound*,
DOI 10.1007/978-3-319-44100-9_3

In parallel with the widespread increase of radiographic imaging modalities, the incidence of thyroid nodules has increased, a large proportion of which are identified incidentally. The incidence of thyroid cancer is also increasing. Consequently, the ability to distinguish characteristics of both benign and malignant nodules has become increasingly recognized and has been the subject of a vast number of research studies, review articles, and lectures.

The American Thyroid Association (ATA) guidelines for the management of thyroid nodules and thyroid cancer have mirrored the developing medical literature on thyroid ultrasound, with increasing emphasis on the sonographic characteristics of thyroid nodules and their relevance to clinical thyroidology. The first version of these guidelines, published in 2006, mentions ultrasound characteristics of thyroid nodules a total of five times [1]. The 2009 ATA guidelines make 14 different references to the ultrasound characteristics of thyroid nodules [2], and a review newly released 2015 ATA guidelines mentions ultrasound characteristics of thyroid nodules and thyroid cancer an incredible 100 times [3]. As previously mentioned, thyroid ultrasound reports from radiology departments commonly lack these vital sonographic descriptions, limiting their value in clinical practice. Among many possible explanations, it may be either that these salient characteristics are not considered important or that an understanding of their relevance is not well appreciated by the interpreting radiologist.

Inherent to the understanding of thyroid ultrasound imaging is a background in anatomy, physiology, pathology, and the physics of sonography. Ultrasound/sonographic pattern recognition is a vital skill which can be developed with proper training and strict adherence to a consistent, systematic approach.

In an effort to better educate the forthcoming generation of endocrinologists in thyroid ultrasonography, the American Association of Clinical Endocrinologists (AACE), with the forethought and diligent efforts of H. Jack Baskin, MD, and Daniel S. Duick, MD, developed an extensive thyroid sonography training program as part of the Endocrine University® Program, held annually at Mayo Clinic—Rochester, Minnesota. Since its inception in 2002, Endocrine University® has trained more than 3000 endocrine fellows in performance of thyroid, neck, and parathyroid ultrasound [4]. Surgeons, furthermore, have access to continuing medical education (CME) via the American College of Surgeons (ACS). Since 2002, the ACS Thyroid and Parathyroid Ultrasound Course has granted verification of ultrasound knowledge and skill at Level 2 designation (only higher category is Level 3 of "proctor ready") by the Accreditation Council for Continuing Medical Education (ACCME). The ACS course has both written exam and hands-on practical ultrasound skills testing components. Nearly 1000 surgeons have availed themselves of this educational opportunity that, while not an independent certification mechanism, affords a level of CME that is important to become an informed practitioner of thyroid and parathyroid ultrasound in patient care and relevant toward obtaining certification (https://www.facs.org/education/accreditation/verification/ultrasound/exported#thyroid).

As the practice of medicine has evolved, third-party payers, the federal government, and other licensing agencies have increased regulations and qualifications necessary for imaging procedures by non-radiologist clinicians. For this reason, the preemptive development of a certification program became necessary. To accomplish such a certification for office-based endocrinologists, a comprehensive program had to be developed to meet the compliance standards of the National Commission for Certifying Agencies (NCCA) [4].

Through the efforts of H. Jack Baskin, MD, Daniel S. Duick, MD, Donald Jones (CEO of American Association of Clinical Endocrinologists (AACE)), Carmine Valente (CEO of American Institute of Ultrasound in Medicine (AIUM)), and Lenny Greenbaum, MD (former president of AIUM), a mutual agreement was reached in the development and acceptance of the Endocrine Certification in Neck Ultrasound (ECNU) program based on 18 nationally recognized compliance standards [4].

The American Association of Clinical Endocrinologists (AACE) education arm, the American College of Endocrinology, instituted the ECNU program in 2008. Since its inception, more than 400 physicians have been certified in thyroid/parathyroid/neck ultrasonography. At present, ECNU is the only certification route available to endocrinologists. In recognition of the reality that other clinicians also perform thyroid and parathyroid ultrasound, certification via ECNU is available to eligible specialties including surgery and pathology.

3.3 Endocrine Certification in Neck Ultrasound (ECNU) Credential

Endocrine Certification in Neck Ultrasound (ECNU) was developed primarily in response to an increasing number of insurance carriers mandating either physician certification and/or practice accreditation as a condition of reimbursement [5]. To satisfy these conditions, ECNU certification is recognized by the American Institute of Ultrasound in Medicine (AIUM), one of the preeminent accreditation bodies for ultrasound practices. AIUM recognizes individuals who achieve the ECNU credential as sufficiently trained in neck ultrasonography. AIUM allows those with the ECNU credential to be directors of ultrasound laboratories and apply for AIUM practice accreditation [5]. This will be discussed further in the AIUM section of this chapter.

The ECNU certification is an objective assessment, ensuring that a physician has the prerequisite knowledge to practice competently in the field of thyroid, neck, and parathyroid sonography [5].

The ECNU Certification Committee is comprised of ECNU-certified practicing endocrinologists and exists to assure that the process for ECNU certification and the significance of this credential remain relevant to the practicing endocrinologist. The ECNU certification process has different routes available to endocrinologists, endocrinology fellows/trainees, or endocrine surgeons in training, cytopathologists, endocrine surgeons, otolaryngologists/head and neck surgeons, and radiologists [5].

As a prerequisite to beginning the ECNU certification process, attestation of performing at least 100 ultrasound studies is required (70 diagnostic ultrasound examinations and 30 ultrasound-guided FNA procedures (UGFNA)). For fellows—in training—at least 50 ultrasound studies (35 diagnostic ultrasounds and 15 UGFNA) are required at the time of initial application, with the attestation that the remaining 50 ultrasound studies will be carried out within the next 12 months after the written comprehensive certification exam (CCE) or before completing fellowship training. Additionally, 15 h of CME credit is required from one or more basic thyroid ultrasound courses within the prior 3 years [5].

The ECNU certification is composed of two primary components, the comprehensive certification exam (CCE) and the Validation of Competency Process (VCP).

The ECNU comprehensive certification exam (CCE) is a 100-question exam, administered over a 2 h period in proctored testing centers. The examination is designed to assess a candidate's knowledge of relevant anatomy, physiology, pathology, and ultrasound physics.

The comprehensive certification exam (CCE), broken down by content, includes the following topics:

- Principles of ultrasound imaging 15 %
- Neck anatomy 15 %
- Thyroid pathology 34 %
- Parathyroid pathology 10 %
- Lymph node pathology 10 %
- Ultrasound-guided fine needle aspiration (USGFNA) 16 %

The ECNU Certification Committee has relied upon practicing physician sonographers for exam question content and illustrative cases [5].

Following notification of a passing score on the comprehensive certification exam (CCE), the candidate is then eligible for the Validation of Competency Process (VCP), which involves submission of ultrasound reports generated by the candidate from patients from his/her medical practice. This component of the certification process is designed to ensure quality and competence in performance of neck ultrasound and proof of the candidate's ability to generate a high quality, meaningful report. Cases and images for VCP submission must be collected within a 2-year window, beginning from 1 year prior to and ending 1 year following successful completion of the CCE [5].

A total of 15 cases are required for the Validation of Competency Process (VCP). The first five diagnostic thyroid nodule cases are due within 3 months of passing the CCE to ensure that the candidate is following the proper reporting components as outlined in the Candidate Handbook and to provide verification that the candidate is actively pursuing certification, a prerequisite for reimbursement by some insurance companies. These five nodule reports must also include submission of 13 standard images adhering to the 2013 AIUM practice guideline for the performance of a thyroid and parathyroid ultrasound examination. The remaining ten cases are due within 1 year of passing the CCE [6]. The second portion of the Validation of Competency Process (VCP) includes the following items [5]:

- Two parathyroid adenoma cases
- Two malignant lymph node cases
- One case of Hashimoto's thyroiditis
- Five ultrasound-guided biopsy cases

The ECNU Validation of Competency Process (VCP) has received some scrutiny for the requirement of the two lymph node and two parathyroid cases. Although this may be challenging to some candidates, it is determined that any physician performing an adequate number of neck ultrasound studies should not have difficulty identifying two malignant nodes and two parathyroid glands during the 2 year window of case collection. Remember, the ECNU credential signifies competency and quality. Not all seeking ECNU certification will achieve it.

A complete review of the requirements for the VCP cases is found in the ECNU handbook. As most endocrinology fellows have had little or no experience with writing ultrasound reports, the AACE ECNU Reference CD, available complimentary upon request from the ECNU Certification Coordinator, includes a full presentation on authoring ultrasound reports, a PowerPoint® framework for case submission and the official ECNU thyroid schematic cartoon. Examples of ECNU case submissions are also included and recommended for review [7].

Upon submission, the Validation of Competency Process (VCP) cases are reviewed by the physician sonologists of the ECNU Certification Committee for quality and consistency based on the requirements in the ECNU handbook. This process is designed to be a constructive, individualized analysis of the candidate's work. It is the hope of the ECNU Certification Committee that the candidate will benefit from the review and take heed of the advice of the reviewers. At times, VCP submissions may require revision to achieve a passing score. Upon successful completion of the VCP, the candidate is awarded the VCP designation, certificate, and lapel pin, and their name is added to a registry of ECNU-certified physicians.

Consistent with all present aspects of medicine, ECNU certification requires recertification at 10 year intervals. As the first cycle of ECNU-certified physicians will not require recertification until 2018, this process may potentially be revised, with the intent to assure relevancy to the practicing physician. At present, ECNU recertification requires these steps [5]:

1. Performing a minimum of 70 diagnostic ultrasound examinations and 30 USGFNA procedures annually
2. Written attestation of the total number of all diagnostic ultrasounds and UGFNA during the preceding year
3. Documentation of a minimum of 15 h of approved CME during each 3 year cycle, with at least 50 h of approved CME during the 10 year cycle
4. Pass the recertification exam

3.4 American Institute of Ultrasound in Medicine (AIUM) Practice Accreditation

Whereas ECNU certifies an individual physician's ability and performance, American Institute of Ultrasound in Medicine (AIUM) Practice Accreditation is a demonstration of the global competency/consistency in all aspects of ultrasound practice operation including:

- Personnel education, training, and experience
- Document storage and record keeping
- Policies and procedures safeguarding patients, ultrasound personnel, and equipment
- Instrumentation
- Quality assurance
- Case studies

This is a voluntary accreditation process that allows a practice to demonstrate meeting or exceeding national standards in both the performance and interpretation of ultrasound studies. AIUM Practice accreditation cycle is 3 years. Like the ECNU Validation of Competency Process (VCP), the AIUM accreditation includes peer review of cases and insight into a different dynamic of review from the accreditation standpoint [8].

Following completion of the ECNU certification process, certificants are advised to take advantage of the "fast track" to AIUM practice accreditation. First and foremost, the ECNU credential is accepted by the AIUM as having adequate training in thyroid/parathyroid ultrasound. First time applicants for AIUM accreditation have the advantage of a discounted accreditation fee and are not required to submit case studies as long as the AIUM practice accreditation application is made within 12 months of achieving ECNU certification [8].

Alternatively, a physician may seek practice accreditation if the physician(s) in the practice has completed the required training specified in the training guidelines for physicians who evaluate and interpret diagnostic thyroid/parathyroid ultrasound examinations. Depending on physician background, this training guideline determines the number of cases as well as the number of CME credits needed to apply for accreditation [8].

The AIUM "Standards and Guidelines for Accreditation of Ultrasound Practices" specifically outlines accreditation, ultrasound practice personnel, the role of physician director of ultrasound, reaccreditation, and yearly volume requirements. This document also reviews requirements for final reports, preliminary reports, and most importantly policies and procedures safeguarding patients, ultrasound personnel, and equipment. Additionally standards are set forth including the need for policies and procedures regarding patient identification, precautions for invasive procedures, incident reporting, patient confidentiality, the ALARA principle ("as low as reasonably achievable" with regard to radiation exposure), quality assurance, document storage, and record keeping [9]. The quality assurance specifically addresses on-going monitoring of ultrasound personnel performance. As an example of on-going documentation of quality assurance activities, the physician who performs the ultrasound examination and generates a report for a patient who ultimately undergoes surgery should periodically correlate the surgical pathology findings with the sonographic findings. A simple form may suffice for this exercise (see Fig. 3.1).

Ultrasound equipment maintenance is an important component of AIUM practice accreditation. All ultrasound machines must be in good operating condition, with documentation of calibration and servicing at least once a year [9]. Additionally, the AIUM has very specific guidelines addressing cleaning of probes between patients and proper high-level disinfection. A background and knowledge of these guidelines is imperative to all who perform ultrasound studies [10].

Specific guidelines do exist for performance of thyroid and parathyroid ultrasound examinations, as outlined by practice parameters from the American College of Radiology, the American Institute of Ultrasound in Medicine, the Society of Pediatric Radiology (SPR), and the Society of Radiologists in Ultrasound (SRU) [11]. An inherent understanding of these practice parameters is critical to obtaining and maintaining practice accreditation.

Little has been written about authoring thyroid/parathyroid ultrasound reports [12, 13]. Minimal training other than experience is available to practicing clinicians. Many clinicians will quickly master probe positioning and even FNA biopsy. However, when moving from patient to paper, many clinicians will demonstrate significant difficulty with consistency and quality. Hence, the Validation of Competency Process

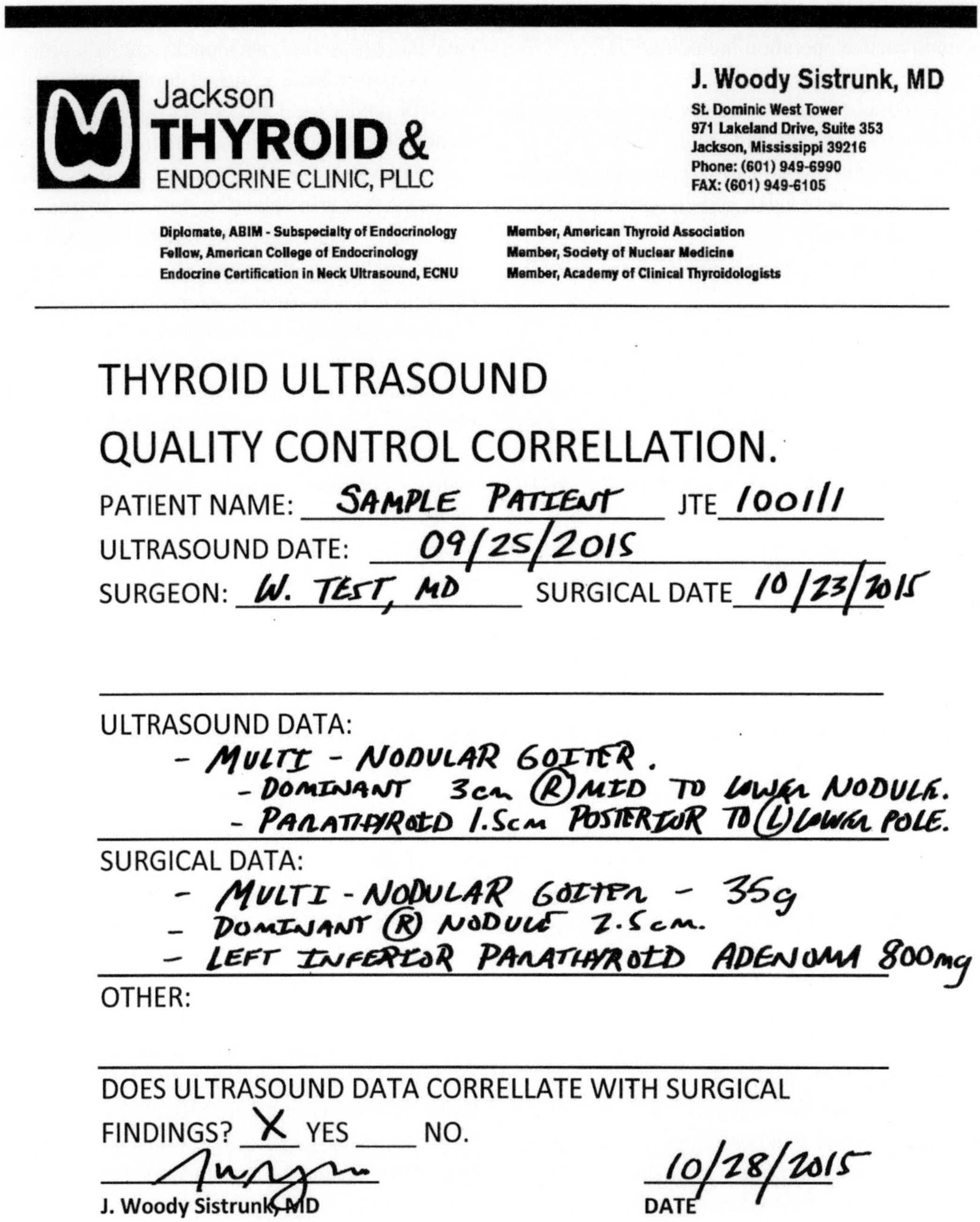
Jackson THYROID & ENDOCRINE CLINIC, PLLC

J. Woody Sistrunk, MD
St. Dominic West Tower
971 Lakeland Drive, Suite 353
Jackson, Mississippi 39216
Phone: (601) 949-6990
FAX: (601) 949-6105

Diplomate, ABIM - Subspecialty of Endocrinology
Fellow, American College of Endocrinology
Endocrine Certification in Neck Ultrasound, ECNU

Member, American Thyroid Association
Member, Society of Nuclear Medicine
Member, Academy of Clinical Thyroidologists

THYROID ULTRASOUND
QUALITY CONTROL CORRELLATION.

PATIENT NAME: SAMPLE PATIENT JTE 100111
ULTRASOUND DATE: 09/25/2015
SURGEON: W. TEST, MD SURGICAL DATE 10/23/2015

ULTRASOUND DATA:
- MULTI - NODULAR GOITER.
- DOMINANT 3cm (R) MID TO LOWER NODULE.
- PARATHYROID 1.5cm POSTERIOR TO (L) LOWER POLE.

SURGICAL DATA:
- MULTI - NODULAR GOITER - 35g
- DOMINANT (R) NODULE 2.5cm.
- LEFT INFERIOR PARATHYROID ADENOMA 800mg

OTHER:

DOES ULTRASOUND DATA CORRELLATE WITH SURGICAL FINDINGS? X YES ____ NO.

J. Woody Sistrunk, MD

10/28/2015
DATE

Fig. 3.1 Sample form correlating the surgical pathology findings with the sonographic findings

(VCP) portion of the ECNU process requires proof of proficiency in reporting the ultrasound procedure. The AIUM practice guideline for documentation of an ultrasound exam explicitly sets forth the necessary components of a comprehensive ultrasound report. Both normal and abnormal findings should be documented. A clear description of the findings must be presented in an organized fashion for adequate documentation as well as communication with the referring physician or surgeon, if needed. Variations from normal should be clearly designated. Pertinent pathology should be described effectively. A succinct impression including applicable recommendations is also vital. In the event of nonroutine results, a system should be in place to communicate these results to the referring physician [12]. Reports of the ultrasound-guided procedure should include a description of the target lesion, needle gauge, the number of passes made and complications from the procedure [12].

3.5 Conclusion

In conclusion, the Endocrine Certification in Neck Ultrasound (ECNU) program provides a certification pathway for clinicians who specialize in the management of thyroid and parathyroid disease to become recognized experts in thyroid and parathyroid sonography. Additionally, the ECNU-certified physician may receive accreditation of his/her practice by AIUM and become the laboratory director for that clinic or facility. With these credentials, physicians and their practices become recognized for excellence in thyroid and parathyroid sonography.

Acknowledgments We greatly acknowledge the review of this chapter for content by Nickie Mizell, ECNU Certification Coordinator and by Therese Cooper BS, RDMS, AIUM Director of Accreditation.

References

1. Cooper DS, Doherty GM, Haugen BR, Kloos RT, Lee SL, Mandell SJ, et al. Management guidelines for patients with thyroid nodules and differentiated thyroid cancer. Thyroid. 2006;16(2):109–42.
2. Cooper DS, Doherty GM, Haugen BR, Kloos RT, Lee SL, Mandell SJ, et al. Revised American Thyroid Association management guidelines for patients with thyroid nodules and differentiated thyroid cancer. Thyroid. 2009;19(11):1167–214.
3. Haugen BR, Bible KC, Doherty G, Mandel SJ, Nikiforov YE, Pacini F, Randolph G, Sawka A, Schlumberger M, Schuff KG, Sherman SI, Sosa JA, Steward D, Tuttle RM, Wartofsky L. 2015 American Thyroid Association management guidelines for adult patients with thyroid nodules and differentiated thyroid cancer. Thyroid. 2016;26:1.
4. Baskin HJ, Duick DS. Vignette: thyroidology, ultrasonography, ECNU and AACE. American Association of Clinical Endocrinologists First Messenger. Vol. 23, No. 4. July/August 2014:3.
5. aace.com [Internet]. Jacksonville: 2015 Endocrine Certification in Neck Ultrasound Candidate Handbook and Application. [Version 2015.] Available from https://www.aace.com/files/ecnu_program_candidate_handbook.pdf.
6. American Institute of Ultrasound in Medicine [Internet]. Laurel, MD: 2013 AIUM Practice Guideline For the performance of a Thyroid and Parathyroid Ultrasound Examination. Available from: https://www.aium.org/resources/guidelines/thyroid.pdf
7. Sistrunk JW. Endocrine Certification in Neck Ultrasound (ECNU) Reference CD [CD-ROM]. Jacksonville: American Association of Clinical Endocrinologists; 2015.
8. American Institute of Ultrasound in Medicine [Internet]. Laurel, MD: Training Guidelines for Physicians Who Evaluate and Interpret Diagnostic Thyroid/Parathyroid Ultrasound Examinations. Approved 04/10/2013. Available from: http://www.aium.org/officialStatements/52.
9. American Institute of Ultrasound in Medicine [Internet]. Laurel, MD: Standards and Guidelines for Accreditation of Ultrasound Practices. [Approved 11/02/2014.] Available from: http://www.aium.org/officialStatements/26.
10. American Institute of Ultrasound in Medicine [Internet]. Laurel, MD: Guidelines for Cleaning and Preparing External- and Internal-use Ultrasound Probes Between Patients. [Approved 04/02/2014.] Available from: http://www.aium.org/officialStatements/57.
11. American College of Radiology, American Institute of Ultrasound in Medicine, Society of Pediatric Radiology (SPR) and the Society of Radiologists in Ultrasound (SRU). [Internet]. Reston, VA: Practice Parameter for the Performance of a Thyroid and Parathyroid Examination. [Amended 2014 (Resolution 39).] Available from: http://www.acr.org/~/media/7405C05D0E3B451788A8DF885BAAC41E.pdf.
12. American Institute of Ultrasound in Medicine (AIUM). AIUM practice guideline for documentation of an ultrasound examination. J Ultrasound Med. 2014;33:2219–24. doi:10.7863/ultra.33.12.2219. Available from http://www.aium.org/resources/guidelines/documenation.pdf.
13. Su HK, Dos Reis LL, Lupo MA, Milas M, Orloff LA, Langer JE, Brett EM, Kazam E, Lee SL, Minkowitz G, Alpert EH, Dewey EH, Urken ML. Striving toward standardization of reporting of ultrasound features of thyroid nodules and lymph nodes: a multidisciplinary consensus statement. Thyroid. 2014;24(9):1341–9.

Part II

Ultrasound Technology

Selection and Setup of Ultrasound in Point-of-Care Medical Practice

4

R. Mack Harrell and Allan Golding

4.1 Introduction

The concept of in-office neck ultrasound for the care of thyroid and parathyroid patients was born in the 1980s when endocrinology pioneers on opposite sides of the United States, Dr. Jack Baskin in Orlando, Florida, and Dr. Dan Duick in Phoenix, Arizona (and a handful of others), began performing routine neck ultrasound evaluations on patients in their endocrine clinics. Over the past 35 years, the art of in-office neck ultrasonography has evolved dramatically to become an important cornerstone of care for patients with neck nodules, thyroid cancer, and hyperparathyroidism. Along the way, other specialties involved in thyroid and parathyroid care have joined the ultrasound revolution, including endocrine surgeons, otolaryngologists, and pathologists. To support and validate this paradigm change in care delivery, the American Association of Clinical Endocrinologists (AACE) began offering neck ultrasound certification testing in 2008 and named this program Endocrine Certification in Neck Ultrasonography (ECNU). To date, over 400 physicians across the world have completed ECNU certification and of those, more than 100 have had their office ultrasound labs certified by the American Institute of Ultrasound in Medicine (AIUM). The purpose of this chapter is to summarize the insights gained from 35 years of outpatient ultrasound suite design with particular emphasis on the space and technologic needs of endocrinologists, endocrine surgeons, and otolaryngologists.

We come to this chapter with several inherent biases, which derive from our clinical experience:

1. Endocrine ultrasound is best implemented by a trained and certified physician holding the US transducer and recording carefully selected images in real time.
2. Endocrine ultrasound requires a unique environment to maximize patient-physician communication. Such an environment should facilitate careful clinical history taking by the physician prior to and during the ultrasound evaluation, thereby, dramatically improving the utility and relevance of the US procedure.
3. The endocrine ultrasound experience presents an unparalleled educational opportunity for the patient and his/her family, and the environment for this experience must maximize comfort and

R.M. Harrell, M.D., F.A.C.P., F.A.C.E., E.C.N.U. (✉)
Department of Endocrine Surgery, Memorial Health Systems, 1150 N. 35th Ave Suite 200, Hollywood, FL 33021, USA
e-mail: rmharrell1@aol.com

A. Golding, M.D., F.A.C.E., E.C.N.U. (✉)
Department of Endocrine Surgery, Memorial Physician Group, 1150 N 35th Ave Suite 200, Hollywood, FL 33021, USA
e-mail: agolding@mhs.net

M. Milas et al. (eds.), *Advanced Thyroid and Parathyroid Ultrasound*,
DOI 10.1007/978-3-319-44100-9_4

image visibility for patients, families, and the imaging physician.

4. Crisp image resolution is essential to the three points listed above, and to that end, every certified neck ultrasound physician should keep up with current imaging techniques and make sure that their office equipment includes appropriate transducers, adequate microprocessing capability, up-to-date image optimizing algorithms and software, and carefully placed flat panels of sufficient size to facilitate patient and family viewing.
5. Despite adherence to all of the above, physicians have accomplished nothing if we do not concisely record the salient points of the patient encounter and the key findings of the US procedure in the medical record along with a plan for further care. Additionally, it is the imager's responsibility to disseminate that documentation to other physicians involved in the patient's care.

Embarking to develop the thyroid/parathyroid imaging space is an exciting and demanding undertaking. Imaging expands the depth of our involvement with endocrinology patients and demands a complete rethinking of practice scope and flow. For some endocrinologists who deliver diabetes care for a majority of their practice volume, becoming an endocrine ultrasonographer may not be practical or affordable. Imaging and biopsy visits require dedicated time and cannot be accomplished in 10–15 min slots. A practice flow set up for diabetes care or postoperative care with physician extenders and limited physician face time will not work well for parathyroid and thyroid cancer care. Significant soul-searching, financial analysis, and genuine dedication to the art and science of endocrine imaging are absolutely necessary before embarking on an office neck ultrasound pathway. However, if all the necessary elements are integrated into the office environment, the personal and professional rewards of on-site office imaging can be substantial.

4.2 Space

In the modern era, clinical exam room space has become increasingly constricted and dominated by the need for advanced electronic medical record (EMR) technology. Deployment constraints for electronic interfaces have decreased physician-patient eye contact and eroded the intimacy of the clinical encounter. Given these limitations, ultrasound physicians should attempt to find space for their ultrasound procedure rooms that maximizes patient comfort and intimacy while minimizing congestion. For our purposes, an optimal procedure room is set up to enclose an ultrasound console, an exam table, two chairs, an EMR console on a suspension arm, one or two sinks and countertops (remember that on-site cytologic adequacy testing requires a clean and a dirty sink by CLIA regulations—Clinical Laboratory Improvement Amendments), staining station, microscope, camera and laptop (for recording of on-site photomicrograms), two floating Mayo tables for biopsy accessories, and two flat panel televisions for patient education and physician sight-line optimization. This particular version of a full service thyroid/parathyroid procedure room requires an allotment of 150–200 square feet of exam room space, a space commitment that many physicians may find difficult to make (Fig. 4.1). The setup can be adapted to smaller space sizes—the goal of accomplishing the exam and procedure can be met but obviously limitations exist related to comfortable movement around the room space. In such cases, many creative solutions can be applied to enhance the overall patient experience, such as by using another room for patient discussion and consultation.

Without on-site cytologic assessment, the second sink and countertop are not needed, thus eliminating 30–50 square feet of unnecessary countertop and bringing the total square footage down to 100–150 square feet (Fig. 4.2).

4.3 Ultrasound Equipment

Although sterilizable touchscreen, portable iPad-like US devices have gained some traction in the surgical community for intraoperative use, most endocrinologic ultrasonographers prefer traditional console devices for a single office or a portable laptop device with convenient plug and play platforms for multiple office use. Several issues must be considered prior to purchase:

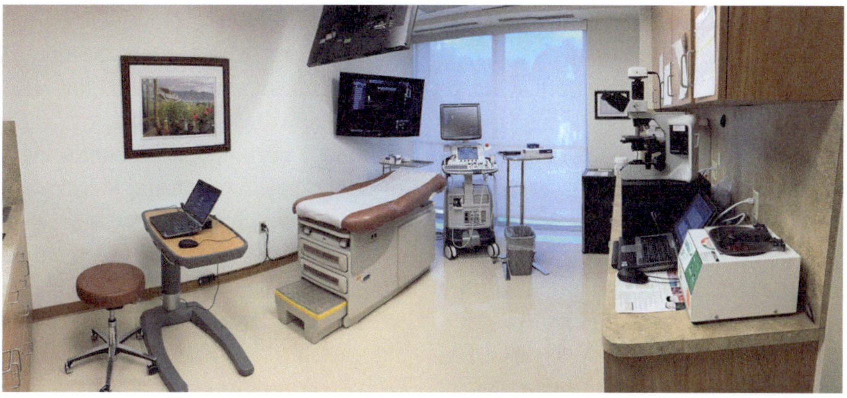

Fig. 4.1 Layout for 15 × 12 ft left-handed ultrasound procedure suite including on-site cytologic adequacy assessment. Note that clean and dirty sinks are required for CLIA licensing along with microscope and digital photography recording on the second laptop to the right

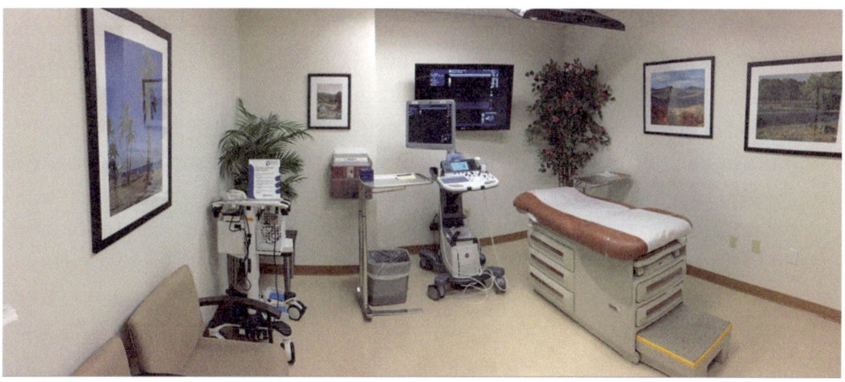

Fig. 4.2 Layout for 14 × 12 ft right-handed ultrasound procedure suite without on-site cytology assessment. Only a single sink is required and the wall flat panel is mounted at the head of the exam table rather than cross-table based on physician preference. The small flat panel with the ultrasound console is used for family display and education. The flat panel on the ceiling is for patient education

1. Does my allocated space accommodate the footprint of my ultrasound of choice?
2. Are the ergonomics of my device and device location customizable for my specific needs (i.e., customizable for handedness, with multifunction foot pedals for taking biopsy images when my hands are otherwise occupied)?
3. Do I have the correct transducers for thyroid, lymph node (LN), and parathyroid imaging and thyroid, parathyroid, and lymph node fine-needle aspiration (FNA)? For example, a flat 3–4 cm linear transducer packed with piano key-arrayed piezoelectric elements may suffice, but matrix array probes provide more piezoelectric elements per square millimeter of transducer face and often yield the sharpest central neck imaging. Lymph node (LN) imaging and biopsy may be best accomplished with more compact and maneuverable hockey stick transducers with fewer piezoelectric elements.
4. Do I have the advanced technology that I need built into my device (e.g., color and/or power Doppler, video clip capture, virtual convex imaging) for structures that are larger than your transducer, strain vs. shear wave elastography for assessment of tissue stiffness, conventional linear array vs. matrix array transducer (discussed above), beam steering for difficult parallel technique FNAs, needle

guidance software, crossbeam image enhancement, and easily controllable and customizable imaging protocols with on/off switches for different imaging needs.
5. Will my ultrasound device power the wall-mounted flat panels I need for ergonomic cross-table viewing and the ceiling flat panel my patient needs for education? If not, can I purchase a compatible image splitter with a signal booster to power both flat panels?
6. Can my ceiling monitor bracket be mounted into concrete or steel for maximum patient safety? Do ceiling lights or air-conditioning vents interfere with ceiling flat panel placement? Are there enough electrical outlets on the room walls and in the ceiling to minimize power cord length?
7. Is there reporting software built into my machine that facilitates the incorporation of my measurements into detailed ultrasound reports along with automatically calculating nodule and LN volume for long-term follow-up?
8. Does the US machine technology allow for simple, on screen, side-by-side comparison of old images and measurements with new ones?

Obviously, machine and room choice are the focal points for most entry-level ultrasonographers, but there is much more to an endocrine imaging practice than putting an ultrasound machine in an appropriate workspace. This theme in the literature does not receive enough attention; an editorial article published in 2011 by Nagarkatti et al. remains a relevant and practical resource to review for additional details ("Overcoming obstacles to setting up office-based ultrasound for evaluation of thyroid and parathyroid diseases") [1].

4.4 Outfitting the Room

Room setup is essential to physician and patient satisfaction. The exam pedestal table and ultrasound device must be situated to accommodate the physician's handedness and to allow the patient and physician to have ergonomic single visual field viewing of ultrasound images for teaching and needle guidance purposes. We have found that placement of a 36–42″ flat panel TV on a tilting ceiling mount affords the best image viewing for patients. Optimization of the physician viewing experience is accomplished by a second wall-mounted 36–42″ flat panel TV on a flexible metallic arm so that the patient's neck, the biopsy needle, and the ultrasound image are all easily included in a single narrow visual field (see Fig. 4.3). Mounting of the flat panels should be handled by experienced video technicians, and the ceiling mount must be bolted into the concrete above any false ceiling materials and plugged into a ceiling outlet. For crisp video on two external monitors, many ultrasound devices require image splitters with signal amplification. Your video technician should be able to handle this installation and perform the necessary image optimization for your flat panel TVs.

Image storage can be handled in several ways. Internal storage on the ultrasound machine is optimal because it enables easy comparison of US images from one year to the next. Because US devices have limited storage capability and hard drive function deteriorates as more data accumulates, a second backup plan is required. Many physicians use external hard drives or DVDs for this purpose, but the optimal backup alternative is the connection to your local hospital's picture archiving and communication system (PACS), if such connectivity can be arranged. PACS storage is reliable, practical, and economical, and it allows other physicians affiliated with your hospital direct access to the images of patients they send to you for care. Hospitals will frequently install your cabling and PACS wall sockets, while handling maintenance costs for you as a practice enhancement, but the terms of such arrangements are negotiated on a case-by-case basis. Finally, cloud-based sharing software is emerging that can be loaded onto newer ultrasound machines. This software allows immediate sharing of patient images on multiple devices (computers, iPads, smartphones) by enrolled physicians. Cloud sharing reimbursement usually involves a fixed cost per patient imaging encounter.

4.5 Interventional Endocrinology

The sub-subspecialty of procedural endocrinology has evolved over the past 35 years from thyroid imaging and thyroid biopsy in the 1980s and

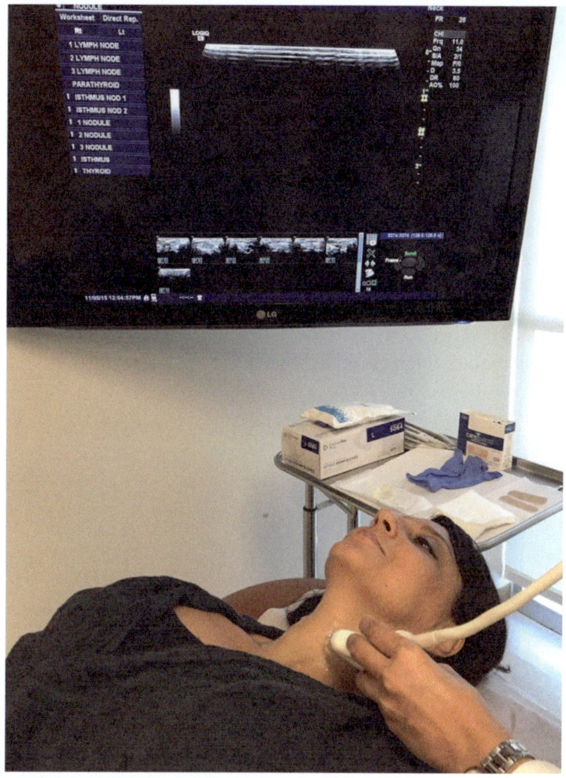

Fig. 4.3 Proper flat panel placement. Note that the sidewall flat panel should be placed so as to allow the transducer, the patient, and the ultrasound image to all comfortably occupy the same visual field

1990s to parathyroid and lymph node imaging and biopsy in the early 2000s and, more recently, has encompassed more invasive modalities of ethanol injection, radiofrequency, and laser ablation of targets such as cystic thyroid nodules, colloid nodules, and malignant lymph nodes. In addition, some physicians have found that on-site Diff-Quik staining and adequacy assessment of FNA smears before sending them for expert cytopathologic interpretation improves FNA technique and makes "non-diagnostic" samples less likely, while other physicians find the moderate complexity CLIA license required for adequacy reimbursement too onerous to justify the time and equipment investment. Incorporation of any or all of these new interventions requires careful space planning and an in-depth knowledge of CLIA regulations.

4.6 FNA and On-Site Adequacy

Fine-needle aspiration biopsy (FNA) of neck masses, thyroid nodules, parathyroid glands, and abnormal lymph nodes (LN) requires adherence to established protocols and careful attention to details. Most physicians prefer to set up their own biopsy trays with disposable supplies rather than using expensive sterilized trays created for hospital use. We prefer using a wheeled stainless steel Mayo table to hold transducer preparation materials: gel and transducer covers on the nursing side of the patient and a second Mayo table on the physician side of the patient, holding 25–27 gauge needles, 10 ml syringes, the biopsy apparatus of choice (e.g., Tao Aspirator®, aluminum needle aspirator gun, three-way stopcock with tubing, and suction syringe), clean glass slides, CytoLyt, molecular marker preservatives, and sealable 95 % ethanol immersion slide holders (Fig. 4.4). This setup allows an assistant to stand comfortably on the side of the procedure pedestal opposite the biopsying physician while preparing and holding the transducer and creating suction, if necessary (Fig. 4.5). We use Diff-Quik® rapid staining techniques (to stain our own adequacy slide(s)), and we wash aspiration material into ThinPrep® CytoLyt Solution (Hologic, Inc., Marlborough, Massachusetts) and molecular marker preservative after each pass. This standard

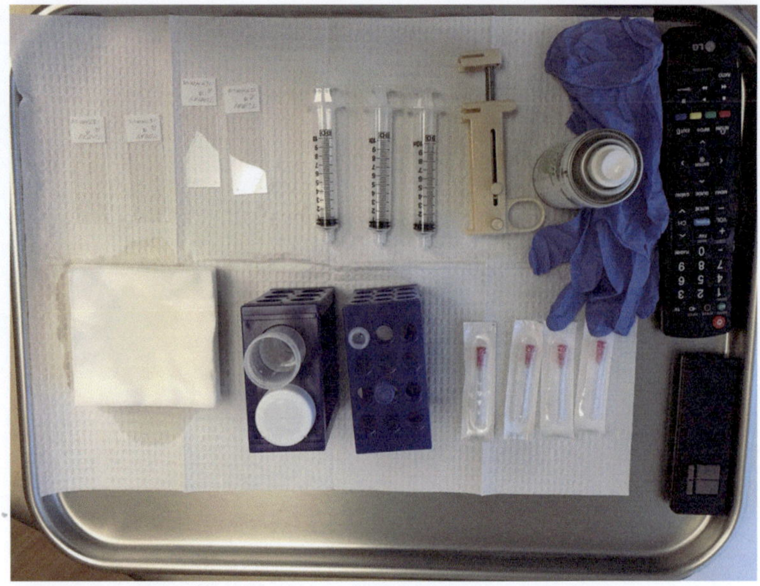

Fig. 4.4 FNA procedure tray layout on a Mayo table. *Top left* proceeding clockwise—(1) four slides for smearing and Diff-Quik on-site microscopic review, (2) three 10 ml syringes, (3) Tao Aspirator®, (4) Spray and Stretch® cold spray for local anesthesia, (5) two non-latex gloves, (6) flat panel controller, (7) roomer light rheostatic controller, (8) four 25 gauge 1.5 in. aspiration needles, (9) RNA preservative for molecular studies, (10) CytoLyt® for liquid-based preservation of aspirate cells, and (11) isopropyl alcohol-soaked 4×4 sponges

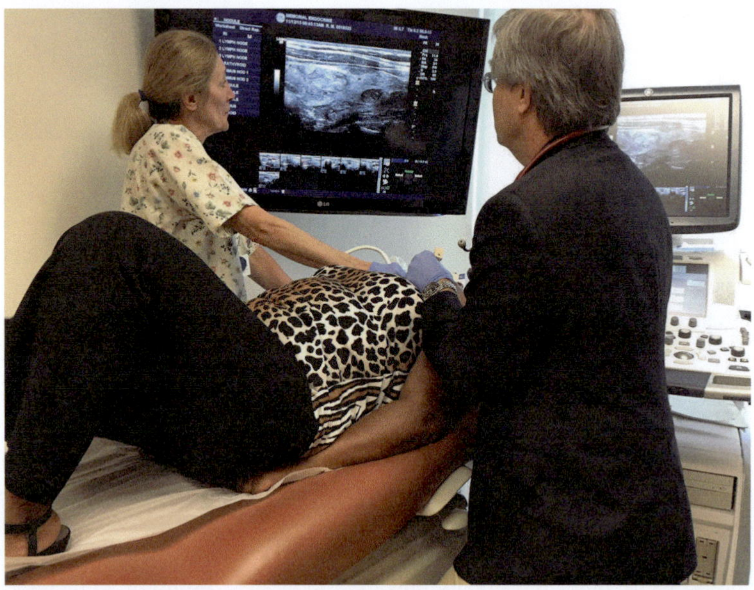

Fig. 4.5 Typical FNA procedural ergonomics for a left-handed biopsying physician and his assistant. Note that the assistant is gloved and holding an US probe covered with a non-latex probe cover the physician performs a parallel technique FNA using the Tao push-button aspirator. All participants are able to visualize the needle passing into the nodule on the wall- or ceiling-mounted flat panel TVs. The procedure table is set at a height that does not require awkward bending on the part of the physician or the assistant

operating procedure allows us to assess adequacy, collect dried stained material for cellular architecture evaluation, collect molecular markers, and send wet-preserved cells for wet technology (CytoLyt with cytospin) Papanicolaou-stained nuclear morphology assessment on each needle pass (Fig. 4.4).

No aspiration biopsy material is wasted, as we perform adequacy assessment of our Diff-Quik® stained material at the bedside, capture and save a photomicrograph of pertinent cells on the Diff-Quik® slide (Fig. 4.6), and then send the slide, CytoLyt® container, and molecular markers container to our preferred cytopathologist. In the midst of an FNA procedure, we typically have three to five people in our procedure room including the patient, a family member, a cytology technician, a nurse to prepare and hold the transducer, and the biopsying physician, a situation which requires every bit of the 150–200 square feet allocated for procedure suite construction (see Fig. 4.1). Elimination of

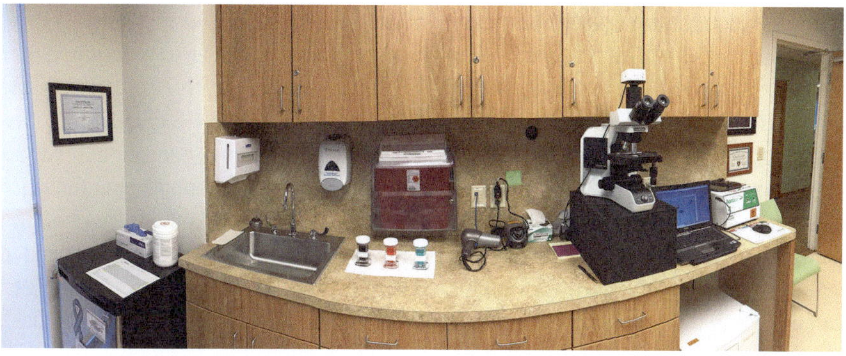

Fig. 4.6 Layout for on-site staining station, microscopic adequacy review, and laptop computer capture of adequacy documentation images. On-site adequacy testing requires a moderate complexity CLIA license (left wall), a clean and dirty sink (clean sink on opposite wall), Diff-Quik staining materials (*indigo*, *red*, and *sea blue* staining containers), sharps disposal container, ergonomically mounted microscope with digital camera atop, and a laptop computer for image storage. Centrifuge to the far right is for FNA needle wash PTH, thyroglobulin, and calcitonin specimens (some labs prefer separation of RBCs from supernatant prior to transport)

on-site assessment speeds up the biopsy process and diminishes space requirements as mentioned earlier (Fig. 4.2). In light of mandatory moderate CLIA license regulations, personnel requirements, and extra space and equipment needs, many capable imaging endocrinologists and surgeons choose to perform FNA without on-site adequacy analysis in their procedure suites.

4.7 FNA for Needle Wash

Modern endocrine imaging often requires FNA for needle wash analysis of parathyroid candidate lesions (measurement of parathyroid hormone, PTH) and lateral LN's (measurement of thyroglobulin and calcitonin). Reference labs like Esoterix and Quest have tissue-validated assays for these proteins and specific requirements for wash volumes and handling. Some physicians centrifuge the wash specimens to remove red blood cells and others do not, depending on their reference lab specifications (Fig. 4.6). Remember that while your accredited office lab may have CLIA-approved assays for serum PTH, thyroglobulin, and calcitonin, these assays need special validation for tissue wash specimens before accepting their results as final. Saline is not serum, and matrix effects may detract from the credibility of unvalidated office lab needle wash results. The key point is to find out your reference lab's specific requirements for these specimens and adhere to these rules assiduously.

4.8 Thyroid Nodule and Lymph Node Ablation

Percutaneous ethanol injection (PEI) can be an effective technique to ablate recurrent, symptomatic thyroid cysts, hyperfunctioning thyroid nodules, and locally recurrent metastatic lymph nodes.

For simple ablation PEI procedures, we use 1.5″ 25 gauge needles connected to 20 ml syringes via 33″ (3.9 mL) IV extension tubing, 5 ml vials of 98 % sterile medical grade ethanol, and a nurse assistant. Ethanol is drawn into the syringe, and the IV tubing is "primed" to eliminate air from the tubing. After careful isopropyl alcohol prep and 1 % lidocaine anesthesia, the procedure needle is then placed in the target lesion (with a prior FNA to establish benignity) under ultrasound guidance by the physician. When the needle tip is confirmed to be properly positioned in the nodule or lymph node, the nurse assistant is asked to inject small volumes of ethanol with the syringe.

For combination procedures in which a thyroid cyst is first aspirated to create space and then injected with 98 % medical grade ethanol, we use a 22 or 25 gauge needle connected to a 20 ml syringe via an IV extension set with two injection ports. Ethanol is drawn into a second syringe and set aside. After an isopropyl alcohol prep and the introduction of subcutaneous 1 % lidocaine local anesthesia, the therapy needle is then placed in the cyst by the physician under ultrasound guidance. When proper placement of the needle tip is confirmed, the nurse assistant is asked to pull back on the syringe and the cyst is drained to near completion. Without changing the position of the needle, the nurse assistant then injects a predetermined volume of ethanol through the second injection port on the IV extension tubing (Fig. 4.7).

Radiofrequency and laser ablation techniques are rarely used in the United States due to device unavailability, high cost, and lack of definitive Food and Drug Administration (FDA) approval for thyroid and lymph node use. Discussion of these techniques is beyond the intended scope of this chapter.

4.9 Summary

In closing, the decision to become an office US imager and proceduralist is not a simple one for endocrinologists, endocrine surgeons, and otolaryngologists. The training necessary for competence is extensive. ECNU certification and American Institute of Ultrasound Medicine (AIUM) US suite accreditation are likely to be required for reimbursement by most payers in the very near future. Certification and accreditation requirements demand a lifelong educational commitment to imaging study. Additionally, the financial outlay for proper construction and outfitting of an ultrasound interventional suite is not trivial, and the service contracts for equipment maintenance are expensive. Finally, endocrinologists may find that ultrasound practice alters the traditional workflow in their offices to such a degree that a majority commitment to diabetes care may no longer be practical or possible.

These caveats aside, ultrasound procedural practice can be a highly rewarding way to enhance the care that you provide for your thyroid and parathyroid patients. With the high prevalence of both thyroid and parathyroid disease in the United States, there is a significant need for physicians with ultrasound imaging and procedural skills. It is our hope that this chapter gives practitioners in endocrinology, otolaryngology, and endocrine surgery a realistic appreciation of the training, equipment, space, and personal dedication required for entry into the new patient-centered practice of office-based endocrine ultrasound medicine.

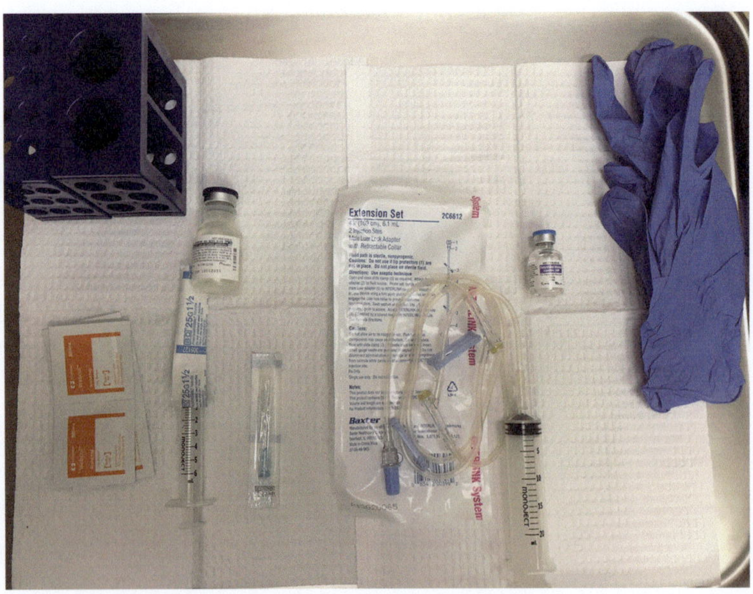

Fig. 4.7 Ethanol injection tray layout on a Mayo table. *Top left* proceeding clockwise—(1) test tube holder, (2) 1 % lidocaine for injection, (3) dehydrated ethanol (98 %) for injection, (3) two non-latex gloves, (4) IV extension tubing with two injection ports connected to a 20 ml syringe, (5) 6 cm^3 syringe with 25 gauge needle, and (6) isopropyl alcohol-saturated prep pads

Reference

1. Nagarkatti SS, Mekel M, Sofferman RA, Parangi S. Overcoming obstacles to setting up office-based ultrasound for evaluation of thyroid and parathyroid diseases. Laryngoscope. 2011;121(3):548–54. doi:10.1002/lary.21391.

5 Principles of Ultrasound and Applied Ultrasound Physics Relevant for Advanced Sonographers

Lawrence T. Kim

5.1 Principles of Sound Waves

Sound waves are a form of transmission of energy and, unlike light, require a medium for transmission. As sound energy moves through a medium, molecules are compressed in a wave-like fashion. The alternating compression and rarefaction of the molecules can be expressed mathematically as a sine wave (Fig. 5.1). The wavelength is defined as the physical length between two successive peaks of the sine wave. Sound frequency is measured in Hertz, where 1 Hertz equals 1 cycle per second. The audible sound spectrum extends from approximately 20 Hz at the lower end to 20 kHz at the upper end. Sound waves above the audible range are called ultrasound.

The velocity of sound is equal to the frequency times the wavelength ($v = f\lambda$) (Fig. 5.2). Unlike light waves, the velocity of sound wave propagation is a property of the medium. Air, which is relatively low in density, has a relatively low sound velocity. Water and the various organs and soft tissues of the body, which are comprised primarily of water, have higher sound velocities. Very dense solids such as the bone have a much higher sound velocity. Ultrasound machines for medical imaging are calibrated for the velocity of sound waves in soft tissue. Sound waves that enter air (as in the trachea) or bone will not generate an interpretable echo because of the large difference in the timing of the echo (Table 5.1).

Sound power is the amount of energy striking a point over a unit of time and is measured in Watts. Sound intensity is the measure of the amount of energy being transmitted through a given area and is expressed in Watts per meter squared. The threshold of human hearing is approximately 1×10^{-12} W/m^2 and is defined as 0 decibel (dB). The decibel scale is logarithmic (dB = 10log(x)). Therefore, a doubling of sound intensity equals a dB change of approximately 3 (10log(2)). Sound intensity is related to pressure amplitude by the equation:

$$I = \frac{p^2}{2pc}$$

where p = pressure amplitude, ρ (rho) = density of the medium, and c = sound velocity. Therefore, doubling the pressure amplitude will quadruple the intensity.

Sound intensity decreases with distance from the source according to the inverse square law. As the distance from the source increases, the sound intensity decreases by the distance squared. Therefore, doubling the distance will decrease the sound intensity by a factor of 4 (Fig. 5.3).

L.T. Kim, M.D., F.A.C.S. (✉)
Division of Surgical Oncology, Department of Surgery, University of North Carolina,
170 Manning Dr., CB # 7213, Chapel Hill, NC 27599-7213, USA
e-mail: Lawrence_Kim@med.unc.edu

M. Milas et al. (eds.), *Advanced Thyroid and Parathyroid Ultrasound*,
DOI 10.1007/978-3-319-44100-9_5

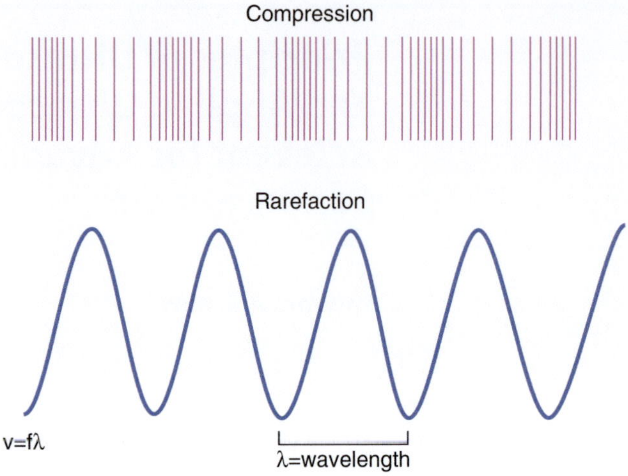

Fig. 5.1 As sound energy moves through a medium, it causes compression and rarefaction of the molecules comprising the medium as depicted by the *line* drawing. This is expressed mathematically as a *sine* wave

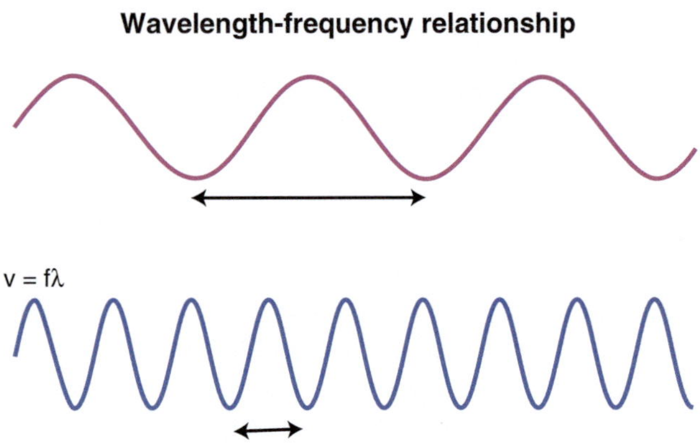

Fig. 5.2 Velocity (V, or often noted as c) = frequency (in cycles/second) × wavelength (λ, distance/cycle). For a given velocity (determined by the medium), a higher frequency is accompanied by a shorter wavelength. The *top* sine wave represents sound with a longer wavelength and lower frequency as compared with the *bottom* sine wave which depicts a higher frequency wave with shorter wavelength

In medical ultrasound, sound power is a fundamental property of the sound wave transmitted from the ultrasound probe. Increasing sound power is similar to turning up the volume on a stereo and can be adjusted on the ultrasound unit. While imaging ultrasound operates well within the safe limits of power output, caution must still be used to avoid unnecessary energy delivery. Thermal injury due to heat transfer has not been reported with diagnostic ultrasound, though it remains a theoretical possibility [1). In practical application in neck ultrasound, sound power is rarely altered. If deep structures cannot be well imaged, increasing the gain or decreasing the frequency of the probe output will usually improve the image [see below).

The propagation of sound is highly influenced by certain characteristics of the medium or mediums through which it travels. Acoustical impedance is one of these and equals density times propagation speed ($Z = \rho v$, where Z = impedance, ρ (rho) = density, and v = propagation speed.). Differences in acoustical impedance account for refraction and reflection at the interface between two media (see below). Another property of the medium that influences sound propagation is its viscosity which affects sound attenuation (a decrease in sound energy). Attenuation is dependent on the viscosity of the medium and the frequency squared of the sound wave and is described mathematically in Stokes' law of sound attenuation:

$$\alpha = \frac{2\eta\omega^2}{3\rho V^3}$$

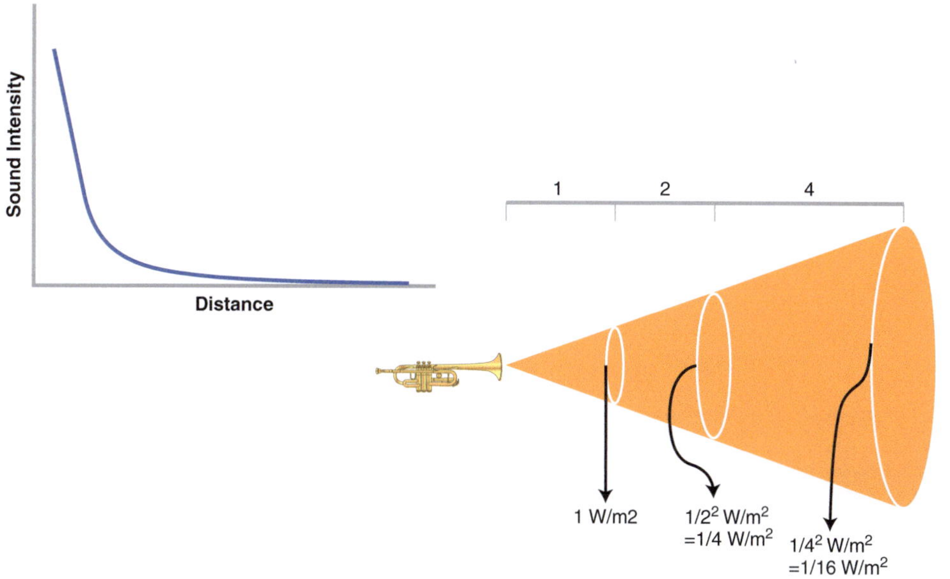

Fig. 5.3 The inverse square law. Sound intensity decreases exponentially as distance increases from the sound source. Sound intensity (*y* axis) decreases exponentially with distance from the source (*x* axis). As distance increases by a factor of 2 sound intensity decreases by a factor of 4

Table 5.1 Velocity of sound in common materials in m/s

Air	340
Water	1500
Fat[a]	1470
Liver[a]	1540
Muscle[a]	1500–1600
Bone[a]	1900–3700

The velocity in air or water is approximate and varies according to temperature and other factors
[a]Values approximated from [4]

where η (eta) is the dynamic viscosity coefficient of the fluid, ω (omega) is the sound's frequency, ρ (rho) is the fluid density, and V is the speed of sound in the medium [3]. Stokes' law is an oversimplification in the case of medical ultrasound, but more complete description is beyond the scope of this text. Notice that the attenuation of sound (α) increases exponentially as frequency increases. This fact has important implications in understanding the limitations of high-frequency ultrasound probes for assessing structures deep within the body. Attenuation values [α (alpha)] have been determined empirically for a number of tissues and are typically expressed in dB/cm [4].

The effect of frequency in choice of medical ultrasound probes can be seen with a simple example. Calculation of attenuation over a given distance can be done by this simple equation:

$$\text{Attenuation}(\text{dB}) = \alpha(\text{dB}/\text{cm}) \times d(\text{cm})$$

Using Stokes' law we can see that doubling the frequency (ω (omega)) will increase α (alpha) by a factor of 4. In the above equation let's compare the effects of doubling a probe frequency, from 5 to 10 MHz. If attenuation equals α for a 5 MHz probe, then attenuation for the 10 MHz probe will equal 4α (alpha). In other words, for any given distance from the probe, attenuation will be four times greater when probe frequency is doubled.

In summary we see that as distance increases away from a sound source, sound intensity decreases by the inverse square law. In addition attenuation causes exponential loss of sound energy, with losses occurring more rapidly for higher frequencies. So the sound-striking objects that are relatively distant from the source is of much lower intensity than that striking objects close to the source. Therefore, echoes coming

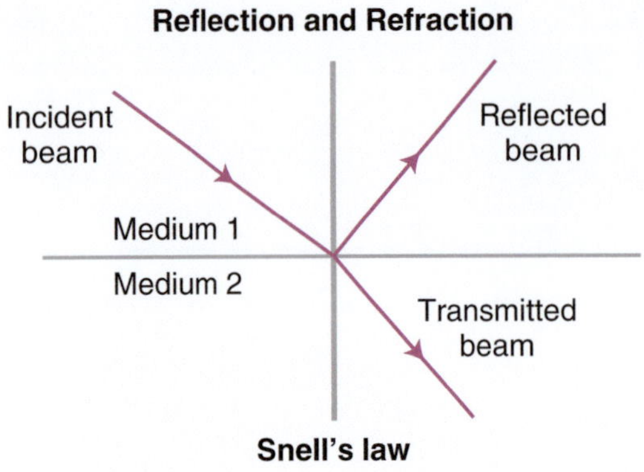

Fig. 5.4 Snell's law. As a sound wave strikes the interface between tissues with different acoustical impedance, some sound waves are refracted and others are reflected. At a critical angle all of the waves will be reflected

from those distant sources are correspondingly weaker.

Echoes are the result of reflected sound energy returning to the probe and must be detected to provide imaging details of an object. Transmission of the sound waves is also necessary to penetrate into tissues that lie deeper in the body. As noted above, differences in acoustical impedance between media accounts for interfaces that both reflect and refract the sound waves according to Snell's law (Fig. 5.4). When sound travels through soft tissues with relatively similar acoustic impendences, such as subcutaneous fat and muscle, some echoes are reflected back to the probe but much of the sound is transmitted deeper into the body, allowing imaging of the deeper tissues until eventually the sound beam is diminished to the point that echoes are inaudible to the probe. If sound travels through acoustically dissimilar tissues, such as air and subcutaneous fat, nearly all of the beam would be reflected back at the interface and very little would be transmitted. For this reason, acoustic coupling gel, a substance with acoustic properties similar to water, is applied to the skin surface when performing medical ultrasound. High-intensity echoes (from intense reflection) which appear bright white on the imaging screen are termed "echogenic," whereas those which are poorly reflective appear darker. Reflectors can generally be described as a diffuse (reflecting echoes in many different directions, such as a bicycle reflector) or specular (reflecting echoes primarily in a single direction, such as a mirror) [2]. Most tissues are diffuse reflectors.

5.2 How Medical Ultrasound Devices Work

Ultrasound for use in medical imaging was investigated beginning in the 1940s. During the 1950s and 1960s, a number of advances were made allowing the first medical imaging. In 1972 grayscale imaging was developed and during the 1970s ultrasound imaging became widely available in medical centers. As ultrasound technology and computing power has improved, ultrasound units have become smaller, faster, and cheaper allowing dispersal into hospitals and clinics worldwide [5].

Medical ultrasound devices work by taking advantage of the piezoelectric effect. When certain crystals are placed into an electromagnetic field, the molecular dipoles align and change the physical shape of the crystal allowing conversion of the electromagnetic field into mechanical energy. This process also works in reverse, whereby the mechanical energy caused by sound striking the piezoelectric crystal will create an electrical current (Fig. 5.5). Quartz is a naturally occurring piezoelectric crystal, but most used in medical ultrasound devices are synthetic, ceramic compounds such as lead zirconate titanate.

Current ultrasound equipment consists of a piezoelectric element which is divided into strip sections, each narrower than a piece of hair and each attached to electrodes. The piezoelectric elements are housed within a handheld device called a probe. The probe both emits sound and captures the reflected sound waves, converting the reflected sound into an electric current that is analyzed by a computer to create the image. The term "transducer" refers to the ability of the device to convert one form of energy into another and technically refers to the piezoelectric element but is commonly used to refer the entire probe. Ultrasound probes are constructed in a variety of sizes and shapes to suit the anatomical purpose to which they are designed. Each probe

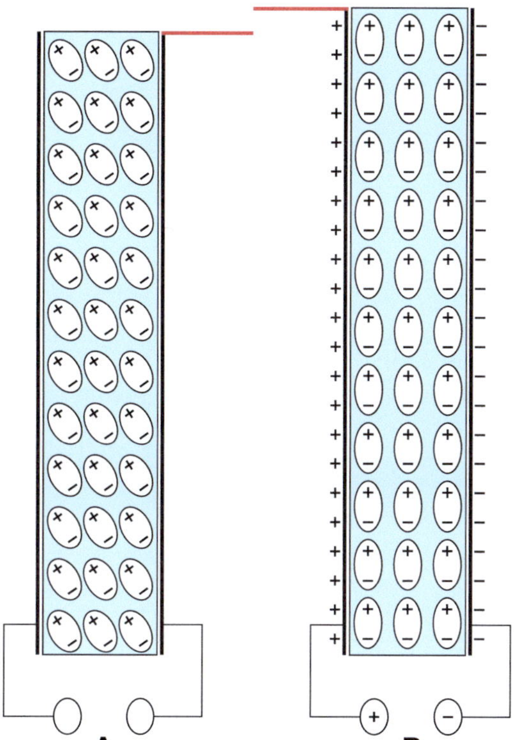

Fig. 5.5 The piezoelectric effect. When a piezoelectric crystal is placed in an electromagnetic field, the molecular dipoles align causing a physical change in the shape of the crystal. An alternating electric current will cause distortions in the shape of the crystal, thereby converting electrical energy into mechanical energy and vice versa. From R. Sofferman and A. Ahuja, Ultrasound of the Thyroid and Parathyroid Glands. Springer 2012

has an outer acoustic lens that helps to focus the emitted sound into a defined slice to improve imaging resolution. For head and neck ultrasound a linear array transducer is most commonly used. When ultrasound is used for imaging, the piezoelectric element spends the vast majority of its time listening for echoes rather than transmitting sound energy. Modern phased array transducers are composed of numerous independent elements that are grouped into sectors. These sectors are arranged so that they fire independently in phases (Fig. 5.6). Phasing of the multiple sectors allows for focusing and steering of the beam. Since each sector generates a sound wave, the addition and subtraction of wave energies as they converge results in the overall wave front. By electronically controlling the timing of sector firing, the beam can be steered and focused [6]. Electronic control of these phased arrays allows the engineer to design transducers that give better overall image quality. (For readers interested in the technical and mathematical aspects of medical ultrasound devices, see [7].)

After sending out a sound pulse, the transducer lists for the resultant echo. Based on the time it takes for the echo to return, the computer will place that echo on the screen at its calculated distance from the probe. The louder the echo, the brighter the dot on the screen. Hence, bright white structures are called "echogenic," while structures that do not generate echoes appear black and are called "anechoic." Based on the results of thousands of pulses and echoes, the computer is able to generate a two-dimensional screen image. "M" mode imaging (M = motion) is a one-dimensional image captured over time. It is used for detecting movement abnormalities, most commonly in cardiac applications. "B" mode (B = brightness) is the familiar 2D grayscale image used in head and neck ultrasound.

As described earlier, echoes returning from distant structures will have markedly diminished strength compared to echoes from structures closer to the probe because of the inverse square law as well as the exponential decrease in sound energy due to attenuation. To correct for this, the computer calculates the time required for the echo to return and uses that to correctly adjust the brightness of the object in the image; the process is called time gain compensation.

Resolution is used informally to describe the clarity of the image. A more formal definition is the ability of the imaging apparatus to display two separate points without merging them. As it pertains to medical ultrasound, there are two types of resolution: axial or longitudinal resolution and lateral resolution. Axial resolution distinguishes objects parallel or in line with the sound beam. Lateral resolution distinguishes objects perpendicular to the beam. Axial resolution is dependent on pulse duration which refers to the length of time that the transducer generates sound. High-frequency sound waves require a shorter pulse duration (e.g., a 5 MHz probe generates 5 cycles

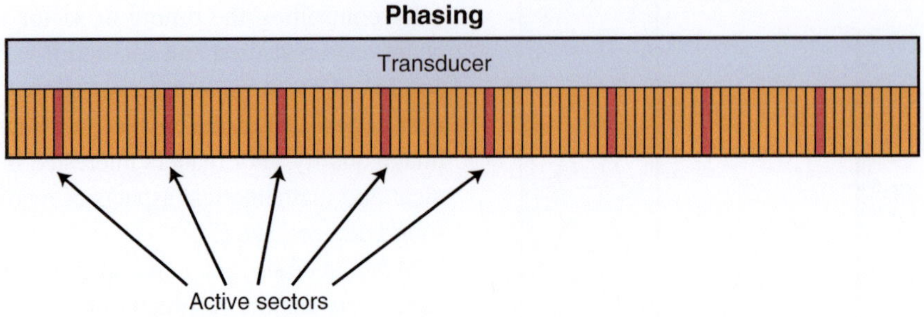

Fig. 5.6 Graphical depiction of an array transducer. A transducer is made up of numerous small, independently controlled crystals. Firing of each crystal can be controlled electronically in "phases" which allow for control of beam shape

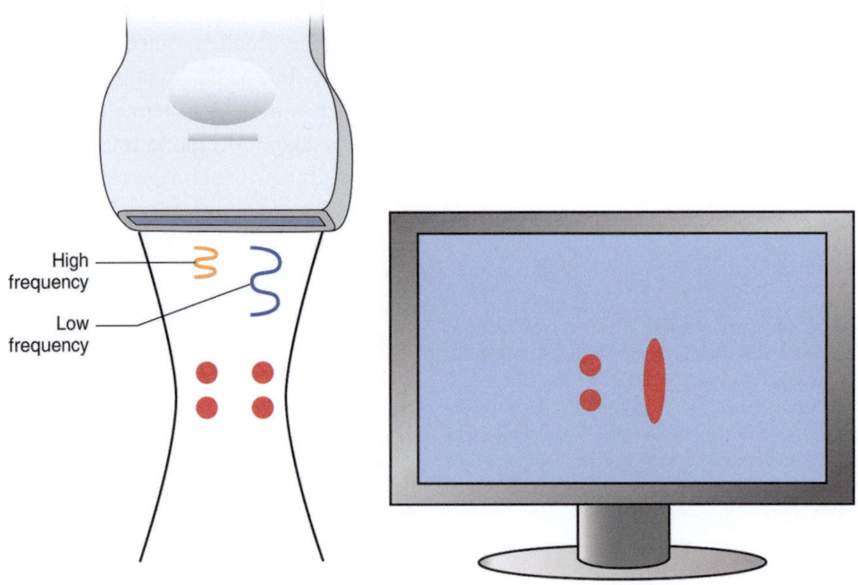

Fig. 5.7 The effect of frequency on resolution. Higher sound frequencies require shorter pulse duration than longer frequencies. As pulse duration shortens, echoes from closely spaced objects along the beam axis become detectable. This results in better axial resolution. Lower frequencies with longer pulse duration result in merging of the two echoes. From R. Sofferman and A. Ahuja, Ultrasound of the Thyroid and Parathyroid Glands. Springer 2012

in 1 μs, whereas a 10 MHz probe generates 10 cycles in the same length of time). If the difference in time between echoes returning from two different objects arranged in parallel is greater than the pulse duration, the objects will then be resolved as separate structures (Fig. 5.7). As the time difference between the returning echoes approaches the pulse duration, the objects will become blurred together. Lateral resolution is highly dependent on beam width. High-frequency probes have a narrower beam width and afford higher resolution. Objects are best seen when imaged in the near field between the probe and the optimal focal zone, called the Fresnel zone. The area more distant to the focal zone where the beams diverge is called the Fraunhofer zone. Ultrasound beams can be focused at different depths, and the position of optimal focus can be controlled and optimized to bring the desired structure into better view (Fig. 5.8). Modern

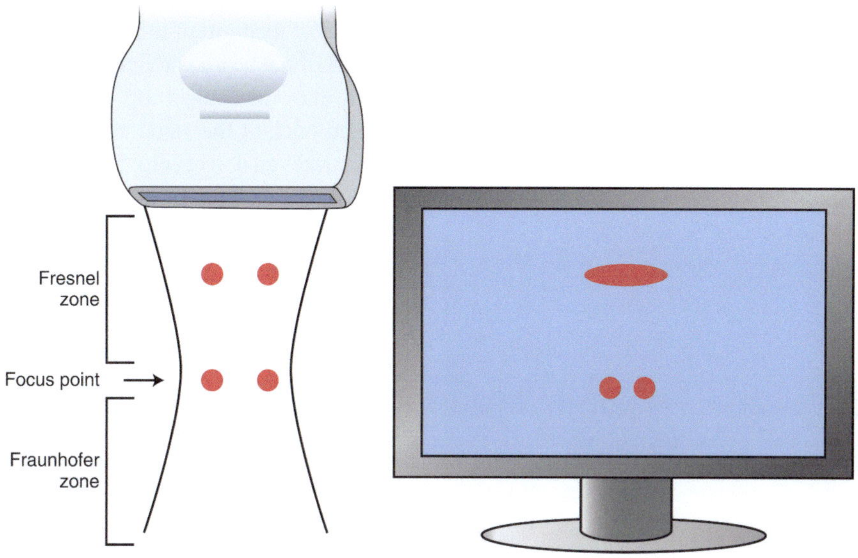

Fig. 5.8 Narrow beam width results in better lateral resolution. Side-by-side objects within the focal zone where the beam width is narrowest are seen as separate objects on the monitor, whereas objects which had a similar distance apart outside of the focal zone are blurred together. From R. Sofferman and A. Ahuja, Ultrasound of the Thyroid and Parathyroid Glands. Springer 2012

machines typically employ more than one focal point or a range of focal points.

A summary of the previous paragraphs brings us to an obvious quandary. Higher resolution ultrasound waves produce better axial resolution but lower penetration due to the effects of attenuation. Lower frequency waves have lower attenuation and therefore better penetration of tissue, but inherently lower resolution. In medical ultrasound, higher frequencies are chosen for superficial structures such as the structures of the neck, breast, and superficial soft tissues. Lower frequencies are chosen for deep structures such as abdominal ultrasound. Typical frequencies for neck ultrasound are in the range of 7.5–18 MHz. Abdominal ultrasound may use frequencies as low as 3.5–5 MHz.

5.3 Physics of Common Artifacts

Artifacts are commonly seen in ultrasound imaging and are a consequence of the physical properties of sound waves. Some artifacts may be helpful in determining the type of medium through which the sound has traveled and, rather than be a hindrance, may provide important diagnostic information.

Enhancement occurs deep to an area of low sound reflection. If sound travels through a region of low reflection, more sound energy is transmitted deep to it and with less than expected attenuation for the distance traveled. Enhancement is seen as an area of unusual brightness and occurs deep to liquid-filled structures such as cysts or large blood vessels but can also occur when sound travels through a relatively homogenous solid structure, such as cartilage (Fig. 5.9).

Shadowing is due to a densely reflective object that reflects essentially all of the sound energy so that no sound is transmitted to the tissues that lie deep to the structure. The image appears black deep to the highly reflecting object. Common sources of shadowing are dense calcifications, bones, kidney or gall bladder stones, or at an air interface (Fig. 5.10).

Reverberation is a common artifact caused by sound waves bouncing back and forth between two parallel highly reflective layers. The probe will detect a prolonged travel time of the returning echo and assume a longer traveling distance. It is seen as a laddering series of echoes. This can be seen within the lumen of blood vessels or cysts (Fig. 5.11). It can also be seen in association with a smooth dense reflector such as a needle.

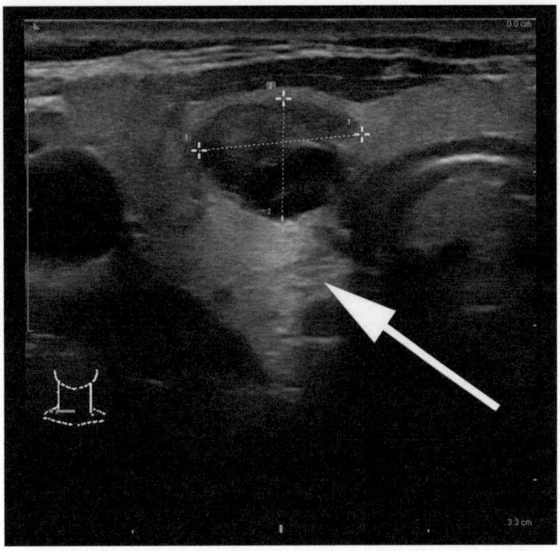

Fig. 5.9 Enhancement seen deep to a hypoechoic thyroid nodule with a cystic component. The area deep to the lesion appears brighter white (*arrow*) compared to adjacent tissue because of more intense echoes. This is because of the unimpeded sound energy being delivered to the tissue

As was mentioned earlier, when sound strikes an object or medium of different acoustic properties, part of the beam is reflected and part is transmitted into the object or medium. Sound is reflected back at the same angle with which the sound strikes an object (Fig. 5.4). As sound energy moves into a medium of different impedance, the transmitted sound wave bends (is refracted) depending on the angle of incidence. Sounds waves encountering a cystic wall or a curved surface at a tangential angle are highly refracted, leading to loss of energy and the formation of a shadow, called an edge artifact. Edge effect can interfere with imaging of objects posterior to the edge of blood vessels in particular (Fig. 5.12).

While not an artifact in the strict sense of the word, reflection can occasionally cause difficulty. A specular reflector such as a needle, if angled so that sound energy is reflected away from the probe, can disappear from view (Fig. 5.13). Some specialized needles are commercially available that are designed to diffusely reflect sound and improve visibility.

Comet tail artifact is a special case of reverberation artifact. It is caused by reverberation occurring between the front and back of a small bright reflector. It is commonly seen in the thy-

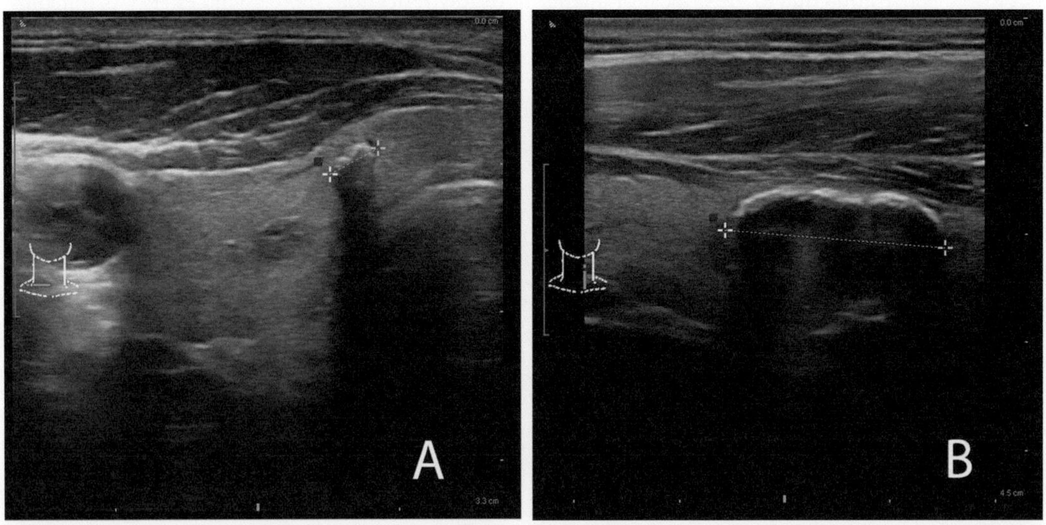

Fig. 5.10 Panel (**a**) shows a calcification (marked by calipers) within the thyroid. Note the shadowing extending deep to the calcification. Panel (**b**) shows a densely calcified capsule of a thyroid nodule. AP dimension of the nodule may not be measurable because of insufficient sound energy reaching beyond the calcification. The shadowing also inhibits visualization of the internal composition of the nodule

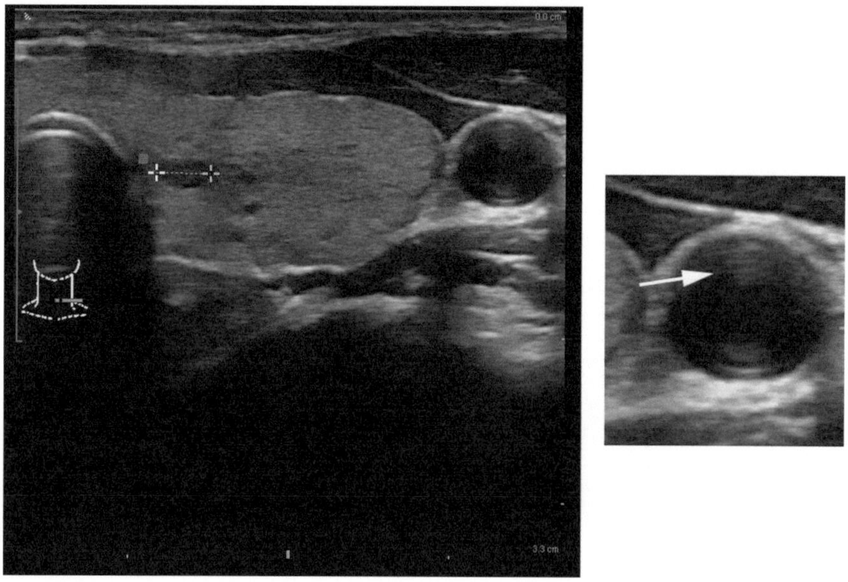

Fig. 5.11 (**a**, **b**) Reverberation artifact seen within the lumen of a carotid artery. Note the ladder pattern due to resonant reverberations (*Arrow*)

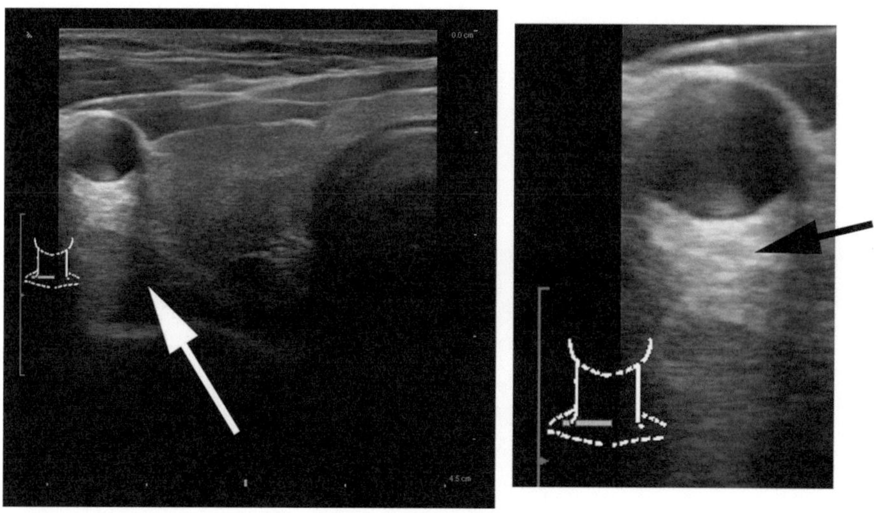

Fig. 5.12 Edge effect seen as two dark streaks extending posteriorly from the edge of the carotid artery (*white arrow*). This is due to the reflection of sound waves according to Snell's law. In the same figure, one can notice the ultrasound beam being focused in its intensity posterior to the carotid artery, appearing as an inverted cone (*black arrow* on magnified image), due to refraction of the sound waves, similar to a lens. Enhancement is also noticeable

roid due to echogenic foci within colloid. With each reverberation some sound energy is released back up to the probe as an echo. The time delay due to the reverberations causes a diminishing triangular cone-shaped echo that looks like a comet's tail (Fig. 5.14).

Ring down artifact is a unique artifact caused by resonance. It occurs when fluid is trapped by tetrahedron of air bubbles. This entrapment allows for resonance to develop. The artifact is seen as a bright long and uninterrupted echo, appearing as a long streak of similar sized short

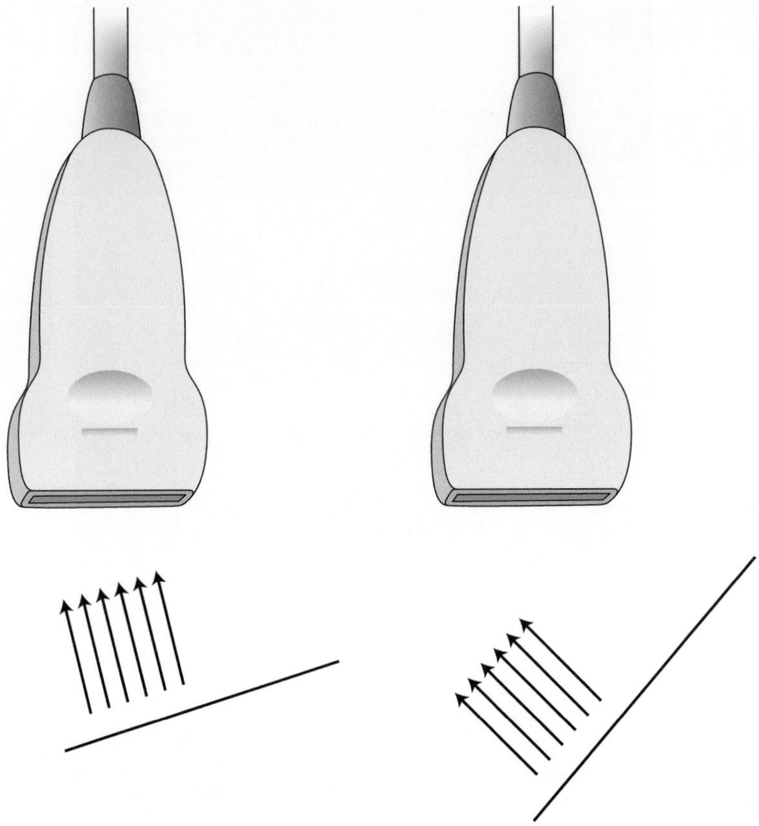

Fig. 5.13 Reflection due to a specular reflector such as a needle can cause most of the sound energy to be reflected away from the probe when the needle is at a steep angle with respect to the transducer. If that occurs, even a densely reflective object may not be visible

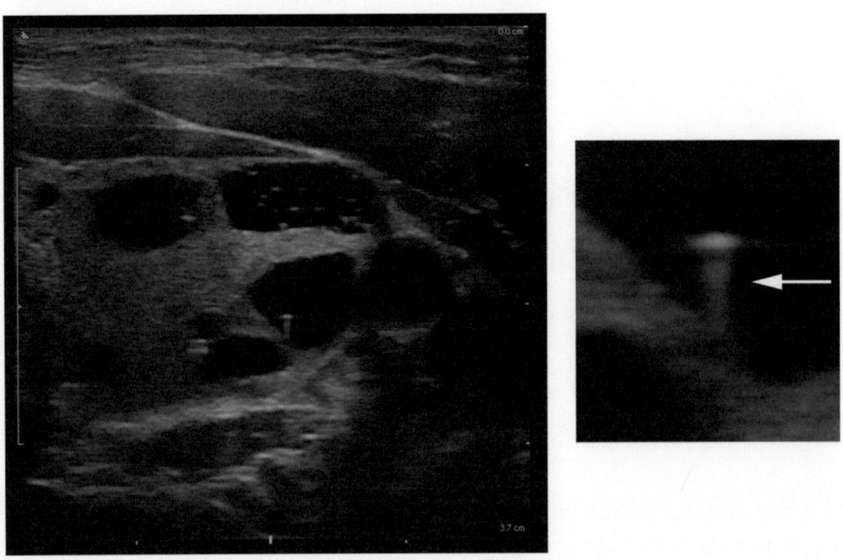

Fig. 5.14 Comet tail artifact. Note the diminishing tail of echoes extending posteriorly from the object. This is best seen in the enlarged view (*inset*, *arrow*). It is a special case of reverberation artifact and typically indicates a benign lesion

lines extending posteriorly from the area of resonance, usually longer than the comet tail artifact. This artifact is relatively rare in the thyroid and parathyroid. It may occasionally be seen in the pharynx or esophagus where bubbles of air and fluid are mixed.

References

1. Zagzebski JA. Essentials of ultrasound physics. St. Louis, MO: Mosby; 1996.
2. Merritt CRB. Physics of ultrasound. In: Rumack CM, Wilson SR, Charboneau JW, Levine D, editors. Diagnostic ultrasound. 4th ed. Philadelphia, PA: Elsevier Mosby; 2011. p. 2–33.
3. Stokes GG. On the theories of the internal friction in fluids in motion, and of the equilibrium and motion of elastic solids. Trans Cambridge Phil Soc. 1845;8(22):287–342.
4. Goss SA, Johnston RL, Dunn F. Comprehensive compilation of empirical ultrasonic properties of mammalian tissues. J Acoust Soc Am. 1978;64(2):423–57.
5. Hagen-Ansert SL. Textbook of diagnostic ultrasonography. 6th ed. St. Louis, MO: Mosby Elsevier; 2006.
6. Zwiebel WJ. Basic ultrasound physics and instrumentation. In: Zwiebel WJ, Sohaey R, editors. Introduction to ultrasound. Philadelphia, PA: Saunders; 1998. p. 2–17.
7. Cobbold RSC. Foundations of biomedical ultrasound. New York, NY: Oxford University Press; 2007.

6 Principles of Color and Power Doppler in Neck Ultrasound Imaging

Nicholas J. Hangiandreou and Nicole L. Strissel

6.1 Introduction

Doppler ultrasound, especially color Doppler imaging, is used extensively in the evaluation of thyroid and parathyroid anatomy and pathology. In this chapter, the principles of the Doppler effect will be discussed and an overview of spectral Doppler methods will be briefly described. Color Doppler imaging will then be discussed in detail, including acquisition methods, characteristics of the images, and artifacts and pitfalls commonly seen when scanning the neck. Power Doppler mode and its relationship to color Doppler will also be described. More detailed explanation of color Doppler physics and technology are available in references [1] and [2], while reference [3] provides more in-depth discussion of artifacts and image optimization techniques.

N.J. Hangiandreou, Ph.D. (✉)
N.L. Strissel, M.S., R.V.T., R.D.M.S. (✉)
Department of Radiology, Mayo Clinic,
200 First Street SW, Rochester, MN 55905, USA
e-mail: hangiandreou@mayo.edu;
strissel.nicole@mayo.edu

6.2 The Doppler Effect

The Doppler effect describes the situation in which a source of waves and a receiver are moving relative to one another. Figure 6.1 shows a particular example where a source of sound waves is moving relative to several different receivers. Although the frequency of the sound emitted by the source is constant, the motion of the sound source will affect the frequency detected by the receivers. The received frequency depends on the position of the receiver with respect to the source and the direction of motion of the source. The receivers "R1," "R2," "R3," and "R4" will each detect different frequencies. In this example, the motion of the source, "S," is directly toward receiver R1 at a velocity "v," effectively squeezing the wave fronts closer together as shown, causing R1 to detect a higher frequency than the transmitted frequency. Motion of the source is directly away from receiver R2, causing wave fronts to be stretched out, resulting in a lower detected frequency by R2. R3, which lies at an angle less than 180° with respect to the source, will also detect a lower frequency than that transmitted but not as low as detected by R2. In the special case where the receiver is at right angles (90°) to the direction of motion (R4), no frequency shift results and the transmitted and received frequencies are equal.

The difference between the detected and transmitted frequencies is called the Doppler

M. Milas et al. (eds.), *Advanced Thyroid and Parathyroid Ultrasound*,
DOI 10.1007/978-3-319-44100-9_6

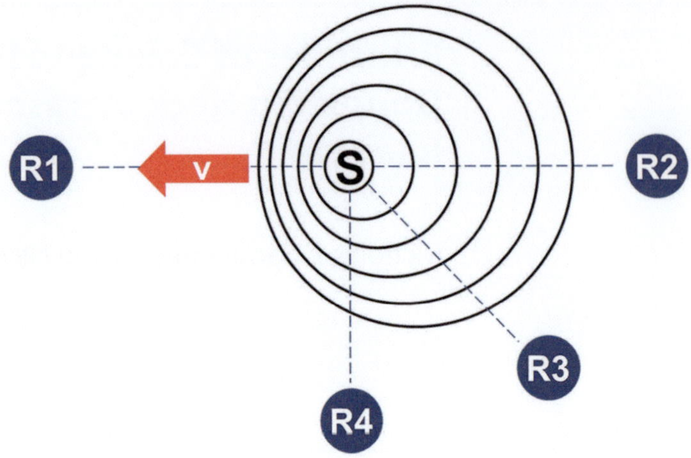

Fig. 6.1 This diagram illustrates the basic idea behind the Doppler effect which describes the situation in which a source of waves ("S") and a receiver ("R1," "R2," "R3," or "R4") are moving relative to one another at a velocity of "v" (*red arrow*). The frequency transmitted by the source and the frequency detected by the receivers are generally all different, depending on the direction of motion and positions of the source and receiver

shift and is directly proportional to the velocity of the source as described by the Doppler equation:

$$\Delta f = \frac{v f_0 \cos(\theta)}{c} \qquad \begin{aligned} &\Delta f: \text{Doppler shift} \\ &v: \text{source velocity} \\ &f_0: \text{source frequency} \\ &\theta: \text{Doppler angle} \\ &c: \text{speed of sound} \end{aligned}$$

(Because of the pulse-echo nature of medical ultrasound, the Doppler equation programmed in ultrasound scanners includes a factor of "2" not reflected in the equation above, indicating that the Doppler shifts detected clinically are twice as large as those predicted by the above equation.) If the source frequency, Doppler angle, and speed of sound propagation in the medium are known, the source velocity can be computed from the measured Doppler shift. The Doppler angle is defined as the angle between the line connecting the source and receiver and the velocity vector (arrow showing the direction of motion). Receivers R1 and R2 have Doppler angles of 0° and 180°, respectively. They will have the greatest possible Doppler shifts but opposite signs, one positive and one negative. The R1 Doppler shift will be positive (since received frequency > transmitted frequency) corresponding to velocity toward the receiver, and the R2 and R3 Doppler shifts will be negative. R4 has a Doppler angle of 90° and a Doppler shift of zero as though no source motion is occurring. Although the Doppler effect can involve the motion of any biologic tissue or fluid, for example, a ureteral jet entering the urinary bladder, the vast majority of clinical radiology applications involve the detection and measurement of vascular flow.

6.3 Duplex/Spectral Doppler Mode

Initial use of the Doppler effect in medical ultrasound was aimed toward rapidly measuring the spectrum of all blood velocities present in a small measurement region or "sample volume." This mode is referred to as spectral, duplex, or pulsed wave Doppler. It produces a real-time graphical scroll of velocity spectra versus time, with ~100 spectra measured each second. A sample measurement of blood velocity in the superior thyroid artery is shown in Fig. 6.2. The horizontal axis of the graph is "time" in units of seconds, and the vertical axis is "velocity" in units of centimeters per second (cm/s). The sample volume is defined by the short yellow lines in the two-dimensional (2D) color Doppler image above the spectral graph and is positioned by the sonographer at the desired measurement location in the 2D image. The ultrasound pulse direction (solid white line through the sample volume) and the blood flow direction indicator (dashed blue line traversing

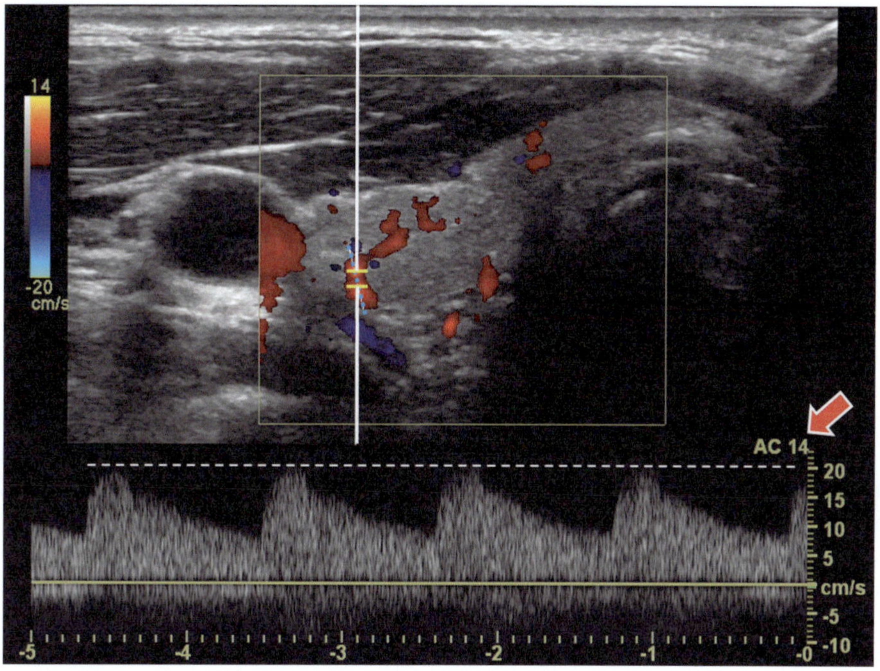

Fig. 6.2 This figure shows an example of a duplex Doppler image, with a spectrum obtained from the superior thyroid artery. The *red arrow* indicates the Doppler angle, here 14°. The *dashed white line* shows the estimated peak systolic velocity of ~20 cm/s

the sample volume) are both also adjusted by the sonographer and define the Doppler angle, displayed as 14° in this image (red arrow).

Each spectrum is acquired from ~100 pulse-echo cycles over a period of ~10 milliseconds (ms), with all pulses aimed through the sample volume along the indicated pulse direction. The detected echoes are typically processed using a fast Fourier transform (FFT) algorithm to compute all components of the velocity spectrum. The entire cross section of the small artery in Fig. 6.2 is contained in the sample volume, resulting in a range of velocities between a peak value that depends on the heart cycle phase down to values near zero which are typically present near the vessel walls. Undesired low-velocity signals caused by slow, soft tissue motion can be removed from the spectrum using the wall filter control. This filter is helpful in eliminating nonvascular artifacts, for example, caused by slow, soft tissue motion around a vessel. However, signals from very slow blood flow can also be removed if the wall filter setting is too high. The brightness of the spectral display can be adjusted using the Doppler gain control. The sensitivity of the velocity axis of the spectral graph can be adjusted using the Doppler scale control (which also adjusts the pulse repetition frequency, PRF). The peak systolic value from the first full waveform cycle is estimated to be ~20 cm/s (horizontal dashed white line). Duplex Doppler is sometimes used in thyroid imaging to demonstrate arterial waveforms, although specific velocity measurements are not typically of interest. When the most accurate velocity measurements are needed, Doppler angles as far as possible from 90° are desirable, since they result in the largest measured Doppler shift signals and the smallest errors in calculated velocities. Doppler angles at or close to 90° will produce very small Doppler shifts and large errors in calculated velocity due to intrinsic spectral broadening effects. The disadvantage of angles near 90° for Doppler can be confusing for the sonographer, as it runs contrary to best practice for grayscale imaging, where incidence angles of 90° often result in the sharpest images. Figure 6.3

shows the Doppler spectral mirror artifact that can occur for Doppler angles near 90°. The spectrum is noisy and demonstrates low velocities replicated on either side of the zero-velocity baseline, as compared with the correctly acquired image in Fig. 6.2. Figure 6.4 illustrates the aliasing artifact which occurs when the highest measured velocity components exceed the upper bounds of the spectral graph (dashed yellow line) and wrap around to appear on the bottom of the graph (solid yellow line). This artifact can be distinguished from true flow away from the probe by noting that it is only an isolated peak that is displayed below the baseline and that this portion of the waveform would "fit" perfectly on the portion of the waveform above the baseline. This artifact may be corrected by adjusting the velocity scale to be less sensitive (which acts to increase the PRF) or shifting the velocity baseline down to fully accommodate the spectra in the upper part of the graph or both as shown in Fig. 6.2.

6.4 Overview of the Color Doppler Image

Figure 6.5 shows an example of a color Doppler image of a typical, normal right thyroid lobe. This is a thin slice, tomographic image typically obtained with a wide bandwidth, high-frequency linear array probe (in this case a 6–15 megaHertz [MHz] linear probe). Color Doppler images of the neck are typically obtained at ~5–15 frames per second (fps). Pixels inside the color box (yellow) are either rendered in color where flowing blood is detected or in grayscale for static soft tissues. Velocity is color-coded according to the color bar shown at the left side of the image (red arrow). The color scale control (which adjusts the PRF) determines the velocity measurement sensitivity, and the specific velocity values that correspond to the top and bottom of the color bar are 10 cm/s and −10 cm/s, respectively, in this example (red arrow). Pixel color indicates estimated mean blood velocity and direction of flow, with the upper portion of the color bar representing flow toward the probe (usually reds and yellows) and the bottom half representing flow away from the probe (usually blue). The color scale may be inverted by the user in some cases, but the upper part of the color bar will always represent flow toward the probe. Zero velocity is indicated by the black region in the center of the color scale. Shown at the ends of the color bar are maximum mean velocity values corresponding for each flow direction. It is important to recognize that these values are accurate only for flow directions directly toward or away from the probe, with a Doppler angle of 0 (or 180) degrees. As flow direction and thus Doppler angle are not specified by the user in color Doppler mode and velocity directions will typically vary across the image plane, color-coded mean velocity values in these images are not usually considered to be highly accurate. If accurate measurements of velocity are needed, duplex Doppler mode should be used. Pixels outside of the color box are all shown in grayscale regardless of the presence of flowing blood. Color and duplex Doppler modes are complementary: The color Doppler image shows less accurate velocity information from multiple locations across a large spatial region, while the duplex Doppler mode measures accurate velocity information in a single small spatial location.

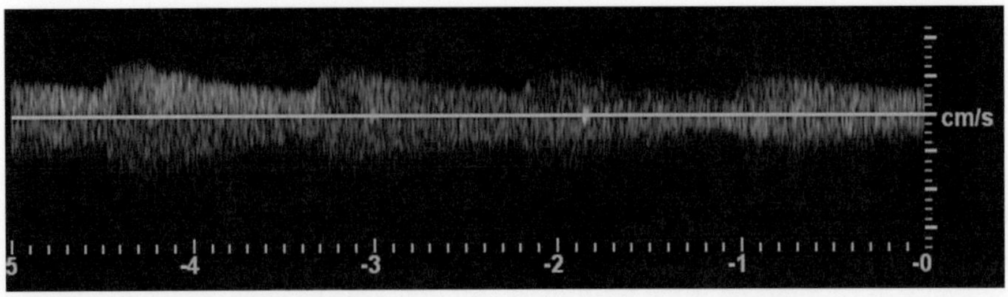

Fig. 6.3 The Doppler spectrum shown here illustrates the Doppler spectral mirror artifact

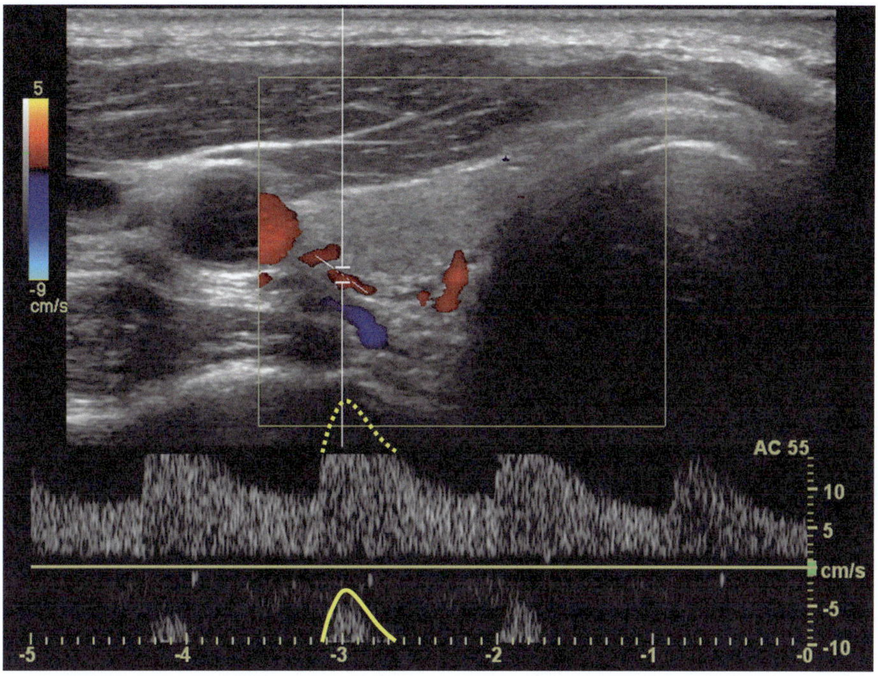

Fig. 6.4 The Doppler spectrum shown in this image illustrates the aliasing artifact. The *dashed yellow line* indicates the part of the velocity spectrum cut off due to the aliasing artifact, and the *solid yellow line* shows the actual location of these high-velocity signals in the wrong location in the spectral display

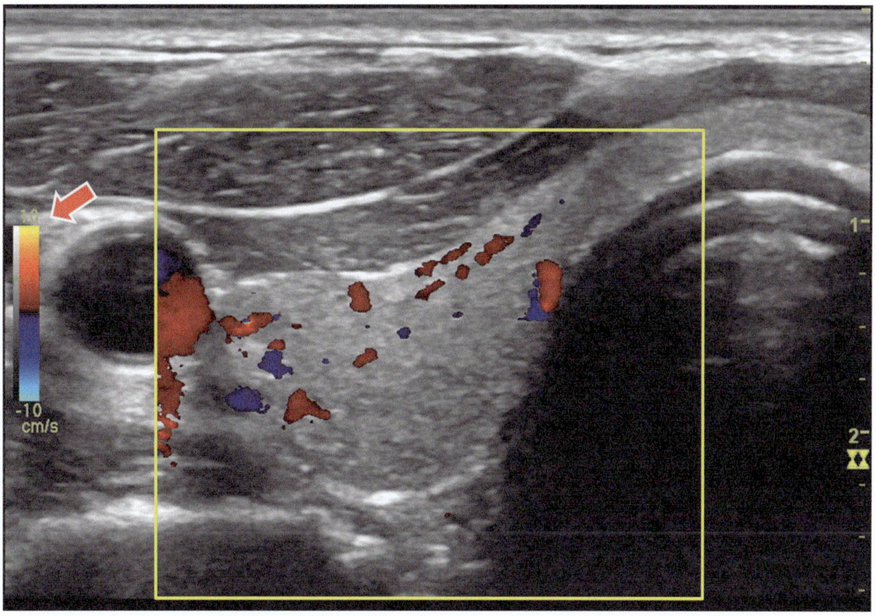

Fig. 6.5 This figure shows an example of a color Doppler image of the right lobe of a normal thyroid gland. The *red arrow* indicates the color scale value and the color bar

6.5 Color Doppler Image Acquisition

Figure 6.6 illustrates some key aspects of the color Doppler image acquisition process. Since these images are composites of grayscale anatomical information and color-coded mean velocity information, two different sets of ultrasound pulses are used. "Grayscale pulses" are aimed parallel to the edges of the image (black arrow). These pulses use the highest available transmit frequency that can penetrate to the specified image depth. An entire set of grayscale pulses is used to span the entire field of view and acquire the 2D grayscale image. "Velocity pulses" are directed parallel to the edges of the color box specified by the sonographer (yellow arrow). The color box can be steered to obtain Doppler angles that better demonstrate flow, in which case the grayscale and velocity pulses will not be parallel to one another. The velocity pulses will typically have transmit frequencies that are significantly lower than those used for the grayscale pulses, in order to minimize the effects of attenuation on the very weak echoes reflected from blood. Transmit frequencies for both sets of pulses may be adjusted.

As shown in Fig. 6.6, the color box can be visualized as an array of Doppler sample volumes. A set of ~10 pulses are directed down each column of sample volumes ("color line") to determine the mean velocity in each one, as compared with the ~100 pulses used for each spectrum in duplex mode as discussed earlier. This limited pulse-echo data set is not sufficient to determine all velocity components (e.g., peak velocity), but autocorrelation algorithms can be used to determine velocity mean, direction, variance, and power. However, the limited number of velocity pulses per color line allows higher color Doppler frames rates to be obtained. The density of velocity pulses across the color box is also reduced as compared with the grayscale pulses to promote higher color Doppler frame rates. However, this also results in limited color spatial (lateral) resolution. Sets of velocity pulses are used to interrogate all of the color lines across the full color box, thus estimating mean velocity at all locations within the color box. Depending on the color Doppler frame rate and the heart rate of the patient, ~3–15 frames may be obtained during each heart cycle, so pulsatile blood flow changes

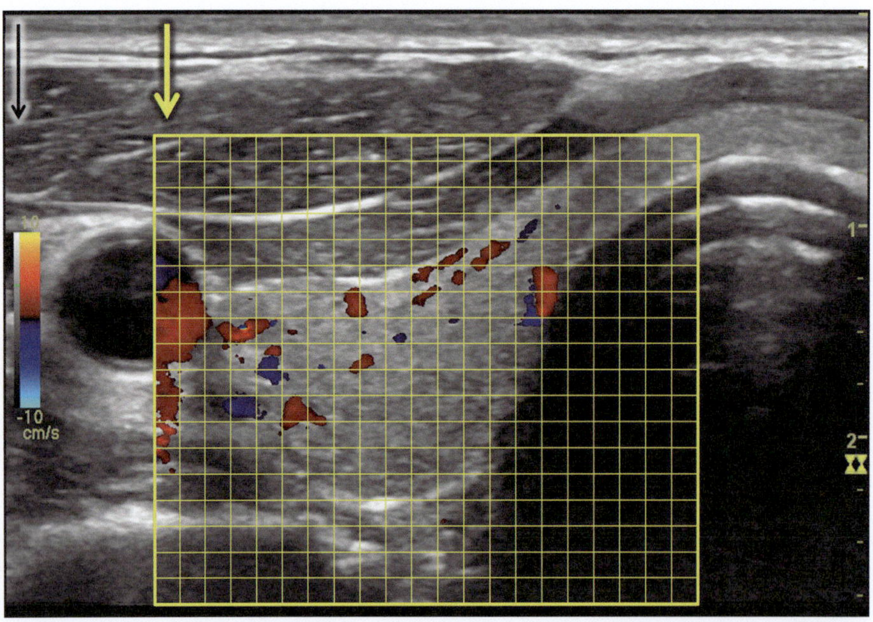

Fig. 6.6 Color Doppler image showing the color box as comprised of an array of Doppler sample volumes (*yellow grid*, not drawn to scale). Also shown are grayscale (*black arrow*) and velocity (*yellow arrow*) pulse directions

may be observed in a sequence of color Doppler images.

After acquisition of all grayscale and velocity echoes for an image, the scanner must analyze all locations inside the color box to determine if flowing blood is present. If so, color-coded velocity information is displayed. Otherwise soft tissue is assumed to be present and grayscale information is shown. This blood-tissue discrimination algorithm considers multiple variables that may include mean velocity, velocity variance, spectral power, and echo amplitude. Different aspects of the blood-tissue discrimination process are often integrated with controls that may be adjusted by the system user to reduce artifacts and optimize image appearance, e.g., wall filter, color gain, and color write priority.

6.6 Color Doppler Limitations and Artifacts

There are several limitations of color Doppler that can negatively impact the use of this mode when scanning the thyroid. One limitation that has already been alluded to involves *low frame rates*. Color Doppler frame rate is most strongly affected by the color box width and depth. Figure 6.7 shows two image examples with different color box sizes. The smaller color box in Fig. 6.7a results in a frame rate of 10 fps, while the larger color box in Fig. 6.7b reduces this to 7 fps. The *aliasing artifact*, described earlier for duplex Doppler, can also occur in color Doppler mode as shown in Fig. 6.8. Aliasing appears as colored regions that include a mix of colors from both sides of the color bar, as seen in the vessel indicated by the red arrow (as well as other vessels) in Fig. 6.8a. Reducing the color scale sensitivity can reduce the incidence of aliasing resulting in vessels with consistent color appearance, as indicated by the red arrow in Fig. 6.8b. *Color dropout* refers to situations where color in a vessel should be demonstrated but is absent. This can be caused by several factors. If the Doppler angle for some vessels is near 90°, detected Doppler frequency shifts will be small and will correspond to low velocities in both directions, as shown in Fig. 6.3 for duplex Doppler mode. The average of these velocity signals will be very near zero, suggesting the absence of blood flow, so color may not be present at this vessel location. Improperly adjusted scan controls, such as color gain (analogous to the spectral Doppler gain discussed earlier), color scale (color mapping sensitivity), and wall filter (which removes low-velocity components from the color display as described earlier for duplex Doppler) can cause this lack of color signal. Color dropout examples caused by poor control settings are shown in Fig. 6.9. Figure 6.9a represents a properly acquired image, while Figs. 6.9b–d demonstrate reduced flow due to a high color scale value, a low color gain setting, and a high wall filter value, respectively. Slow flow and small vessels are especially prone to color dropout. *Blooming artifact*, also referred to as *color bleed*, describes

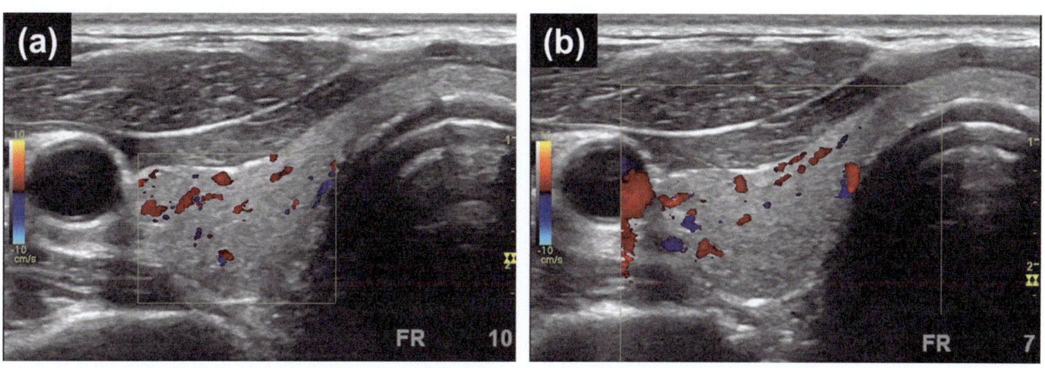

Fig. 6.7 These two figures show the influence of color box size and depth on color Doppler frame rate. The images in (**a**) and (**b**) have frame rates of 10 and 7 frames per second, respectively

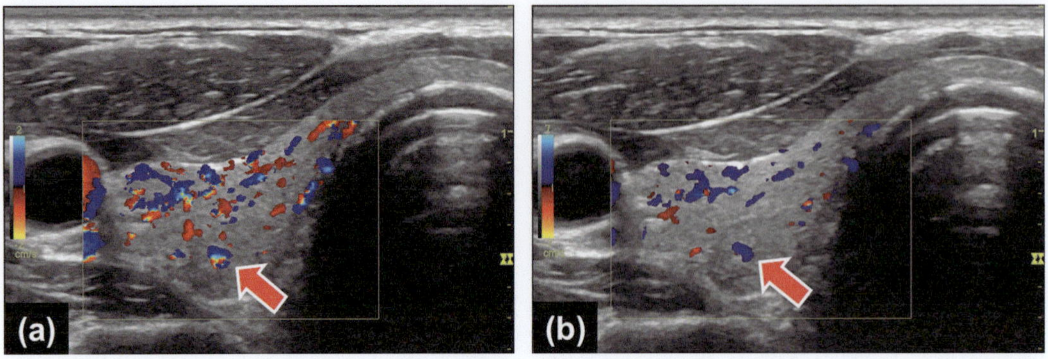

Fig. 6.8 Color Doppler aliasing is shown in (**a**). Panel (**b**) shows this artifact corrected by increasing the color scale. The *red arrows* in both panels indicate the same vascular structure shown in each of the images

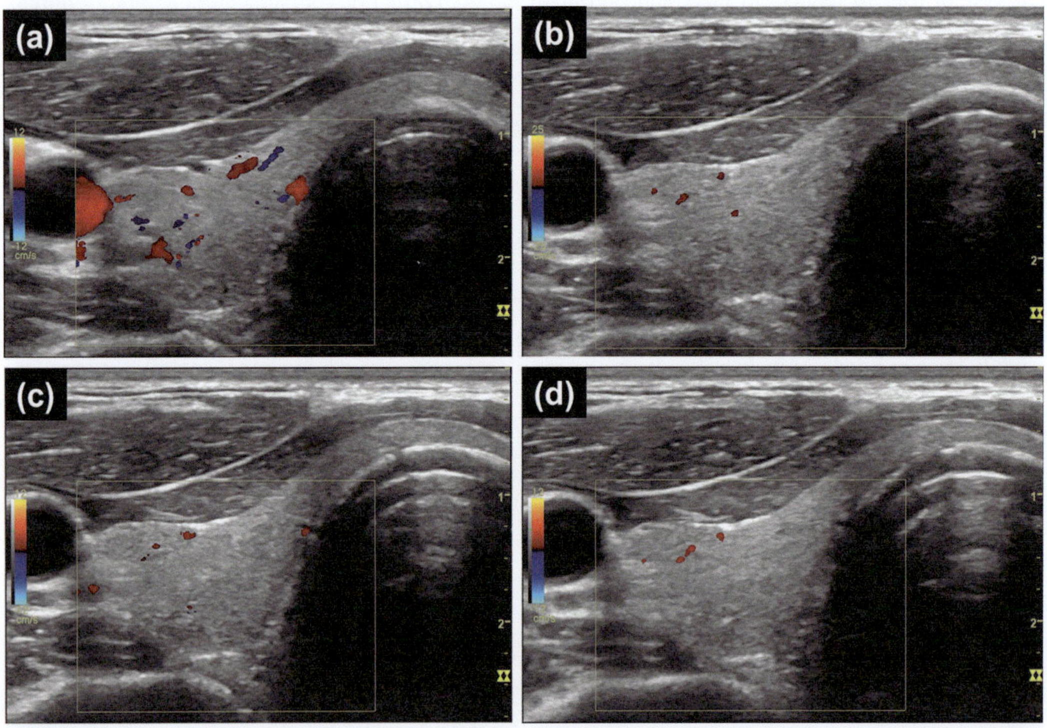

Fig. 6.9 Color dropout is shown in (**b**), (**c**), and (**d**), caused by improper adjustment of the image controls. Panel (**a**) shows a properly acquired image for comparison. In (**b**) the color scale has been set too high (to a value of 25 cm/s). In (**c**) the color gain value is too low, while in (**d**) the wall filter value is too high

the situation in which color from a vessel extends outside of the vascular space to the vessel wall and other soft tissues. This artifact is typically caused by improperly adjusted scan controls, including color gain, color write priority (which preferentially colors pixels with low, blood-like echo amplitudes), and wall filter. An example of color bleed caused by an incorrectly elevated color gain setting is shown in Fig. 6.10b, as compared to the correctly acquired image in Fig. 6.10a. Finally, *flash artifact* is commonly seen as one or more large regions of color appearing over soft tissues or hypoechoic shadowed image regions. This artifact is caused by gross motion of the

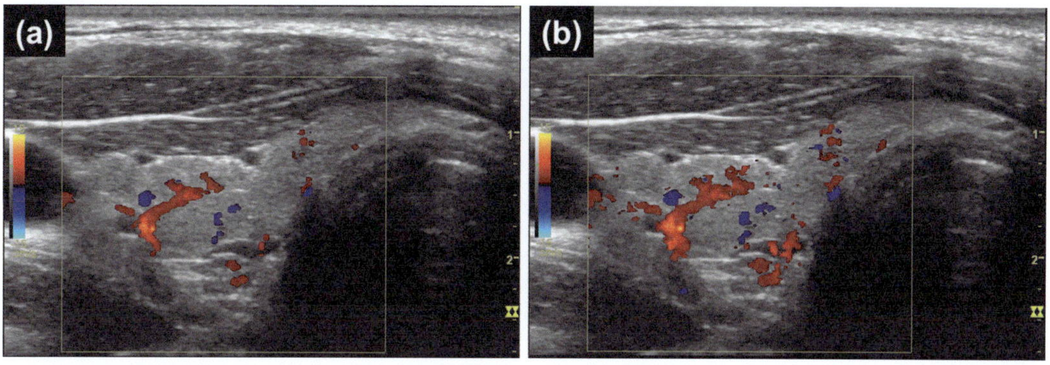

Fig. 6.10 Color blooming (or bleed) artifact caused by poor adjustment of the color gain control is shown in (**b**), as compared with the properly acquired image in (**a**)

patient or probe or by tissue vibration (e.g., caused by the patient speaking). Examples of flash artifact are shown in Fig. 6.11. Figure 6.11a shows a properly acquired image, and Fig. 6.11b–d shows examples of flash artifact caused by a patient cough, the patient swallowing, and the patient talking, respectively. Modern scanners may provide a specific "flash filter" control to reduce the incidence of this artifact.

6.7 Power Mode Doppler Imaging

Power (or energy) mode Doppler imaging is a variation of color Doppler that is sometimes used, especially when increased sensitivity to the presence of slow flow is needed. Figure 6.12a shows an example of a power Doppler image along with the corresponding color Doppler image in Fig. 6.12b. The power Doppler image does not color-code mean velocity information as in color Doppler mode but rather codes the power of the Doppler spectrum. Spectral power is computed by the autocorrelation algorithm (used also to compute mean velocity for color Doppler mode). The power value is associated with the amount of moving blood that is present at each location in the image and does not include any information about mean velocity or flow direction. This can be seen by comparing the color pixels in the color and power mode images in Fig. 6.12. The color bar shown in the power mode image also reflects this difference and demonstrates only an orange-yellow color scheme. Since flow direction is not shown in power mode images, the aliasing artifact will also not be demonstrated. The noise properties of the power signal promote improved visualization of slow velocity signals, and sensitivity is further improved by increasing the number of pulse-echo cycles per image and increasing the level of frame averaging. The latter changes also tend to reduce the power Doppler frame rate, as compared with color Doppler, and make power mode more prone to flash artifact. The increased sensitivity to slow flow allows power mode Doppler to more reliably demonstrate vessels even when the Doppler angle is near 90°. The power mode image in Fig. 6.12 does demonstrate greater vascularity as compared with the corresponding color mode image, but, as with all of the image comparisons in this chapter, it is important to recognize that there will be some variability in the depiction of vasculature due to breathing motion and heart cycle phase variability. Although initially introduced to improve overall sensitivity to slow flow, the observed advantages of power Doppler as compared with color Doppler on modern ultrasound imaging systems will generally vary between commercial products. Hybrid modes such as directional power Doppler are also available on some scanners.

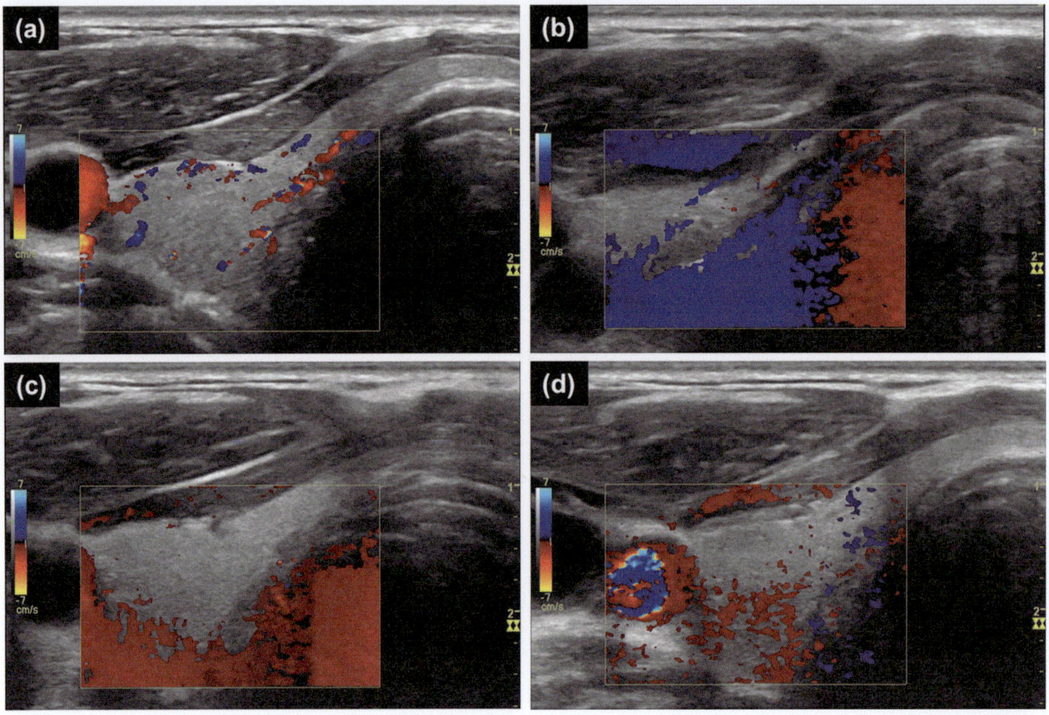

Fig. 6.11 Flash artifact is shown in (**b**), (**c**), and (**d**), caused by patient coughing, swallowing, and talking, respectively. Panel (**a**) shows an image without artifact for comparison

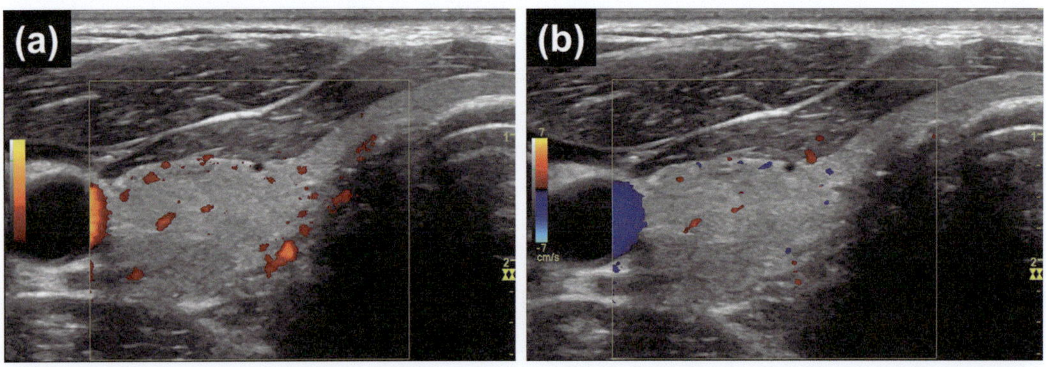

Fig. 6.12 An example of a power (or energy) mode Doppler image is shown in (**a**), compared with the corresponding color Doppler image shown in (**b**)

References

1. Hoskins P, Martin K, Thrush A, editors. Diagnostic ultrasound physics and equipment. 2nd ed. New York, NY: Cambridge University Press; 2010.
2. Gill R. The physics and technology of diagnostic ultrasound: a practitioner's guide. Sydney, NSW: High Frequency Publishing; 2012.
3. Rubens DJ, Bhatt S, Nedelka S, Cullinan J. Doppler artifacts and pitfalls. Radiol Clin N Am. 2006;44(6):805–35.

3D Ultrasound

7

Dina Elaraj

7.1 Introduction

Ultrasound is the most widely used imaging modality in the evaluation of thyroid and parathyroid disease. The most commonly used technique involves the use of a high frequency transducer and the capture of two-dimensional (2D) grayscale images. These images can provide information regarding thyroid gland size and appearance; presence, size, and appearance of thyroid nodules; and presence, size, and location of abnormal parathyroid glands. In addition, 2D ultrasound is the preferred imaging modality to evaluate the cervical lymph nodes in a patient with thyroid cancer and can give information regarding lymph node size, shape, appearance, and location.

The imaging characteristics of thyroid nodules and cervical lymph nodes on 2D ultrasound are used to increase or decrease the clinical suspicion of malignancy. Ultrasound characteristics of thyroid nodules that are associated with malignancy include hypoechogenicity, microcalcifications, and irregular margins [1]. Ultrasound characteristics of malignant cervical lymph nodes include enlarged size, round shape, microcalcifications, cystic change, loss of hilar architecture, and increased peripheral flow [2–5]. Although some of these features have very high positive predictive value in detecting malignancy, they are not 100% specific, and many thyroid cancers and metastatic nodes may lack these features, lowering their sensitivity. Furthermore, the assessment of vascularity using 2D ultrasound has been subject to high interobservor variability, which is likely a reflection of the inhomogeneous vascular pattern of thyroid nodules and lymph nodes, as well as that the choice of the plane for evaluation is operator dependent. Because of these limitations, adjuncts and alternatives to 2D ultrasound have been developed and studied.

An alternative to gray scale 2D ultrasound is three-dimensional (3D) ultrasound, with or without the addition of intraveneous contrast agents [6, 7, 21]. These techniques have been used for the assessment of thyroid cancer margins and vascular flow patterns in both thyroid nodules and cervical lymph nodes. 3D ultrasound has also proven to be more accurate than 2D ultrasound in the determination of overall thyroid gland volume and nodule volume.

D. Elaraj, M.D., F.A.C.S. (✉)
Section of Endocrine Surgery, Department of Surgery, Northwestern University Feinberg School of Medicine, 676 N. St. Clair Street, Suite 650, Chicago, IL 60611, USA
e-mail: delaraj@nm.org

7.2 Technical Aspects of Three-Dimensional (3D) Ultrasound

The application of 3D imaging in the neck is largely related to evaluation of the thyroid gland, with very limited literature regarding 3D ultra-

M. Milas et al. (eds.), *Advanced Thyroid and Parathyroid Ultrasound*,
DOI 10.1007/978-3-319-44100-9_7

sound for the evaluation of parathyroid disease [8]. The most extensive application of 3D ultrasound technology has been in the field of obstetrics and gynecological imaging [9] For example, the 3D view of the fetus allows the best evaluation of fetal anatomy and provides information not available on the 2D views. Other applications include breast imaging [10], brachytherapy seed implantation for patients with prostate cancer [11], estimation of urinary bladder volumes [12], and echocardiography [13].

Images displayed in three dimensions are either reformatted from 2D images produced by a conventional ultrasound transducer with a one-dimensional (1D) array (Fig. 7.1) or generated directly in real time by an ultrasound transducer with a 2D array (Fig. 7.2). Conventional 1D transducers are more commonly used than 2D arrays because they are less expensive and require less specialized technology. They do, however, require rapid or gated scanning techniques in order to avoid motion artifact [14]. Two scanning methods exist: automated capture and freehand capture [14, 15]. Automated capture involves attaching the transducer to a mechanical scanning device which then moves the transducer. 2D images are acquired at predefined intervals. Disadvantages of this approach include device bulkiness and higher cost because it is a motor controlled system and will also have maintenance costs. Freehand capture involves movement of the transducer by the ultrasonographer. The transducer has an attachment that provides information regarding orientation and angulation which allows for 3D image reconstruction after data acquisition. In contrast to data acquisition using transducers with 1D arrays, transducers with 2D arrays allow the transducer to remain stationary and the scanning to be done electronically by sweeping an ultrasound beam composed of volumes shaped like pyramids or cones over the anatomic structure of interest (Fig. 7.2) [14, 15]. The returned echoes are processed to produce 3D images in real time.

Once the data acquisition has been completed, images can then be displayed in either B-mode (gray scale) or Doppler using a variety of display techniques. The most common display techniques are (1) multiplanar reformatting, (2) volume rendering, and (3) surface rendering [14, 15]. Multiplanar reformatting is the most common display technique and displays planar cross-sectional images that resemble conventional 2D ultrasound images but are extracted from the 3D

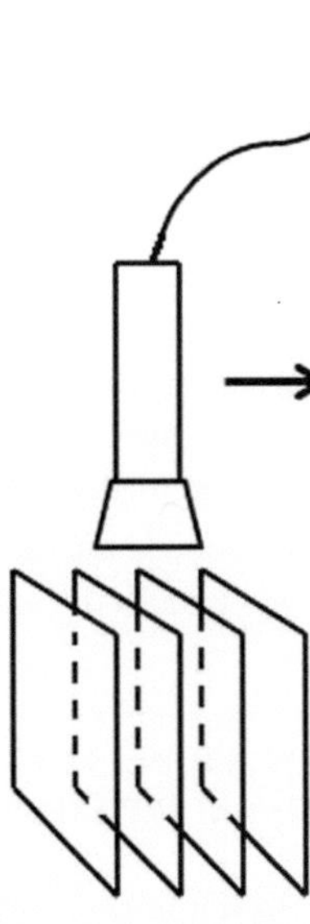

Fig. 7.1 Multiple two-dimensional (2D) ultrasound images produced by sweeping a conventional one-dimensional (1D) ultrasound transducer over an anatomic structure of interest. The 2D images can be reformatted to display images in three dimensions (3D)

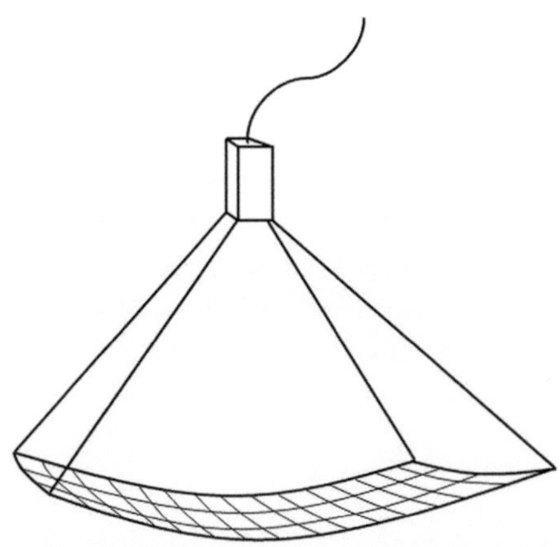

Fig. 7.2 Ultrasound transducer with a two-dimensional (2D) array remains stationary while electronically sweeping the ultrasound beam over an anatomic structure of interest. The three-dimensional (3D) images are generated in real time

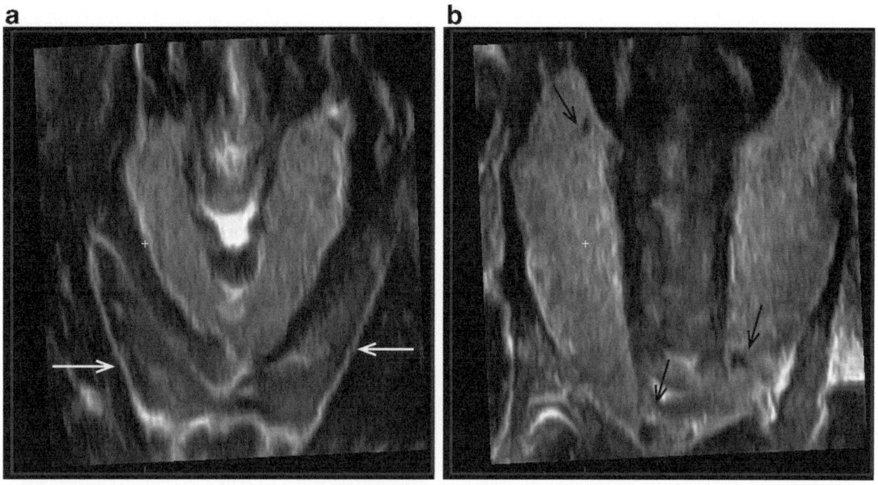

Fig. 7.3 Multiplanar reconstruction 3D images of the thyroid in the coronal plane are show anteriorly at the level of the isthmus and thyroid cartilage (*arrows*) in (**a**) and more posteriorly in (**b**). Several small cystic nodules are noted (*arrows*) in (**b**)

image (Fig. 7.3). The 2D planes are shown with 3D cues. The orthogonal plane view displays three perpendicular planes simultaneously, and the cube view shows the 3D image as a polyhedron which represents the boundaries of the reconstructed volume [14]. Each plane can be manipulated relative to any of the other planes. The polyhedron in the cube-view display technique can be rotated in any direction. The volume rendering display technique shows the entire 3D image projected onto a 2D plane. The surface rendering display technique only displays an image of the surfaces of structures. Some of these display techniques can also be combined.

3D ultrasound has advantages and disadvantages compared with 2D ultrasound (Table 7.1) [15]. Advantages of 3D ultrasound include that it stores all data continuously, it allows for a more rapid examination/faster data acquisition because it is not necessary for the ultrasonographer to select single images to save, and data can be manipulated to display images in any plane or produce 3D reconstructions, which allows for the assessment of exact spatial relationships. 3D ultrasound with Doppler can also allow for a more accurate assessment of the vascularity of a structure, as it can evaluate the vessels during a 360° rotation of the volume rather than rely on the ultrasonographer's choice of the plane for the evaluation of vascularity. The main disadvantage of 3D ultrasound compared with 2D ultrasound is that 3D ultrasound may have inferior image quality because of the lower resolution of the extracted planes from volume data [16]. In addition, 3D ultrasound images require large data sets and computational requirements to process and display the data and may be subject to motion and reconstruction artifacts.

Applications of 3D ultrasound technology in the evaluation of thyroid disease can broadly be divided into three categories: risk assessment of thyroid nodules for malignancy, preoperative assessment of extrathyroidal extension of thyroid cancers, and thyroid volume calculations for radioactive iodine administration.

7.3 Risk Assessment of Thyroid Nodules for Malignancy

Thyroid nodules are common in the general population, especially in women. The risk of malignancy in a thyroid nodule is 7–15 %, and the most accurate and cost-effective way to distinguish between a benign and a malignant thyroid nodule is fine-needle aspiration (FNA) biopsy [1]. Nodules are selected for FNA biopsy based on their size and appearance on 2D ultrasound. The

Table 7.1 Comparisons between two-dimensional (2D) and three-dimensional (3D) ultrasound

2D ultrasound	3D ultrasound
Superior image quality	Inferior image quality because of the lower resolution of the extracted planes from volume data
Images not subject to motion artifact	Images may be subject to motion and reconstruction artifact
Smaller data set	Larger data set
Stores only images that the ultrasonographer selects	Stores all data continuously
Slower data acquisition	Faster data acquisition
Some views impossible to achieve because of restrictions related to patient anatomy or position	Data can be manipulated to display images in any viewing plane
Comparisons of structures over time dependent on images selected to be saved	Permits comparisons of full data sets over time which may lead to more accurate follow-up
There is interobserver variability in the evaluation of thyroid echogenicity, borders, and volume	There is better interobserver reproducibility in the evaluation of thyroid echogenicity, borders, and volume
Thyroid volume calculations are operator dependent: the ultrasonographer must find the perfect angle and location of the transducer to measure three perpendicular axes	Thyroid volume calculations are not operator dependent
Thyroid volume calculations are an estimate based on a regular geometric shape (i.e., each thyroid lobe is assumed to be an ellipsoid)	Thyroid volume calculations are more exact (sum of cross-sectional areas of each 2D image multiplied by the interslice distance)

American Thyroid Association (ATA) recommends FNA biopsy of nodules ≥1 cm with intermediate or high suspicion for malignancy based on sonographic pattern (hypoechoic, irregular margins, microcalcifications, evidence of extrathyroidal extension, taller-than-wide shape) and of nodules ≥1.5 cm with low suspicion for malignancy based on sonographic pattern (isoechoic, hyperechoic, partially cystic with eccentric solid areas) [1]. Nodules ≥2 cm that are spongiform or partially cystic without any suspicious features may be biopsied or observed [1].

While most thyroid nodules are benign, 2–25 % of FNA biopsy results are in an indeterminate category (atypia/follicular lesion of undetermined significance, follicular neoplasm/suspicious for follicular neoplasm, suspicious for malignancy) [1]. Although most nodules that have indeterminate cytology will ultimately prove to be benign [17, 18], many patients are referred for surgery for definitive diagnosis. Therefore, any technique that can either diminish the concern for malignancy and avoid FNA biopsy, or be applied after an indeterminate cytology result may help to reduce the need for thyroidectomy for definitive diagnosis of a benign thyroid nodule.

3D ultrasound may be able to refine the selection of thyroid nodules for FNA biopsy by more clearly demonstrating nodule characteristics such as overall shape, margins, and vascular patterns compared with static 2D imaging (Fig. 7.4). In a study of 71 nodules, 16 of which were malignant, evaluated with 3D ultrasound with power Doppler, Slapa and colleagues found the following features associated with malignancy: ill-defined border in multiplanar reformation mode, lobulated shape of the nodule in the c-plane (the plane parallel to the ultrasound probe), and the density of central vascularization within the lowest or highest ranges [19]. The combination of these three features was demonstrated to have a sensitivity of 100 % and a specificity of 60–69 % for the assessment of malignancy, and the application of these criteria for selection of nodules to undergo FNA biopsy would have decreased the number of biopsies from 71 to 38 without missing a malignant nodule [19]. Similarly, Li and colleagues found that irregular shape of a thyroid nodule on 3D ultrasound had high sensitivity (91 %) and specificity (88 %) in identifying malignant thyroid nodules in a study of 103 nodules, 53 of which were malignant [20]. In three cases (one benign and two malignant), the shape of the thyroid nodule was deemed to be regular on 2D but irregular on 3D ultrasound [20].

The evaluation of thyroid nodule vascularity by 3D ultrasound may also be useful in the evalu-

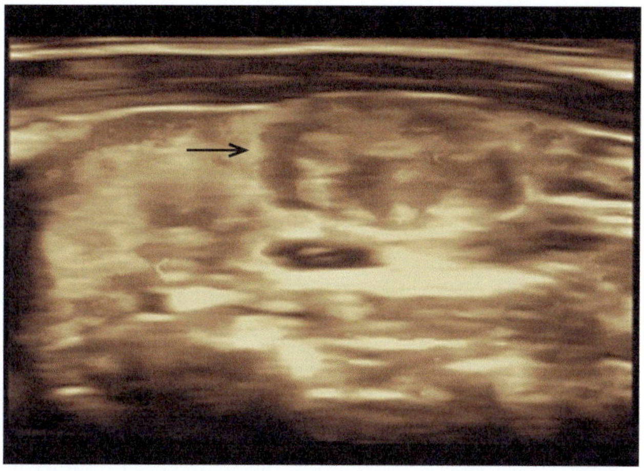

Fig. 7.4 Sagittal surface-rendered reconstructed 3D image shows a lobulated border along the superior border of the nodule (*arrow*)

ation of a thyroid nodule for malignancy within certain subtypes of nodules. Molinari and colleagues studied 20 nodules with features of malignancy on 2D ultrasound (hypoechogenicity, microcalcification, irregular margins), 15 of which were follicular neoplasms and 10 of which were malignant [21]. 3D ultrasound with an IV contrast agent demonstrated that the malignant nodules had statistically higher vascular density, number of vascular trees, number of branching nodes, and vascular tortuosity than benign nodules [21]. While the assessment of vascular density of thyroid nodules would probably not change the indication for FNA biopsy, it may increase or decrease the risk of malignancy in a follicular neoplasm, and thus has the potential to influence the choice of operation (diagnostic thyroid lobectomy vs total thyroidectomy).

7.4 Preoperative Assessment of Extrathyroidal Extension of Thyroid Cancers

The most common type of thyroid cancer is papillary thyroid cancer (PTC), comprising approximately 85 % of cases of differentiated thyroid cancer [1]. The treatment of PTCs by the majority of surgeons in the United States is total or near-total thyroidectomy with appropriate lymph node dissection [22]. However, large studies have not shown a difference in outcomes between total or near-total thyroidectomy and thyroid lobectomy for PTCs <1.0 cm, and thus thyroid lobectomy is an acceptable treatment for PTCs <1.0 cm without extrathyroidal extension [23, 24]. Previous studies have shown that extrathyroidal extension is an independent risk factor for cancer recurrence [25] and upstages the T stage from T1 to T3. Therefore, the preoperative identification of extrathyroidal extension may change the extent of thyroidectomy for PTCs <1.0 cm.

Both 2D and 3D thyroid ultrasound have been studied in the preoperative staging of a patient with PTC. Multiple criteria have been evaluated to define extrathyroidal extension on 2D ultrasound including the degree of nodule contact with the adjacent thyroid capsule and disruption of the adjacent capsule [26]. In a study of 221 PTCs ≤1.0 cm, Kwak and colleagues determined that more than 25 % contact with the adjacent capsule had the highest accuracy in predicting the extrathyroidal extension of the cancer using 2D ultrasound [26]. One limitation of this study is that the degree of contact was measured by visual analysis of the radiologist, which can be subjective. Gweon and colleagues studied 79 PTCs with a mean size of 0.98 cm (range 0.5–3.6 cm) by 2D ultrasound, with 3D ultrasound performed if the PTC was seen to abutting the thyroid capsule [16]. Using the definition of extrathyroidal extension as more than 25 % of the perimeter of the lesion in contact with the thyroid capsule, this study found that 3D ultrasound had higher sensitivity than 2D ultrasound for the detection of extrathyroidal extension but similar accuracy

[16]. There was moderate interobserver agreement among three radiologists for 3D ultrasound versus only fair-to-moderate interobserver agreement for 2D ultrasound [16]. Thus, 3D ultrasound may have an advantage over 2D ultrasound in the preoperative evaluation of extrathyroidal extension of PTC, and may therefore influence the surgeon to perform total thyroidectomy for PTCs <1.0 cm if extrathyroidal extension is seen on the preoperative ultrasound.

7.5 Thyroid Volume Calculations

One treatment option for patients with hyperthyroidism (Graves' disease or one or multiple toxic nodules) is radioactive iodine. Dosage protocols are based on measurements of thyroid volume and radioactive iodine uptake; therefore, the accuracy of the measurement of thyroid volume is important. Multiple methods exist to estimate thyroid volume including ultrasound, scintigraphy, and cross-sectional imaging modalities such as magnetic resonance imaging (MRI) and computed tomography (CT).

2D ultrasound is the most frequently used modality to estimate thyroid volume and is based on assuming each thyroid lobe to be an ellipsoid. The ultrasonographer measures the largest diameter of three perpendicular axes of each lobe, and the volume of each lobe is calculated using the standard formula for the volume of an ellipsoid: $\text{volume} = (\pi/6) \times \text{length} \times \text{width} \times \text{depth}$. This method, however, may result in errors in volume calculations of up to 30 % [27, 28] which is thought to be related to irregular contours of the gland not being able to be approximated by a regular geometric shape. Therefore, 3D ultrasound techniques have been studied to measure thyroid volume.

Studies comparing 2D and 3D ultrasound measurement of thyroid gland and thyroid nodule volume have shown that 3D ultrasound results in more accurate volume calculations compared to 2D ultrasound. In a study of 18 thyroid-shaped phantoms evaluated by 2D ultrasound, 3D ultrasound, CT, and MRI, Freesmeyer and colleagues found that 3D ultrasound was superior to 2D ultrasound and essentially equivalent to CT and MRI for thyroid volumetry [29]. Similarly, in a prospective study of 27 patients who had thyroid volume calculated by 2D ultrasound, 3D ultrasound, and submersion after thyroidectomy (volume of water displaced by the surgical specimen), Malago and colleagues found that the median difference in volume was underestimated by 29 % by 2D ultrasound and by only 6 % by 3D ultrasound [28]. In addition to advantages related to accuracy of thyroid volume calculations, 3D ultrasound has been demonstrated to have lower interobserver and intraobserver variability in the evaluation of thyroid volume compared to 2D ultrasound [30, 31]. Therefore, the use of 3D ultrasound for thyroid volumetry may result in more accurate dosing of radioactive iodine for patients with hyperthyroidism.

7.6 Summary

In summary, 3D ultrasound has been studied in the evaluation of various thyroid conditions in order to overcome limitations of conventional 2D ultrasound related to the 2D display, user dependency, and interobserver variability. 3D ultrasound may be able to refine the selection of thyroid nodules for FNA biopsy beyond criteria currently in use based on 2D ultrasound characteristics. Furthermore, 3D ultrasound may have an advantage over 2D ultrasound in the preoperative evaluation of extrathyroidal extension of papillary thyroid cancer and may, therefore, influence the extent of thyroidectomy. Lastly, 3D ultrasound may be able to more accurately quantify thyroid volume, therefore allowing for more accurate radioactive iodine dosing for patients with hyperthyroidism. Limitations to 3D ultrasound are related to the technique used to acquire images, motion and reconstruction artifact, image quality, and computational requirements needed to process large data sets quickly.

References

1. Haugen BR, Alexander EK, Bible KC, Doherty GM, Mandel SJ, Nikiforov YE, et al. 2015 American Thyroid Association Management Guidelines for adult patients with thyroid nodules and differentiated thyroid cancer: the American Thyroid Association guidelines task force on thyroid nodules and differentiated thyroid cancer. Thyroid. 2016;26(1):1–133.
2. Kuna SK, Bracic I, Tesic V, Kuna K, Herceg GH, Dodig D. Ultrasonographic differentiation of benign from malignant neck lymphadenopathy in thyroid cancer. J Ultrasound Med. 2006;25(12):1531–7. quiz 8-40.
3. Rosario PW, de Faria S, Bicalho L, Alves MF, Borges MA, Purisch S, et al. Ultrasonographic differentiation between metastatic and benign lymph nodes in patients with papillary thyroid carcinoma. J Ultrasound Med. 2005;24(10):1385–9.
4. Leboulleux S, Girard E, Rose M, Travagli JP, Sabbah N, Caillou B, et al. Ultrasound criteria of malignancy for cervical lymph nodes in patients followed up for differentiated thyroid cancer. J Clin Endocrinol Metab. 2007;92(9):3590–4.
5. Ivanac G, Brkljacic B, Ivanac K, Huzjan R, Skreb F, Cikara I. Vascularisation of benign and malignant thyroid nodules: CD US evaluation. Ultraschall Med. 2007;28(5):502–6.
6. Spiezia S, Farina R, Cerbone G, Assanti AP, Iovino V, Siciliani M, et al. Analysis of color Doppler signal intensity variation after levovist injection: a new approach to the diagnosis of thyroid nodules. J Ultrasound Med. 2001;20(3):223–31. quiz 33.
7. Zhang B, Jiang YX, Liu JB, Yang M, Dai Q, Zhu QL, et al. Utility of contrast-enhanced ultrasound for evaluation of thyroid nodules. Thyroid. 2010;20(1):51–7.
8. Miyabe R. Three-dimensional ultrasonography before minimally invasive focused parathyroidectomy: the importance of coronal images. Surg Today. 2009;39(2):98–103.
9. Pretorius DH, Borok NN, Coffler MS, Nelson TR. Three-dimensional ultrasound in obstetrics and gynecology. Radiol Clin North Am. 2001;39(3):499–521.
10. Lee MC, Gonzalez SJ, Lin H, Zhao X, Kiluk JV, Laronga C, et al. Prospective trial of breast MRI versus 2D and 3D ultrasound for evaluation of response to neoadjuvant chemotherapy. Ann Surg Oncol. 2015;22(9):2888–94.
11. Hrinivich WT, Hoover DA, Surry K, Edirisinghe C, Montreuil J, D'Souza D, et al. Three-dimensional transrectal ultrasound guided high-dose-rate prostate brachytherapy: a comparison of needle segmentation accuracy with two-dimensional image guidance. Brachytherapy. 2016;15(2):231–9.
12. Riccabona M, Nelson TR, Pretorius DH, Davidson TE. In vivo three-dimensional sonographic measurement of organ volume: validation in the urinary bladder. J Ultrasound Med. 1996;15(9):627–32.
13. Nosir YF, Fioretti PM, Vletter WB, Boersma E, Salustri A, Postma JT, et al. Accurate measurement of left ventricular ejection fraction by three-dimensional echocardiography. A comparison with radionuclide angiography. Circulation. 1996;94(3):460–6.
14. Fenster A, Downey DB, Cardinal HN. Three-dimensional ultrasound imaging. Phys Med Biol. 2001;46(5):R67–99.
15. Downey DB, Fenster A, Williams JC. Clinical utility of three-dimensional US. Radiographics. 2000;20(2):559–71.
16. Gweon HM, Son EJ, Youk JH, Kim JA, Park CS. Preoperative assessment of extrathyroidal extension of papillary thyroid carcinoma: comparison of 2- and 3-dimensional sonography. J Ultrasound Med. 2014;33(5):819–25.
17. Cibas ES, Ali SZ. The Bethesda System for reporting thyroid cytopathology. Am J Clin Pathol. 2009;132(5):658–65.
18. Baloch ZW, Fleisher S, LiVolsi VA, Gupta PK. Diagnosis of "follicular neoplasm": a gray zone in thyroid fine-needle aspiration cytology. Diagn Cytopathol. 2002;26(1):41–4.
19. Slapa RZ, Jakubowski WS, Slowinska-Srzednicka J, Szopinski KT. Advantages and disadvantages of 3D ultrasound of thyroid nodules including thin slice volume rendering. Thyroid Res. 2011;4(1):1.
20. Li WB, Zhang B, Zhu QL, Jiang YX, Sun J, Yang M, et al. Comparison between thin-slice 3-D volumetric ultrasound and conventional ultrasound in the differentiation of benign and malignant thyroid lesions. Ultrasound Med Biol. 2015;41(12):3096–101.
21. Molinari F, Mantovani A, Deandrea M, Limone P, Garberoglio R, Suri JS. Characterization of single thyroid nodules by contrast-enhanced 3-D ultrasound. Ultrasound Med Biol. 2010;36(10):1616–25.
22. Haigh PI, Urbach DR, Rotstein LE. AMES prognostic index and extent of thyroidectomy for well-differentiated thyroid cancer in the United States. Surgery. 2004;136(3):609–16.
23. Bilimoria KY, Bentrem DJ, Ko CY, Stewart AK, Winchester DP, Talamonti MS, et al. Extent of surgery affects survival for papillary thyroid cancer. Ann Surg. 2007;246(3):375–81. discussion 81-4.
24. Haigh PI, Urbach DR, Rotstein LE. Extent of thyroidectomy is not a major determinant of survival in low- or high-risk papillary thyroid cancer. Ann Surg Oncol. 2005;12(1):81–9.
25. Wada N, Nakayama H, Suganuma N, Masudo Y, Rino Y, Masuda M, et al. Prognostic value of the sixth edition AJCC/UICC TNM classification for differentiated thyroid carcinoma with extrathyroid extension. J Clin Endocrinol Metab. 2007;92(1):215–8.
26. Kwak JY, Kim EK, Youk JH, Kim MJ, Son EJ, Choi SH, et al. Extrathyroid extension of well-differentiated

papillary thyroid microcarcinoma on US. Thyroid. 2008;18(6):609–14.
27. van Isselt JW, de Klerk JM, van Rijk PP, van Gils AP, Polman LJ, Kamphuis C, et al. Comparison of methods for thyroid volume estimation in patients with Graves' disease. Eur J Nucl Med Mol Imaging. 2003;30(4):525–31.
28. Malago R, D'Onofrio M, Ferdeghini M, Mantovani W, Colato C, Brazzarola P, et al. Thyroid volumetric quantification: comparative evaluation between conventional and volumetric ultrasonography. J Ultrasound Med. 2008;27(12):1727–33.
29. Freesmeyer M, Wiegand S, Schierz JH, Winkens T, Licht K. Multimodal evaluation of 2-D and 3-D ultrasound, computed tomography and magnetic resonance imaging in measurements of the thyroid volume using universally applicable cross-sectional imaging software: a phantom study. Ultrasound Med Biol. 2014;40(7):1453–62.
30. Lyshchik A, Drozd V, Schloegl S, Reiners C. Three-dimensional ultrasonography for volume measurement of thyroid nodules in children. J Ultrasound Med. 2004;23(2):247–54.
31. Schlogl S, Andermann P, Luster M, Reiners C, Lassmann M. A novel thyroid phantom for ultrasound volumetry: determination of intraobserver and interobserver variability. Thyroid. 2006;16(1):41–6.

8 Elastography: Applications and Limitations of a New Technology

Manish Dhyani, Changtian Li, Anthony E. Samir, and Antonia E. Stephen

8.1 Introduction

Thyroid nodules have been reported in up to 50 % of the population, and they are most common in women >65 years of age [1–3, 8]. Ultrasound is widely used as the primary imaging modality in the diagnosis and evaluation of thyroid nodules. There are several ultrasound features that correlate with malignancy, including the presence of microcalcifications, marked hypoechogenicity, "taller-than-wide" shape, irregular margins, and intranodular vascularization at Doppler [3–5, 9]. These features, although helpful in selecting nodules for biopsy, are not able to reliably detect or exclude malignancy with a high degree of confidence [6–10]. As a result, fine-needle aspiration biopsy (FNAB) is the next step to determine if a thyroid nodule is benign or malignant. However, even FNAB has inherent limitations and up to 15–30 % of FNAB samples are not conclusive (indeterminate) and cannot be clearly diagnosed as benign or malignant [3, 11]. These indeterminate nodules are often subjected to repeat biopsy with molecular testing or referred for diagnostic lobectomy. Molecular testing on biopsy samples, although an important advance in the workup of thyroid nodules, also has limitations with regard to estimating malignancy risk and can also be quite expensive [12, 13]. Thyroidectomy for patients with indeterminate nodules, although often required due to nodule size or local compressive symptoms, perhaps could be avoided in selected circumstances if the malignancy risk could be more accurately assessed.

Elastography is a novel ultrasound-based technique that has been shown to have considerable success in identifying malignant thyroid nodules [14]. There are two kinds of elastography currently in use for thyroid nodules in clinical practice: strain elastography and shear wave elastography. The objective of this chapter is to review the application of elastography in thyroid nodules and discuss its potential utility and limitations.

M. Dhyani, M.D. • A.E. Samir
Department of Radiology, Harvard Medical School, Massachusetts General Hospital, 55 Fruit Street, White 270, Boston, MA 02114, USA
e-mail: dhyani.manish@mgh.harvard.edu

C. Li, M.D., Ph.D.
Department of Ultrasound, Chinese PLA General Hospital, The Southern Building, 28th Fuxing Road, Haidian District, Beijing 100853, China
e-mail: liction4995@163.com

A.E. Stephen, M.D. (✉)
Department of Surgery, Harvard Medical School, Massachusetts General Hospital, Yawkey 7B, 55 Fruit Street, Boston, MA 02114, USA
e-mail: astephen@partners.org

M. Milas et al. (eds.), *Advanced Thyroid and Parathyroid Ultrasound*,
DOI 10.1007/978-3-319-44100-9_8

8.2 Strain Elastography

Strain elastography is a technique that assesses the elastic nature of tissues by analyzing the tissue strain and deformation in response to compression [15, 16]. It requires either an external mechanical force, such as palpation with the ultrasound probe, or an internal endogenous force such as cardiovascular movements from nearby vessels, resulting in an axial displacement of the tissue. Tissue deformation from the applied or endogenous stress is measured and visualized before and after tissue compression. The measured tissue stiffness for the region of interest (ROI) is assessed relative value to the surrounding tissues and is displayed using a color scale [17–19]. The elastographic image can then be visualized on the screen side by side with a conventional B-mode image. A limitation of this technique is that it provides a relatively qualitative elastography measurement and can be user dependent with regard to the amount of compression applied.

8.3 Shear Wave Elastography

In an attempt to overcome the limitations of strain elastography, shear wave elastography was developed as a quantitative assessment of tissue elasticity. It is based on the velocity of shear wave propagation through tissues, as generated by an acoustic pulse from an ultrasound probe. Because shear wave elastography is dependent on the radiation force from the ultrasound probe and not external compression by an ultrasonographer, this technique is generally thought of as less operator dependent and more reproducible [20, 21]. There are two available methods for shear wave thyroid elastography: the supersonic shear wave and the acoustic radiation force impulse (ARFI) [22]. The supersonic shear wave technique uses focused ultrasonic beams that propagate through the ROI, and ARFI uses short-duration acoustic pulses to excite the tissues within the ROI [14]. The ARFI technique of shear wave elastography has been studied in thyroid nodules and confirmed as a valid technique in estimating malignancy [23–29].

8.4 The Application of Elastography for Thyroid Nodules

Both strain and shear wave elastographies have been studied with regard to their characterization of thyroid nodules. Overall the results have been encouraging but not uniformly positive when analyzing the ability of these techniques to estimate the risk of malignancy. With regard to strain elastography, a 2010 meta-analysis, which included eight studies and 639 nodules, noted a mean sensitivity and specificity of 92 % and 90 %, respectively [30]. Another meta-analysis published in 2013 included 24 studies and 3531 thyroid nodules in 2624 patients and compared the performance of strain elastography to conventional ultrasound features in predicting malignancy [31]. They noted a better performance from strain elastography and concluded that the newer technique increased the accuracy of conventional ultrasound. Other studies, however, have been less encouraging. For example, Moon et al. 2012 did not note an improvement in detection of malignancy with the addition of strain elastography over conventional ultrasound alone [32].

To assess the overall performance of shear wave elastography for diagnosis of benign and malignant thyroid nodules, several meta-analyses were conducted. Lin et al. included 15 studies and 1867 thyroid nodules and reported the pooled sensitivity and specificity of SWE as 84.3 and 88.4 % [33]. In Zhang et al., a total of 698 thyroid nodules in 469 patients were studied and the sensitivity and specificity were 84 and 90 % [34].

Additional studies have specifically examined the diagnostic value of elastography in thyroid nodules with indeterminate FNAB results, which is the group of thyroid nodule patients for whom this technique could be most useful. Rago et al. studied a total of 142 nodules with real-time strain elastography and reported a sensitivity and specificity of 96.8 % and 91.8 %, respectively, for the exclusion of malignancy in nodules that demonstrated a highly elastography (lowest degree of stiffness) score [35]. A study by Garino et al. included 108 patients, all with indeterminate thyroid nodules, and noted a 76 % sensitivity and 88 % specificity for the detection of malignancy [36].

In a study by Samir et al., 35 patients with indeterminate biopsy results (including "atypia of unknown significance" (AUS), "follicular lesion of undetermined significance" (FLUS), "follicular nodule or suspicion for follicular neoplasm" (SFN), or "Hurthle cell neoplasm or suspicion for Hurthle cell neoplasm" (SHN)) were studied with shear wave elastography, and nodules with higher median SWE tissue Young modulus estimates were found to be associated with malignancy. The area under the ROC curve was 0.81 for differentiating malignant nodules from benign ones, and the sensitivity and specificity were 82 % and 88 %, respectively, with a cutoff value of 22.3 kPa [14]. Other studies have had more varied results; Lippolis et al. reported a very low specificity of 6 % in indeterminate nodules subjected to elastography [37]. In conclusion, elastography did provide useful information in the diagnosis of indeterminate thyroid nodules, but elastography alone cannot be used to definitively exclude malignancy in thyroid nodules.

8.5 Limitations of Elastography in the Evaluation of Thyroid Nodules

8.5.1 Operator Dependence

As described above, a key limitation of elastography, in particular the strain method, is examiner dependence. Elastography studies must be performed by experienced operators who are trained in the specific techniques and understand the equipment and scoring systems. For this reason, elastography may not be widely available. Although shear wave elastography is a more operator-independent and reproducible method, the external pressure applied on the neck of the patient may affect the elasticity values. Due to the nonlinear elastic effect, the stiffness of tissues rises with the increase in the pressure applied [38]. For more precise stiffness values, a force-controlled device should be used. See Fig. 8.1 for a demonstration of variable elastography measurements in the same tissue with different applied force.

8.5.2 Thyroid Inflammation

Inflammation and fibrosis are very common in the thyroid gland and often coexist with thyroid nodules. The influence of concomitant thyroiditis on the elasticity of thyroid nodules is still a matter of debate. According to some authors, Hashimoto's thyroiditis, or chronic autoimmune thyroiditis, does not significantly affect the coexisting nodules' stiffness [39–41]. However, acute or subacute thyroiditis may cause more significant changes in elasticity of the thyroid parenchyma in general and therefore may influence the elasticity measurement of coexistent thyroid nodules [42]. Therefore, postponing the evaluation of the nodule stiffness until complete recovery from acute or subacute thyroiditis is recommended [43]. Figure 8.2 represents a shear wave elastogram of a patient who was diagnosed with a benign follicular adenoma (oncocytic type) in the setting of chronic lymphocytic (Hashimoto's) thyroiditis. As seen in the image, the SWE value of 28.55 kPa would qualify this subject as a malignant nodule based on the cutoff value of 22.3 kPa proposed by Samir et al. [14].

8.5.3 Cyst Fluid and Calcifications

The fluid within a thyroid nodule may affect the elasticity measurements. Interestingly, the stiffness of benign nodules with a cystic component was higher than solid ones [40, 44]. This finding may be related to the pressure exerted by the liquid contained in the cystic compartment [44]. The presence of both micro- and macrocalcifications may influence the stiffness of thyroid nodules. In particular, macrocalcifications around or within a nodule may lead to a significant increase in elasticity (Fig. 8.3). In nodules with both types of calcifications, the influence might be more pronounced [40]. Due to the possibility of a false-positive result, thyroid nodules with coarse calcifications may not be suitable for elastographic examination [45].

It may be possible to perform the quantitative measurements by placing the ROI on the target

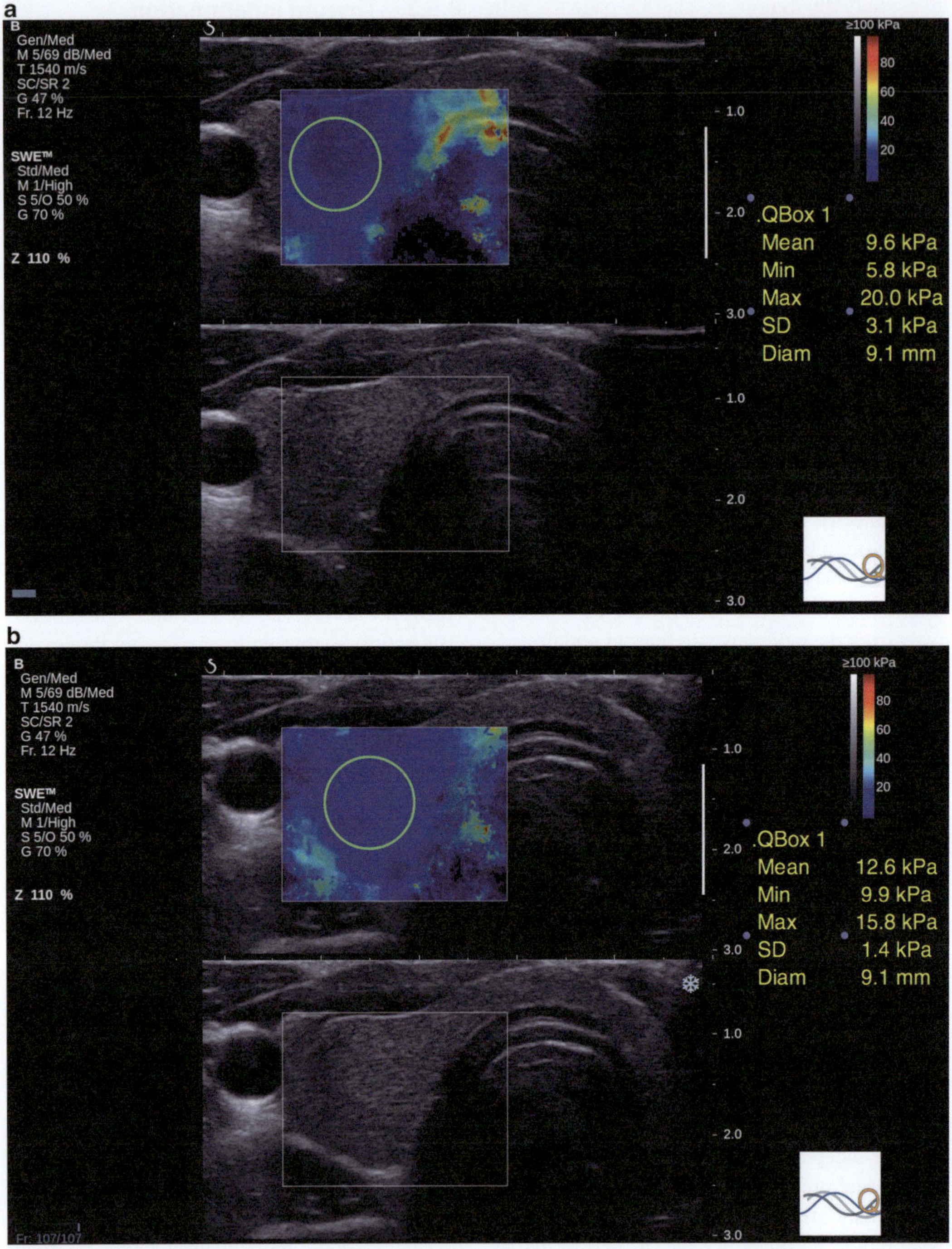

Fig. 8.1 (**a**, **b**) SWE values of 9.6 and 12.6 kPa in a normal thyroid using 3 N and 5 N of force, respectively

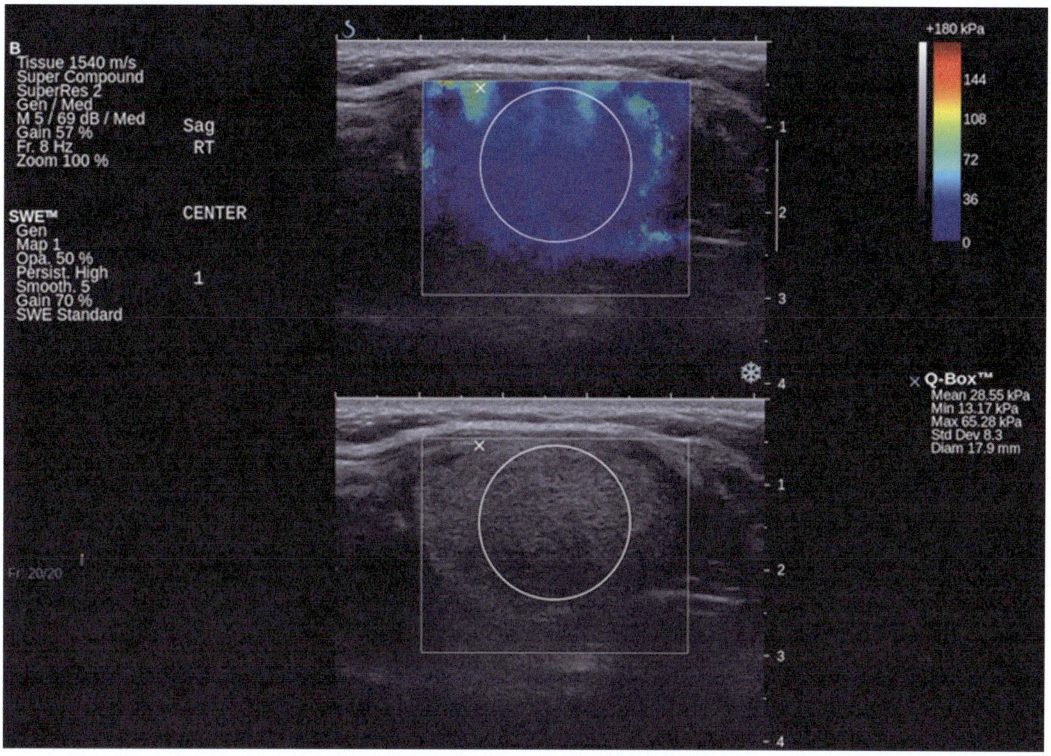

Fig. 8.2 A 50-year-old female with a right thyroid nodule that was suspicious for a Hurthle cell neoplasm on FNA. The elastogram shows a SWE value of 28.55 kPa. The patient underwent a total thyroidectomy, and the nodule was a benign follicular adenoma (oncocytic type) in the setting of chronic lymphocytic (Hashimoto's) thyroiditis

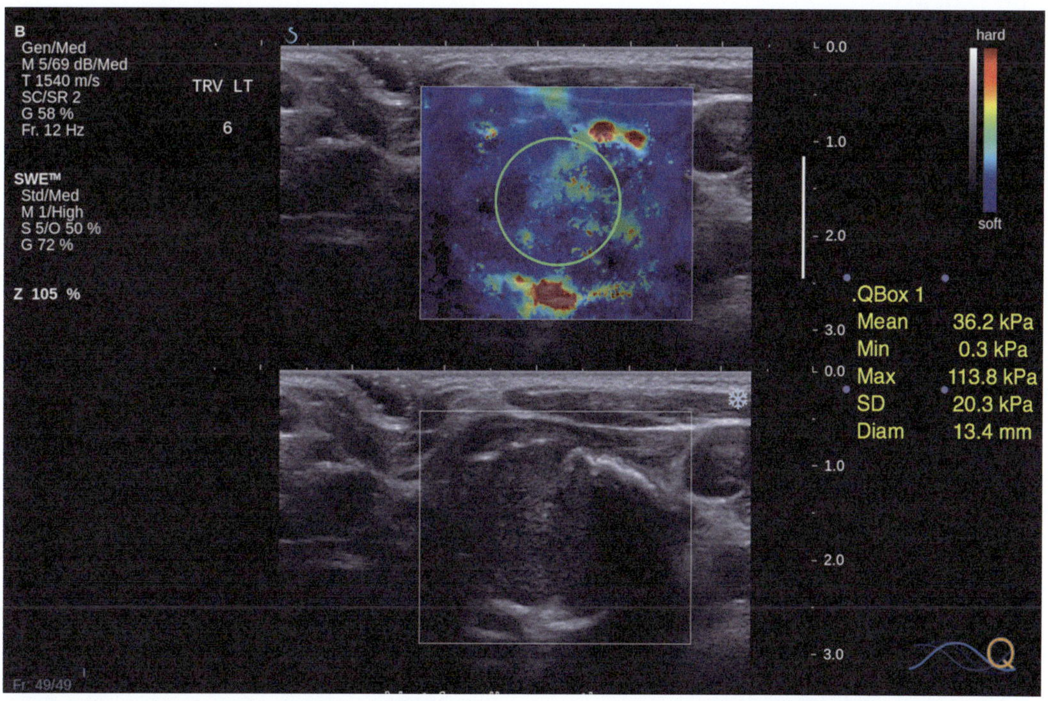

Fig. 8.3 A 85-year-old female with a left thyroid nodule measuring 2.6 cm, FLUS on FNA. The final pathology after surgery was a benign Hurthle cell adenoma with extensive calcification. As seen in the elastogram, the calcification causes significant elasticity increase

nodule with the calcified or cystic areas avoided; however, this may not be feasible when the solid area is less than the sampling size of ROI.

8.6 Conclusions

In conclusion, elastography is a relatively noninvasive test that could increase the specificity of conventional ultrasound in the differentiation between malignant and benign thyroid nodules. Furthermore, the combination of this technique and conventional ultrasound may be a valuable tool in the identification of nodules that require FNAB and in nodules with indeterminate or nondiagnostic cytology. However, the general limitations described above should be acknowledged. It may be that the best and most appropriate application of elastography in the diagnosis of thyroid nodules will be as a complement to conventional ultrasound and FNAB with genetic testing [46].

References

1. Hegedus L, Bonnema SJ, Bennedbæk FN. Management of simple nodular goiter: current status and future perspectives. Endocr Rev. 2003;24(1):102–32.
2. Tumbridge WM, Evered DC, Hall R, et al. The spectrum of thyroid disease in a community: the Whickham survey. Clin Endocrinol (Oxf). 1997;7:481–93.
3. Frates MC, Benson CB, Charboneau JW, et al. Management of thyroid nodules detected at US: society of radiologists in ultrasound consensus conference statement 1. Radiology. 2005;237(3):794–800.
4. Haugen BR, Alexander EK, Bible KC, et al. 2015 American Thyroid Association management guidelines for adult patients with thyroid nodules and differentiated thyroid cancer. Thyroid. 2016;26(1):1–133.
5. Dhyani M, Faquin W, Lubitz CC, Daniels GH, Samir AE. How to interpret thyroid fine-needle aspiration biopsy reports: a guide for the busy radiologist in the era of the Bethesda classification system. Am J Roentgenol. 2013;201(6):1335–9.
6. Russ G, Royer B, Bigorgne C, Rouxel A, Bienvenu-Perrard M, Leenhardt L. Prospective evaluation of thyroid imaging reporting and data system on 4550 nodules with and without elastography. Eur J Endocrinol. 2013;168(5):649–55.
7. Shuzhen C. Comparison analysis between conventional ultrasonography and ultrasound elastography of thyroid nodules. Eur J Radiol. 2012;81(8):1806–11.
8. Reiners C, Wegscheider K, Schicha H, et al. Prevalence of thyroid disorders in the working population of Germany: ultrasonography screening in 96,278 unselected employees. Thyroid. 2004;14(11):926–32.
9. Iannuccilli JD, Cronan JJ, Monchik JM. Risk for malignancy of thyroid nodules as assessed by sonographic criteria: the need for biopsy. J Ultrasound Med. 2004;23(11):1455–64.
10. Friedrich-Rust M, Meyer G, Dauth N, et al. Interobserver agreement of Thyroid Imaging Reporting and Data System (TIRADS) and strain elastography for the assessment of thyroid nodules. PLoS One. 2013;8(10):e77927.
11. Asteria C, Giovanardi A, Pizzocaro A, et al. US-elastography in the differential diagnosis of benign and malignant thyroid nodules. Thyroid. 2008;18(5):523–31.
12. Faquin WC. Can a gene-expression classifier with high negative predictive value solve the indeterminate thyroid fine-needle aspiration dilemma? Cancer Cytopathol. 2013;121(3):116–9.
13. Alexander EK, Kennedy GC, Baloch ZW, et al. Preoperative diagnosis of benign thyroid nodules with indeterminate cytology. N Engl J Med. 2012;367(8):705–15.
14. Samir AE, Dhyani M, Anvari A, et al. Shear-wave elastography for the preoperative risk stratification of follicular-patterned lesions of the thyroid: diagnostic accuracy and optimal measurement plane. Radiology. 2015;277:565.
15. Kwak JY, Kim EK. Ultrasound elastography for thyroid nodules: recent advances. Ultrasonography. 2014;33(2):75–82.
16. Ophir J, Cespedes I, Ponnekanti H, Yazdi Y, Li X. Elastography: a quantitative method for imaging the elasticity of biological tissues. Ultrason Imaging. 1991;13(2):111–34.
17. Sarvazyan A, Hall TJ, Urban MW, Fatemi M, Aglyamov SR, Garra BS. An overview of elastography – an emerging branch of medical imaging. Current Med Imaging Rev. 2011;7(4):255.
18. Aguilo MA, Aquino W, Brigham JC, Fatemi M. An inverse problem approach for elasticity imaging through vibroacoustics. IEEE Trans Med Imaging. 2010;29(4):1012–21.
19. Itoh A, Ueno E, Tohno E, et al. Breast disease: clinical application of US elastography for diagnosis 1. Radiology. 2006;239(2):341–50.
20. Rago T, Santini F, Scutari M, Pinchera A, Vitti P. Elastography: new developments in ultrasound for predicting malignancy in thyroid nodules. J Clin Endocrinol Metab. 2007;92(8):2917–22.
21. Tanter M, Bercoff J, Athanasiou A, et al. Quantitative assessment of breast lesion viscoelasticity: initial

clinical results using supersonic shear imaging. Ultrasound Med Biol. 2008;34(9):1373–86.
22. Zhang YF, Xu HX, He Y, et al. Virtual touch tissue quantification of acoustic radiation force impulse: a new ultrasound elastic imaging in the diagnosis of thyroid nodules. PLoS One. 2012;7:e49094.
23. Zhang Y-F, He Y, Xu H-X, et al. Virtual touch tissue imaging on acoustic radiation force impulse elastography a new technique for differential diagnosis between benign and malignant thyroid nodules. J Ultrasound Med. 2014;33(4):585–95.
24. Zhang Y-F, Liu C, Xu H-X, et al. Acoustic radiation force impulse imaging: a new tool for the diagnosis of papillary thyroid microcarcinoma. Biomed Res Int. 2014;2014:416969.
25. Bojunga J, Dauth N, Berner C, et al. Acoustic radiation force impulse imaging for differentiation of thyroid nodules. PLoS One. 2012;7(8):e42735.
26. Xu J-M, Xu H-X, Xu X-H, et al. Solid hypo-echoic thyroid nodules on ultrasound: the diagnostic value of acoustic radiation force impulse elastography. Ultrasound Med Biol. 2014;40(9):2020–30.
27. Xu J-M, Xu X-H, Xu H-X, et al. Conventional US, US elasticity imaging, and acoustic radiation force impulse imaging for prediction of malignancy in thyroid nodules. Radiology. 2014;272(2):577–86.
28. Liu B-J, Xu H-X, Zhang Y-F, et al. Acoustic radiation force impulse elastography for differentiation of benign and malignant thyroid nodules with concurrent Hashimoto's thyroiditis. Med Oncol. 2015;32(3):1–9.
29. Zhang F-J, Han R-L, Zhao X-M. The value of virtual touch tissue image (VTI) and virtual touch tissue quantification (VTQ) in the differential diagnosis of thyroid nodules. Eur J Radiol. 2014;83(11):2033–40.
30. Bojunga J, Herrmann G, Meyer S, et al. Real-time elastography for the differentiation of benign and malignant nodules: a meta-analysis. Thyroid. 2010;20(10):1145–50.
31. Razavi SA, Hadduck TA, Sadigh G, et al. Comparative effectiveness of elastographic and b-mode ultrasound criteria for diagnostic discrimination of thyroid nodules: a meta-analysis. Am J Roentgenol. 2013;200(6):1317–26.
32. Moon HJ, Sung JM, Kim EK. Diagnostic performance of gray-scale US and elastography in solid thyroid nodules. Radiology. 2012;262(3):1002–13.
33. Lin P, Chen M, Liu B, Wang S, Li X. Diagnostic performance of shear wave elastography in the identification of malignant thyroid nodules: a meta-analysis. Eur Radiol. 2014;24(11):2729–38.
34. Zhang B, Ma X, Wu N, et al. Shear wave elastography for differentiation of benign and malignant thyroid nodules a meta-analysis. J Ultrasound Med. 2013;32(12):2163–9.
35. Rago T, Scutari M, Santini F, et al. Real-time elastosonography: useful tool for refining the presurgical diagnosis in thyroid nodules with indeterminate or nondiagnostic cytology. J Clin Endocrinol Metab. 2010;95(12):5274–80.
36. Garino F, Deandrea M, Motta M, et al. Diagnostic performance of elastography in cytologically indeterminate thyroid nodules. Endocrine. 2014;49(1):175–83.
37. Lippolis P, Tognini S, Materazzi G, et al. Is elastography actually useful in the presurgical selection of thyroid nodules with indeterminate cytology? J Clin Endocrinol Metab. 2011;96(11):E1826–30.
38. Bhatia KS, Tong CS, Cho CC, Yuen EH, Lee YY, Ahuja AT. Shear wave elastography of thyroid nodules in routine clinical practice: preliminary observations and utility for detecting malignancy. Eur Radiol. 2012;22(11):2397–406.
39. Magri F, Chytiris S, Capelli V, et al. Shear wave elastography in the diagnosis of thyroid nodules: feasibility in the case of coexistent chronic autoimmune Hashimoto's thyroiditis. Clin Endocrinol (Oxf). 2012;76(1):137–41.
40. Szczepanek-Parulska E, Woliński K, Stangierski A, Gurgul E, Ruchała M. Biochemical and ultrasonographic parameters influencing thyroid nodules elasticity. Endocrine. 2014;47(2):519–27.
41. Gietka-Czernel M, Kochman M, Bujalska K, Stachlewska-Nasfeter E, Zgliczyński W. Real-time ultrasound elastography-a new tool for diagnosing thyroid nodules. Endokrynol Pol. 2010;61(6):652–7.
42. Ruchała M, Szmyt K, Sławek S, Zybek A, Szczepanek-Parulska E. Ultrasound sonoelastography in the evaluation of thyroiditis and autoimmune thyroid disease. Endokrynol Pol. 2014;65(6):520–31.
43. Nishihara E, Hirokawa M, Ohye H, et al. Papillary carcinoma obscured by complication with subacute thyroiditis: sequential ultrasonographic and histopathological findings in five cases. Thyroid. 2008;18(11):1221–5.
44. Bhatia K, Rasalkar D, Lee Y, et al. Cystic change in thyroid nodules: a confounding factor for real-time qualitative thyroid ultrasound elastography. Clin Radiol. 2011;66(9):799–807.
45. Vorländer C, Wolff J, Saalabian S, Lienenlüke RH, Wahl RA. Real-time ultrasound elastography—a noninvasive diagnostic procedure for evaluating dominant thyroid nodules. Langenbecks Arch Surg. 2010;395(7):865–71.
46. Andrioli M, Persani L. Elastographic techniques of thyroid gland: current status. Endocrine. 2014;46(3):455–61.

Part III

Thyroid Ultrasound: Anatomy and Fundamental Features

Normal Thyroid Appearance and Anatomic Landmarks in Neck Ultrasound

9

Peter J. Mazzaglia and Liudmila Muraveika

An excellent working knowledge of cross-sectional head and neck anatomy will facilitate head and neck ultrasound performance (Fig. 9.1).

Knowing the relevant anatomic structures and their relationships to each other will make learning and performing thyroid and parathyroid ultrasound more straightforward and enjoyable. Being able to expertly and confidently conduct and interpret the ultrasound exam will also set your patients' minds at ease.

Exams should follow a standard and sequential approach. Proper patient positioning will lift the thyroid up above the clavicles and allow the ultrasonographer to obtain a more complete exam. This is achieved by placing a shoulder roll under the patient in the supine position, which achieves moderate neck extension. The best place to begin the exam is in the midline directly over the trachea, as it is the easiest landmark to identify by physical exam. A high-frequency probe is preferred for head and neck ultrasound, as it provides excellent image resolution of the structures of interest, which are usually no more than 5–6 cm deep. When saving images, the laterality and orientation of each image should be clearly labeled.

The trachea has a characteristic appearance caused by the echogenic cartilage rings that surround the anterior and lateral aspects of this otherwise hollow tube (Fig. 9.2, Video 9.1). Placing the probe transversely directly over the trachea, one will quickly see the very bright hyperechoic stripes corresponding to the tracheal cartilage rings. Moving the probe in a caudal direction from the thyroid cartilage, one first encounters the cricoid cartilage, then followed by a number of cartilage rings. The patient's body habitus and neck length will determine how many rings can be seen, but it is usually not more than a couple before the manubrium is encountered. The lumen of the trachea itself appears nearly black, as it is a hollow structure, which does not reflect any of the ultrasound waves passing through it. There are internal echoes present in the lumen that occur as an artifact related to the cartilage rings. The most superficial structures encountered are the skin and subcutaneous tissue (Fig. 9.3). The dermis is the most superficial layer. It is 1–2 mm in thickness and has a similar echogenicity to the thyroid gland. Just deep to it is a layer of subcutaneous

Electronic supplementary material: The online version of this chapter (doi:10.1007/978-3-319-44100-9_9) contains supplementary material, which is available to authorized users. Videos can also be accessed at http://link.springer.com/chapter/10.1007/978-3-319-44100-9_9.

P.J. Mazzaglia, M.D. (✉)
Rhode Island Hospital, The Warren Alpert School of Medicine, Brown University, University Surgical Associates, 2 Dudley St., Providence, RI 02905, USA
e-mail: peterjmazzaglia@gmail.com

L. Muraveika, M.D., P.H.D.
Department of Surgery, Stanford University Medical Center, 3181 Berryessa Street, Apt#2, Palo Alto, CA 94303, USA
e-mail: liudmila.muraveika@me.com

M. Milas et al. (eds.), *Advanced Thyroid and Parathyroid Ultrasound*,
DOI 10.1007/978-3-319-44100-9_9

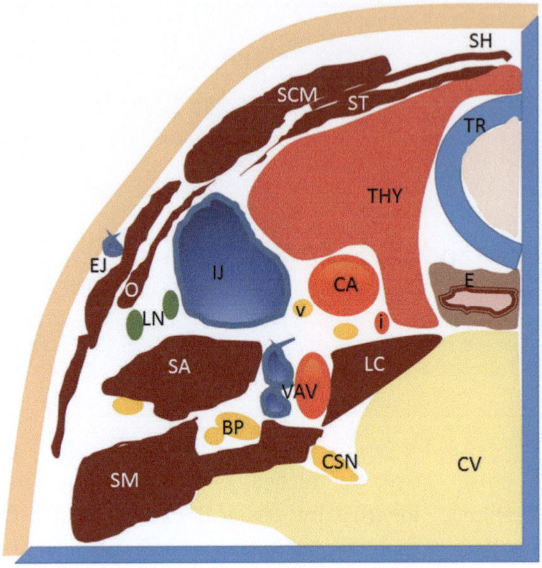

Fig. 9.1 Transverse anatomy of the neck through the thyroid

Fig. 9.2 Trachea in cross section

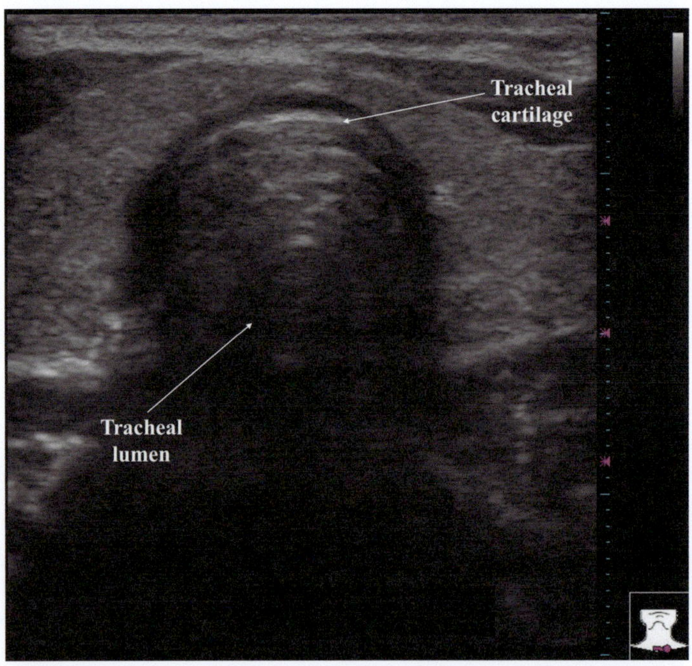

fat, its width variable according to the patient's body habitus. The echogenicity of this fatty layer is brighter than the dermis and is starkly contrasted with the muscle layers that lie beneath it. To either side of the midline, just below the subcutaneous fat, lie the strap muscles, specifically the sternohyoid more superficially and medial and the sternothyroid, deeper and more lateral. In the transverse view, each of them is the shape of a convex lens. They are quite hypoechoic relative to the overlying fat and underlying thyroid, and each is enveloped by a fine white line. The deeper ster-

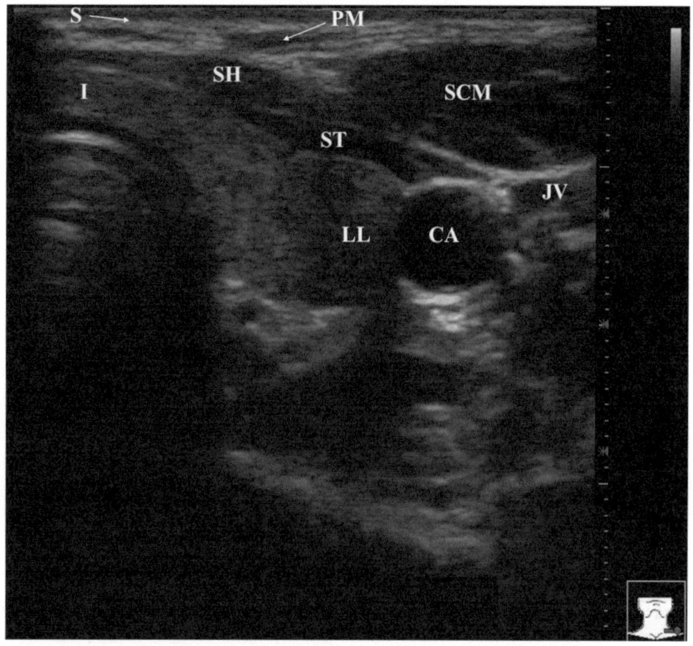

Fig. 9.3 Axial image of superficial structures. S = skin, PM = subcutaneous fat, SH = sternohyoid muscle, ST = sternothyroid muscle, SCM = sternocleidomastoid muscle, I = isthmus of the thyroid, LL = left lobe of the thyroid, CA = common carotid artery, JV = internal jugular vein

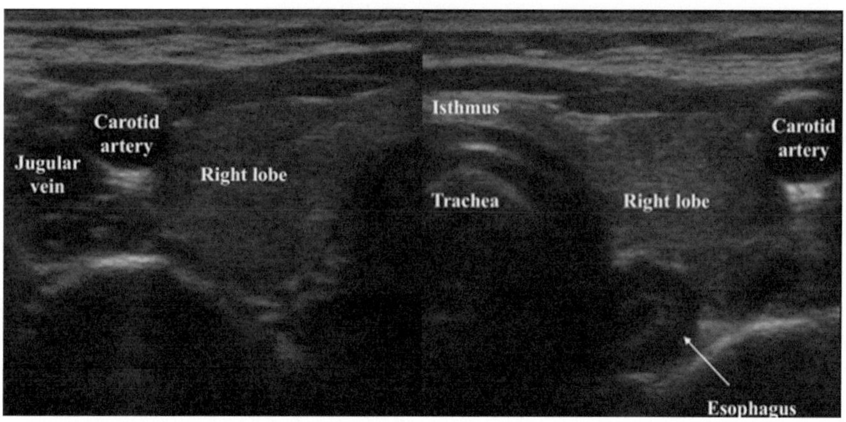

Fig. 9.4 Axial view through the thyroid and adjacent structures

nothyroid extends from the sternum up to the thyroid cartilage, and the more superficial sternohyoid is essentially seen the entire length of the neck, as it inserts upon the hyoid bone.

Immediately posterior to the strap muscles sits the thyroid gland (Fig. 9.4). Its two lobes straddle the trachea, connected by the narrow isthmus. The normal thyroid gland is homogeneous in echotexture. It appears hyperechoic as compared to the overlying strap muscles. Each lobe sits snuggly between the trachea medially and the carotid artery laterally. The two lobes normally appear as mirror images of each other and usually are quite similar in size. Because the esophagus normally resides slightly to the left of the midline, it is frequently seen as an additional structure posterior to the left thyroid lobe (Fig. 9.5).

The contours of the thyroid are usually very smooth and quite discrete. Each lobe is bordered by the trachea medially, strap muscles anteriorly, and the carotid artery laterally. Posteriorly, there is the fat and lymphatic tissue that fills the central compartment between the spine and the thyroid. Because that tissue does not lie within any

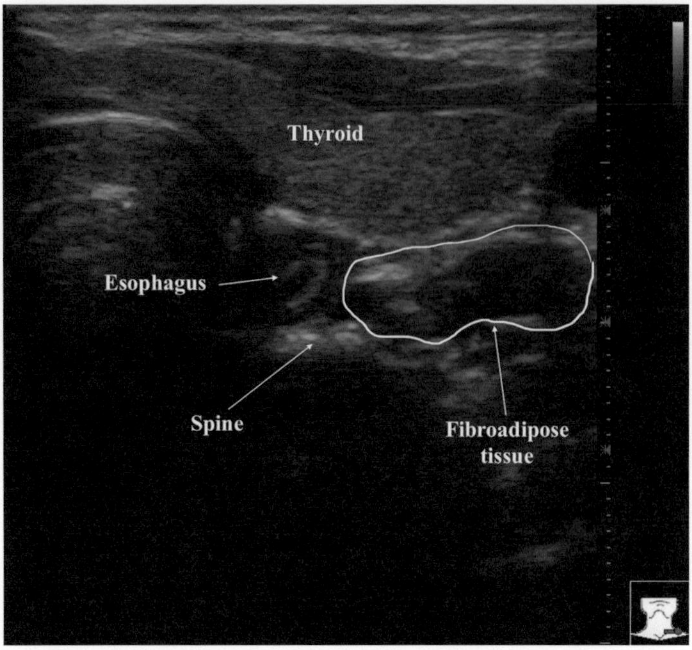

Fig. 9.5 Structures found posterior to the thyroid

defined structure, the posterior border of the thyroid is often less well defined. The fatty tissue behind the thyroid usually appears heterogeneous and can be darker or brighter than the overlying thyroid parenchyma.

Thyroid size varies from patient to patient, but in general, in adults, the width (*W*) or transverse diameter and depth (*D*) or anterior-posterior diameter are quite similar, generally between 1.5 and 2.5 cm. The height or length (*L*) of the thyroid lobe is typically 4–5 cm. The thickness (anterior-posterior diameter) of the isthmus is usually less than 5 mm. In most patients the normal lobes are quite similar in size; however, rarely there will be a rather undeveloped lobe unilaterally. The measurement of the thyroid lobes and focal lesions should be performed in a standard fashion, and the order should be specified, so that comparisons of nodules and sizes of lobes can be made. For example, these authors report the dimensions as $W \times D \times L$, whereas many ultrasound labs will report dimensions as $D \times W \times L$. Many sonographers will obtain the width and depth of the thyroid on a transverse view (Fig. 9.6). The length (superior to inferior) is always obtained from the sagittal view (Fig. 9.7), and when the lobe demonstrates an irregular shape, many sonologists will also obtain the depth measurement on the sagittal view, placing the cursors at the widest portion of the lobe.

If the volume of a thyroid lobe needs to be calculated, this can easily be done using the formula: width × depth × length × 0.479.

Cervical lymph nodes are easily seen during neck sonography. The normal lateral compartment nodes are typically easily seen, especially the larger normal submandibular (level II) nodes (Fig. 9.8), but it is relatively uncommon to see the normal, much smaller lymph nodes in the central compartment. Minimally enlarged and reactive central compartment nodes are however commonly seen in patients with Hashimoto's thyroiditis. Normal parathyroid glands are also not typically seen as they are small and echogenic, blending in with the fibrofatty connective tissue. The submandibular gland itself is homogeneous and shares an echotexture usually identical to that of the thyroid. It is located just beneath the jaw and above the carotid bifurcation.

The most prominent vessels in the neck are the carotid artery and the internal jugular vein, and they lie just lateral to the thyroid lobe (Fig. 9.9). They are just posterior to the lateral aspect of the strap muscles and the medial aspect

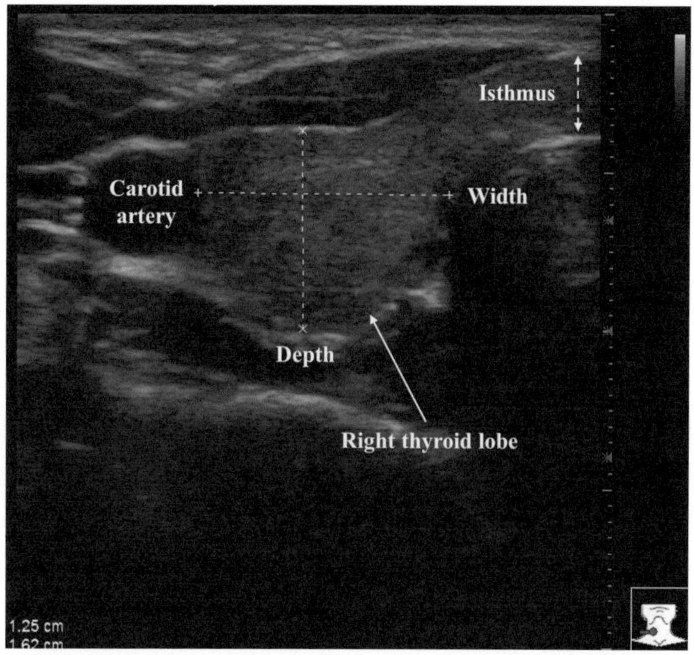

Fig. 9.6 Measurement of width and depth of the right lobe on the transverse view

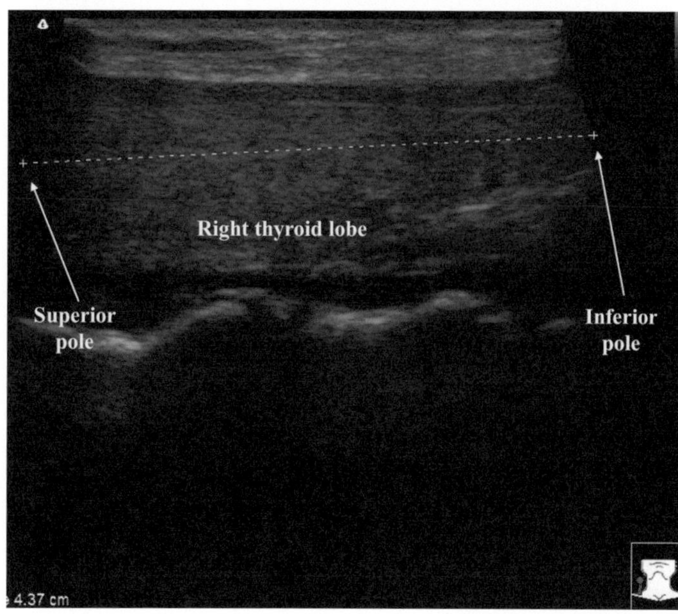

Fig. 9.7 Measurement of length of the right lobe in sagittal view

of the much larger sternocleidomastoid. In the axial view, the carotid is medial, usually abutting the thyroid, and is circular in cross section. Lateral to it lies the jugular vein, which is usually larger, more oval, and completely compressible with the ultrasound probe. Within the artery, there may be luminal calcifications in patients with atherosclerotic disease, and these tend to be most prominent at the carotid bifurcation. They appear as bright white plaques along the inner arterial wall. If observed carefully, a valve can often be seen within the jugular vein just before it joins the subclavian. The paper-thin valve leaflets will appear fluttering within the lumen.

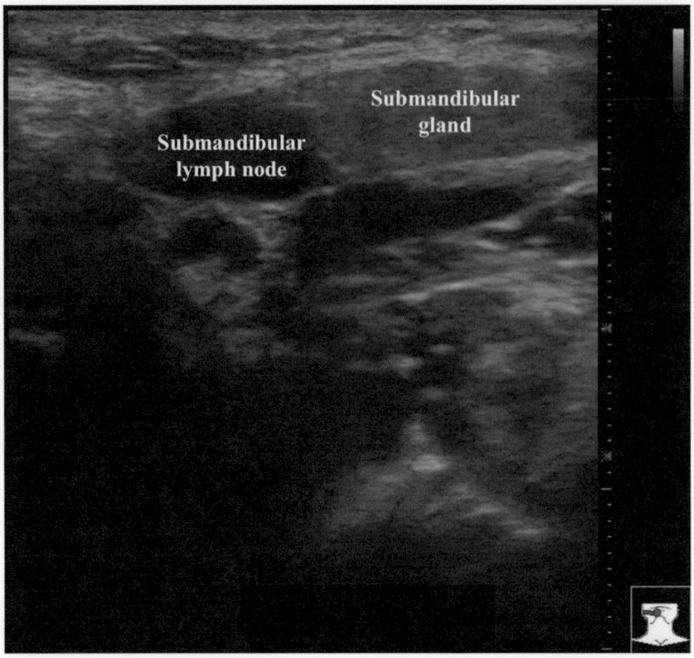

Fig. 9.8 Normal submandibular gland and lymph node

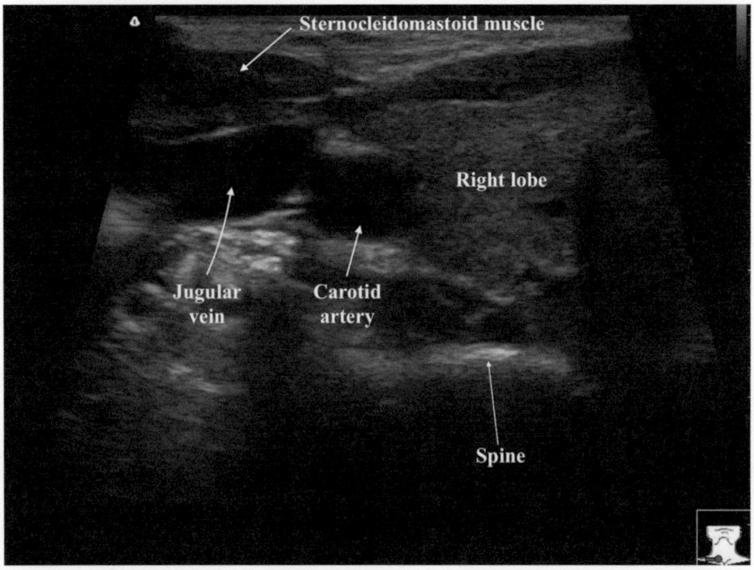

Fig. 9.9 Vasculature-transverse view

The posterior structures in the neck are less well defined and not readily discerned from each other. Beginning medially, the spine is the most posterior structure visible (Fig. 9.9). It is directly behind the trachea and can be seen extending bilaterally behind the thyroid lobes. It appears as a very hyperechoic white linear or curvilinear structure due to the near-complete reflection of the ultrasound waves as they strike the bone interface. Usually there is a layer of hypoechoic tissue between the spine and the posterior aspect of the thyroid, consisting of fat and lymphatics in the paratracheal space (Fig. 9.5). Normally, the esophagus can be clearly seen sitting in the groove between the trachea and the spine on the left. It appears as a slightly irregular concentric

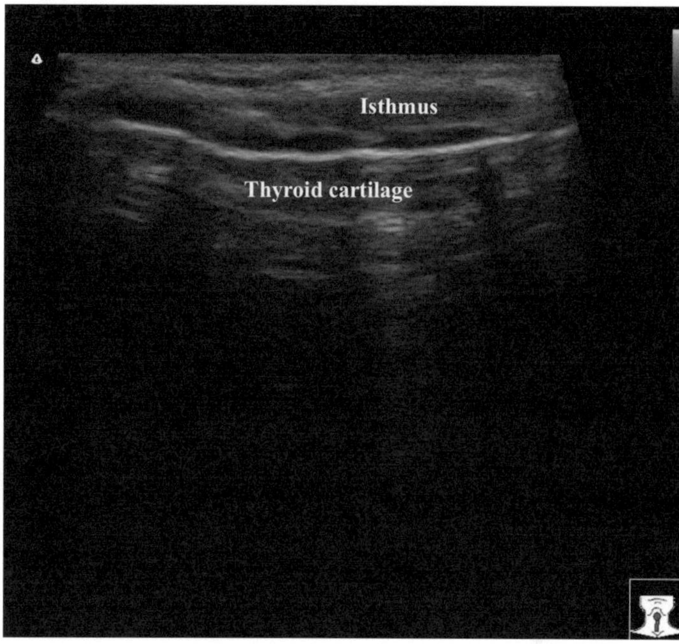

Fig. 9.10 Sagittal view of thyroid isthmus and tracheal rings

circle or oval in the transverse view. The two rings visible correspond to the outer serosa and the inner mucosa (Fig. 9.5). Many times the esophagus is in direct contact with the posterior aspect of the thyroid, and it should not be mistaken for a hypoechoic thyroid nodule. It is somewhat mobile, and its location can sometimes be shifted to the right of the midline. Its identity can be confirmed by observing the mucosal layer while having the patient swallow. When the wave of peristalsis passes, the mucosa will undulate and shimmer slightly.

Newer sonographers may find examining the neck in the transverse orientation easier to grasp than in the sagittal orientation (Videos 9.1 and 9.2). The best way to examine a structure in the sagittal view is to place the probe in a transverse orientation directly over the structure and then to rotate the probe 90° clockwise. When imaging a thyroid lobe, be careful to keep the center of the probe over the center of the lobe being examined while rotating. It is very easy to end the rotation with the probe either medial or lateral to the target structure, and it can be a bit disorienting since we are not as accustomed to this view. Simply move the probe slightly medially or slightly laterally, and your thyroid lobe will come back into view. Once the 90° clockwise rotation is performed, the superior aspect of the lobe will be on the left-hand side of the screen image, and the inferior aspect will be to the right. This convention of superior to the left and inferior to the right should always be followed, so as to minimize any confusion.

When examining the neck in the sagittal view, you will come across the following structures. In Fig. 9.10 the probe is directly over the isthmus, which shows up as a very narrow strip of homogeneous tissue that is hyperechoic relative to the overlying strap muscles and underlying trachea. The tracheal cartilages can be seen individually deep to the isthmus as small oval structures in the anterior wall of the trachea. Moving laterally, you will next encounter the thyroid lobe (Fig. 9.7), which will appear almond shaped with its superior pole to the left and inferior pole to the right (Video 9.3). On the left, you should be able to see the hypoechoic longitudinal tube behind the thyroid, which is the esophagus in long axis. Just lateral to the thyroid will be an easily identifiable, long, tubular structure corresponding to the carotid artery, and of course the jugular vein will be just lateral to that (Fig. 9.11).

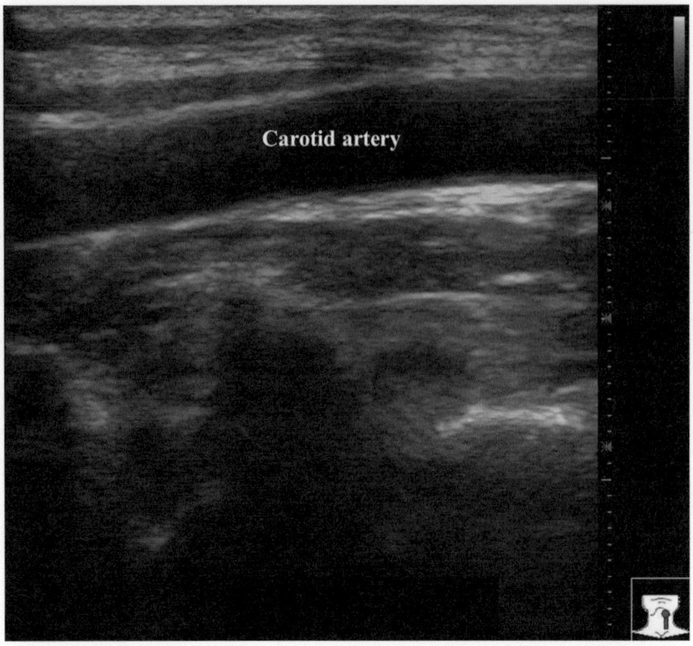

Fig. 9.11 Sagittal view of carotid artery

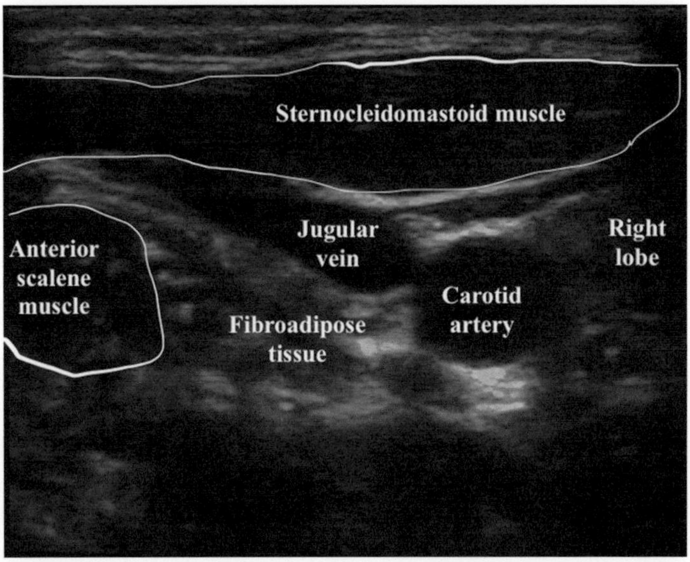

Fig. 9.12 Lateral compartment structures

It is important to extend the imaging beyond the lateral border of the thyroid, into the lateral neck compartment which contains muscles, lymphatics, and fatty tissue (Fig. 9.12). The sternocleidomastoid is quite close to the skin, and in cross section, it is a large dark oval, varying in size significantly from person to person. It is present from the clavicle all the way to the mastoid process, and the carotid and jugular are just deep to it in the inferior two thirds of the neck. The anterior and middle scalene muscles are hypoechoic structures seen on axial imaging deep to the sternocleidomastoid muscle. Because of this deeper location, resolving their borders is not as clear as the more superficial strap muscles. Also there is often a significant amount of

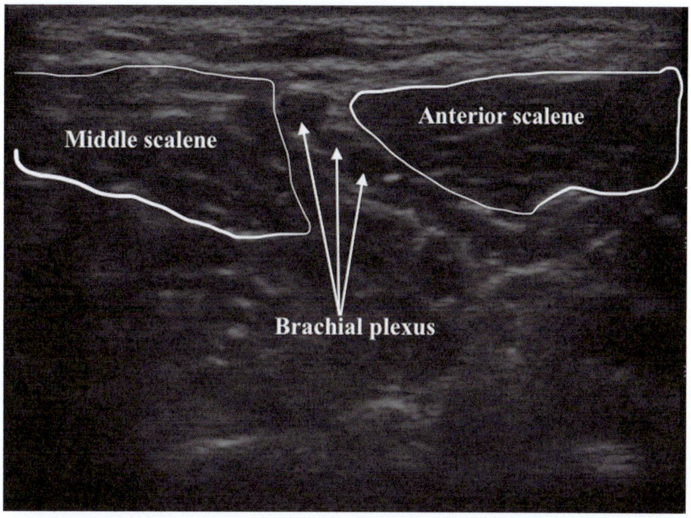

Fig. 9.13 Brachial plexus

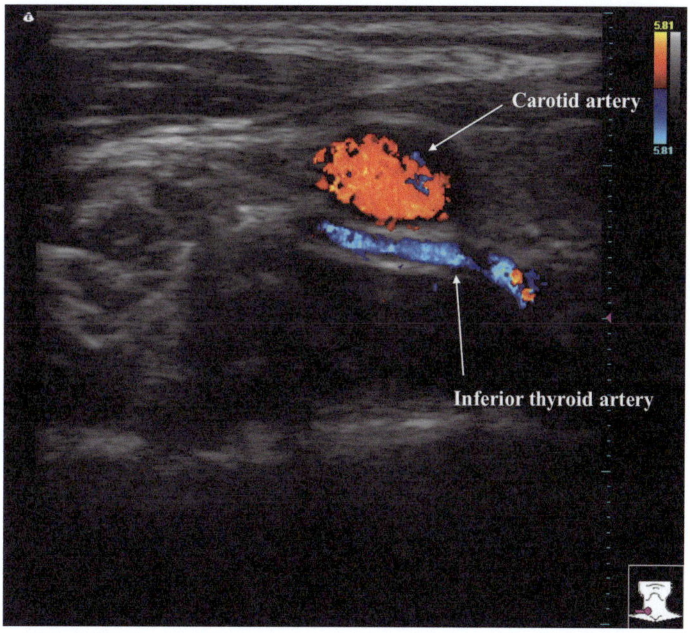

Fig. 9.14 Color Doppler flow of the right neck

fat and lymphatic tissue between them and the overlying SCM. Between the anterior and middle scalene muscles on axial view lie the fascicles of the brachial plexus. They appear as a stack of small circular hypoechoic structures (Fig. 9.13).

Color Doppler images of the neck are useful for distinguishing blood vessels from small nodules or lymph nodes and for assessing vascular patterns of flow in thyroid nodules, parathyroid gland, and lymph nodes. When the color Doppler function is used, the color will be displayed within the color box within the image where flow or motion is detected (Fig. 9.14). In this figure the inferior thyroid artery which passes behind the carotid sheath from lateral to medial before branching out to supply the thyroid and parathyroid glands can be seen behind the right thyroid lobe. Sometimes it may be difficult to distinguish a small vessel from a lymph node or parathyroid, and the use of the Doppler function can be quite helpful in making this distinction.

The superior thyroid artery originates from the external carotid artery, and its terminal branches can be seen feeding the superior pole of the thyroid. The inferior thyroid artery originates from the thyrocervical trunk, and its terminal branches enter the thyroid posteriorly in its mid-portion. Regarding the vascularity of the thyroid parenchyma itself, it is not generally necessary or helpful to examine a normal thyroid lobe with Doppler imaging. In general, the parenchyma of each lobe should have a moderate amount of flow that is evenly distributed (Video 9.4). Since the gain function on the ultrasound machine can be used to enhance or diminish the apparent volume of flow, no true assessments about vascularity should be made.

10 Feature Illustration: Echogenicity, Composition, and Shape

Jill E. Langer

10.1 Echogenicity

The echogenicity of a thyroid nodule refers to its brightness relative to the normal thyroid parenchyma. Normal parenchyma appears homogeneously hyperechoic or relatively bright on sonography related to the high number of acoustic interfaces within the normal follicles of the thyroid gland. The echogenicity of a nodule is described relative to this bright background of the normal thyroid as either (a) hypoechoic meaning darker than the normal thyroid (Fig. 10.1), (b) hyperechoic meaning brighter than the normal thyroid (Fig. 10.2), or (c) isoechoic meaning equal in echogenicity compared to the normal thyroid (Fig. 10.3). Many nodules have regions of varying echogenicity and may be described by the dominant echogenicity (e.g., predominantly hypoechoic), or when there is no dominant pattern, as heterogeneous in echogenicity (Fig. 10.4). For nodules that are partially cystic, the echogenicity of the solid part should be used to describe the nodule's echogenicity, and cystic components are considered anechoic, meaning devoid of echoes, with hypoechoic used only in reference to solid components of a nodule [1].

Most thyroid cancers appear dark or hypoechoic as compared with thyroid parenchyma due to their highly cellular composition. Histologically, the increased cellularity and cellular compaction present in classic papillary thyroid cancer and medullary thyroid cancer produces less acoustic interfaces than micro-follicles and therefore typically causes these lesions to appear hypoechoic compared with surrounding normal thyroid tissue [2, 3] (Fig. 10.1). However, not all neoplasms of the thyroid are hypoechoic in appearance. Follicular neoplasms, including a benign follicular adenoma, a follicular carcinoma, or a follicular variant of papillary cancer, are composed of small micro-follicles with variable amounts of colloid. Therefore, the echogenicity of these follicular-predominant carcinomas and adenomas is less commonly hypoechoic and instead is much more commonly isoechoic or hyperechoic compared with the parenchyma [4, 5] (Figs. 10.2 and 10.3). Additionally, many benign nodules will also appear hypoechoic. Since benign nodules are much more common than malignant nodules, a nodule that is hypoechoic but otherwise lacks

Electronic supplementary material: The online version of this chapter (doi:10.1007/978-3-319-44100-9_10) contains supplementary material, which is available to authorized users. Videos can also be accessed at http://link.springer.com/chapter/10.1007/978-3-319-44100-9_10.

J.E. Langer, M.D. (✉)
Department of Radiology, The Perelman School of Medicine at the University of Pennsylvania, 3400 Spruce Street, Philadelphia, PA 19104, USA
e-mail: jill.langer@uphs.upenn.edu

M. Milas et al. (eds.), *Advanced Thyroid and Parathyroid Ultrasound*, DOI 10.1007/978-3-319-44100-9_10

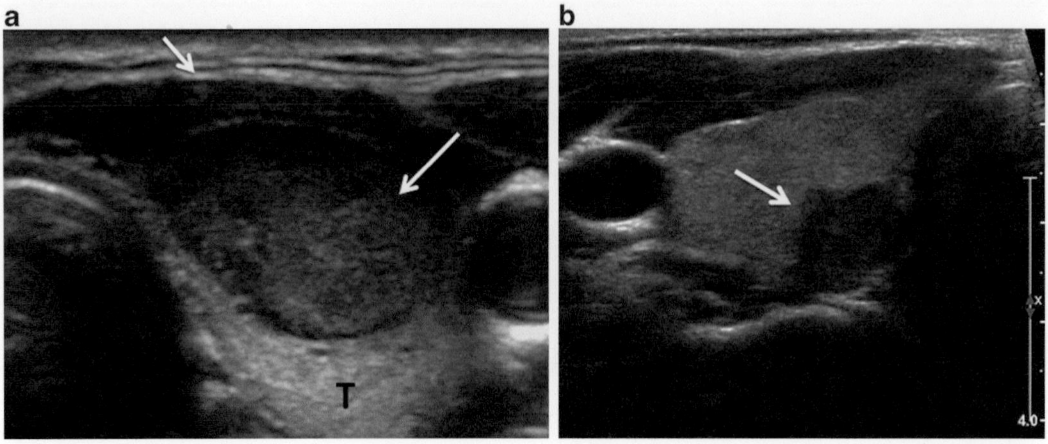

Fig. 10.1 Hypoechoic nodules. (**a**) Transverse view of the thyroid demonstrates a nodule (*long white arrow*) that is hypoechoic or darker than the surrounding thyroid parenchyma (T) but slightly less hypoechoic than the overlying neck musculature (*short arrow*). This nodule proved to a benign hyperplastic nodule on FNA. (**b**) Transverse view of the right lobe of the thyroid in a different patient demonstrates a hypoechoic nodule which proved to be a papillary thyroid carcinoma. A lobulated border is noted in this lesion

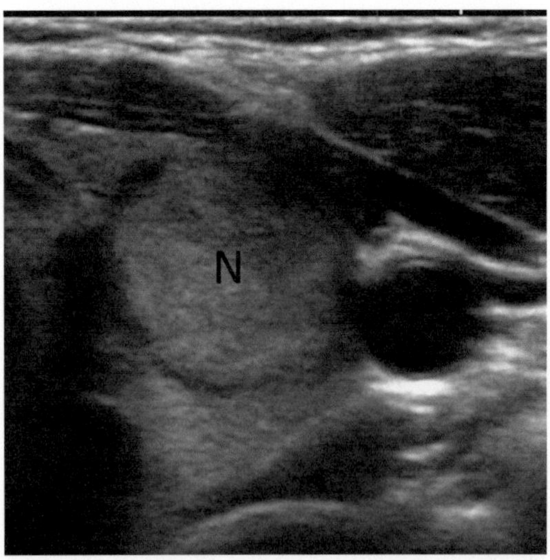

Fig. 10.2 Hyperechoic nodule. Transverse view of the left lobe of the thyroid shows a nodule (N) which proved to be a follicular variant of papillary carcinoma which is hyperechoic relative to the thyroid parenchyma

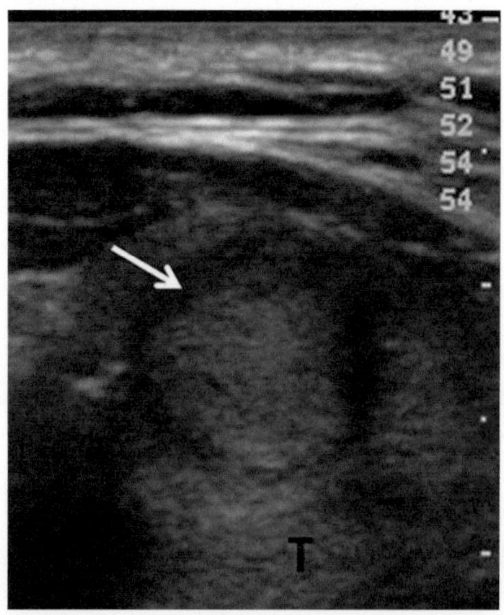

Fig. 10.3 Isoechoic nodule. Transverse view of the left lobe of the thyroid shows a solid nodule (*arrow*) with echogenicity relatively similar to the background parenchyma (T) which proved to be a follicular variant of papillary carcinoma

any additional features associated with malignancy will statically most likely be benign. Hypoechogenicity, as a unique characteristic of a nodule, is therefore only a moderately sensitive finding for malignancy, with a reported median sensitivity of about 80 %. The reported specificity of hypoechogenecity for malignancy varies greatly depending on the histological subtypes of cancers in the population studied as well as the association of hypoechogenecity with other features and has been reported to range from 36 to 92 % [2, 3, 6–8]. Some authors have identified a sonographic feature called “marked hypoechogenicity” that describes a nodule with echogenicity that is darker than the surrounding strap muscles [7–9]. Compared to nodules that are hypoechoic with respect to parenchyma but not as hypoechoic as strap muscles, marked hypoechogenicity is less sensitive for identification of thyroid cancer, approximately 41 % sensitive, but much more specific, typically over 90 % [6, 8] (Fig. 10.5).

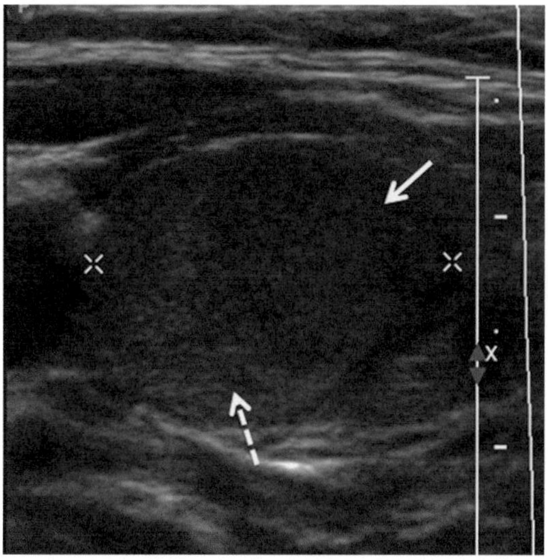

Fig. 10.4 Mixed echogenicity. Transverse view of the right lobe of the thyroid shows a nodule outlined by calipers. The more medial portion of the nodule (*straight line arrow*) is hypoechoic, and the more lateral portion (*dashed arrow*) is brighter and isoechoic with the thyroid parenchyma

The assessment of echogenicity is subjective and tends to have only fair to moderate interobserver reproducibility even among expert observers (Kappa values 0.3–0.5) [7, 10, 11]. Echogenicity can be altered by differing sonographic techniques including changes in the overall gain and transducer frequency. Additionally, in patients with autoimmune thyroid disease such as Hashimoto's thyroiditis, the echogenicity of the parenchyma is much more heterogeneous in appearance making classification of the nodule's echogenicity more subjective.

10.1.1 Composition

Nodule composition describes the amount or proportion of solid soft tissue and fluid in a nodule. Nodules can be described as (a) solid, meaning composed entirely or nearly entirely of soft tissue with only a few small scattered cystic spaces (Fig. 10.6); (b) predominantly solid, meaning that soft tissue components comprise at least 50 % or greater of the volume of the nodule (Fig. 10.7); (c) predominantly cystic meaning that soft tissue components comprise less than

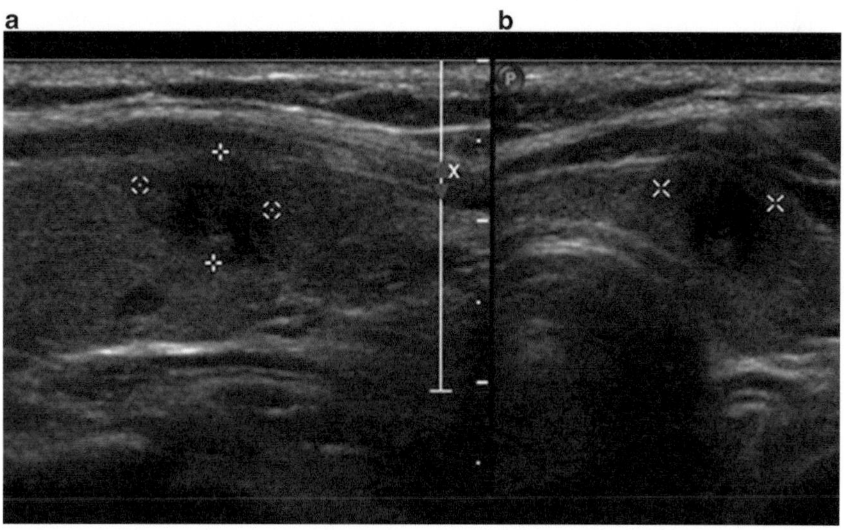

Fig. 10.5 Markedly hypoechoic nodule. Split screen sagittal (**a**) and transverse (**b**) view of a thyroid gland shows a markedly hypoechoic nodule with echogenicity darker than the overlying musculature which proved to be a papillary thyroid cancer. This degree of hypoechogenicity carries a higher specificity for malignancy than hypoechogenicity less than the musculature

50 % of the volume of the nodule (Fig. 10.8); or (d) entirely cystic, meaning fluid filled without appreciable solid component (Fig. 10.9). Some authors have used numerical percentages of cystic or solid elements to describe nodule composition, most commonly by quartiles [1, 12].

Thyroid cancers are most commonly solid or nearly entirely solid and are more likely to be solid than benign nodules [1–9] However, because benign nodules outnumber malignant ones, this feature carries a relatively low specificity for malignancy as an isolated feature. It is estimated that a solid nodule has a 15–27 % likelihood of being malignant [12]. Although there is some subjectivity in reporting the degree of cystic change present in a nodule, the interobserver agreement for reporting solid nodule consistency is reported to be quite high [10, 11].

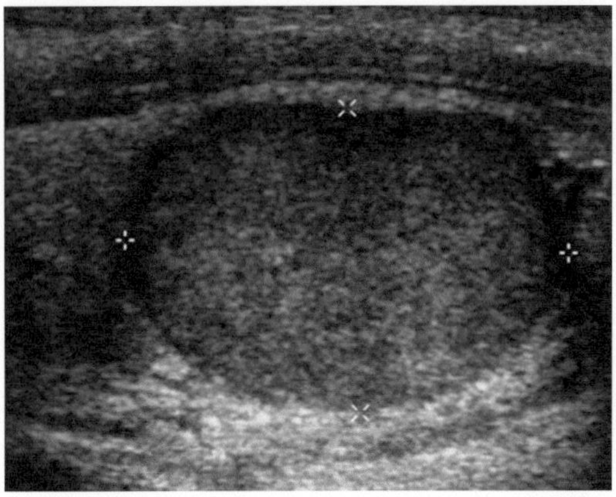

Fig. 10.6 Solid composition. Sagittal view of the left lobe shows an entirely solid, hypoechoic nodule which proved to be a follicular adenoma

Cystic change within a nodule is very common [1, 6]. Hyperplastic nodules contain abundant colloid which appears cystic on sonography, and neoplasms may undergo cystic degeneration or necrosis, producing cystic areas [13]. It is uncommon for cancers to have a predominantly cystic appearance with a recent study of partially cystic nodules showing a 6.1 % prevalence of malignancy among predominately cystic nodules [14]. When evaluating a partially cystic nodule for malignancy risk, the evaluation should concentrate on the solid component. Features concerning for a malignant cystic nodule include a solid component that is hypoechoic, is lobulated, has an irregular border, and/or contains calcifications (Fig. 10.10 and Video 10.1). If the solid component is eccentrically (peripherally) located within a partially cystic nodule and the margin of the solid component has an acute angle with the wall of the nodule, the risk for malignancy is also increased (Video 10.2). Conversely, if the solid component is isoechoic, is centrally located within the nodule or, if peripheral, lacks an acute angle with the nodule wall, or has a

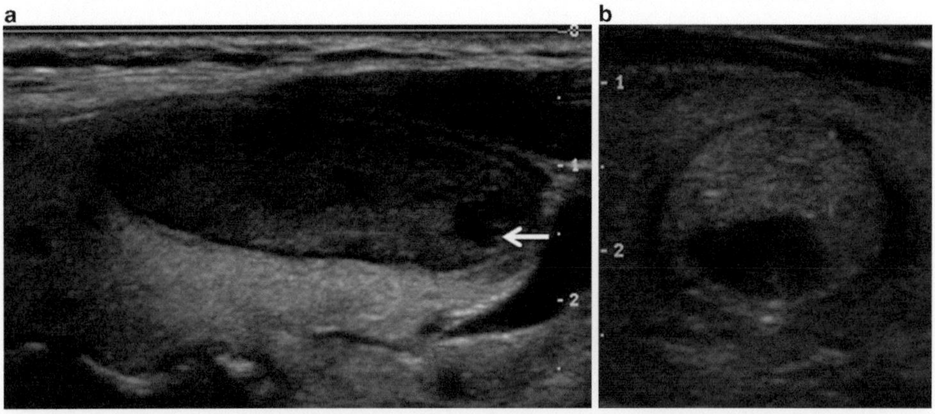

Fig. 10.7 Predominantly solid composition. (**a**) Sagittal view of the left lobe shows a predominantly solid, hypoechoic nodule with a few small cystic regions (*arrow*) which proved to be benign on biopsy. When there are very few cystic regions as in this nodule, some sonologists may classify this nodule as solid. (**b**) Transverse view of the right lobe of the thyroid shows a predominantly solid, hyperechoic nodule with cystic regions occupying less than 50 % of the volume of the nodule

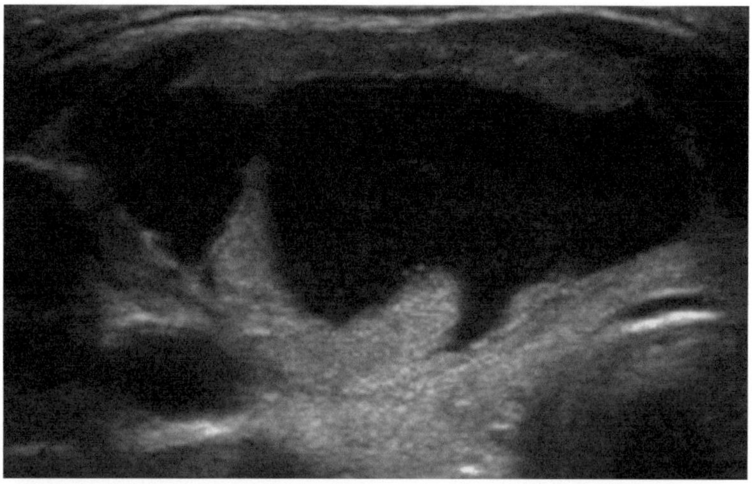

Fig. 10.8 Predominately cystic composition. Transverse view of the right lobe of the thyroid shows a predominantly cystic, nodule with cystic regions occupying greater than 50 % of the volume of the nodule

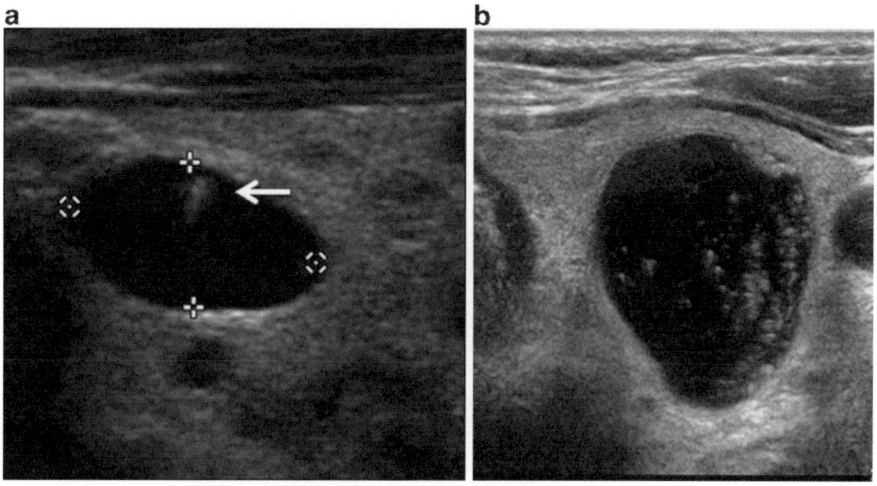

Fig. 10.9 Entirely cystic composition. (**a**) This nodule (*outlined* by *calipers*) is completely anechoic without an identifiable solid component. A small echogenic focus (*arrow*) is related to colloid reverberation artifact. This most likely represents either a colloid cyst or less likely a true cyst of the thyroid and is considered benign. (**b**) Transverse view of the left lobe of the thyroid in a different patient shows a cystic nodule multiple echogenic foci representing colloid

smooth margin, the nodule is likely benign (Figs. 10.8 and 10.11) [12, 15].

Purely cystic nodules and the nodules with a spongiform appearance have a very low risk of malignancy. Moon et al. [7] defined a spongiform appearance as one in which the nodule has multiple microcytic areas that occupy more than 50 % of the nodule volume and found that only 1 of the 360 thyroid cancers appeared spongiform in their series (Fig. 10.12 and Video 10.3). Bonavita et al. [16] used spongiform to mean tiny spaces involving the entire nodule and found all 210 nonvascular nodules with this sonographic appearance to be benign. Current biopsy guidelines recognize pure cystic and spongiform nodules as very low risk for malignancy, and the size cutoff for FNA of such lesions is more lenient (if performed at all) than for intermediate- and high-risk sonographically appearing nodules. Often, comet-tail artifact, representing reverberation of sound waves caused by inspissated colloid, is

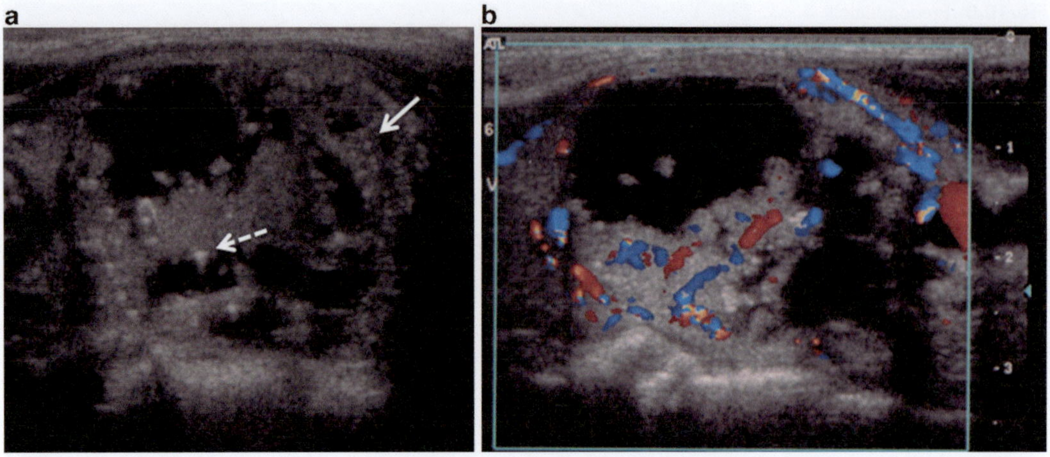

Fig. 10.10 Cystic papillary thyroid carcinoma. (**a**) Transverse and (**b**) sagittal color Doppler images of this cystic papillary thyroid carcinoma show the solid competent to be frond-like, to be lobulated, and to have marked vascular flow. Multiple echogenic foci are noted, some of which show reverberation artifact (*dashed arrow*) and are likely are colloid, while others are punctate without reverberation (*arrow*) and are suggestive of calcifications

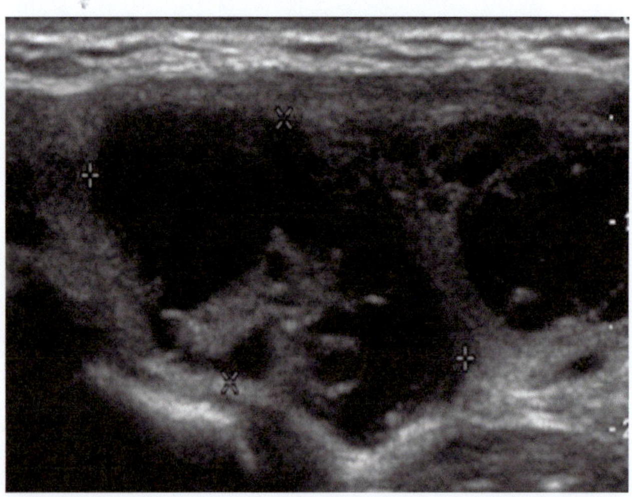

Fig. 10.11 Benign cystic nodules. The solid component of this cystic nodule is isoechoic to the parenchyma, with straight margins and spongiform in appearance, typical of a benign cystic nodule

present in both entirely cystic appearing and spongiform nodules. It is worth noting that colloid may be present in both benign and malignant nodules. As noted above, very few thyroid cancers will be predominantly cystic and may contain colloid, but these cystic carcinomas will often have another suspicious US feature such as frond-like solid tissue and/or calcifications [14] (Fig. 10.10).

10.2 Taller-Than-Wide Shape

A taller-than-wide shape is defined as a ratio of >1 of the anteroposterior diameter to the transverse diameter when measured in the transverse plane (Fig. 10.13). Disproportionate growth in the anteroposterior dimension is considered an aggressive growth pattern across rather than within the normal tissue planes and is thought to

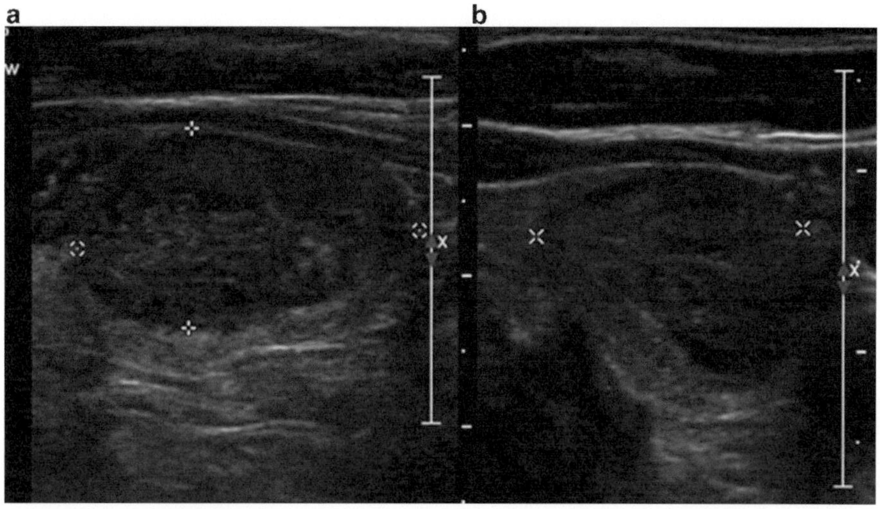

Fig. 10.12 Spongiform appearance of a nodule. Split screen sagittal (**a**) and transverse (**b**) shows a nodule with interspersed cystic spaces throughout occupying more than 50 % of the nodule. This appearance has been termed spongiform and carries and extremely low risk for malignancy

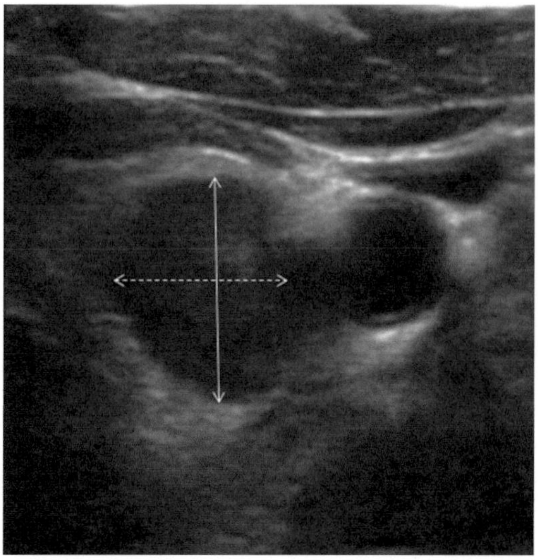

Fig. 10.13 Taller-than-wide shape. This 12 mm papillary cancer is hypoechoic and solid and is noted to have a greater anterior-posterior length than width (*dashed arrow*) on this transverse image, a finding termed taller-than-wide shape. This feature carries a relatively high specificity for thyroid cancer and is most commonly noted in small cancers

correspond to decreased compressibility of tumor as compared with parenchyma [12]. This finding was first observed when performing ultrasound exams of breast carcinomas [8] and when applied to thyroid nodule evaluation was similarly found to be a feature of thyroid malignancy. This finding is not very sensitive but has specificity ranging from 82 to 93 % and is most commonly noted in smaller cancers, under 1 cm [17–20].

In studies that specify how measurements are made, there are no significant differences comparing transverse or longitudinal imaging planes for determining the ratio [17].

10.3 Conclusions

Nodule echogenicity, composition and shape are key features that aid the assessment of the risk of thyroid malignancy. Whereas most thyroid cancers are both solid and hypoechoic, many benign nodules will also have this appearance, and some cancers, especially follicular-derived lesions, are usually hyperechoic, lowering the specificity of these features. Taller-than-wide shape and marked hypoechogenicity are highly specific features of carcinoma but are not present in the majority of tumors. Analysis of partially cystic nodules is directed at assessing the appearance of the solid component for suspicious features such as nodularity, calcification, and irregular margins. Spongiform appearance and entirely cystic nodules carry a very low likelihood of malignancy, avoiding the need for biopsy in most cases.

References

1. Frates MC, Benson CB, Charboneau JW, Cibas ES, Clark OH, Coleman BG, Cronan JJ, Doubilet PM, Evans DB, Goellner JR, Hay ID, Hertzberg BS, Intenzo CM, Jeffrey RB, Langer JE, Larsen PR, Mandel SJ, Middleton WD, Reading CC, Sherman SI, Tessler FN. Management of thyroid nodules detected at US: Society of Radiologists in Ultrasound consensus conference statement. Radiology. 2005;237:794–800.
2. Papini E, Guglielmi R, Bianchini A, Crescenzi A, Taccogna S, Nardi F, Panunzi C, Rinaldi R, Toscano V, Pacella CM. Risk of malignancy in nonpalpable thyroid nodules: predictive value of ultrasound and color-Doppler features. J Clin Endocrinol Metab. 2002;87:1941–6.
3. Frates MC, Benson CB, Doubilet PM, Kunreuther E, Contreras M, Cibas ES, Orcutt J, Moore Jr FD, Larsen PR, Marqusee E, Alexander EK. Prevalence and distribution of carcinoma in patients with solitary and multiple thyroid nodules on sonography. J Clin Endocrinol Metab. 2006;91:3411–7.
4. Jeh SK, Jung SL, Kim BS, Lee YS. Evaluating the degree of conformity of papillary carcinoma and follicular carcinoma to the reported ultrasonographic findings of malignant thyroid tumor. Korean J Radiol. 2007;8:192–7.
5. Kim DS, Kim JH, Na DG, Park SH, Kim E, Chang KH, Sohn CH, Choi YH. Sonographic features of follicular variant papillary thyroid carcinomas in comparison with conventional papillary thyroid carcinomas. J Ultrasound Med. 2009;28:1685–92.
6. Haugen BR, Alexander EK, Bible KC, Doherty GM, Mandel SJ, Nikiforov YE, et al. 2015 American Thyroid Association Management Guidelines for adult patients with thyroid nodules and differentiated thyroid cancer: the American Thyroid Association guidelines task force on thyroid nodules and differentiated thyroid cancer. Thyroid. 2016;26(1):1–133.
7. Moon WJ, Jung SL, Lee JH, Na DG, Baek JH, Lee YH, Kim J, Kim HS, Byun JS, Lee DH. Benign and malignant thyroid nodules: US differentiation--multicenter retrospective study. Radiology. 2008;247:762–70.
8. Kim EK, Park CS, Chung WY, et al. New sonographic criteria for recommending fine-needle aspiration biopsy of nonpalpable solid nodules of the thyroid. AJR Am J Roentgenol. 2002;178:687–91.
9. Ahn SS, Kim EK, Kang DR, Lim SK, Kwak JY, Kim MJ. Biopsy of thyroid nodules: comparison of three sets of guidelines. AJR Am J Roentgenol. 2010;194:31–7.
10. Choi SH, Kim EK, Kwak JY, Kim MJ, Son EJ. Interobserver and intraobserver variations in ultrasound assessment of thyroid nodules. Thyroid. 2010;20:167–72.
11. Wienke JR, Chong WK, Fielding JR, Zou KH, Mittelstaedt CA. Sonographic features of benign thyroid nodules: interobserver reliability and overlap with malignancy. J Ultrasound Med. 2003;22:1027–31.
12. Grant EG, Tessler FN, Hoang JK, et al. Thyroid ultrasound reporting lexicon: white paper of the ACT thyroid imaging, reporting and data system (TIRADS) Committee. J Am Coll Radiol. 2015;12:1272–9.
13. Malhi H, Beland MD, Cen SY, et al. Echogenic foci in thyroid nodules: significance of posterior acoustic artifacts. AJR Am J Roentgenol. 2014;203(6):1310–6.
14. Henrichsen TI, Reading CC, Charboneau JW, et al. Cystic change n thyroid carcinoma: prevalence and estimated volume in 360 carcinomas. J Clin Ultrasound. 2010;38:361–6.
15. Kim DW, Lee EJ, In HS, Kim SJ. Sonographic differentiation of partially cystic thyroid nodules; a prospective study. AJNR Am J Neuroradiol. 2010;31:1961–6.
16. Bonavita JA, Mayo J, Babb J, Bennett G, Oweity T, Macari M, Yee J. Pattern recognition of benign nodules at ultrasound of the thyroid: which nodules can be left alone? AJR Am J Roentgenol. 2009;193:207–13.
17. Moon HJ, Kwak JY, Kim EK, Kim MJ. A taller-than-wide shape in thyroid nodules in transverse and longitudinal ultrasonographic planes and the prediction of malignancy. Thyroid. 2011;21:1249–53.
18. Chen SP, Hu YP, Chen B. Taller-than-wide sign for predicting thyroid microcarcinoma: comparison and combination of two ultrasonographic planes. Ultrasound Med Biol. 2014;40:2004–11.
19. Ren J, Liu B, Zhang LL, et al. A taller-than-wide shape is a good predictor of papillary thyroid carcinoma in small solid nodules. J Ultrasound Med. 2015;34:19–26.
20. Kim HG, Moon HJ, Kwak JY, Kim EK. Diagnostic accuracy of the ultrasonographic features for subcentimeter thyroid nodules suggested by the revised American Thyroid Association guidelines. Thyroid. 2013;23:1583–90.

11 Feature Illustration: Thyroid Nodule Margins and Extrathyroidal Extension and Invasion

Mira Milas, Dubravka Milas Tollison, and Zvonimir Luka Milas

11.1 Overview

The terms margin and contour have been used somewhat interchangeably in current literature to refer to the boundary of a discreet thyroid nodule identified by ultrasound (US) [1–9]. The boundary exists between the physical composition of the thyroid nodule and the surrounding parenchyma of the thyroid gland. This is an important concept to keep in mind because margins and contour can also describe the external surface of the thyroid gland. Margins are also the vocabulary term used by pathologists and surgeons mostly to describe the interface between diseased organs and surrounding normal anatomical structures and tissue. The scenarios where the external margins or surface of the thyroid gland, as an organ, appear as a diffusely irregular or infiltrative process both on pathological review and on sonography are rare and include anaplastic thyroid cancer, primary thyroid lymphomas and metastases from other primary malignancies, and occasionally, a discreet nodule that is malignant but has completely replaced the parenchyma of a thyroid lobe. Therefore, this chapter will *not* consider those scenarios but rather focus on the clinical patient presentations that occur routinely with respect to evaluation of discreet nodules.

US features are not meant to be used in isolation as criteria to guide biopsy decisions or diagnostic interpretation. This is because the reliability and accuracy of each feature are insufficiently high for these overall clinical goals [6–8, 10]. For example, in a recent study, 99 % of benign thyroid nodules and 62 % of malignant nodules had well-circumscribed margins [11].

Multiple studies have suggested that margins alone cannot accurately predict the presence of thyroid malignancy, giving rise to classification schemes such as via TIRADS and ATA over recent years [10, 12–14]. This is a fundamental

Electronic supplementary material: The online version of this chapter (doi:10.1007/978-3-319-44100-9_11) contains supplementary material, which is available to authorized users. Videos can also be accessed at http://link.springer.com/chapter/10.1007/978-3-319-44100-9_11.

M. Milas, M.D., F.A.C.S. (✉)
Department of Surgery and the Endocrinology & Metabolism Institute, University of Arizona College of Medicine – Phoenix, Banner - University Medical Center Phoenix, 1441 North 12th Street, 2nd floor, Phoenix, AZ 85006, USA
e-mail: Mira.Milas@bannerhealth.com

D.M. Tollison, M.D.
Department of Family Medicine, Class of 2001, Banner - University Medical Center Phoenix, University of Arizona College of Medicine – Phoenix, 1300 North 12th Street, Phoenix, AZ 85006, USA
e-mail: dmtollison@gmail.com

Z.L. Milas, M.D., F.A.C.S.
Department of Surgery, Levine Cancer Center at the Carolinas Medical Center, University of North Carolina Chappell Hill, 1021 Morehead Medical Dr. #3259, Charlotte, NC 28204, USA
e-mail: zvonimir.milas@carolinashealthcare.org

M. Milas et al. (eds.), *Advanced Thyroid and Parathyroid Ultrasound*,
DOI 10.1007/978-3-319-44100-9_11

concept pointed out consistently by other authors in this textbook in the sections of feature illustration and pattern recognition: individual features in general, and margins in particular, are but one of several considerations that contributes to assessment of the type of disease, which should be the ultimate goal of clinicians using ultrasound.

Margin description is essential to include in a formal ultrasound report [1, 2, 10]. The following scenarios of thyroid nodule margins illustrate the spectrum of possible descriptions. As in the literature and daily vernacular, the term "margin" and "contour" will likely be interwoven while referring to the following illustrations. Surgical photos are likewise provided as a means of a pictorial essay showing how, in many cases, there is direct correlation between sonographic appearance and actual physical features of thyroid nodules.

11.2 Nodule Margins and Contour

The boundary of a thyroid nodule can be classified along a spectrum from smooth and well-defined to infiltrative. While thyroid ultrasound topics are generously represented in the literature, margins as an isolated topic, or precise subject of reviews, are rare. The definitions and illustrations provided here are a compilation from published guidelines and the authors' personal experience. Therefore, it may be helpful to imagine the relevant terminology along the novel schematic introduced here as a visual aid and considered along with various descriptive terms provided below as synonyms for margin features (Fig. 11.1). The schematic starts with the image of a thin line. The thin line is meant to represent the border (in a two-dimensional relationship) or boundary (three dimensional) between a nodule and the surrounding thyroid parenchyma. The line can be smooth (straight) or jagged (notched, wavy, saw-toothed, frizzy). The line can be thin or thick. The path of the line may change over distances or the visual spatial relationship seen either in two-dimensional or three-dimensional ultrasound imaging. That path may stay as a simple, familiar, and regular shape (circle/oval or sphere/ellipsoid) or take gradual or sudden turns (giving rise to geometric segments, sections, projections, or lobules). In sections of that path, the line may vary in smoothness or thickness. It may be difficult to tell that whether in fact there is a "line": the area where the echogenicity of the nodule encounters the echogenicity of the surrounding thyroid may be ambiguous, fuzzy,

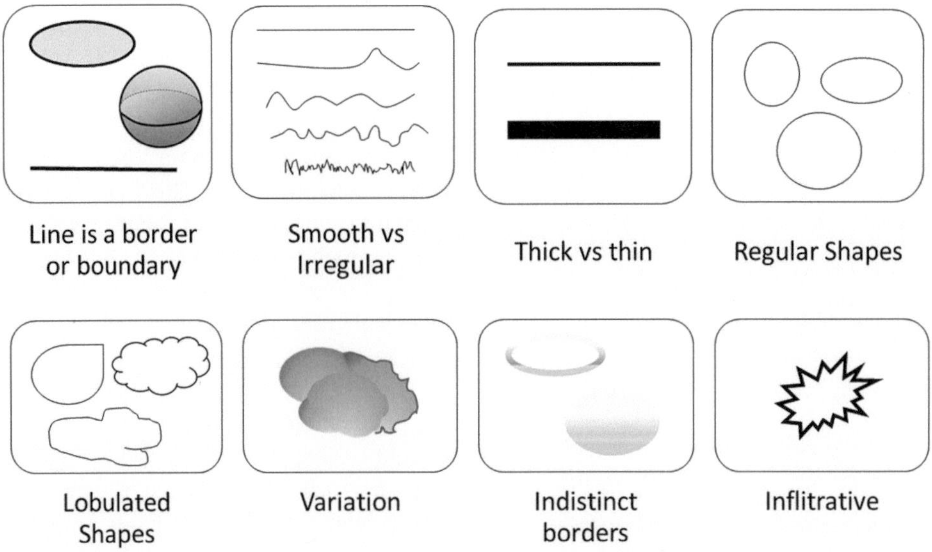

Fig. 11.1 Visual schematic of margin features applicable to thyroid nodules

blurry, vague, indistinct, and unclear. Finally, it may be possible to tell that the line encroaches into territory where biologically and anatomically it should not go, disturbing and interfering with spatial planes.

It is relevant at this point to clarify an important concept that particularly strikes novice sonographers and trainees in residency and fellowship when first realized and that sometimes escapes appreciation by physicians even with advanced experience. Namely, the distinction between follicular adenomas and follicular carcinomas exists at the level of the nodule margin (Fig. 11.2a, b), *not at the level of the thyroid gland capsular margin*. Capsular invasion of follicular carcinomas is histologically detected at the margin that surrounds the nodule; vascular and lymphatic invasion can be present at that same margin and also within the nodule [15]. This is in contrast to extrathyroidal extension: in Fig. 11.2c, d, papillary thyroid cancer (PTC) cells are seen nestled beyond the thyroid border but not beyond the pathological inked margin. Figure 11.2e demonstrates these relationships in an ultrasound image.

In terms of margins, therefore, there are visual (artistic) and linguistic (poetic) challenges of trying to clarify and codify the pathology of thyroid disease as detected by an imaging modality like ultrasound. The figures and videos in this chapter are all ultrasound cine clips to emphasize the point that margins are spatially continuous and that a single, still image cannot represent the entire contour of the nodule.

11.2.1 Completely Smooth and Well-Defined Margins

Thyroid cysts represent the classical version of a margin that is completely smooth. The interface between the liquid composition of the cyst provides stark contrast to the solid thyroid parenchyma, and thus the ultrasound wave physics translate that contrast into a hyperechoic thin line as the border (Fig. 11.3). The terms well-defined and well-circumscribed are likewise interchangeably used. The connotation of these terms is that it is visually clear to see the margin and to appreciate that there is a distinct structure (nodule) embedded within surrounding thyroid parenchyma. The contour of the structure can be readily traced on the ultrasound monitor. Representative images and cine clips of both cystic and solid nodules with smooth margins are shown in Video 11.1a–e.

11.2.2 Lobulated Margins

This describes the geometric path of the margin, resulting in forms that make the nodule appear to have curved or wavy additional segments. The actual line of the margin can vary in thickness and smoothness and even display infiltrative characteristics. Insufficient data have been reported to know the independent risk of malignancy when a lobulated margin is observed in the presence or absence of other features. Representative surgical images (Fig. 11.4) (medullary thyroid carcinoma) and cine clips of nodules with lobulated margins are shown in Video 11.2a–e.

11.2.3 Irregular Margins

The appearance of anything but a smooth border raises the concern for *potential* malignancy. The assessment that a margin is irregular implies that an actual border can be detected (in contrast to an indistinct border). There are varying manifestations of irregular margins. Some can appear smooth for the majority of the circumference or contour but have an area where the line is jagged; other nodules have a jagged margin at all points. Careful assessment of the entire margin of the nodule is therefore necessary as illustrated in Video 11.3. The majority of the nodule has a well-defined margin, but the inferior aspect is irregular and jagged. In the ATA classification, the presence of an irregular and jagged margin sorts the nodule into a high risk of malignancy category and in TIRADS, at least into category 4 [10, 12–15].

The relationship between echogenicity of the nodule and degree of irregularity of its margins is

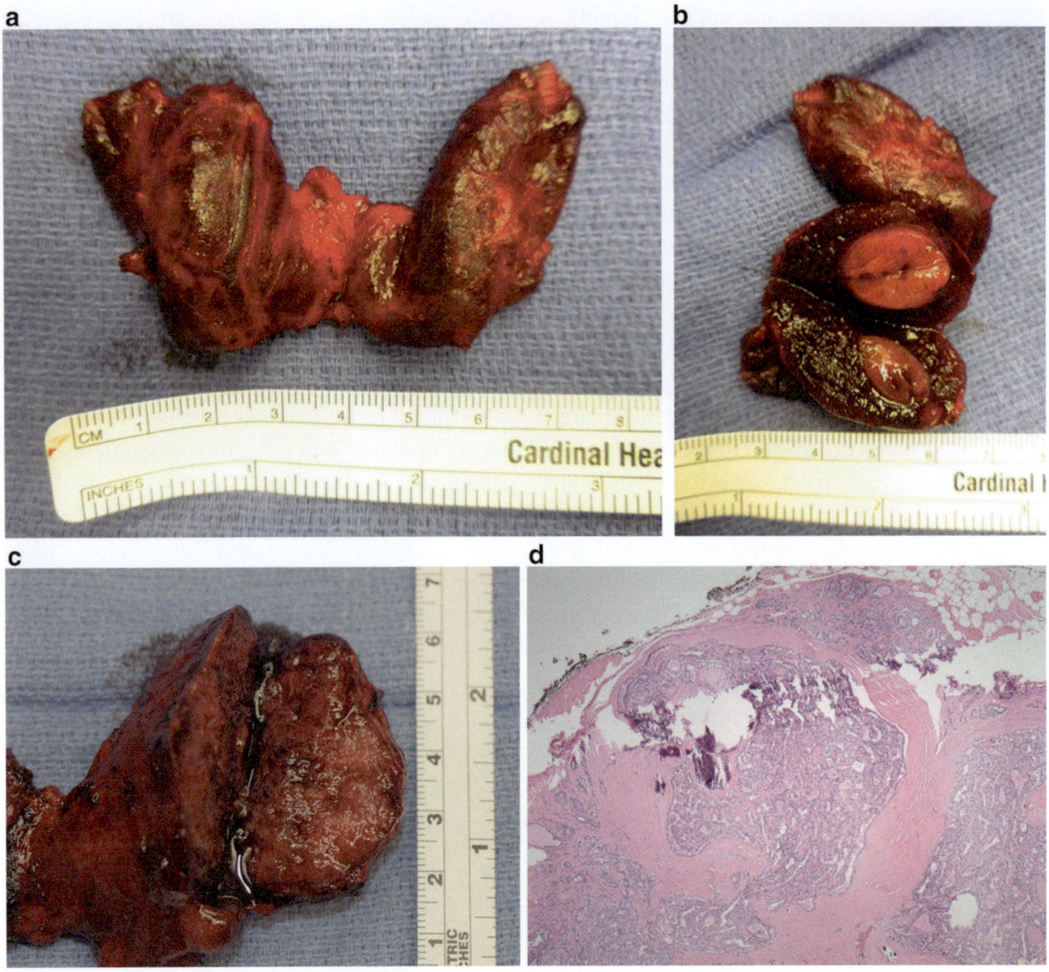

Fig. 11.2 Surgical total thyroidectomy specimen seen intact (**a**) and sectioned (**b**) to reveal a benign follicular adenoma (tan oval) surrounded by reddish normal thyroid parenchyma. It is this interface between the edge of the adenoma and the thyroid that represents the margin visible by ultrasound and also the border at which vascular or capsular invasion would indicate a follicular carcinoma. In contrast, a large papillary thyroid cancer is shown within the left thyroid lobe (**c**) to have an irregular periphery that extends up the surface of the thyroid gland, leaving no intervening normal thyroid tissue. Microscopic view (**d**) shows that the papillary thyroid cancer extends outside the thyroid capsule into the perithyroidal fat (white foamy material in *top right corner*) and up to the histologic margin (the think *black inked line* visible along the *top* of tissue). Thus, there are different applications of the term "margin" in relation to nodules and thyroid specimen. (**e**) Margins of nodules versus pathologic margins of surgical specimens. *Yellow dotted lines* are size caliper markings of a small thyroid nodule. The *blue line* circling the nodule indicates the margin that is relevant for the pathologist in distinguishing follicular adenomas from follicular carcinomas. The *arrows* outline the capsule of the thyroid gland, which serves as the pathologic margin of a routine thyroidectomy specimen. Shown are two ultrasound views (E1) and a surgical specimen view (E2)

not fully understood by most experts, mainly due to lack of data, so as to allow clear classification into an ATA or TIRADS category [10, 12–15]. This combination has not been formally assigned to a risk of malignancy pattern or classification. While hyperechogenicity mostly favors a benign nodule, and irregular borders are generally exceptionally rare with benign nodules, the combination of these features has unknown diagnostic associations.

e1

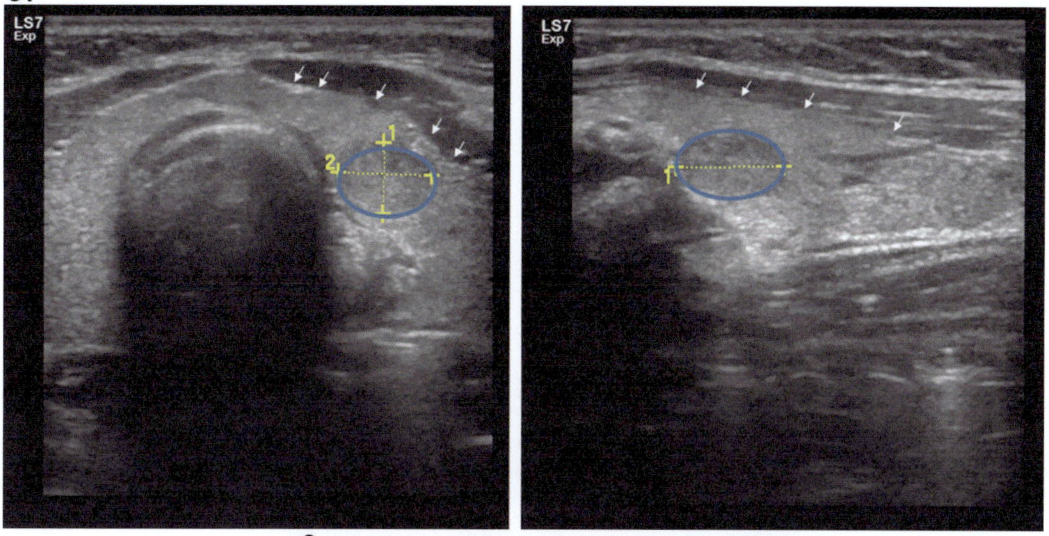

e2

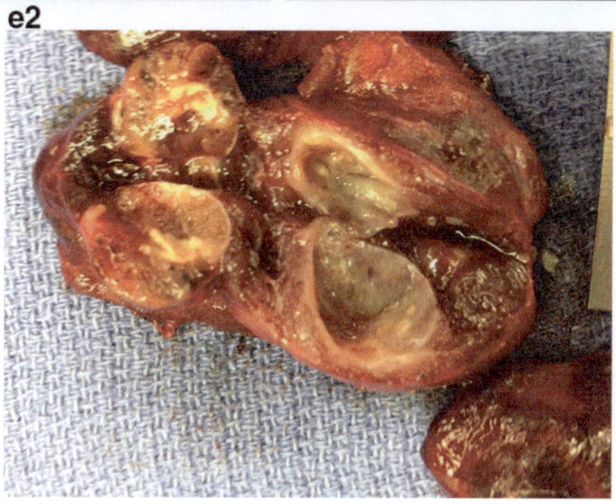

Fig. 11.2 (continued)

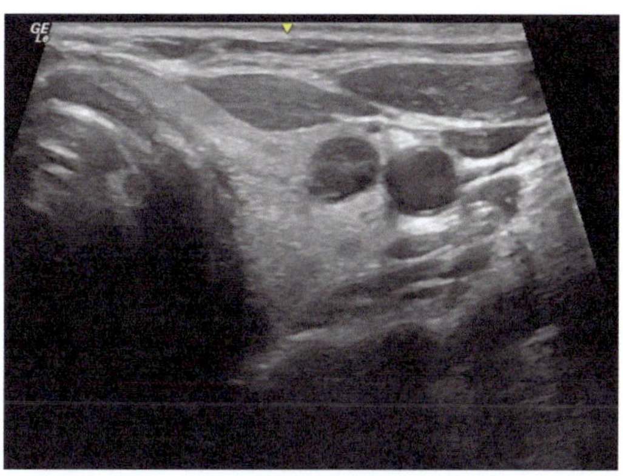

Fig. 11.3 Example of a cystic nodule in the left lobe adjacent to the common carotid artery that has a smooth cyst wall

Representative cine clips of a variety of irregular margins are shown in Videos 11.2e and 11.4a–f and Fig. 11.5.

11.2.4 Indistinct or Poorly Defined Margins

The pathologic correlation to this feature is related to the invasive nature of malignant cells which gradually encroach into normal surrounding tissues. Because cancers can have a desmoplastic, fibrotic texture which is unevenly distributed along those lines of invasion, the interface with normal thyroid parenchyma can

a b

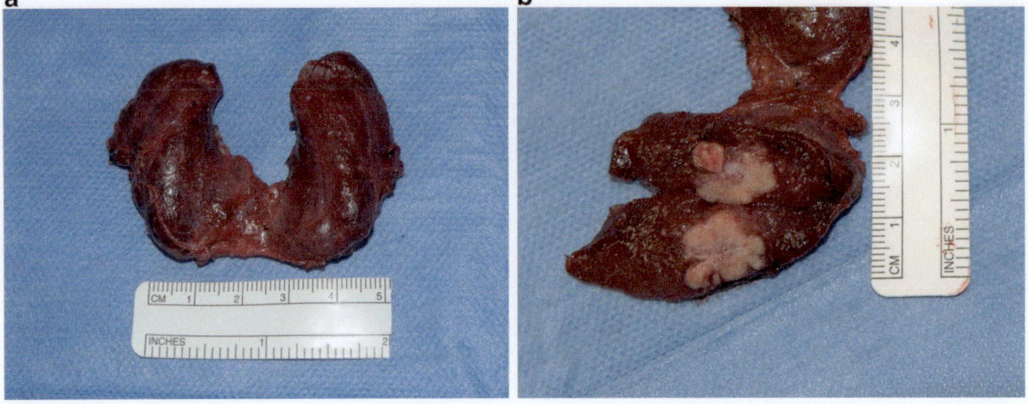

Fig. 11.4 Lobulated margins in medullary thyroid carcinoma (**a**—intact pathological specimen, **b**—sectioned lobe)

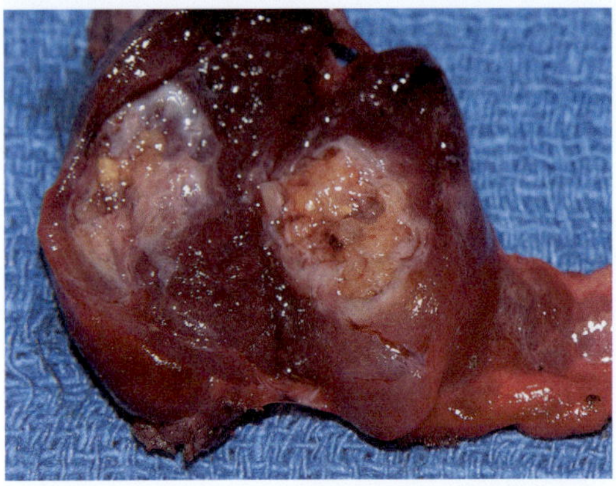

Fig. 11.5 Surgical specimen of nodule (known papillary thyroid cancer) with irregular margins (see also Video 11.4a–f)

appear blurred. Representative images and cine clips of a variety of these clinical scenarios are shown in Video 11.5a–g. However, since hyperplastic nodules represent a local disruption of the follicular architecture of the thyroid, it is common for these begin nodules to also have a poorly defined margin along a portion of the nodule (Video 11.5f). The typical spongiform appearance of these nodules and the absence of other sonographic features of malignancy, such as all solid consistency and calcifications, help to distinguish these nodules from malignancy.

11.2.5 Infiltrative Margins

This type of margin is the sonographic demonstration of a malignant process in the vast majority of cases. The border of a nodule is clearly seen to involve areas of normal thyroid parenchyma in a way that is not an architectural distortion but invasion along unnatural anatomical directions. In contrast, a benign process, even a large benign nodule, may displace normal anatomical shapes or efface the overlying tissue, but the two structures remain distinct or, in surgical terms, respect anatomical boundaries.

Representative images and cine clips of a variety of these clinical scenarios, all cytologically or histologically confirmed malignancies, are shown in Video 11.6a–c. Thyroiditis, especially subacute thyroiditis, may have infiltrative margins, as the inflammatory process extends unevenly throughout the gland and, if nodular and focal, may mimic a malignancy.

11.2.6 Halo

As its name implies, this term describes the specific appearance of the entire circumference of the border between a nodule and the surrounding thyroid parenchyma. Namely, the ultrasound detects a sonolucent (anechoic, black) rim that is distinct and that surrounds an isoechoic or hyperechoic nodule [1–5]. By definition, it would be difficult to detect this sonolucent rim around a hypoechoic nodule. Physically and pathologically, it represents a capsule of thick fibrous, collagenous material that is often rich with vasculature. Variations of these features abound as well in terms of halo thickness, degree of irregularity, intensity of vascularity on color Doppler imaging, and continuity around a nodule. There is some evidence-based information to suggest lower risk of malignancy with thin and regular halos and higher risk of malignancy with thick and irregular halos and that variably thick halos are more likely to be associated with follicular variants of papillary thyroid carcinoma [1–5, 10, 16].

Representative images and cine clips of a variety of these clinical scenarios are shown in Video 11.7a–e.

11.2.7 Artifacts and Challenging Scenarios of Contour Evaluation

It is not always possible to evaluate the margins of a nodule because of sonographic artifacts, edge artifacts, and other limitations that are beyond the control of the sonographer. One example is the presence of a calcified margin. While calcifications in general were addressed in an earlier chapter, case illustrations in this chapter show the posterior acoustic shadowing that results from eggshell calcifications and prevents imaging of the remainder of the nodule margin (Videos 11.2c, 11.7, and 11.8c–e).

11.3 Extrathyroidal Extension

Extrathyroidal extension (ETE) of thyroid malignancy ranges from microscopic to grossly invasive. In contrast to the margin features above that describe the interface between a nodule and the surrounding thyroid gland, extrathyroidal extension is suspected when a malignant thyroid nodule can be seen to have grown through the thyroid capsule and beyond the thyroid gland [17]. A sonographic assessment to determine the possible presence of extrathyroidal extension should be performed by carefully assessing the integrity of the thyroid capsule overlying the nodule.

11.3.1 Absence of Extrathyroidal Extension

Representative images and cine clips of nodules, varying in proximity to the external capsule of the thyroid gland, are shown to illustrate the clinical scenarios where extrathyroidal extension is *absent* (Videos 11.5g, 11.6b, and 11.8a).

11.3.2 Suspected Extrathyroidal Extension

Representative images and cine clips of nodules with suspected extrathyroidal extension are shown to illustrate different clinical scenarios in relationship to overlying strap muscles and the deep posterior edge of the thyroid gland in the paratracheal space (Video 11.8b–g). When the edge of the nodule is irregular and located at the deepest posterior border of the thyroid gland so that a normal rim of the thyroid tissue is not seen on ultrasound, concern exists about possible tumor proximity to the path of the recurrent laryngeal nerve (Fig. 11.6). It is important to note any voice changes on history and physical exam and perform laryngeal ultrasound or direct laryngoscopy as appropriate.

11.4 Extrathyroidal Invasion

This feature is the most severe version of extrathyroidal extension and may be suspected on the basis of clinical signs (hoarseness, fixed and immobile mass, abnormal cervical lymphadenopathy) even prior to acquiring ultrasound images. It is really only possible to characterize this feature as absent or present and then to note whether the invasive features are suspected or definitely seen on ultrasound. The most significant clue is loss of normal architectural shapes (e.g., with tracheal rings, strap muscle, and their hyperechoic fascial lining). Noticing such changes, even if subtle, may change clinical action preoperatively (e.g., to obtain additional cross-sectional imaging such as with a CT scan when this might not otherwise have been done)

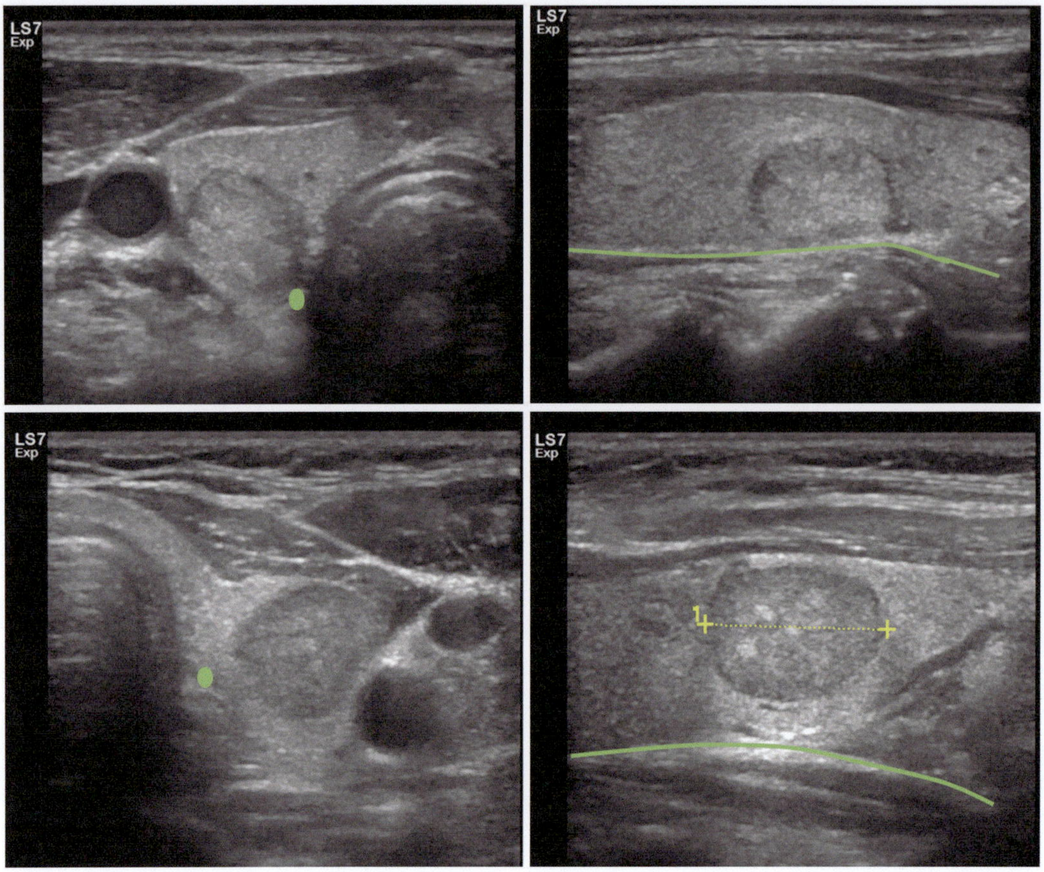

Fig. 11.6 Anatomical pathway of the recurrent laryngeal nerve (green) in relation the thyroid. The top panel shows a thyroid nodule in the right lobe in transverse and longitudinal views, with a closer proximity than the nodule in the left lobe (bottom panels)

and intraoperatively. It allows both the physicians and the patient to prepare for possible greater extent of disease and minimize surprises, allowing for a more thoughtful assessment of risks and benefits of treatment. Representative cine clips are shown in Video 11.9a, b and correlated with the surgical specimen. In this case, the findings are not subtle. The curved, bright hyperechoic arc of the tracheal rings is distorted by a thyroid mass that spans across the isthmus. Anteriorly, the strap muscled likewise are almost indistinguishable. These ultrasound findings predicted the severity of thyroid cancer, as seen in the surgical specimen; the ultrasound information allowed the operative plan to address the disease comprehensively at the time of the initial surgery, in this case to include tracheal resection (Fig. 11.7).

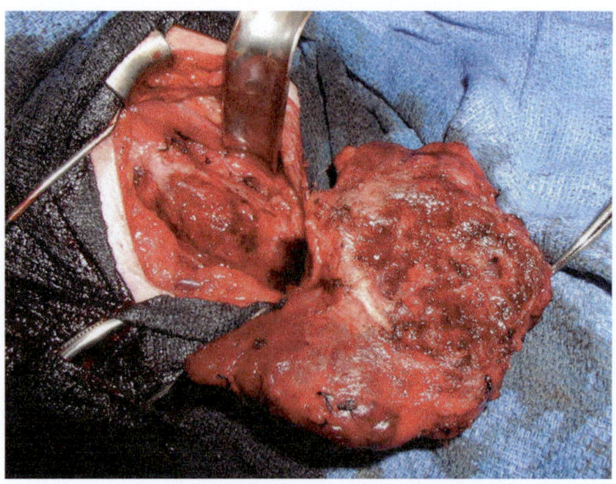

Fig. 11.7 Surgical specimen of this papillary thyroid cancer, showing the protrusion of tumor through the posterior surface of the isthmus. There is residual cancer on the anterior surface of the trachea that extended transmurally into the lumen. Involved rings of the trachea were resected and the trachea reconnected

11.5 Conclusions

Margins are an essential feature to describe about thyroid nodules and these details should be included routinely in ultrasound reports. A spectrum of characteristics are detectable and inform about potential risks of malignancy.

References

1. American Institute of Ultrasound in Medicine; American College of Radiology; Society for Pediatric Radiology; Society of Radiologists in Ultrasound. AIUM practice guideline for the performance of a thyroid and parathyroid ultrasound examination. J Ultrasound Med. 2013;32:1319–29.
2. Su HK, Dos Reis LL, Lupo MA, Milas M, Orloff LA, Langer JE, Brett EM, Kazam E, Lee SL, Minkowitz G, Alpert EH, Dewey EH, Urken ML. Striving toward standardization of reporting of ultrasound features of thyroid nodules and lymph nodes: a multidisciplinary consensus statement. Thyroid. 2014;24(9):1341–9.
3. Xie C, Cox P, Taylor N, LaPorte S. Ultrasonography of thyroid nodules: a pictorial review. Insights Imaging. 2016;7(1):77–86.
4. Ginat DT, Butani D, Giampoli EJ, Patel N, Dogra V. Pearls and pitfalls of thyroid nodule sonography and fine-needle aspiration. Ultrasound Q. 2010;26(3):171–8.
5. Solbiati L, Osti V, Cova L, Tonolini M. Ultrasound of thyroid, parathyroid glands and neck lymph nodes. Eur Radiol. 2001;11:2411–24.
6. Papini E, Guglielmi R, Bianchini A, Crescenzi A, Taccogna S, Nardi F, Panunzi C, Rinaldi R, Toscano V, Pacella CM. Risk of malignancy in nonpalpable thyroid nodules: predictive value of ultrasound and color-Doppler features. J Clin Endocrinol Metab. 2002;87:1941–6.
7. Wienke JR, Chong WK, Fielding JR, Zou KH, Mittelstaedt CA. Sonographic features of benign thyroid nodules interobserver reliability and overlap with malignancy. J Ultrasound Med. 2003;22:1027–31.
8. Schlumberger MJ. Papillary and follicular thyroid carcinoma. N Engl J Med. 1998;338:297–306.
9. Yoon JH, Kim EK, Kwak JY, Moon HJ, Kim GR. Sonographic features and ultrasonography-guided fine-needle aspiration of metastases to the thyroid gland. Ultrasonography. 2014;33(1):40–8.
10. ATA. 2015 Revised American Thyroid Association management guidelines for patients with thyroid nodules and differentiated thyroid cancer: the American Thyroid Association (ATA) Guidelines Taskforce on thyroid nodules and differentiated thyroid cancer. Thyroid. 2016;19:1167–214.
11. Zhang J, Liu BJ, Xu HX, Xu JM, Zhang YF, Liu C, Wu J, Sun LP, Guo LH, Liu LN, Xu XH, Qu S. Prospective validation of an ultrasound-based thyroid imaging reporting and data system (TI-RADS) on 3980 thyroid nodules. Int J Clin Exp Med. 2015;8(4):5911–7.
12. Horvath E, Majlis S, Rossi R, Franco C, Niedmann JP, Castro A, Dominguez M. An ultrasonogram reporting system for thyroid nodules stratifying cancer risk for clinical management. J Clin Endocrinol Metab. 2009;94:1748–51.
13. Park J-Y, Lee HJ, Jang HW, Kim HK, Yi JH, Lee W, Kim SH. A proposal for a thyroid imaging reporting and data system for ultrasound features of thyroid carcinoma. Thyroid. 2009;19:1257–64.
14. Kwak JY, Han KH, Yoon JH, Moon HJ, Son EJ, Park SH, Jung HK, Choi JS, Kim BM, Kim E-K. Thyroid imaging reporting and data system for US features of nodules: a step in establishing better stratification of cancer risk. Radiology. 2011;260:892–9.
15. Zhang JZ, Hu B. Sonographic features of thyroid follicular carcinoma in comparison with thyroid follicular adenoma. J Ultrasound Med. 2014;33(2):221–7.
16. Yoon JH, Kim EK, Hong SW, Kwak JY, Kim MJ. Sonographic features of the follicular variant of papillary thyroid carcinoma. J Ultrasound Med. 2008;27(10):1431–7.
17. Yi YS, Kim SS, Kim WJ, Bae MJ, Kang JH, Choi BG, Jeon YK, Kim BH, Lee BJ, Wang SG, Kim IJ, Kim YK. Comparison of two- and three-dimensional sonography for the prediction of the extrathyroidal extension of papillary thyroid carcinomas. Korean J Intern Med. 2016;31(2):313–22.

12 Feature Illustration: Hyperechoic Foci and Calcifications

Harshawn Malhi and Edward G. Grant

12.1 Introduction

Echogenic foci within thyroid nodules are commonly seen on ultrasound [1, 2]. In the past, many authors had assumed that any echogenic foci in thyroid nodules were calcifications [2]. Large echogenic foci which have posterior shadowing can be confidently diagnosed as calcifications. However, small echogenic foci without shadowing may represent punctate calcifications, which are found in psammoma bodies and are highly associated with papillary thyroid cancer, but may also be seen in non-calcified nodules, representing the back wall of small cystic spaces or inspissated crystals within colloid-containing nodules. Since benign, colloid-containing nodules are the most common type of thyroid nodule, the majority of small echogenic foci are most likely to be present within a benign nodule, rather than a thyroid cancer. Attempting to characterize thyroid nodules by sonographic features is important to help determine if a thyroid nodule is concerning for a malignancy, thus warranting further evaluation with biopsy or is benign appearing and not necessarily requiring a biopsy. Typical malignant features of thyroid nodules on ultrasound include entirely solid consistency, markedly hypoechoic echogenicity, taller-than-wide shape, irregular or infiltrating borders, and calcifications. Calcifications within thyroid malignancies may be large and produce distal acoustic shadowing but may also be small echogenic foci, less than 1 mm, and not associated with shadowing. Benignity is associated with nodules that are purely or predominately cystic or have a spongiform appearance [3–6]. These types of benign nodules often contain abundant colloid and non-shadowing echogenic foci. It is imperative to correctly characterize echogenic foci in nodules as their specific appearance will influence the decision to perform a biopsy. This chapter will describe the different examples of echogenic foci seen in thyroid nodules on ultrasound.

Echogenic foci can be subclassified into five categories:

1. Punctate echogenic foci with no posterior artifact
2. Echogenic foci with small comet-tail artifacts ($\leq$1 mm long)
3. Echogenic foci with large comet-tail artifacts (>1 mm long)
4. Internal echogenic foci with acoustic shadowing
5. Peripheral echogenic foci with acoustic shadowing

H. Malhi, M.D. (✉) • E.G. Grant, M.D. (✉)
Department of Radiology, Keck Hospital of USC, University of Southern California, 1500 San Pablo Street, #2250, Los Angeles, CA 90033, USA
e-mail: harshawn.malhi@usc.edu; edgrant@usc.edu

M. Milas et al. (eds.), *Advanced Thyroid and Parathyroid Ultrasound*,
DOI 10.1007/978-3-319-44100-9_12

12.2 Punctate Foci with No Posterior Artifact

Punctate foci in the thyroid nodule with no posterior artifact are the most common type of echogenic foci [2]. Previously, the literature considered all of these foci to represent microcalcifications (defined as calcifications <1 mm). However, some of these foci are thought to represent a bright echo reflected from the back wall of tiny cystic spaces in colloid-containing nodules [1] (see Fig. 12.1). In fact, an earlier study explored the origins of similar punctate echogenic foci in the ovary and concluded that, indeed, they are often the result of specular reflections from the back walls of tiny unresolved cysts [7]. As mentioned above, some echogenic foci may also represent inspissated crystals in colloid-containing nodules.

The significance in trying to differentiate between actual microcalcifications and back walls of cysts or colloid crystals is that the presence of microcalcifications is one of the most specific features of malignancy. Microcalcifications in malignant thyroid nodules are psammoma bodies, which are 10–100-μm round laminar crystalline calcific deposits (see Fig. 12.2). They are found in 29–59 % of all primary thyroid carcinomas, most

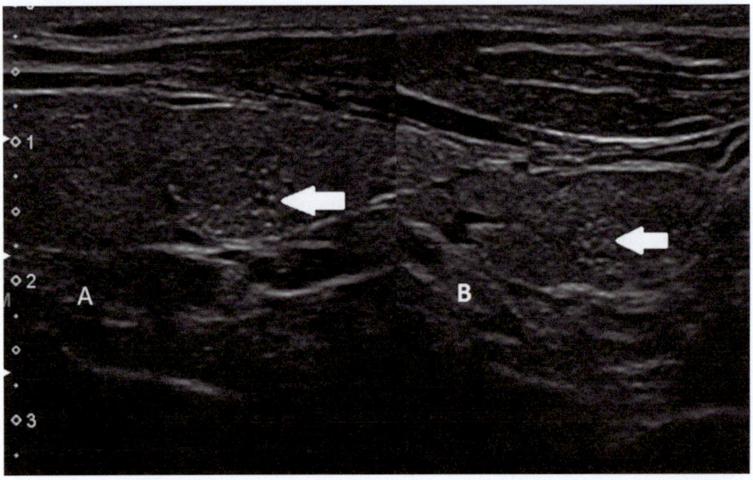

Fig. 12.1 Longitudinal (**a**) and transverse (**b**) ultrasound images of the right thyroid lobe. 56-year-old male with a predominately solid-appearing thyroid nodule measuring approximately 2 cm containing punctate echogenic foci with no posterior acoustic artifact (*arrows*). Biopsy finding was benign colloid nodule (Bethesda II), suggesting that the foci are the back wall of colloid cysts

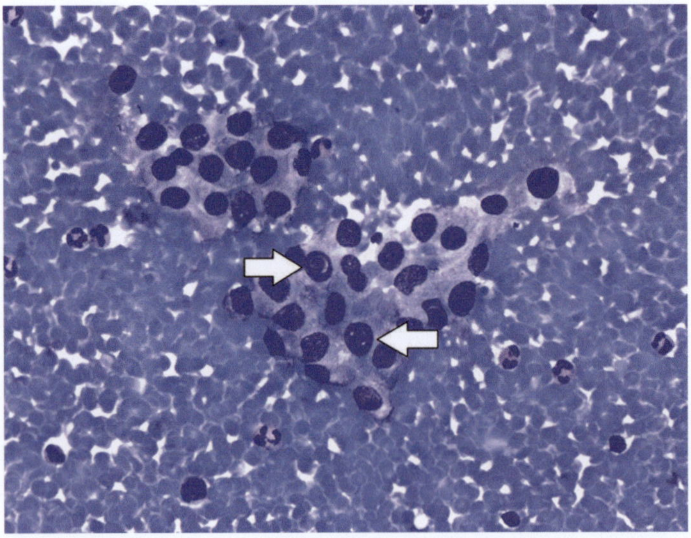

Fig. 12.2 Micrograph of psammoma bodies (*arrows*) in papillary thyroid cancer

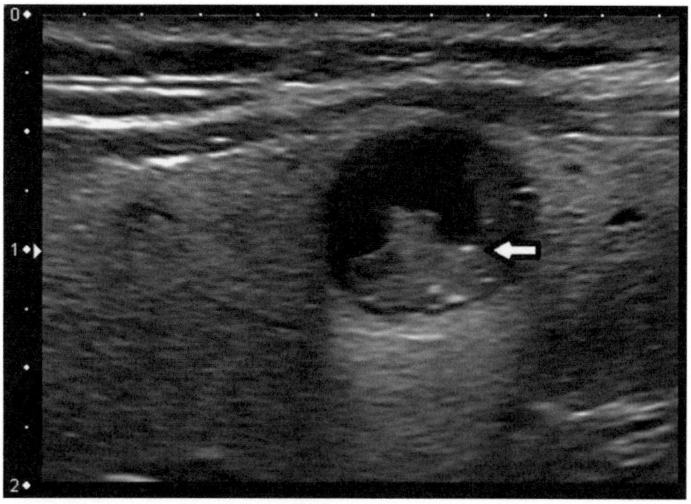

Fig. 12.3 Ultrasound image of a partially cystic/solid 1 cm thyroid nodule containing punctate foci with no posterior acoustic artifact (*arrow*) in a 54-year-old female. Biopsy finding was suspicion of papillary carcinoma (Bethesda V), which was confirmed at subsequent surgery

commonly in the papillary type. The presence of microcalcifications has been noted in follicular and anaplastic thyroid carcinomas as well as in benign conditions such as follicular adenoma and Hashimoto's thyroiditis. On ultrasound, microcalcifications appear as punctate rounded hyperechoic foci without acoustic shadowing [8–10] [see Fig. 12.3] and may be difficult or impossible to differentiate from benign entities mentioned above such as cyst back walls or colloid. Therefore, an analysis of the presence or absence of the other sonographic features associated with malignancy (such as all solid consistency and infiltrating borders) is helpful in the decision to pursue FNA when this type of echogenic foci is noted.

12.3 Echogenic Foci with Small Comet-Tail Artifacts (≤1 mm Long)

A comet-tail artifact is a form of reverberation artifact between two reflective interfaces resulting in closely spaced reflective echoes. The returning sequential echoes may be so close together that individual signals are difficult to perceive, with the later echoes decreasing in amplitude secondary to attenuation. On ultrasound, this is displayed as an artifact with decreased width and signal strength and manifests as a triangular, tapered shape [1, 11, 12] [see Fig. 12.4 and Chap. 5].

Traditionally, all echogenic foci with a comet-tail artifact were thought to be a strong sign of benignity. This is because the artifact was thought to be arising from the inspissated crystals of benign colloid nodules [1, 2, 12]. A recent study however has shown that the rate of malignancy of nodules containing echogenic foci with small (<1 mm) comet-tail artifact was similar to those without acoustic artifact (around 15 %) [2]. This finding suggests that some malignant microcalcifications may also demonstrate small comet-tail artifact. This is supported by the literature that shows several forms of calcifications in a variety of organs and of various sizes demonstrate comet-tail artifact [13]. Why some microcalcifications presumably demonstrate small comet-tail artifacts while others do not is unclear but may in part be related to factors such as ultrasound machine settings (e.g., spatial compounding, frame averaging, speckle reduction), transducer frequency, scanning operator variability, and other technical factors. Again, based on these findings, the additional parenchymal characteristics of the nodule need to be closely evaluated in helping to determine if biopsy of the nodule is warranted.

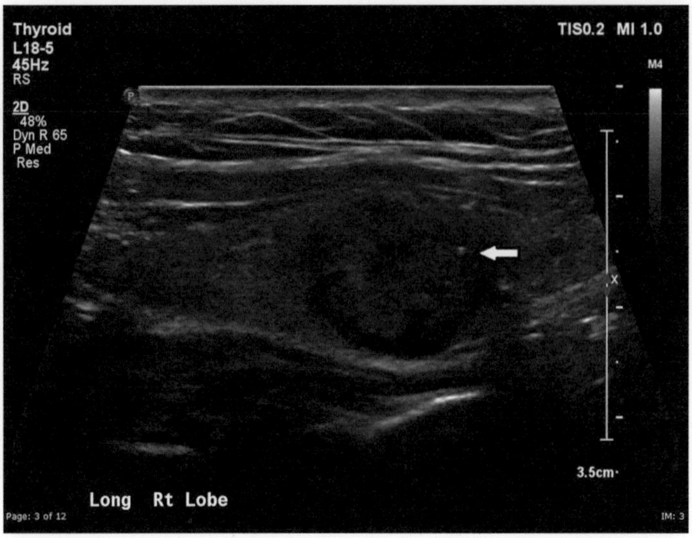

Fig. 12.4 Ultrasound image of an irregular margined, predominately solid, and hypoechoic 1.8-cm right thyroid lobe nodule in a 48-year-old female. Echogenic foci with small (<1 mm) comet-tail artifact are present (*arrow*). Biopsy finding was suspicious of papillary carcinoma (Bethesda V), which was confirmed at subsequent surgery

12.4 Echogenic Foci with Large Comet-Tail Artifact (>1 mm)

A recent study demonstrated a very low rate of malignancy (3.9 %) in nodules possessing echogenic foci with large (>1 mm) comet-tail artifact as compared to other echogenic foci. This suggests that these artifacts are most likely secondary to those seen with inspissated colloid crystals in benign colloid nodules. An older study described the comet-tail artifact as a benign feature in avascular cystic nodules likely related to colloid and determined four patterns of the artifact in colloid cysts. In their series, nodules with one of these features showed 100 % sensitivity and specificity for benignity [12]. Thus, a thyroid nodule containing echogenic foci with large comet-tail artifacts in a primarily cystic nodule suggests benignity and may preclude the need for biopsy [2] [see Fig. 12.5].

12.5 Internal Echogenic Foci with Posterior Acoustic Shadowing

Echogenic foci associated with posterior acoustic shadowing are true thyroid calcifications. In order to cause the shadowing, the calcification is typically larger than 1 mm in size and often much larger and can be quite variable in shape [see Fig. 12.6]. Pathologically they represent fragmented plates, spicules, or granular deposits of calcium within fibrous septa in the thyroid gland parenchyma and/or nodules. In the literature, these foci are commonly referred to as "macro-" or "coarse" calcifications and are thought to be dystrophic calcifications secondary to tissue necrosis. The ACR committee on thyroid ultrasound in their recent publication of a Thyroid Imaging Reporting and Data System (TIRADS) chose the term macrocalcification for this type of echogenic focus [14, 15]. They can be seen in multinodular goiter but also in solitary thyroid nodules. Approximately 15 % of nodules with these calcifications harbor malignancy. Of note, these are the most common type of echogenic foci in medullary type of thyroid cancer [2, 3, 8, 10].

12.6 Peripheral Echogenic Foci with Posterior Acoustic Shadowing

These echogenic foci also are true calcifications and are curvilinear in shape, occurring along the periphery of nodules and are associated with posterior shadowing [see Fig. 12.7a, b]. In the literature, these peripheral calcifications are fre-

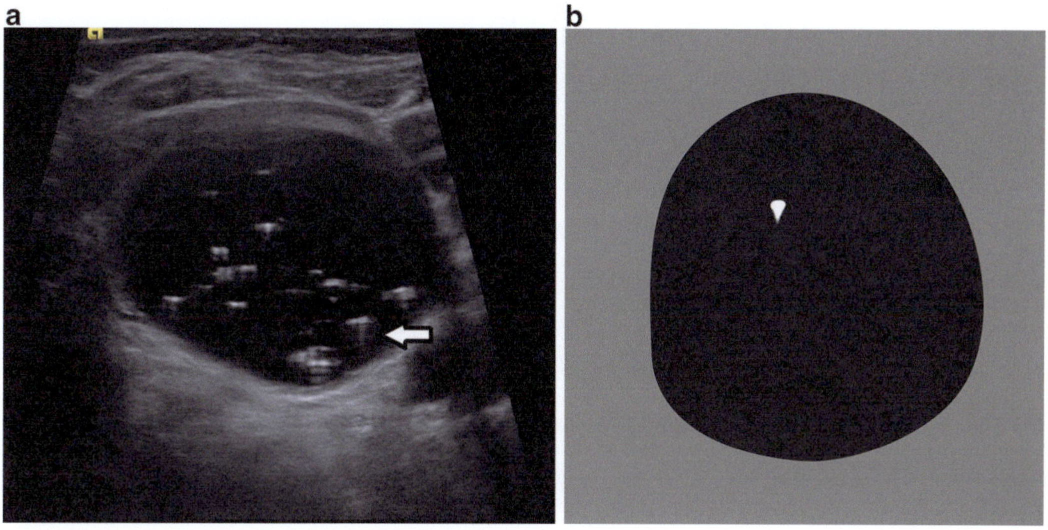

Fig. 12.5 (**a**) Ultrasound image of the left thyroid lobe in a 61-year-old woman shows a cystic 2.6-cm nodule containing several echogenic foci with large (>1 mm) posterior comet-tail artifacts (*arrow*). Biopsy finding was benign colloid nodule (Bethesda II). (**b**) Schematic representation of the *inverted triangle* associated with large comet-tail artifact (Image courtesy of Matthew Skalski, medical illustrator, University of Southern California)

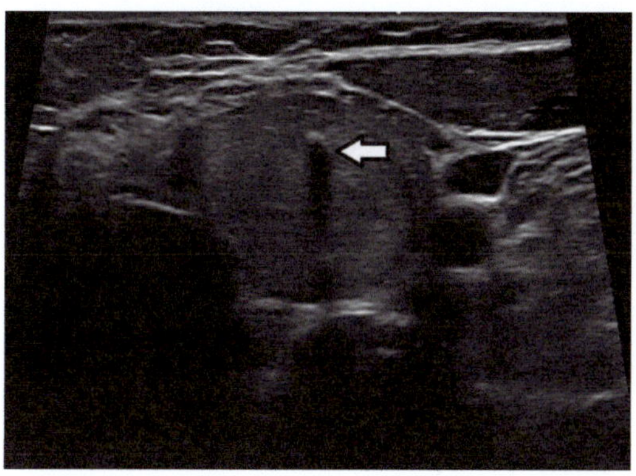

Fig. 12.6 Ultrasound image of a left 2.8-cm solid hyperechoic thyroid nodule in a 59-year-old female. Central shadowing clumped parenchymal calcification is noted (*arrow*). Biopsy finding was benign colloid nodule with Hurthle cell changes (Bethesda II)

quently referred to as "rim" calcifications or "eggshell" calcifications when smooth and regular and extend around the entire nodule. Frequently, the extent of posterior shadowing precludes further evaluation of the internal parenchymal features of the nodule. In fact, in some instances, attempting a biopsy of these nodules is nearly impossible if the periphery is completely circumscribed by calcification. As seen with large internal macrocalcifications, the presence of these foci is associated with an increased risk of malignancy, as compared to nodules without echogenic foci [2]. Nodules that have peripheral calcifications that are irregular in thickness or an interrupted peripheral calcification with soft tissue extending through the rim are highly likely to be malignant [16] [Figs. 12.8 and 12.9].

12.7 Nodules Possessing More than One Type of Echogenic Foci

Nodules frequently contain more than one type of echogenic foci. In a recently published paper, almost half of nodules with echogenic foci contained more than one subtype. After nodules with large comet-tail artifacts were excluded, the chance that malignancy was present increased by a factor of 1.48 for every additional type of focus seen. This suggests that nodules with more than one type of high-risk focus have a greater chance of harboring malignancy and, as such, should be approached more aggressively in regard to performing a biopsy [2, 8, 10] [see Fig. 12.10].

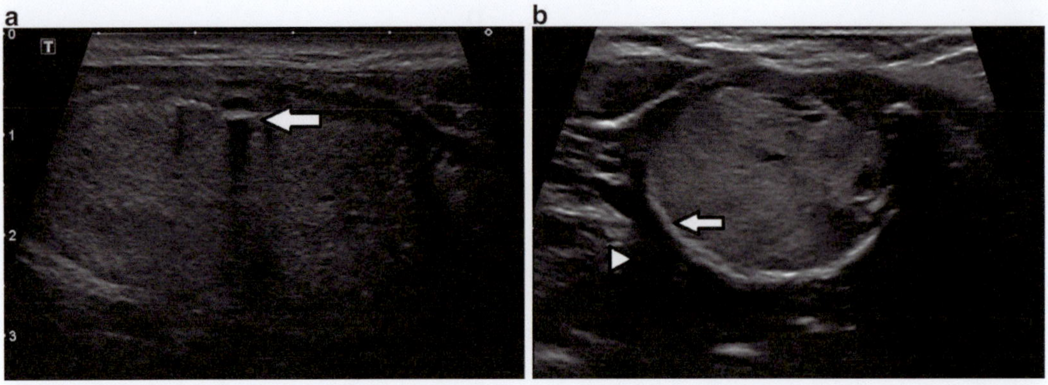

Fig. 12.7 (**a**) Longitudinal ultrasound image of the left thyroid lobe in a 71-year-old female shows a 4-cm predominately solid nodule. Peripheral calcifications with posterior shadowing (*arrow*) are present. Biopsy finding was benign colloid nodule (Bethesda II). (**b**) Ultrasound image of a predominately solid right thyroid lobe nodule in a 48-year-old female. "Eggshell" rim calcifications (*arrow*) are present with posterior shadowing (*arrowhead*). Patient deferred biopsy

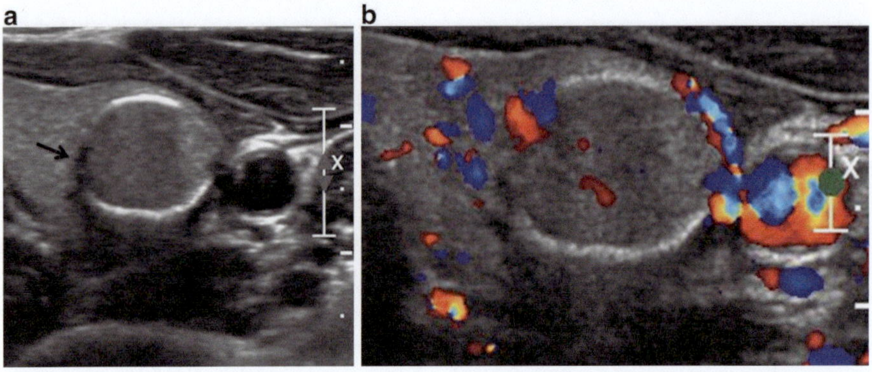

Fig. 12.8 Ultrasound images of the left lobe in a 52-year-old woman show a nodule with thin rim or eggshell calcinations that is interrupted along the lateral aspect (*arrow*). (**b**) Color Doppler showed internal vascularity consistent with a solid consistency. Biopsy finding was follicular variant of papillary thyroid carcinoma

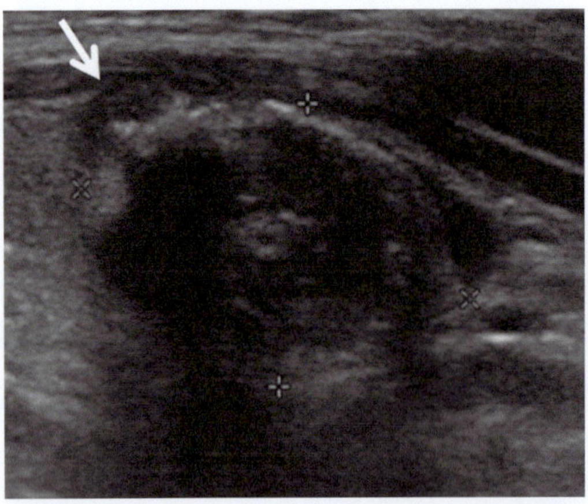

Fig. 12.9 Longitudinal ultrasound image of the left thyroid lobe in a 43-year-old woman shows a nodule (*outlined* by *calipers*) with peripheral calcifications that are irregular in thickness and interrupted by soft tissue extending through the calcifications (*arrows*). Biopsy finding was papillary thyroid carcinoma

12.7.1 Pitfalls

Punctate echogenic foci, usually over 1 mm in size and without distal acoustic shadowing, have been observed to develop following FNA in benign cystic nodules that lacked these features prior to biopsy, most commonly in nodules that dramatically had decreased in size on follow-up imaging (Reference [17]/Koo). Similar echogenic foci have also been observed in nodules that undergo spontaneous involution (Reference [18]/Kim). Although larger than 1 mm, these echogenic foci may be misinterpreted to be microcalcifications if earlier images of the nodule are not available to appreciate the natural history of the benign-appearing nodule's involution [Fig. 12.11]. This

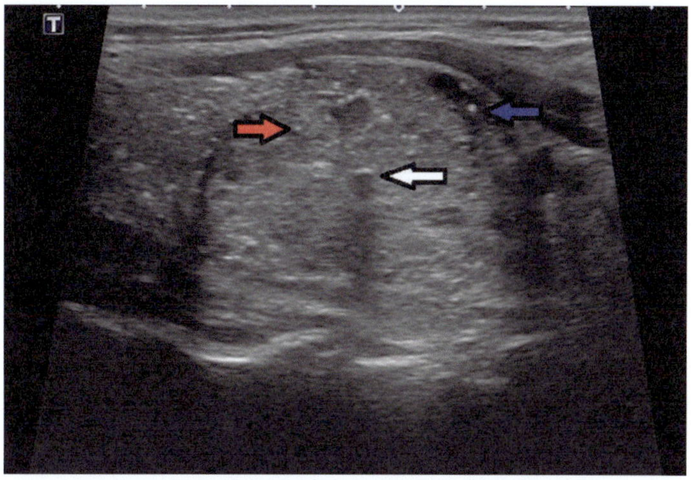

Fig. 12.10 Ultrasound image of a solid left thyroid lobe nodule measuring 4 cm in this 31-year-old male. Combination of echogenic foci is present including punctate foci with no posterior artifact (*red arrow*), foci with small comet-tail artifact (*blue arrow*), and course central calcifications with posterior shadowing (*white arrow*). Biopsy finding was papillary carcinoma (Bethesda VI), which was confirmed at subsequent surgery

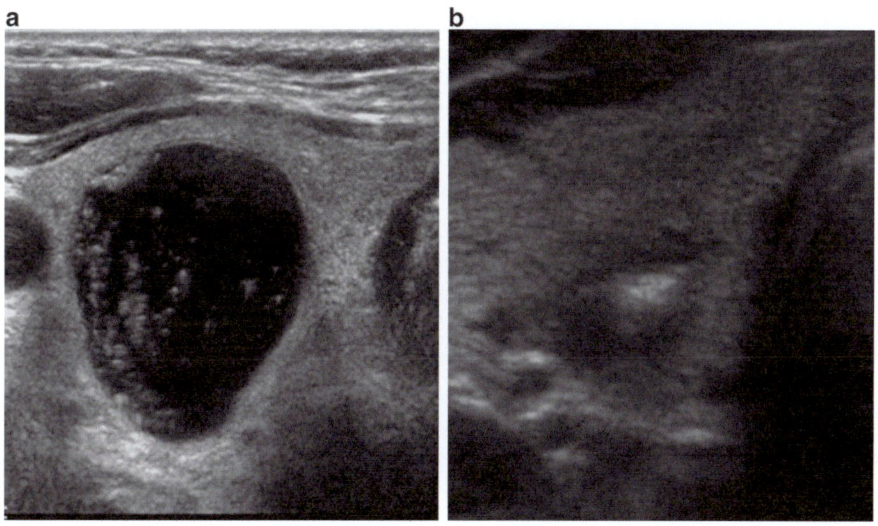

Fig. 12.11 (**a**) Ultrasound image of a predominately cystic, colloid-containing right thyroid lobe nodule in a 61-year-old female. (**b**) Follow-up imaging 5 months later shows interval spontaneous involution of the nodule. The colloid material has now coalesced centrally and acoustic shadowing is evident posterior to the nodule. The irregular margins of the collapsed cystic nodule and the central echogenic focus are both mimics of papillary thyroid carcinoma

misinterpretation is also compounded by the tendency of the involuting nodule to have an irregular shape and to have distal acoustic shadowing caused by the uneven edges of the nodule surface, which can also be interpreted as suspicious features. The authors speculated that the echogenic foci were the result of cellular debris, cholesterol and keratin, and potentially aggregated colloid crystals which clumped together as the fluid component of the nodule diminished.

12.8 Conclusion

The presence of echogenic foci within thyroid nodules is important in that their specific imaging characteristics can help determine if the nodule is benign versus malignant. It is important to note that not all punctate foci without posterior artifact will be psammomatous (malignant) microcalcifications and that some may represent the back wall of a cyst or inspissated crystals seen in benign colloid nodules. Nodules with small comet-tail artifacts are indeterminate and should be evaluated with caution. Nodules with large comet-tail artifacts, especially those in the setting of a cystic nodule, are almost always invariably benign. Biopsy can clearly be avoided in most of these lesions, unless there are other compelling features present. Evaluation of nodules with foci demonstrating posterior acoustic shadowing is more straightforward in that these do represent true thyroid macrocalcifications. These do have an increased association with malignancy but not to the extent seen with microcalcifications. While important, none of these echogenic foci should be evaluated in isolation; rather, the additional parenchymal features of the nodule (i.e., solid vs benign, irregular vs smooth walled, etc.) should also be taken into consideration when determining if further nodule evaluation with biopsy is warranted.

References

1. Beland MD, Kwon L, Delellis RA, Cronan JJ, Grant E. Nonshadowing echogenic foci in thyroid nodules: are certain appearances enough to avoid thyroid biopsy? J Ultrasound Med. 2011;30:753–60.
2. Malhi H, Beland MD, Cen SY, et al. Echogenic foci in thyroid nodules: significance of posterior acoustic artifacts. AJR Am J Roentgenol. 2014;203(6): 1310–6.
3. Frates MC, Benson CB, Charboneau JW, et al. Management of thyroid nodules detected at US: Society of Radiologists in Ultrasound consensus conference statement. Radiology. 2005;237:794–800.
4. Gharib H, Papini E, Paschke R, et al. American Association of Clinical Endocrinologists, Associazione Medici Endocrinologi, and European Thyroid Association medical guidelines for clinical practice for the diagnosis and management of thyroid nodules. Endocr Pract. 2010;16:468–75.
5. Kim EK, Park CS, Chung WY, et al. New sonographic criteria for recommending fine-needle aspiration biopsy of nonpalpable solid nodules of the thyroid. AJR. 2002;178:687–91.
6. Bonavita JA, Mayo J, Babb J. Pattern recognition of benign nodules at ultrasound of the thyroid: which nodules can be left alone? AJR Am J Roentgenol. 2009;193:207–13.
7. Muradali D, Colgan T, Hayeems E, Burns PN, Wilson SR. Echogenic ovarian foci without shadowing: are they caused by psammomatous calcifications? Radiology. 2002;224:429–35.
8. Hoang JK, Lee WK, Lee M, Johnson D, Farrell S. US features of thyroid malignancy: pearls and pitfalls. RadioGraphics. 2007;27:847–60.
9. Moon WJ, Jung SL, Lee JH, et al. Benign and malignant thyroid nodules: US differentiation—multicenter retrospective study. Radiology. 2008;247:762–70.
10. Nachiappan AC, Metwalli ZA, Hailey BS, Patel RA, Ostrowski ML, Wynne DM. The thyroid: review of imaging features and biopsy techniques with radiologic-pathologic correlation. Radiographics. 2014;34(2):276–93.
11. Feldman MK, Katyal S, Blackwood MS. US artifacts. Radiographics. 2009;29(4):1179–89.
12. Ahuja A, Chick W, King W, Metreweli C. Clinical significance of the comet-tail artifact in thyroid ultrasound. J Clin Ultrasound. 1996;24:129–33.
13. Tchelepi H, Ralls PW. Color comet-tail artifact: clinical applications. AJR. 2009;192(1):11–8.
14. Kwak JY, Han KH, Yoon JH, et al. Thyroid imaging reporting and data system for US features of nodules: a step in establishing better stratification of cancer risk. Radiology. 2011;260(3):892–9.
15. Grant EG, Tessler FN, Hoang JK, et al. Thyroid ultrasound reporting lexicon: white paper of the ACR Thyroid Imaging, Reporting and Data System (TIRADS) Committee. J Am Coll Radiol. 2015;12:1272.
16. Park YJ, Kim JA, Son EJ, Youk JH, Kim EK, Kwak JY, Park CS. Thyroid nodules with macrocalcification: sonographic findings predictive of malignancy. Yonsei Med J. 2014;55:339–44.
17. Koo JH, Shin JH, Han B, Ko EY, Kang SS. Cystic thyroid nodules after aspiration mimicking malignancy. Sonographic characteristics. J Ultrasound Med. 2010;29:1415–21.
18. Kim SS, Kim MR, Mok JY, et al. Benign cystic nodules may have ultrasonographic features mimicking papillary thyroid carcinoma during interval changes. Endocr J. 2011;58:633–8.

13 Feature Illustration: Vascularity

William D. Middleton

13.1 Nodular Lesions

There are certain situations where color Doppler clearly assists in the evaluation of thyroid nodules. The use of color Doppler may aid in distinguishing a predominantly cystic nodule from a vascular structure within or adjacent to the thyroid gland. In the setting of an isoechoic, solid nodule, the detection of peripheral vascularity can be helpful in confirming that a nodule is really present (Fig. 13.1). It can also help in defining the extent of the nodule and thus in accurately measuring the nodule. Color Doppler can also be useful in the assessment of complex cystic nodules that have internal regions of increased echogenicity. It is useful both for diagnosis and for targeting a biopsy to determine if the echogenic portion of a mixed cystic and solid nodule merely represents internal debris or hemorrhage or represents a true solid component. If the solid-appearing component has no detectable blood flow, it is often clotted blood, which can usually be confirmed by noting mobility while scanning the patient in an upright or decubitus position (Figs. 13.2 and 13.3). To improve the diagnostic yield, FNA of avascular components should be avoided in lieu of solid components with detectable vascularity.

The value of color Doppler in distinguishing benign and malignant nodules is much less certain. Many investigators have analyzed the degree and pattern of vascularity in thyroid nodules. Most have shown that intranodular vascularity is statistically more likely to be detected in malignant nodules (Fig. 13.4) than in benign nodules (Fig. 13.5). Unfortunately, they have also shown that malignant nodules have a range of vascular patterns as well as a range of degrees of vascularity (Fig. 13.6). In addition, benign nodules have been shown to have a broad range of vascular patterns and degrees, including hypervascular internal flow (Fig. 13.7). The amount of overlap in the vascularity of benign and malignant nodules substantially limits the value of vascularity in the differentiation of these nodules.

Table 13.1 summarizes the results of a number of studies that had histologic proof and specifically determined the statistics of nodule vascularity independent of gray-scale findings [1–12]. Most have divided flow patterns into peripheral and intranodular. The definition of flow that increases the risk of malignancy varies but included (1) any detectable peripheral or intranodular flow, (2) any detectable intranodular flow, (3) isolated or predominant intranodular flow, and (4) marked intranodular flow. Using these different criteria, the sensitivity, specificity, positive

W.D. Middleton, M.D. (✉)
Mallinckrodt Institute of Radiology, Washington University School of Medicine,
510 South Kingshighway Blvd., Saint Louis, MO 63110, USA
e-mail: middletonb@wustl.edu

M. Milas et al. (eds.), *Advanced Thyroid and Parathyroid Ultrasound*,
DOI 10.1007/978-3-319-44100-9_13

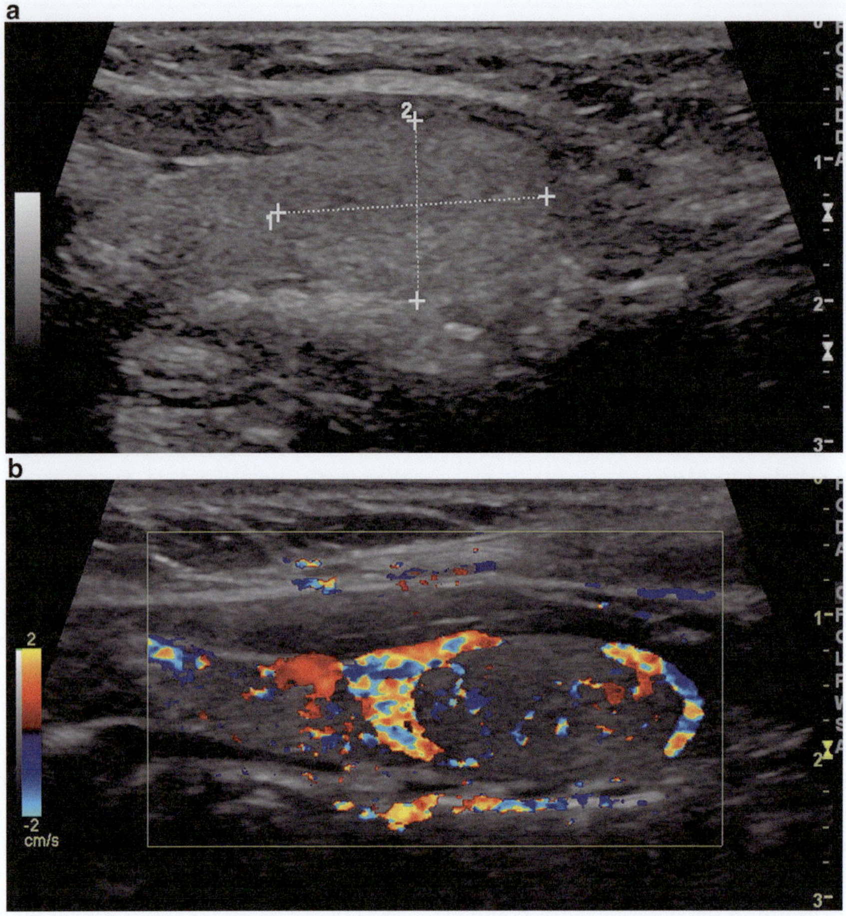

Fig. 13.1 Value of color Doppler with isoechoic nodules. (**a**) Longitudinal gray-scale view shows a solid isoechoic nodule that is very difficult to visualize and measure. (**b**) Longitudinal color Doppler view shows perinodular blood flow that defines the margin of the nodule

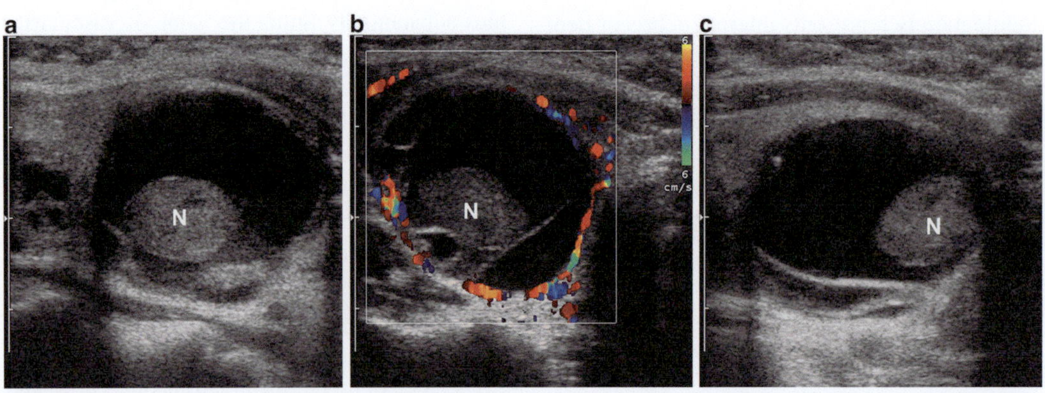

Fig. 13.2 Value of color Doppler with cystic nodules containing eccentric solid components. (**a**) Longitudinal gray-scale view shows a predominantly cystic nodule that has what appears to be a solid mural nodule (N). Because of this solid component, this patient had been scheduled for FNA. (**b**) Transverse color Doppler view shows lack of blood flow in the apparent solid mural nodule. This suggests the solid lesion may be a luminal blood clot and not a mural nodule. (**c**) Longitudinal view with the patient in the upright position shows that the avascular solid component has moved to the inferior portion of the cyst, confirming that it is mobile and not a mural nodule. In this case, FNA was canceled

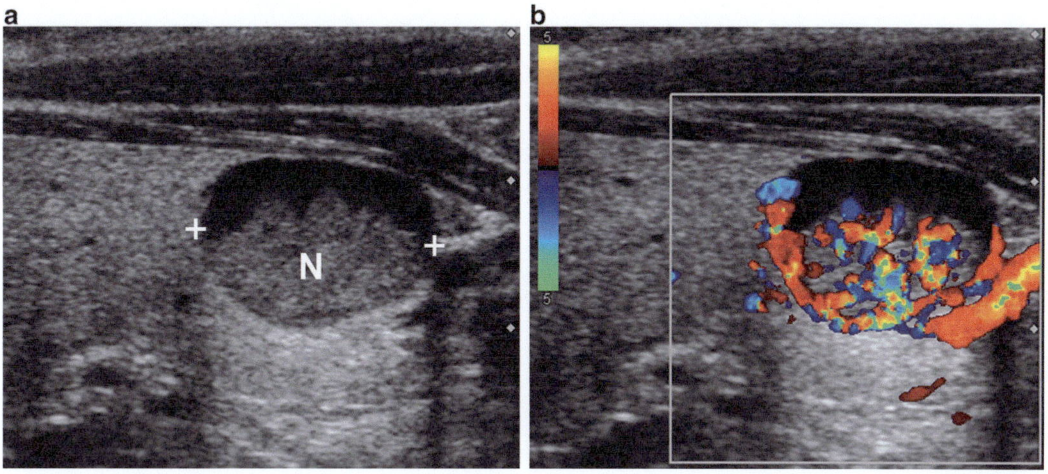

Fig. 13.3 Value of color Doppler with cystic nodules containing eccentric solid components. (**a**) Longitudinal gray-scale view shows a nodule (*cursors*) with a cystic component in the nondependent portion and a solid component (N) in the dependent portion. The differential diagnosis based on this image is a cyst with dependent debris or clot versus a cyst with a solid eccentric mural nodule. (**b**) Corresponding color Doppler view shows intense hypervascularity in the solid component, confirming it is a mural nodule. Cytology was interpreted as a follicular lesion of undetermined significance

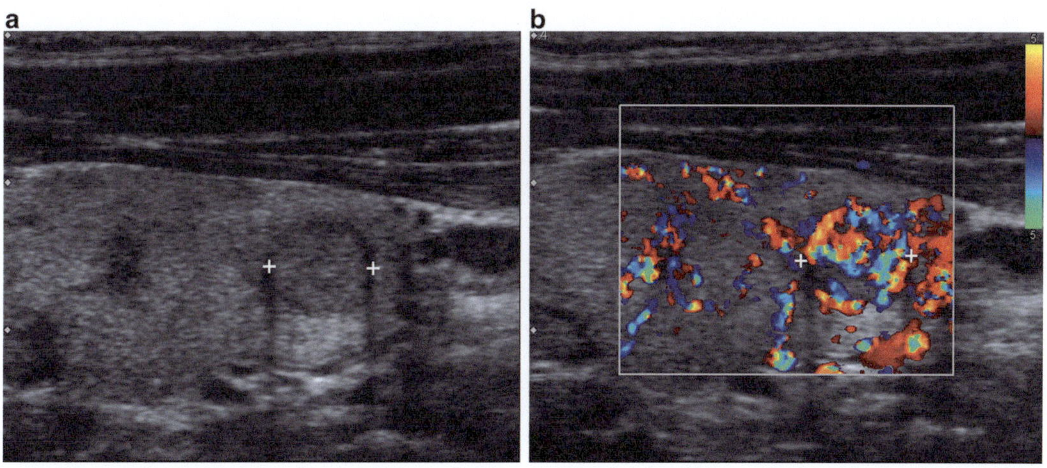

Fig. 13.4 Papillary thyroid cancer with hypervascular intranodular blood flow. (**a**) Longitudinal gray-scale view shows an intermediate suspicion, entirely solid, slightly hypoechoic smoothly marginated nodule (*cursors*) with refractive shadowing and no calcifications. (**b**) Corresponding color Doppler view shows marked intranodular blood flow

predictive value, and negative predictive values ranged from 15 to 75 %, 34 to 96 %, 6 to 61 %, and 28 to 97 %, respectively. In addition to the statistics mentioned above, one can use an odds ratio to compare the risk of malignancy of a positive result (for instance, intranodular flow) to the risk of malignancy of a negative result (for instance, no intranodular flow). A ratio of 5 would indicate that a nodule with intranodular flow was five times more likely to be malignant than a nodule without intranodular flow. As Table 13.1 shows, the odds ratios ranged from 0.2 to 9.4. In most cases the odds ratio was less than 2. In a study that included 31 malignant nodules, Papini

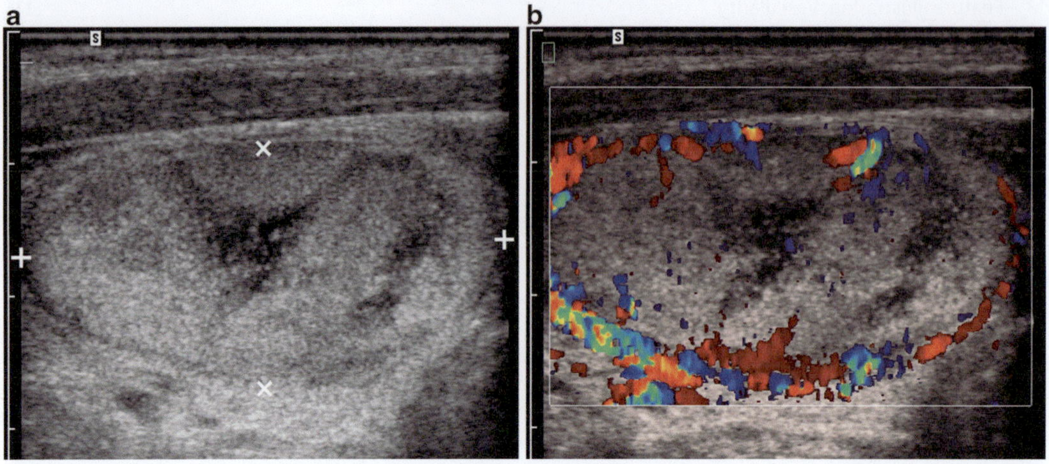

Fig. 13.5 Benign nodular hyperplasia with predominantly peripheral flow. (**a**) Longitudinal gray-scale view shows a low suspicion, almost entirely solid, isoechoic, smoothly marginated nodule (*cursors*) with no calcifications. (**b**) Corresponding color Doppler view shows abundant peripheral flow and almost no central flow

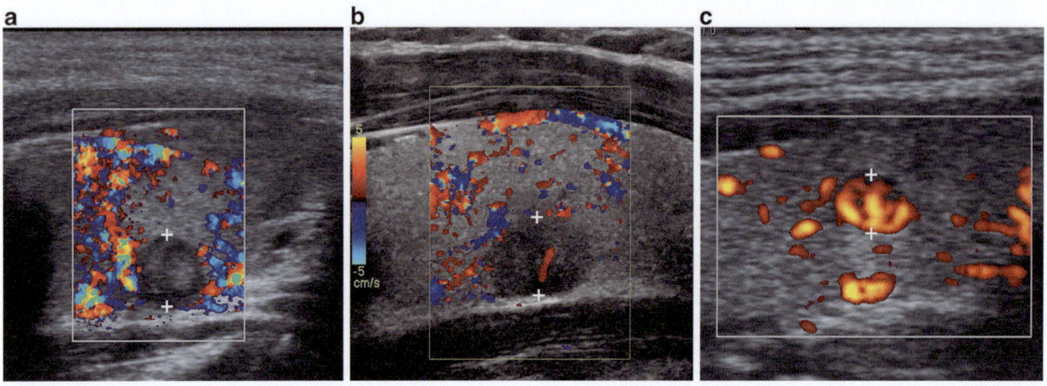

Fig. 13.6 Spectrum of vascularity in malignant thyroid nodules. (**a**) Papillary thyroid cancer (*cursors*) with no detectable blood flow. (**b**) Papillary thyroid cancer (*cursors*) with minimal internal blood flow. (**c**) Medullary thyroid cancer (*cursors*) with hypervascular internal blood flow

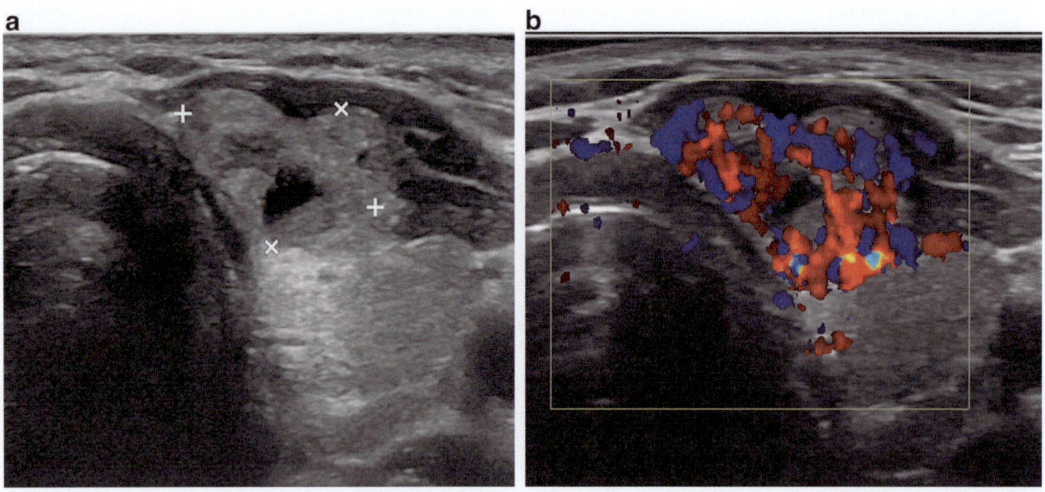

Fig. 13.7 Benign nodular hyperplasia with hypervascular internal blood flow. (**a**) Transverse gray-scale view shows an intermediate suspicion, lobulated, predominantly solid, slightly hypoechoic smoothly marginated nodule (*cursors*) with no calcifications. (**b**) Corresponding color Doppler view shows hypervascular internal blood flow

Table 13.1 Relationship to the pattern of nodular blood flow and risk of malignancy

Study	Criteria used	# of nodules	% malignancy	Sens (%)	Spec (%)	PPV (%)	NPV (%)	Odds ratio	Conclusion
Sharma 2011 [8]	Detectable flow anywhere	67	23 (16/67)	75	60.80	37.50	88.60	3.3	Not helpful
Rosario 2015 [12]	Intranodular flow	1502	10.6 (160/1502)	70	36	11.50	91.00	1.28	Not helpful
	Isolated or predominant intranodular flow	1502	10.6 (160/1502)	15	96	31.60	90.50	3.3	Not helpful
Cappelli 2006 [4]	Intranodular flow	6135	4.6 (284/6135)	62	50	5.60	96	1.4	? Not included in final recommendations
Popowicz 2009 [6]	Intranodular flow	316	8.5 (27/316)	51.90	56.70	8.90	92.70	1.2	Not helpful
Rago 1998 [1]	Marked intranodular flow	104	28.8 (30/104)	49	67	34	78	1.5	Not helpful
Brito 2014 [11]	Increased central flow	7578		48	53				Not helpful
Papini 2002 [2][a]	Intranodular flow	402	7.7 (31/402)	74 (23/31)	80.8 (300/371)	24.50	97.40	9.4	Helpful—included in recommendations
Frates 2003 [3]	Extensive intranodular flow	209	15.3 (32/209)	43.80	85.30	35.00	85.30	2.4	Limited usefulness
	Small to moderate or greater intranodular flow	209	15.3 (32/209)	62.50	57.10	20.80	79.50	1	Limited usefulness
Lyshchik 2007 [5]	Intranodular flow (all nodules)	86	53.5 (46/86)	65.20	52.50	61.20	56.80	1.4	Qualitative analysis of vascularity was not helpful
	Intranodular flow (nodules <2 cm)	43	67.4 (29/43)	65.50	85.70	90.50	54.50	2	Qualitative analysis of vascularity was not helpful
	Intranodular flow (nodules >2 cm)	43	39.5 (17/43)	64.70	34.60	49.30	60.00	1.23	Qualitative analysis of vascularity was not helpful
Lee 2011 [9]	Predominant intranodular	191	37.7 (72/191)	11.1	94.1	53.3	63.6	1.5	Not useful
Ozel 2012 [10]	Any intranodular	363	6.10 (22/363)	63.6	34	10.1	96.4	2.8	Useful
Moon 2010 [7]	Any flow	1083	24.8 (269/1083)	40.1	43	18.9	68.5	0.6	Negative correlation between vascularity and malignancy
	Intranodular flow	1083	24.8 (269/1083)	16.7	69.3	15.3	28.4	0.21	Negative correlation between vascularity and malignancy

Sens = sensitivity, Spec = specificity, PPV = positive predictive value, NPV = negative predictive value
[a]Nonpalpable nodules 8–15 mm

et al. had the highest odds ratio of 9.4 using any intranodular flow as the criterion [2]. In this study, intranodular flow had a 24.5 % risk of malignancy and no intranodular flow had a 2.6 % risk of malignancy.

In a recent study of 1342 benign and 160 malignant nodules (malignant rate of 10.6 %), suspicious flow was defined in two different ways [12]. Intranodular flow of any degree regardless of the presence or degree of peripheral flow had an odds ratio of 1.28 and a positive predictive value of 11.5 %. Intranodular flow without peripheral flow or exceeding peripheral flow had an odds ratio of 3.3 and a positive predictive value of 31.6 %. The authors concluded that Doppler evaluation of blood flow was not helpful.

In another large study of 5851 benign and 284 malignant nodules (malignant rate of 4.6 %), intranodular flow of any degree was considered suspicious for malignancy [4]. Using this criterion, the odds ratio was 1.4 and the positive predictive value was 5.6 %. Doppler findings were not included in the final recommendations of this study.

In a study of 814 benign and 269 malignant nodules (malignant rate of 24.8 %), suspicious flow was defined in two different ways [7]. In both cases there was actually a negative correlation with malignancy.

A meta-analysis of studies including 7578 nodules used increased intranodular flow as the criterion for malignancy and found a sensitivity of 48 % and a specificity of 53 % [11]. The authors did not conclude that analysis of vascularity was helpful.

In a slightly different analysis, Phuttharak compared the results of gray-scale findings alone versus the combination of gray-scale and Doppler findings [13]. Central hypervascularity that exceeded flow in the remainder of the nodule was considered suspicious for malignancy. The sensitivity, specificity, positive predictive value, and negative predictive value were 80 % (4/5), 84.6 % (22/26), 50 % (4/8), and 95.7 % (22/23), respectively, for gray-scale findings alone and 40 % (2/5), 96.2 % (25/26), 66.7 % (2/3), and 89.3 % (25/28) for combined gray-scale and Doppler findings. The authors concluded that Doppler findings were useful since they improved the specificity and the positive predictive values, albeit with a loss of sensitivity. A significant limitation of this study was the low number of nodules that were analyzed (only 31 total nodules and only five malignant nodules).

There is some data that suggests Doppler flow patterns may add clinically useful information for nodules that have been aspirated and have cytology indicative of follicular lesions of undetermined significance or atypia of undetermined significance [14–17]. Approximately 15–20 % of these indeterminate lesions ultimately are shown to be malignant. Currently there are no gray-scale sonographic features that assist in separating the benign and malignant nodules in this category. However, intranodular vascularity has been shown in several studies to be more closely associated with malignancy (Fig. 13.8). Sensitivity, specificity, positive predictive value, and negative predictive value range from 80 to 86 %, 39 to 90 %, 23 to 51 %, and 90 to 97 %, respectively. The odds ratio for a positive result ranges from 2.8 to 17.7. Table 13.2 shows the results of several studies that had histologic proof and specifically determined the statistics of nodule vascularity independent of gray-scale findings. DeNicola also evaluated measurement of RI values from the nodules and using a cutoff value of less than 0.75 as a sign of malignancy obtained a sensitivity of 40 %, specificity of 97 %, positive predictive value of 67 %, negative predictive value of 92 %, and an odds ratio for a positive result of 8.4 [15]. These results suggest a complimentary role for color Doppler in the management of follicular lesions. However, it is important to realize that in individual patients the presence of central flow (Fig. 13.9) does not ensure that a lesion is malignant and predominantly peripheral flow does not exclude a malignancy.

In summary, Doppler evaluation of nodule blood flow is much less helpful than gray-scale evaluation. While detection of intranodular vascularity may increase the risk of malignancy minimally, many benign nodules are hypervascular (Figs. 13.7 and 13.9), and the absence of

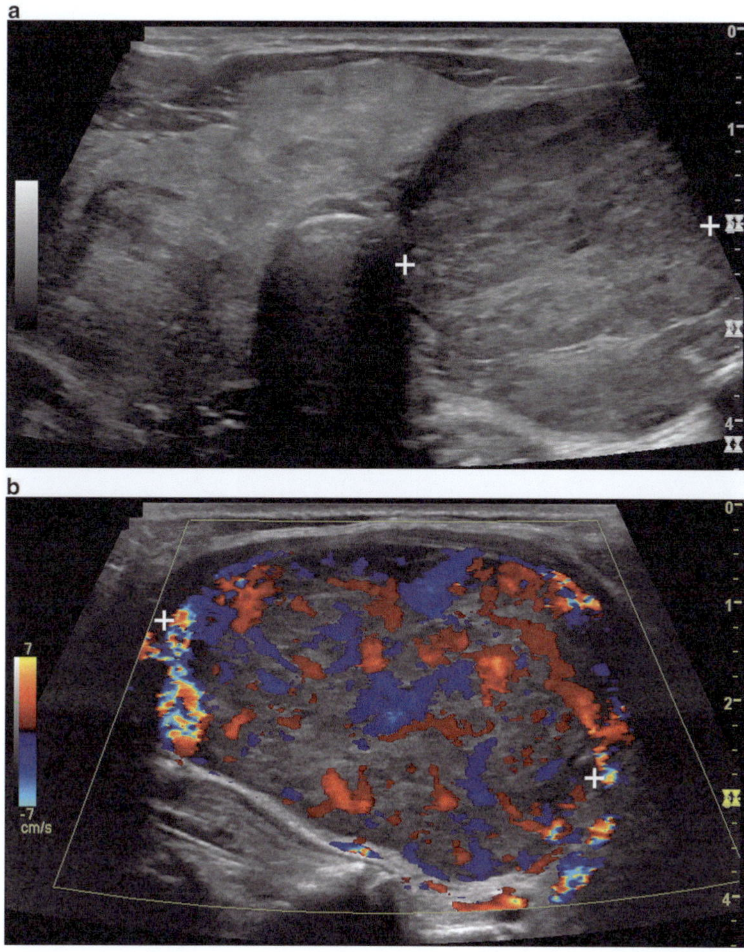

Fig. 13.8 Follicular cancer with predominant central internal blood flow. (**a**) Transverse gray-scale view shows a large, entirely solid, hypoechoic, intermediate suspicion nodule (*cursors*) with smooth margins and no calcifications. (**b**) Longitudinal color Doppler view shows readily detectable blood flow throughout the center of the nodule

Table 13.2 Relationship of the pattern of nodular blood flow and risk of malignancy for nodules with cytologic results of follicular neoplasm, follicular lesions of undetermined significance, or atypia of undetermined significance

Study	Criteria used	# of nodules	% malignancy	Sens (%)	Spec (%)	PPV (%)	NPV (%)	Odds ratio
Iared 2010 [17][a]	Predominant intranodular	457	14.7 (67/457)	85.1	86.2	51.4	97.1	17.7
Choi 2009 [16]	Intranodular flow	114	21.9 (25/114)	84	39	28	90	2.8
DeNicola 2005 [15]	Predominant intranodular	86	11.6 (10/86)	80	90	50	97	17.2
Fukanari 2004 [14]	Intranodular flow	310	14.2 (44/310)	86	52	23	96	5.4

Sens = sensitivity, Spec = specificity, PPV = positive predictive value, NPV = negative predictive value
[a]Meta-analysis

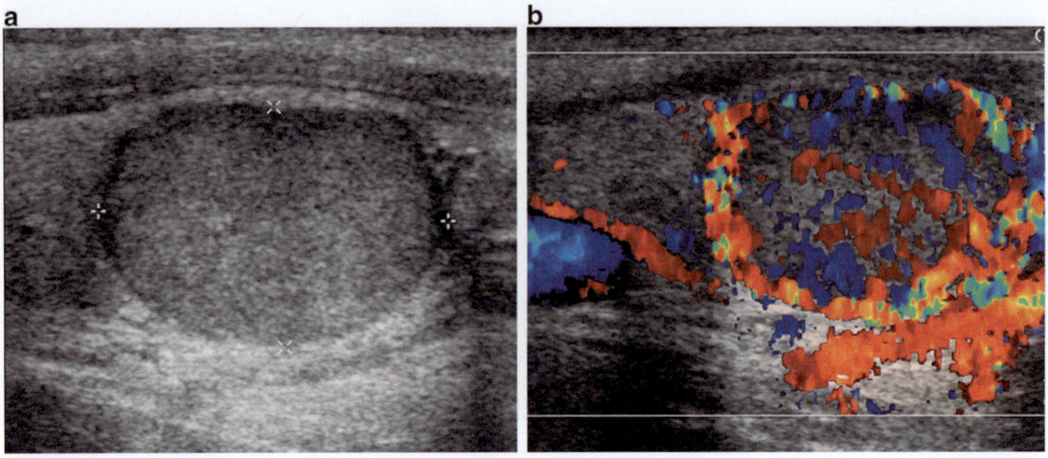

Fig. 13.9 Follicular adenoma with central and peripheral blood flow. (**a**) Longitudinal gray-scale view shows a large, entirely solid, hypoechoic, intermediate suspicion nodule (*cursors*) with smooth margins and no calcifications. (**b**) Longitudinal color Doppler view shows readily detectable blood flow throughout the center and periphery of the nodule

detectable internal flow in no way excludes malignancy (Fig. 13.6). In 2009 the American Thyroid Association guidelines for patients with thyroid nodules included increased intranodular flow as a malignant feature that warranted FNA at a smaller nodule size (along with several well-known gray-scale findings) [18]. The guidelines published in 2015 eliminated this Doppler finding in their recommendations for FNA of a thyroid [19].

13.2 Hyperthyroidism

Distinction of Graves' disease, the most common cause of hyperthyroidism, and thyrotoxicosis caused by destructive thyroiditis (subacute thyroiditis, silent thyroiditis, pregnancy-related thyroiditis) is generally made based on a combination of clinical and laboratory findings. Radioactive iodine uptake and scanning have traditionally been used when imaging is necessary and are generally considered the gold standard. However, radioactive iodine is a relatively expensive and time-consuming examination that cannot be used in pregnancy or in breast-feeding women. Given its widespread availability, ultrasound and Doppler have now assumed an important complimentary role.

Ralls originally recognized the color Doppler hypervascularity of Graves' disease and coined the term "thyroid inferno" (Fig. 13.10) in 1988 [20]. Since then there have been a number of studies showing that there are statistically significant differences in the subjective categorization of Doppler vascularity between Graves' disease and destructive thyroiditis [21, 22] and from other forms of thyroid disease [23] and from euthyroid controls [23]. In a study of 65 patients, Kumar found mild to moderate patchy or diffuse increased flow in 32/34 patients with Graves' disease (sensitivity 94 %) and only 1/31 patients with destructive thyroiditis (specificity 97 %) [21]. Uchida et al. had much less encouraging results [22]. In a study of 215 patients, they found mild or marked increased flow in a patchy or diffuse distribution in 112/194 patients with Graves' disease (sensitivity 58 %) and in 1/21 patients with painless thyroiditis (specificity 95 %).

Given the inconsistent results with subjective analysis of parenchymal blood flow, some investigators have described quantitative techniques for measuring blood flow. These generally use

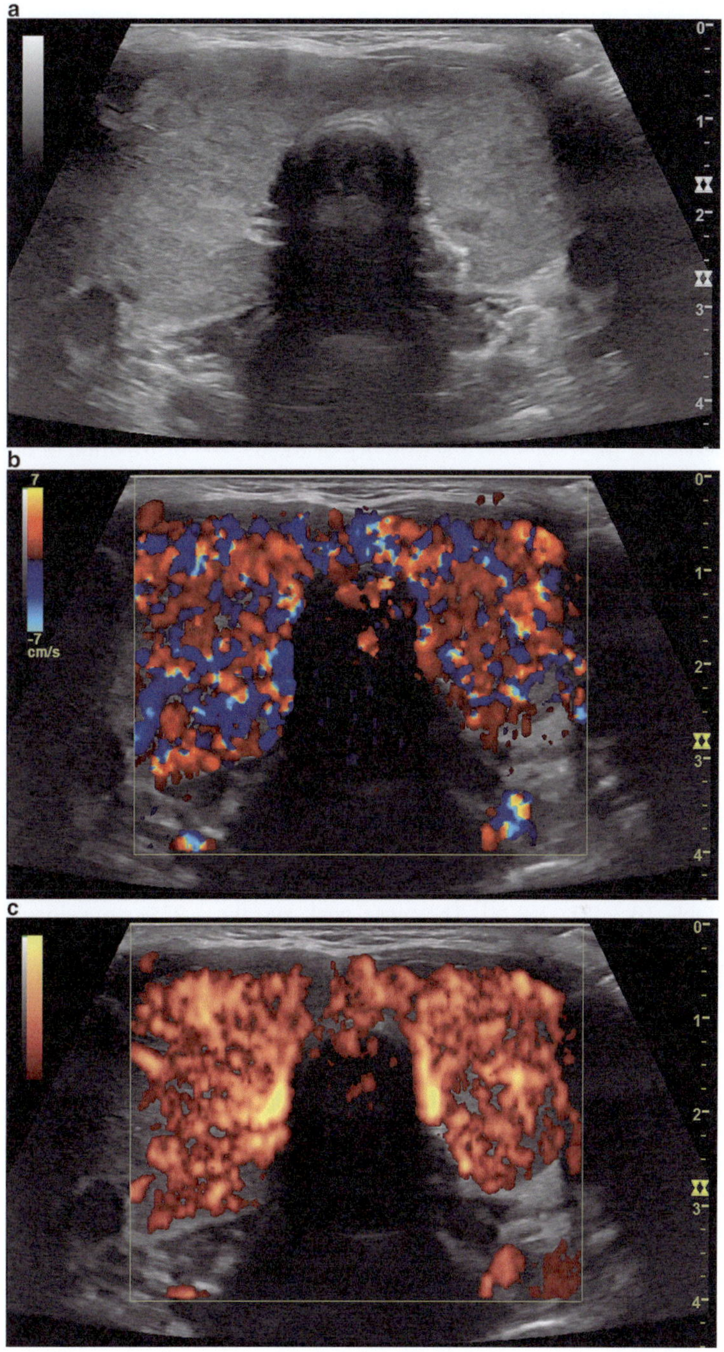

Fig. 13.10 Graves' disease with classic "thyroid inferno" hypervascularity. (**a**) Transverse gray-scale view shows an enlarged thyroid that is slightly hypoechoic and slightly heterogeneous. There are no nodules. (**b**) Corresponding color Doppler view shows intense, homogeneous, diffuse hypervascularity. (**c**) Corresponding power Doppler view shows findings similar to the color Doppler image

software that analyze color or power Doppler images of the thyroid and calculate a percentage of blood flow by comparing the number of pixels with color Doppler signals to the total number of pixels within a selected region of interest. In a study of 114 patients, Ota used proprietary software built in to their ultrasound unit and found mean thyroid total blood flow values of 14.9 % (±6.4 %), 0.8 % (±0.5 %), 0.9 % (±0.7), and 0.8 % (±0.5 %) for Graves' disease, painless thyroiditis, subacute thyroiditis, and normal controls, respectively [24]. Using a cutoff of 4 % resulted in a sensitivity and specificity of 100 %. Using power Doppler and a different quantification method, Banaka also calculated the percent blood flow in the thyroid [25]. In the right lobe, they found values of 24.2 % (±16.3 %), 10.3 % (±7.1 %), 14.7 % (±13.8 %), and 3.7 % (±3.5 %), for Graves' disease, euthyroid Hashimoto's disease, hypothyroid Hashimoto's disease, and normal controls, respectively. Very similar values were obtained in the left thyroid lobe. Using a cutoff value of 7.4 % for the right lobe and 5.6 % for the left lobe, they obtained a sensitivity of 82–89 % and specificity of 85–88 % for distinguishing autoimmune disease (Graves' and Hashimoto's) from normal controls. Although these techniques can theoretically improve on subjective assessment of vascularity, they are cumbersome, very dependent on adjustment of technical parameters, and not uniformly available.

Analysis of arterial waveforms has also received a great deal of attention. Measurement of velocity, flow volume, resistive index, and other parameters have been studied. Most studies have focused on the superior or inferior thyroidal artery. The results from several studies are summarized in Table 13.3 [21, 26–28]. The mean peak systolic velocity in either the ITA or STA ranged from 58 to 78 cm/s, 21 to 33 cm/s, and 17 to 33 cm/s, for Graves' disease, destructive thyroiditis, and euthyroid controls, respectively. Using cutoff values from 30 to 45 cm/s to distinguish Graves' disease from destructive thyroiditis, sensitivity has ranged from 76 to 95 %, and specificity has ranged from 81 to 100 % (Fig. 13.11).

Uchida et al. [22] compared PSV measurements to a subjective grading system of parenchymal blood flow in 194 patients with Graves' disease and 21 with painless thyroiditis. They found 27 patients with Graves' disease who had no parenchymal flow or flow seen as minimal color spots and 55 patients with patchy uneven distribution of flow. Seventy Graves' patients had a mild increased flow in a patchy distribution, and 42 had a marked increase in flow in a diffuse distribution. They concluded that subjective analysis of parenchymal flow was useful in making the diagnosis of Graves' disease when it was clearly increased, but that Graves' disease could not be excluded when parenchymal flow was decreased. Interestingly, in the group of Graves' patients with decreased parenchymal flow, measurement of STA-PSV remained higher than in the patients with painless thyroiditis (41 ± 32 cm/s vs. 27 ± 14 cm/s). Using a cutoff of 30 cm/s, they achieved a sensitivity of 74 % and a specificity of 77 %. A velocity cutoff of 45 cm/s produced a low sensitivity but a positive predictive value and specificity of 100 %.

Table 13.3 Comparison of peak systolic velocity in patients with Graves' disease and destructive thyroiditis

Article	#	Artery studied	Velocity mean: Graves' disease	Velocity mean: Destructive thyroiditis	Velocity mean: Euthyroid controls	Cutoff	Statistics (%)
Zuhur 2014 [27][a]	20	Mean ITA	59 ± 25 (13–146)	21 ± 5 (11–34)	17 ± 4 (7–29)	40 cm/s	Sens 76
							Spec 100
						30 cm/s	Sens 95
							Spec 95
Chen 2012 [28]	220	Mean STA	75 cm/s ± 2.8	33 cm/s ± 2.3	33 cm/s ± 3.5	45.25 cm/s	Sens 80.4
							Spec 81.4
Kumar 2009 [21]	65	Mean ITA	58 ± 13	22 ± 5		40 cm/s	Sens 94
							Spec 100
Uchida 2010 [26]	57	Mean STA	78 ± 36	28 ± 13	21 ± 8	45 cm/s	Sens 84
							Spec 92

ITA = inferior thyroidal, STA = superior thyroidal artery, Sens = sensitivity, Spec = specificity
[a]Pregnant patients with Graves' disease, destructive thyroiditis, and gestational thyrotoxicosis

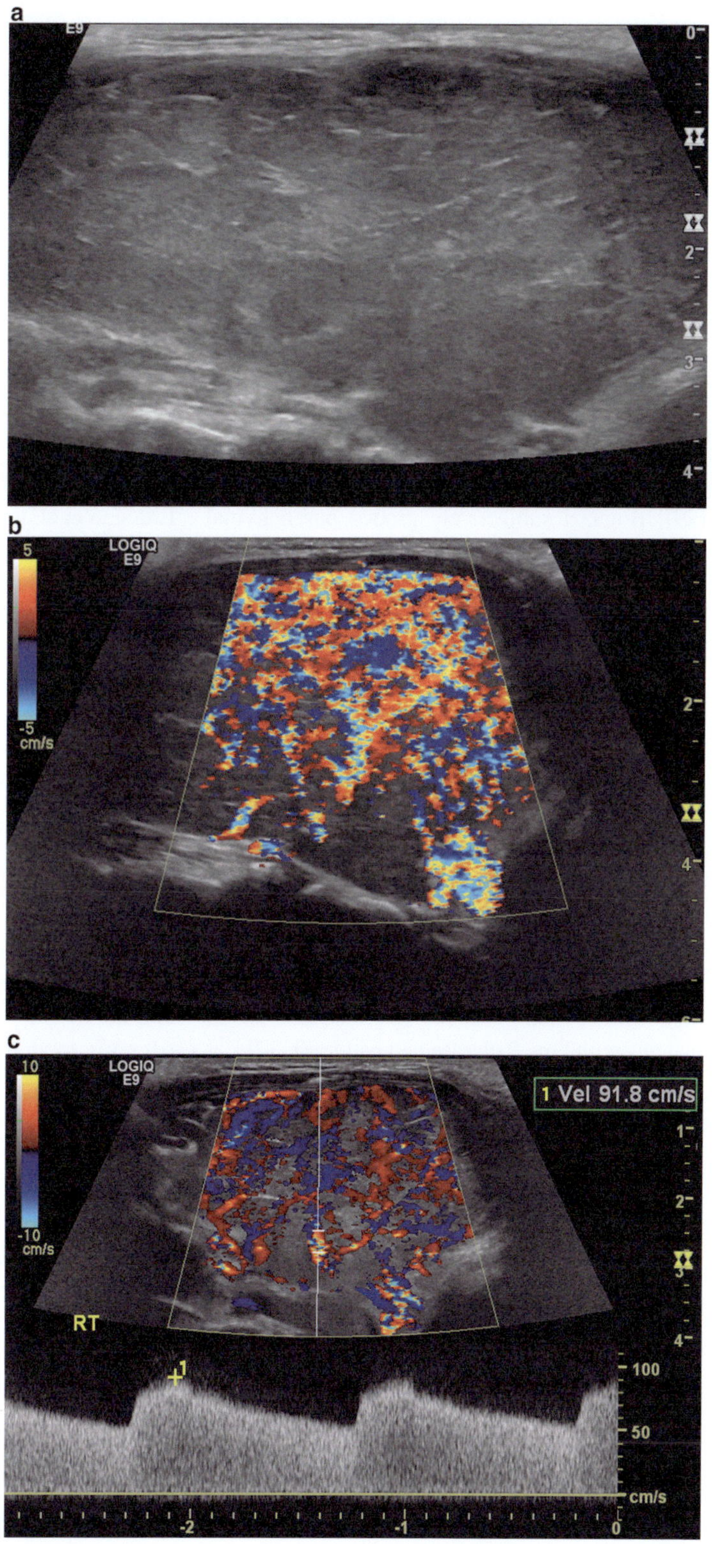

Fig. 13.11 Graves' disease with elevated inferior thyroidal artery peak systolic velocity. (**a**) Longitudinal gray-scale view shows an enlarged thyroid that is heterogeneous and hypoechoic. There are no nodules. (**b**) Corresponding color Doppler view shows intense, homogeneous, diffuse hypervascularity. (**c**) Pulsed Doppler waveform from the inferior thyroidal artery shows an elevated peak systolic velocity of 91.8 cm/s

Doppler analysis has also been shown to be helpful in distinguishing the two different types of amiodarone-induced thyrotoxicosis (AIT) [29, 30]. Type 1 AIT usually occurs in thyroid glands that have preexisting abnormalities such as diffuse or nodular goiters or Graves' disease prior to amiodarone therapy. It is usually treated with thionamides and potassium perchlorate therapy. These glands generally have an abnormal gray-scale appearance and increased parenchymal blood flow. Type 2 AIT is a destructive thyroiditis caused by cytotoxic effects of amiodarone on a normal gland. It is usually treated with glucocorticoids. These glands typically have a relatively normal gray-scale appearance and no vascularity [29]. Bogazzi subjectively graded parenchymal blood flow into four different patterns ranging from no flow or minimal color spots (grade 0) to markedly increased flow (grade 3). Pattern 0 was seen in all 16 untreated patients with type 2 AIT, all nine euthyroid patients on long-term amiodarone treatment, all nine patients with subacute thyroiditis, and all 26 normal controls. Of the 11 patients with type 1 AIT, seven had pattern 1, one had pattern 2, and three had pattern 3 [31]. In a follow-up study, Bogazzi et al. studied 55 patients with AIT. Of the 16 patients with type 1 disease, 13 had patchy parenchymal flow in an uneven distribution, two had mild hypervascularity in a patchy distribution, and one had marked hypervascularity in a diffuse homogeneous distribution. All 39 patients with type 2 disease had pattern 0 [32].

It is almost always easy to differentiate Graves' disease from Hashimoto's thyroiditis based on clinical and laboratory analysis. But patients may have ultrasound scans performed prior to the diagnosis. Since there is overlap in the gray-scale and color Doppler appearance of these conditions, Doppler waveform analysis has been used to help make the distinction.

Table 13.4 Peak systolic velocity measurements (mean and standard deviation) from the inferior thyroidal artery of the right and left lobes in patients with Graves' disease, Hashimoto's thyroiditis, and normal controls [25]

Condition	Right lobe (cm/s)	Left lobe (cm/s)
Euthyroid Hashimoto's thyroiditis	40 (±15)	43 (±14)
Hypothyroid Hashimoto's thyroiditis	52 (±36)	45 (±22)
Graves' disease	83 (±43)	88 (±46)
Normal controls	19 (±9)	20 (±9)

Erdogan et al. measured peak systolic velocity in perithyroidal arteries (not otherwise specified) and found statistically significant differences between Graves' disease (mean velocity in 29 patients = 48 cm/s ± 12) and Hashimoto's thyroiditis (mean velocity in 24 patients = 22 cm/s ± 8) [23]. Banaka et al. measured the peak systolic velocity in the inferior thyroid artery in patients with Graves' disease ($n=29$), hypothyroid Hashimoto's thyroiditis ($n=54$), euthyroid Hashimoto's thyroiditis ($n=70$), and normal controls ($n=48$) [25]. The mean velocities are shown in Table 13.4. There were significant differences between Hashimoto's thyroiditis and Graves' disease and between the entire group of patients and the normal controls. Using a cutoff value of 61 cm/s to distinguish Hashimoto's thyroiditis from Graves' disease, the sensitivity was 83 % and the specificity was 87 %. They found that peak systolic velocities were superior to quantitative measurement of vascularity index and superior to subjective analysis of parenchymal echogenicity (Fig. 13.12). Resistive indices were also calculated on the Doppler waveforms but were not useful.

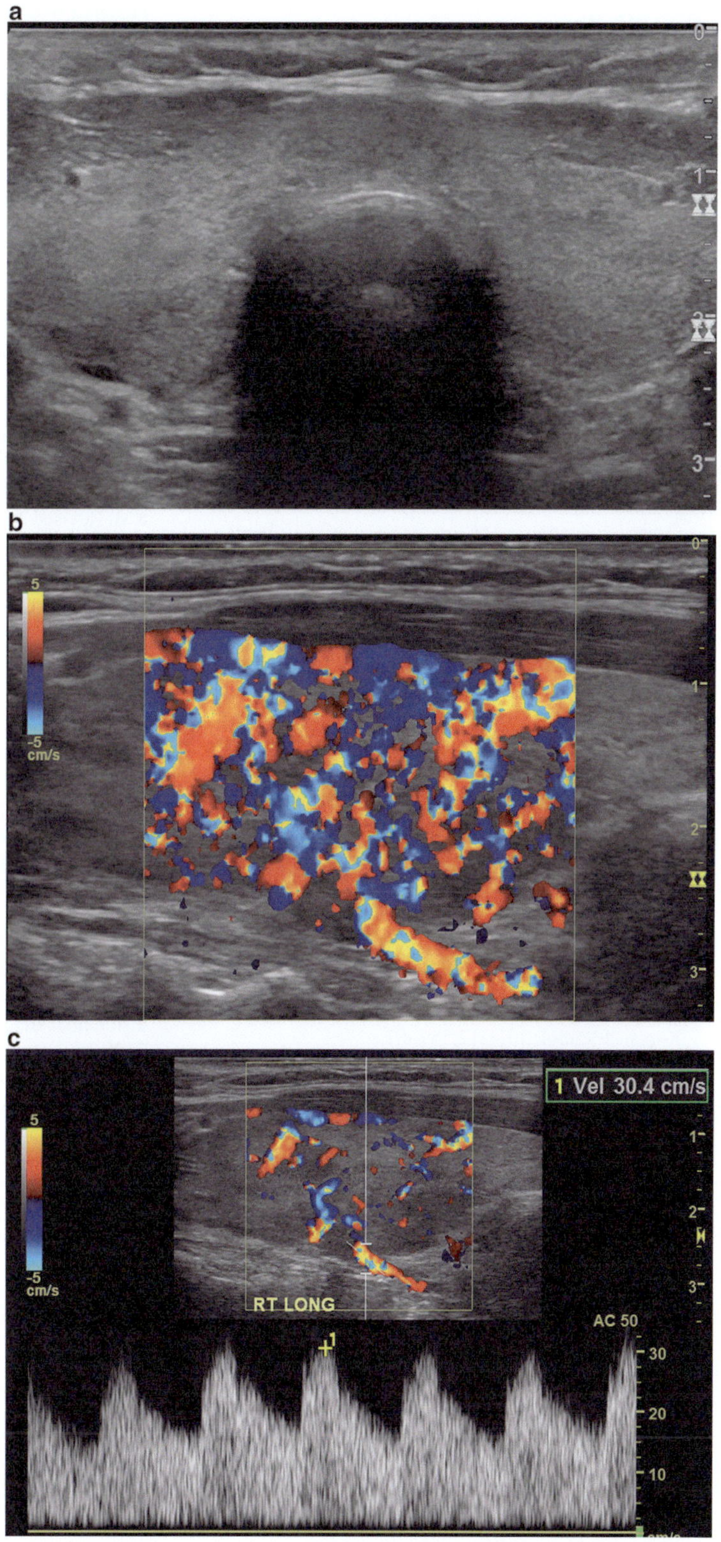

Fig. 13.12 Hashimoto's thyroiditis. (**a**) Transverse gray-scale view shows an enlarged thyroid that is slightly hypoechoic and slightly heterogeneous. There are no nodules. The gray-scale features are consistent with either Hashimoto's thyroiditis or Graves' disease. (**b**) Longitudinal color Doppler view shows intense, homogeneous, diffuse hypervascularity. The color Doppler features are consistent with either Hashimoto's thyroiditis or Graves' disease. (**c**) Pulsed Doppler waveform from the inferior thyroidal artery shows a peak systolic velocity of 30.4 cm/s. This is higher than normal but less than expected for Graves' disease. In this case the arterial velocity suggests Hashimoto's thyroiditis rather than Graves' disease

References

1. Rago T, Vitti P, Chiovato L, De Liperi A, Miccoli P, et al. Role of conventional ultrasonography and color flow-Doppler sonography in predicting malignancy in 'cold' thyroid nodules. Eur J Endocrinol. 1998;138: 41–6.
2. Papini E, Guglielmi R, Bianchini A, Crescenzi A, et al. Risk of malignancy in nonpalpable thyroid nodules: predictive value of ultrasound and color-doppler features. J Clin Endocrinol Metab. 2002;87:1941–6.
3. Frates MC, Benson CB, Doubilet PM, Cibas ES, Marqusee E. Can color Doppler sonography aid in the prediction of malignancy of thyroid nodules. J Ultrasound Med. 2003;22:127–31.
4. Cappelli C, Castellano M, Pirola I, Gandossi E, et al. Thyroid nodule shape suggests malignancy. Eur J Endocrinol. 2006;155:27–31.
5. Lyshchik A, Moses R, Barnes SL, Higashi T, et al. Quantitative analysis of tumor vascularity in benign and malignant solid thyroid nodules. J Ultrasound Med. 2007;26:837–46.
6. Popowicz B, Klencki M, Lewinski A, Slowinska-Klencka D. The usefulness of sonographic features in selection of thyroid nodules for biopsy in relation to the nodule's size. Eur J Endocrinol. 2009;161: 103–11.
7. Moon HJ, Kwak JY, Kim MJ, Son EJ, Kim EK. Can vascularity at power Doppler us help predict thyroid malignancy. Radiology. 2010;255:260–9.
8. Sharma A, Gabriel H, Nemcek AA, Nayar R, Du H, Nikolaidis P. Subcentimeter thyroid nodules: utility of sonographic characterization and ultrasound-guided needle biopsy. AJR Am J Roentgenol. 2011;197: W1123–8.
9. Lee YH, Kim DW, In HS, Park JS, Kim SH, et al. Differentiating between benign and malignant solid thyroid nodules using an US classification system. Korean J Radiol. 2011;12:559–67.
10. Ozel A, Erturk SM, Ercan A, Yilmaz B, Basak T, et al. The diagnostic efficiency of ultrasound in characterization for thyroid nodules: how many criteria are required to predict malignancy? Med Ultrason. 2012;14:24–8.
11. Brito JP, Gionfriddo MR, Nofal AA, Boehmer KR, et al. The accuracy of thyroid nodule ultrasound to predict thyroid cancer: systematic review and meta-analysis. J Clin Endocrinol Metab. 2014;99:1253–63.
12. Rosario PW, da Silva AL, Borges MAR, Calsolari MR. Is Doppler ultrasound of additional value to gray-scale ultrasound in differentiating malignant and benign thyroid nodules. Arch Endocrinol Metab. 2015;59:79–83.
13. Phuttharak W, Somboonporn C, Hongdomnern G. Diagnostic performance of gray-scale versus combined gray-scale with colour Doppler ultrasonography in the diagnosis of malignancy in thyroid nodules. Asian Pac J Cancer Prev. 2009;10:759–64.
14. Fukanari N, Mitsuji Nagahama M, Sugino K, Mimura T, Ito K, Ito K. Clinical Evaluation of Color Doppler Imaging for the Differential Diagnosis of Thyroid Follicular Lesions. World J. Surg. 2004;28: 1261–1265.
15. De Nicola H, Szejnfeld J, Logullo AF, Wolosker AM, et al. Flow pattern and vascular resistive index as predictors of malignancy risk in thyroid follicular neoplasms. J Ultrasound Med. 2005;24:897–904.
16. Choi YJ, Yun JS, Kim DH. Clinical and ultrasound features of cytology diagnoses follicular neoplasm. Endocr J. 2009;56(3):383–9.
17. Iared W, Shigueoka DC, Cristofoli JC, Andriolo R, Atallah AN, et al. Use of color Doppler ultrasonography for the prediction of malignancy in follicular thyroid neoplasms. J Ultrasound Med. 2010;29:419–25.
18. Cooper DS, Doherty GM, Haugen BR, Kloos RT, Lee SL, Mandel SJ, Mazzaferri EL, McIver B, Pacini F, Schlumberger M, Sherman SI, Steward DL, Tuttle RM. Revised American Thyroid Association management guidelines for patients with thyroid nodules and differentiated thyroid cancer. American Thyroid Association (ATA) Guidelines Taskforce on Thyroid Nodules and Differentiated Thyroid Cancer. Thyroid. 2009;19(11):1167–214.
19. Haugen BR, Alexander EK, Bible KC, Doherty GM, Mandel SJ, et al. 2015 American Thyroid Association Management Guidelines for adult patients with thyroid nodules and differentiated thyroid cancer: the American Thyroid Association Guidelines Task Force on thyroid nodules and differentiated thyroid cancer. Thyroid. 2016;26(1):1–133.
20. Ralls PW, Mayekawa DS, Lee KP, Colletti PM, Radin DR, Boswell WD, Halls JM. Color-flow Doppler sonography in Graves disease: "thyroid inferno". Am J Roentgenol. 1988;150(4):781–4.
21. Kumar KVS, Pasupuleti V, Jayaraman M, Abhyuday V, Rayudu R, Modi KD. Role of thyroid Doppler in differential diagnosis of thyrotoxicosis. Endod Prac. 2009;15:6–9.
22. Uchida T, Shigihara N, Takeno K, Komiya K, et al. Characteristics of patients with graves disease and intrathyroid hypovascularity compared to painless thyroiditis. J Ultrasound Med. 2014;33:1791–6.
23. Erdogan MF, Anil C, Cesur M, Baskal N, Erdogan G. Color flow Doppler sonography for the etiologic diagnosis of hyperthyroidism. Thyroid. 2007;17: 223–8.
24. Ota H, Amino N, Morita S, Kobayashi K, Kubota S, Fukata S, Kamiyama N, Miyauchi A. Quantitative measurement of thyroid blood flow for differentiation of painless thyroiditis from Graves' disease. Clin Endocrinol (Oxf). 2007;67(1):41–5.
25. Banaka I, Thomas D, Kaltsas G. Value of the left inferior thyroid artery peak systolic velocity in diagnosing autoimmune thyroid disease. J Ultrasound Med. 2013;32:1969–78.
26. Uchida T, Takeno K, Goto M, Kanno R, et al. Superior thyroid artery mean peak systolic velocity for the

diagnosis of thyrotoxicosis in Japanese patients. Endocr J. 2010;57(5):439–43.
27. Zuhur SS, Ozel A, Kuzu I, Erol RS, Ozcan N, et al. The diagnostic utility of color Doppler ultrasonography, Tc-99m pertechnetate uptake, and TSH-receptor antibody for differential diagnosis of Graves' disease and silent thyroiditis: a comparative study. Endod Prac. 2014;20:310–9.
28. Chen L, Zhao X, Liu H, Wang Y, Li L, Lu B, Li Y, Hu R. Mean peak systolic velocity of the superior thyroid artery is correlated with radioactive iodine uptake in untreated thyrotoxicosis. J Int Med Res. 2012;40: 640–7.
29. Alzahrani AS, Ceresini G, Aldasouqu SA. Role of ultrasonography in the differential diagnosis of thyrotoxicosis: a noninvasive, cost-effective, and widely available but underutilized diagnostic tool. Endod Prac. 2012;18:567–78.
30. Eaton SEM, Euinton HA, Newman CM, Weetman AP, Bennet WM. Clinical experience of amiodarone-induced thyrotoxicosis over a 3-year period: role of colour-flow Doppler sonography. Clin Endocrinol (Oxf). 2002;56:33–8.
31. Bogazzi F, Bartalena L, Brogioni S, Mazzeo S, et al. Color flow Doppler sonography rapidly differentiates type I and type II amiodarone-induced thyrotoxicosis. Thyroid. 1997;7:541–5.
32. Bogazzi F, Martino E, Dell'Unto E, Brogioni S, et al. Thyroid color flow Doppler sonography and radioiodine uptake in 55 consecutive patients with amiodarone-induced thyrotoxicosis. J Endocrinol Invest. 2003;26:635–40.

Part IV

Pattern Recognition of Thyroid Disease Sonographic Presentations

14 The Application of Sonographic Patterns to Risk Stratification of Thyroid Nodules

Susan J. Mandel

14.1 Introduction

Over the last three decades, ultrasound (US) imaging of thyroid nodules has aimed for risk stratification for thyroid cancer to assist with identification of those nodules for which fine-needle aspiration (FNA) biopsy is recommended. Initial reports focused on correlations between individual grayscale features with thyroid cancer and identified relationships with solid composition, hypoechogenicity including marked hypoechogenicity, irregular margins, the presence of microcalcifications, and a taller-than-wide shape [1]. In addition, documentation of increased intranodular vascularity with either color flow or power Doppler imaging was correlated with malignancy in populations with a higher prevalence of follicular rather than papillary cancers [2, 3].

Exclusive reliance on identification of these individual features for FNA decision-making is tempered by two main observations. First, two recent meta-analyses of the extensive literature of observational reports correlating ultrasound features and thyroid cancer detected significant heterogeneity among studies [4, 5]. In part, this may be attributed to significant interobserver variability for accurate sonographic feature classification [1, 6]. In fact, the correct identification of microcalcifications, one of the individual features associated with the highest likelihood of cancer, is correlated to the proficiency of the sonographer, with overcall by less experienced operators [4], potentially leading to inappropriate recommendations for FNA. Second, focus on the individual features is predicated upon the erroneous assumption that these features are present independently of each other; rather, the appearance of some features is highly correlated with others. For example, microcalcifications almost exclusively appear in solid hypoechoic nodules. Similarly, irregular borders, which demarcate the interface between the nodule's echogenicity and the surrounding thyroid, by definition, are generally only apparent in a hypoechoic nodule when the background thyroid echotexture is usually normal. This natural relationship among features leads to the concept of identifying sonographic patterns, specifically defining characteristic nodule appearances that are each composed of a constellation of individual sonographic features simultaneously manifest together.

Currently, there are several systems of sonographic patterns for thyroid nodule risk stratification, developed for the most part by single institutions. They share the fact that pattern recognition is more reproducible among different

S.J. Mandel, M.D., M.P.H. (✉)
Division of Endocrinology, Diabetes and Metabolism, Perelman School of Medicine, University of Pennsylvania, Philadelphia, PA 19104, USA
e-mail: Susan.Mandel@uphs.upenn.edu

M. Milas et al. (eds.), *Advanced Thyroid and Parathyroid Ultrasound*,
DOI 10.1007/978-3-319-44100-9_14

operators [7–9] and is less influenced by physician experience [7]. This is the first step to a more standardized evidence-based approach to FNA decision-making.

14.2 Classification Systems of Sonographic Patterns

In 2005, Reading first introduced the concept of pattern recognition, subtitling his article "A 'Classic Pattern' Diagnostic Approach" [10]. His report described "the classic appearances of some of the commonly encountered benign and malignant nodules that are seen in day-to-day practice." And he foreshadowed that "Although more than half of all thyroid nodules encountered in day-to-day practice will fit into one of the classic categories, this article is not meant to be a complete description of the ultrasound appearances of all conceivable types of thyroid nodule, as many nodules will not fall into one of these specific categories. It is likely that additional classic nodule appearances will be identified over time." Four patterns of nodules requiring FNA and five patterns of nodules for which FNA can be avoided were presented, but the report is qualitative without application and validation in a subset of nodules.

Since then, publications from groups around the world have addressed defining nodule sonographic patterns with associated quantitative risk stratification for malignancy. Validation for these systems varies, retrospective or prospective, generally single group. In addition, over the last 2 years, secondary publications have begun to appear that apply these classification schemes to different populations, for the most part reporting similar results. However, no one system has achieved universal acceptance, leading to some confusion for the practitioners of sonography. The next paragraphs describe the sonographic pattern classification systems most widely referenced in current practice.

The first Thyroid Imaging Reporting and Data System (TIRADS) was developed in 2009 [9] and was based upon the concepts of the original Breast Imaging Reporting and Data System (BIRADS) that defined mammographic categories according to cancer risk. Using pattern recognition, the objective of this TIRADS classification was not only to identify thyroid nodules for FNA but also to define those associated with a negligible malignancy risk such that FNA could be avoided. This original TIRADS system described in 2009 by Horvath et al. defined six categories, with TIRADS 1 normal thyroid, TIRADS 2 benign nodules, TIRADS 3 probably benign nodules, TIRADS 4 suspicion nodules, TIRADS 5 probably malignant nodules, and TIRADS 6 diagnosed malignancy [9]. Therefore, essentially only four main categories apply to nodules, and these (TIRADS 2–5) are characterized by both grayscale and Doppler ultrasound criteria to define ten patterns (Table 14.1). In the defining study of 1097 nodules, all 62 TIRADS 2 nodules were cytologically benign, and the probability of a malignant FNA cytology increased, 3.4 %, 14 %, and 87 %, respectively, in TIRADS 3, 4, and 5. In addition the authors subdivided TIRADS 4 into 4a and 4b with respective malignant cytology risks of 7 and 27 %. Since its inception, the applicability and clinical use of this original TIRADS have been limited in part due to the perceived intricacy of the ten pattern descriptions subgrouped under TIRADS 2–5.

Park proposed thyroid imaging reporting based upon a logistic regression equation to estimate cancer risk that was derived from a database of 1694 nodules with ultrasound imaging and FNA results [11]. Each ultrasound exam was scored according to the absence or presence of 12 ultrasound features which resulted in a five-category scale: thyroid ultrasound (TUS) 1–5. FNA was not recommended for TUS 1 and TUS 2. This system has not been widely adapted again because of the complexity inherent in categorizing multiple sonographic features and entering the score into a logarithmic equation to decide about FNA.

The goal of the second iteration of TIRADS, a system developed in Korea by Kwak et al. in 2011, was to develop a "practical" and less complex TIRADS stratifying malignancy risk and focused on FNA decision-making [12] (Table 14.1). These authors stressed that in

Table 14.1 Published versions of Thyroid Imaging Reporting and Data System (TIRADS) classifications for thyroid nodules

System		TIRADS 2	TIRADS 3	TIRADS 4a	TIRADS 4b	TIRADS 4c	TIRADS 5
Horvath 2009 [9]	Pattern	"Benign"	"Probably benign"	"Undetermined"	"Suspicious"	NA	"Consistent with malignancy"
		Colloid type 1 nodule: anechoic avascular nodule with hyperechoic spots	Hashimoto's pseudonodule: hyper-, iso-, or hypoechoic nodule with peripheral vascularization in Hashimoto's	Simple neoplastic pattern: solid or mixed cystic/solid hyper-, iso-, or hypoechoic nodule with thin capsule	Malignant pattern A: hypoechoic nonencapsulated nodule with irregular shape and margins and penetrating vessels, with or without calcifications		Malignant pattern B: Iso- or hypoechoic nonencapsulated vascular nodule with multiple microcalcifications
		Colloid type 2 nodule: nonencapsulated mixed vascular nodule with hyperechoic spots (spongiform)		DeQuervain pattern: hypoechoic lesion noncalcified with ill-defined margins			Malignant pattern C: Isoechoic mixed nonencapsulated vascular nodule with or without calcifications
		Colloid type 3 nodule: nonencapsulated mixed nodule with isoechoic solid vascular portion with hyperechoic spots		Suspicious neoplastic pattern: hyper-, iso-, or hypoechoic hypervascularized encapsulated nodule with thick capsule containing coarse or microcalcifications			
	Estimated malignancy rate	0 %	<5 %	5–10 %	10–80 %		>80 %

(continued)

Table 14.1 (continued)

System		TIRADS 2	TIRADS 3	TIRADS 4a	TIRADS 4b	TIRADS 4c	TIRADS 5
Kwak 2011 [12]	Pattern	NA	"Probably benign"	"Low suspicion for malignancy"	"Intermediate suspicion for malignancy"	"Moderate concern but not classic for malignancy"	"Highly suggestive of malignancy"
Based upon the presence of five suspicious ultrasound features			Nodule with no suspicious features	Nodule with one suspicious feature	Nodule with two suspicious features	Nodule with three or four suspicious features	Nodule with five suspicious features
1. Solid composition 2. Hypo- or marked hypoechogenicity 3. Irregular or microlobulated margins 4. Microcalcifications 5. Taller-than-wide shape	Estimated malignancy rate		1.7 %	3.3 %	9.2 %	44–72 %	88 %
Russ 2013, 2016 [8, 14]	Pattern	"Benign"	"Very probably benign"	"Low suspicion of malignancy"	"High suspicion of malignancy"	NA	"Effectively certainly malignant"
High suspicion signs defined as		Simple or septated cyst, spongiform nodule, isolated macrocalcification	No high suspicion signs	No high suspicion signs	One or two high suspicion signs, no metastatic lymph nodes		Three to five high suspicion signs and/or the presence of metastatic lymph nodes
1. Taller-than-wide shape 2. Irregular (speculated or microlobulated) borders 3. Microcalcifications 4. Markedly hypoechoic			Iso- or hyperechoic	Mildly hypoechoic			
5. High stiffness with elastography if available	Estimated malignancy rate	0 %	0.25 %	6 %	69 %		100 %

parallel to BIRADS, differentiating category 3 from 4 was crucial because surveillance is recommended for the former and biopsy for the latter. In addition, they also introduced a 4c subcategory. The study included 1658 nodules larger than 1 cm that underwent FNA. In a multivariate analysis, five ultrasound features were associated with malignancy: solid composition, hypo- or marked hypoechogenicity, irregular or microlobulated margins, microcalcifications, and taller-than-wide shape. Using a derived regression equation, cancer risk exponentially increased with the number of suspicious ultrasound features present. With these findings, the authors proposed a new TIRADS classification system: TIRADS 3 no suspicious features, TIRADS 4a one suspicious feature, TIRADS 4b two suspicious features, TIRADS 4c three or four suspicious features, and TIRADS 5 five suspicious features. A main limitation of this classification system was each feature was assigned the same weight even though the authors noted that odds ratios for malignancy of certain features, such as irregular or microlobulated margins and microcalcifications, were higher than those of solid composition and hypoechogenicity. Furthermore, inherent in this type of checklist classification scheme is the assumption that each feature can occur independently of the other four and is therefore just as likely to be the only suspicious finding. For example, TIRADS 4a is defined by only one suspicious feature. This could certainly be solid composition, but it would be highly unlikely that microlobulated or irregular margins would be the one element defining TIRADS 4a nodule because these types of margins virtually always occur in solid hypoechoic or markedly hypoechoic nodules. Hence, a total of three characteristics are present, all of which are highly correlated, and these then define a TIRADS 4c nodule.

Subsequently, the Korean Society of Thyroid Radiology sought to modify the initial Kwak TIRADS system by assigning a different risk score to each suspicious ultrasound feature according to their odds ratios for cancer prediction derived from a multicenter retrospective study [13]. The total score associated with each nodule could then be used to predict malignancy risk. For example, the scores for hypo- versus marked hypoechogenicity were 2 and 6 points, respectively. No risk score was assigned to composition. However, what resulted from this new scheme was no longer a pattern recognition classification; rather, this scoring system reverted to identification of individual sonographic features and has not been widely adopted.

Also recognizing the differing probabilities of malignancy associated with the five ultrasound features, Russ and his colleagues proposed a third TIRADS classification scheme in 2013 [8], now referred to as the French system [14] (Table 14.1). Solid composition was removed from the list of high suspicion sonographic features. In addition, only marked, but not mild, hypoechogenicity was included in the list. High suspicion features were specifically defined as irregular shape, irregular borders, marked hypoechogenicity, microcalcifications, and, if available, high stiffness on elastography, but elastography was not considered prerequisite for this TIRADS classification. Mild hypoechogenicity in the absence of high suspicion features was categorized as TIRADS 4a. The presence of only one or two high suspicion features led to a TIRADS 4b category, but once three or more features were present, the nodule was classified as TIRADS 5. This system was validated in a prospective 2-year study of 4550 nodules (4.5% prevalence of thyroid cancer) that underwent US FNA. In addition, the authors estimated a 34% reduction in the number of FNAs if biopsy was not recommended for stable TIRADS 2 and 3 nodules [8].

Recognizing that the current TIRADS classifications have originated from individual institutions and none have been widely adapted in the United States, the American College of Radiology (ACR) has prioritized development of a TIRADS system, with the ultimate aim of applying it to risk stratification and triage of nodules for FNA or observation [15]. The initial step of the committee charged with this project was to develop a lexicon of defined sonographic features demonstrated to be consistently associated with either benignity or malignancy, which could be used to describe every thyroid lesion. The lexicon contains six ultrasound categories: composition, echogenicity, shape as taller than wide, size based upon maximal diameter, margins, and echogenic foci. Each category contains terms describing the varied appearances within that category, with discussion of the associated malignancy risk. The purpose of the lexicon is to develop a structured method for nodule evaluation and to decrease the variation of thyroid nodule reporting currently seen in the radiology practices in the United States. Although the authors recognized that nodule size is not generally correlated with cancer risk, the purpose of its inclusion is for the future development of ACR Guidelines for thyroid nodule management. The next step of this project, currently underway, includes statistical validation of the lexicon reporting system; therefore, this ACR TIRADS is still under development and not ready for clinical application.

The current 2015 American Thyroid Association (ATA) Management Guidelines for Adult Patients with Thyroid Nodules and Differentiated Thyroid Cancer sought to make pattern recognition more straightforward and reproducible for physicians who perform sonography on patients in their practices [16]. The ATA task force recognized the existence of three competing TIRADS systems, none of which has achieved universal adoption, as well as their perceived complexity by non-radiologists. The ATA Guidelines provide an "atlas" that offers examples of 15 sonographic nodule images and one image of sonographically suspicious lateral cervical lymph node. These 16 images are divided into five defined categories of sonographic patterns with associated cancer risks to triage nodules for FNA with recommendations for either surveillance or FNA with nodule size cutoffs (Fig. 14.1, Table 14.2). The patterns in each category were derived from a graded evidence-based literature review. The benign category includes the pure cyst, and FNA is not recommended, unless performed for therapeutic drainage. The very low suspicion patterns (cancer risk estimate <3 %) are spongiform nodules and mixed cystic solid nodules without high suspicion features defined as irregular (infiltrative, microlobulated) margins, microcalcifications, taller-than-wide shape, interrupted rim calcifications with small extrusive soft tissue component, evidence of extrathyroidal extension, or sonographically suspicious cervical lymph nodes. Low suspicion nodules (cancer risk estimate 5–10 %) include iso- or hyperechoic solid nodules or partially cystic nodules with eccentric solid areas without high suspicion features. Cancer risk increases to 10–20 % for intermediate suspicion nodules that are smoothly marginated, hypoechoic, and solid. The frequency of cancer is highest (>70–90 %) for the high suspicion category that includes solid hypoechoic nodules or solid hypoechoic component of a partially cystic nodule with any of the high suspicion features. Sonographic assessment of cervical lymph nodes is also prerequisite for all imaging as the presence of suspicious lymph nodules mandates FNA of the lymph node regardless of nodule pattern. Recommended FNA size cutoffs are smaller, 1 cm, for the patterns more likely to be associated with cancer and then increase as the likelihood of malignancy decreases, such that for the very low suspicion pattern observation may suffice.

A 2016 publication compared the diagnostic performance of the Korean TIRADS system [12] with the ATA 2015 sonographic patterns in a retrospective analysis of 1293 supracentimetric nodules that underwent US FNA with 234 (18.1 %) detected cancers [17]. Of note, only 44 (3.4 %) nodules could not be classified into one of the ATA patterns and included iso- or hyperechoic nodules with either irregular margins, microcalcifications, or taller-than-wide shape; eight (18.4 %) were cancers. This chapter author (SM), also an author of the ATA Guidelines, appreciates the provided descriptions of the nonclassifiable nodules. The sonographic images incorporated in the ATA Guidelines required evidence-based associations with cancer from literature review. The ATA authors recognized that, although from clinical experience certain patterns indicated high-risk nodules, there was insufficient evidence to include these. Specifically, the excluded patterns were the non-hypoechoic types: isoechoic or hyperechoic nodules with high suspicion features. This 2016

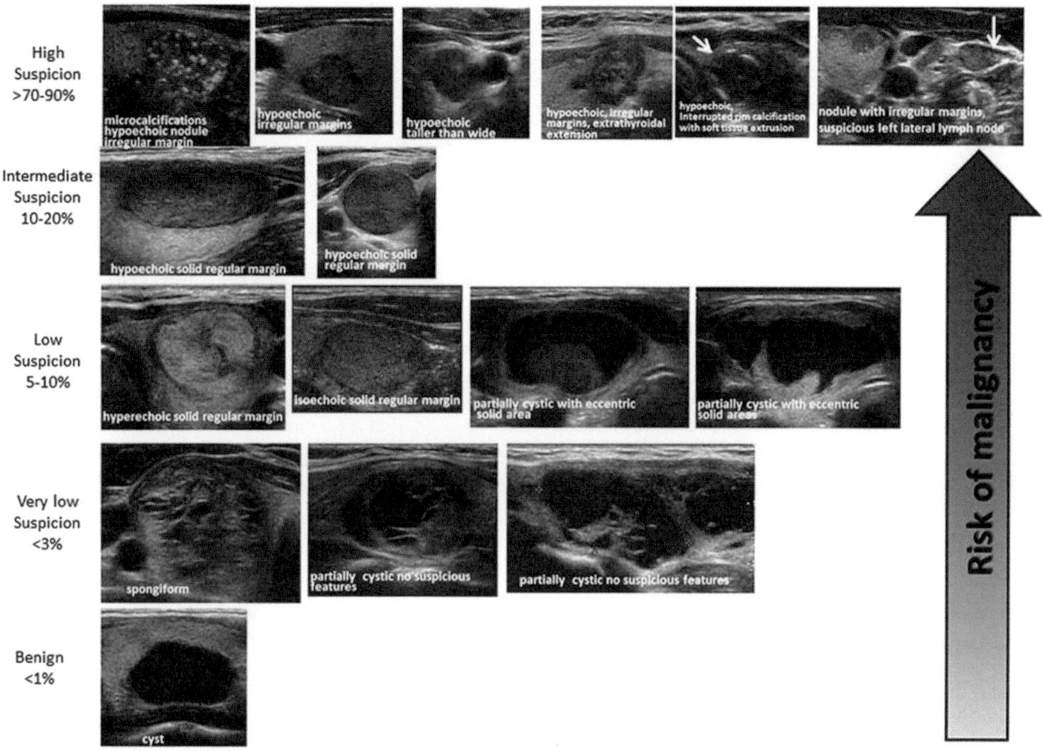

Fig. 14.1 American Thyroid Association nodule sonographic patterns and risk of malignancy

report confirms the significant cancer risk of these patterns, similar to that for ATA intermediate suspicion nodules. Overall, the Korean TIRADS and ATA classifications were highly correlated. In addition, using the classification-specific indications for FNA (TIRADS-FNA for 4a, 4b, 4c, and 5; ATA-FNA based upon pattern and size cutoff), the sensitivity for cancer detection was >95 %, and the yield of cancer was high, diagnosed in about 25 % of all nodules meeting respective FNA criteria. In addition, the negative predictive value was >97 % indicating that the ~25 % of nodules excluded from FNA in both systems are unlikely to be malignant [17].

The most recently introduced pattern scheme originates from the American Association of Clinical Endocrinologists (AACE) in collaboration with the Italian Associazione Medici Endocrinologi (AME) [18]. This is a three-tiered pattern classification, also with recommendation for either surveillance or FNA at size cutoffs determined by cancer risk (Fig. 14.2). Low-risk nodules (cancer risk estimate 1 %) include spongiform nodules and nodules that are more than 50 % cystic nodules without suspicious features. These suspicious features are the same as those identified in the ATA Guidelines, with two differences: only marked, not mild, hypoechogenicity is included and interrupted rim calcifications with a soft tissue excrescence are not. Intermediate risk (cancer risk estimate 5–15 %) includes both mildly hypoechoic and isoechoic solid nodules with either smooth or ill-defined margins and stillness on elastography if available. High-risk lesions (estimated cancer risk 50–90 %) have one of the suspicious features. This three-tiered classification of nodule sonographic patterns is similar to prior systems and telescopes some of the ATA patterns. The AACE/AME three-level system telescopes some of the five levels of the ATA classification as indicated in Table 14.3.

The current landscape of sonographic patterns is confusing; no one classification system is universally accepted, and the ACR will likely

Table 14.2 ATA 2015 sonographic patterns, estimated risk of malignancy, and FNA guidance for thyroid nodules

Sonographic pattern	US features	Estimated malignancy risk (%)	FNA size cutoff (largest dimension)	TIRADS corresponding classification
Benign	Purely cystic nodules (no solid component)	<1	No biopsy[a]	TIRADS 2 Horvath, Kwak, Russ
Very low suspicion	Spongiform or partially cystic nodules *without* any of the sonographic features described in low, intermediate, or high suspicion patterns	<3	Consider FNA at ≥2 cm	TIRADS 2 Horvath, Russ
			Observation without FNA is also a reasonable option	TIRADS 2 or 3 Kwak
Low suspicion	Isoechoic or hyperechoic solid nodule, or partially cystic nodule with eccentric solid areas, *without* microcalcification, irregular margin or extrathyroidal extension, or taller-than-wide shape	5–10	Recommend FNA at ≥1.5 cm	TIRADS 3 Russ TIRADS 4a Horvath, Kwak
Intermediate suspicion	Hypoechoic solid nodule with smooth margins without microcalcifications, extrathyroidal extension, or taller-than-wide shape	10–20	Recommend FNA at >1 cm	TIRADS 4a Horvath, Russ TIRADS 4b Kwak
High suspicion	Solid hypoechoic nodule or solid hypoechoic component of a partially cystic nodule *with* one or more of the following features: irregular margins (infiltrative, microlobulated), microcalcifications, taller-than-wide shape, rim calcifications with small extrusive soft tissue component, evidence of extrathyroidal extension	>70–90[b]	Recommend FNA at ≥1 cm	TIRADS 4b, 5 Horvath, Russ TIRADS 4c, 5 Kwak

US-guided FNA is recommended for cervical lymph nodes that are sonographically suspicious for thyroid cancer
[a]Aspiration of the cyst may be considered for symptomatic or cosmetic drainage
[b]The estimate is derived from high-volume centers; the overall risk of malignancy may be lower given the interobserver variability in sonography
Adapted from Table 6 ref. [16]
Horvath ref. [9], Russ ref. [8], Kwak ref. [12]

introduce its own TIRADS in the near future. There are commonalities among the systems that serve to address the most frequently encountered US appearances of nodules. However, more data is needed to risk stratify nodules that cannot be currently classified in some or all of the systems. This includes nodules with isolated macrocalcifications which may be linear or dystrophic and solid nodules with mixed echogenicity. For example, none of the classification systems address whether a macrocalcification alters the cancer risk of a spongiform or isoechoic smoothly marginated nodule based upon its grayscale parenchymal pattern.

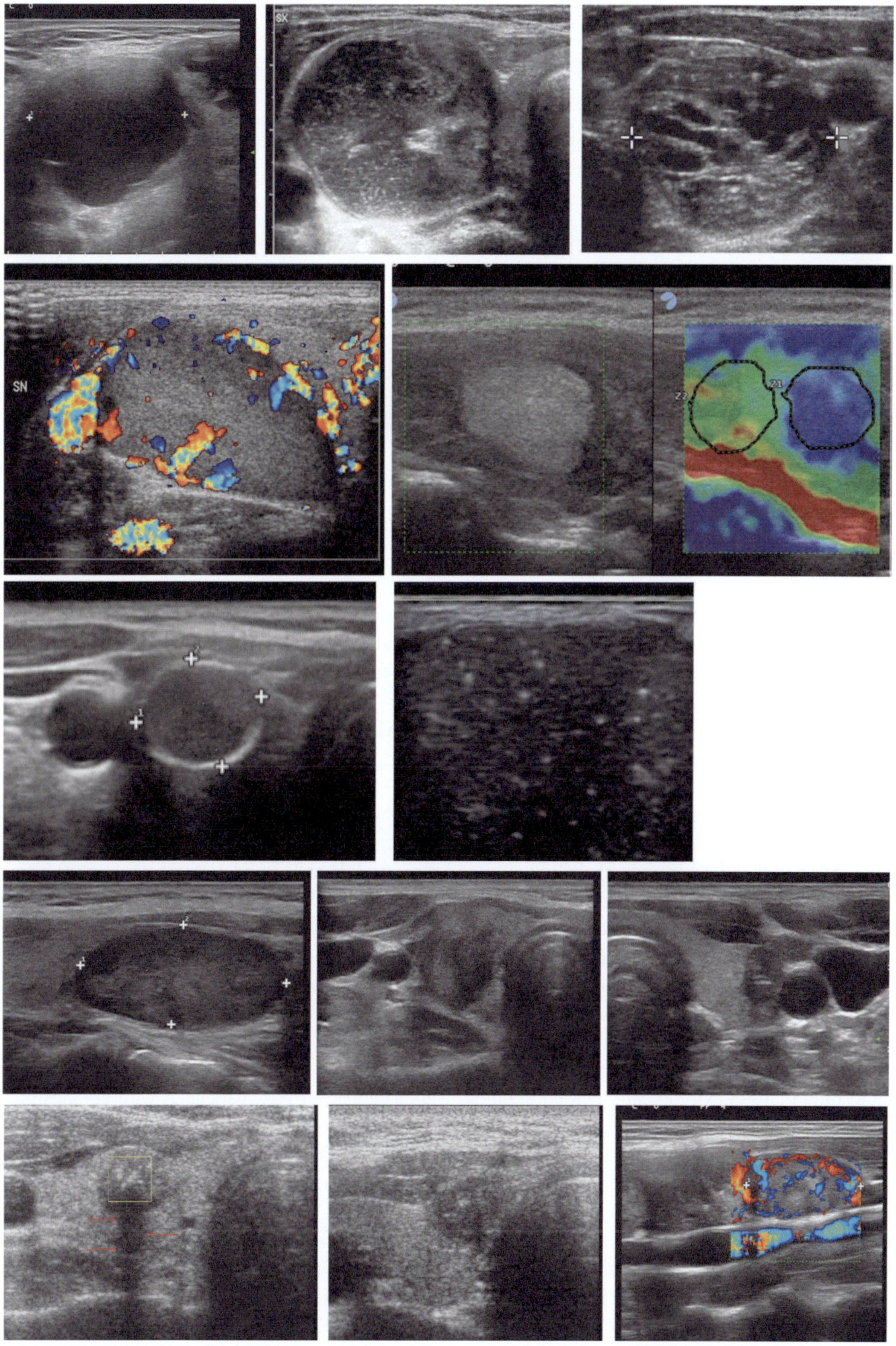

Fig. 14.2 AACE/AME Thyroid Ultrasound Features and Risk of Malignancy. Reprinted from Endocrine Practice, 2016; 22: 622–639, with permission from the American Association of Clinical Endocrinologists

Table 14.3 Comparison of 5-tiered ATA sonographic patterns with 3-tiered AACE/AME risk lesions

ATA 2015 Ref. [16]	AACE/AME 2016 Ref. [18]
Benign Pure cyst	**Low risk** Cysts Most cystic nodules not associated with suspicious US features Isoechoic spongiform nodules
Very low suspicion Spongiform or partially cystic nodules *without* any of the sonographic features described in low, intermediate or high suspicion patterns	
Low suspicion Isoechoic or hyperechoic solid nodule, or partially cystic nodule with eccentric solid areas, *without* microcalcification, irregular margin or extrathyroidal extension, or taller than wide shape	**Intermediate risk** Slightly hypoechoic or isoechoic nodules with ovoid or round shape, with smooth or ill-defined margins May have intranodular vascularity, stiffness on elastography, continuous rim calcifications
Intermediate suspicion Hypoechoic solid nodule with smooth margins *without* microcalcifications, extrathyroidal extension, or taller than wide shape	
High suspicion Solid hypoechoic nodule or solid hypoechoic component of a partially cystic nodule *with* one or more of the following features: irregular margins (infiltrative, microlobulated), microcalcifications, taller than wide shape, rim calcifications with small extrusive soft tissue component, evidence of extrathyroidal extension	**High risk** Nodules with at least one of the following features: Marked hypoechogenicity, speculated or microlobulated margins, microcalcifications, taller than wide shape, extrathyroidal growth

14.3 Application of Sonographic Patterns

With the existence of sonographic pattern classification systems, the question arises of how these can be applied not just to FNA decision-making but to potentially modify cancer risks associated with the Bethesda cytology diagnoses and hence better triage patients for surgery. Prior work has demonstrated that the presence of individual suspicious sonographic characteristics may increase a nodule's cancer risk over that conferred by benign, indeterminate, or nondiagnostic cytologic diagnoses [19–21]. Using the Kwak TIRADS classification, several papers have combined sonographic patterns with cytologic diagnoses to refine a nodule's estimated cancer risk. In a study of 1398 cytologically benign nodules, the false-negative rate based upon cytology alone was only ~1 % for TIRADS 3, 4a, and 4b nodules but was considerably higher, 9.8 % and 22 %, respectively, for TIRADS 4c and 5 nodules [22]. Therefore, repeat US-guided FNA should be considered for benign thyroid nodules with three or more suspicious US features (TIRADS 4c or 5). Similarly, the Kwak TIRADS classification has been shown to modify the cancer risk in nodules with a cytologic diagnosis of follicular neoplasm. Although the overall cancer rate was 24 % for 497 such nodules, risk increased with advanced score—TIRADS 4a 14.3 %, TIRADS 4b 23.1 %, TIRADS 4c 87.5 %, and TIRADS 5 100 % [23]. This may influence recommendations for immediate surgery or extent of surgery versus potential molecular testing. For 294 cytologically nondiagnostic nodules larger than 1 cm, the malignancy rates of TIRADS 3 and 4a were very low, 0.8 and 1.3 %, indicating that repeat FNA is unnecessary. However, for TIRADS 4b, 4c, and 5, the rates were 6.1 %, 14.4 %, and 31 %, respectively, thus suggesting that nodules with more than one suspicious US feature should undergo additional sampling [24].

In addition, TIRADS sonographic patterns may alter the cancer risk associated with nodules that have increased uptake on ^{18}F-fluorodeoxyglucose positron emission/computed tomography (^{18}FDG-PET/CT) scans. Overall, approximately one in three (35 %) ^{18}FDG-PET-positive thyroid nodules proves to be cancerous [25]. In a Korean study of 87 nodules incidentally detected with increased ^{18}FDG uptake, cancer rates of 9 %, 15 %, 39 %, 72 %, and 100 % were reported for TIRADS 3, 4a, 4b, 4c, and 5, respectively [26]. In addition, for these ^{18}FDG-avid nodules, the cancer risk was higher in each TIRADS category compared to the reference risk for that pattern. Hence US FNA should be performed for ^{18}FDG-avid nodules even if no suspicious US features are present, such as in TIRADS 3 nodules.

14.4 Conclusion

Operationalizing the TIRADS system, with decisions about when to recommend FNA, is critical to its performance. Current analyses of the diagnostic performance of the TIRADS systems to identify malignancy, with calculation of sensitivities, specificities, likelihood ratios, diagnostic odds ratios, and receiver-operator curves, are predicated on binary decision-making for FNA based upon a given sonographic pattern without modification by nodule size. This means that a TIRADS 3 nodule does not undergo FNA, but FNA is performed for all TIRADS 4 nodules. However, there are already discrepancies in TIRADS application in practice with some groups performing FNA for TIRADS 3 lesions [27].

In addition, since none of the TIRADS systems to date apply nodule size cutoffs to modify FNA decision-making for a certain TIRADS category, this means that more potentially clinically indolent thyroid cancers representing a reservoir of disease may be diagnosed [28, 29]. These clinically indolent cancers may include subcentimeter classic papillary thyroid cancers that image as TIRADS 4 or 5 [28] or supracentimeter follicular variants of papillary cancers or even noninvasive follicular thyroid neoplasms with papillary-like nuclear features (NIFTP) [30, 31]. The goal of nodule identification for FNA is not simply identification of cancer itself, but rather cancers that are potentially clinically relevant. Therefore, FNA of a higher suspicion TIRADS 4 or TIRADS 5 subcentimeter nodule, in the absence imaging suspicion for extrathyroidal extension or sonographically identified and cytologically confirmed lymph node metastases, may not be considered to have clinical utility as the vast majority of these small cancers do not progress, especially in older individuals [32].

The application of any ultrasound pattern classification to FNA decision-making needs to include more than sonographic risk stratification; nodule size and the clinical context must be considered. For example, a patient may have a personal risks associated with a higher likelihood of thyroid cancer, e.g., neck irradiation during childhood, family history of follicular cell-derived thyroid cancer in two or more first-degree relatives, or a genetic syndrome like Cowden's [16]. Therefore, different size cutoffs for FNA should be applied based upon both sonographic and individualized risk. The clinical utility of the current systems, including consideration of nodule size and patient history, requires prospective and pragmatic validation in other populations. Decision-making by sonographic pattern alone is not sufficient.

References

1. Moon WJ, Jung SL, Lee JH, Na DG, Baek JH, Lee YH, et al. Benign and malignant thyroid nodules: US differentiation--multicenter retrospective study. Radiology. 2008;247(3):762–70.
2. Papini E, Guglielmi R, Bianchini A, Crescenzi A, Taccogna S, Nardi F, et al. Risk of malignancy in non-palpable thyroid nodules: predictive value of ultrasound and color-Doppler features. J Clin Endocrinol Metab. 2002;87(5):1941–6.
3. Cappelli C, Castellano M, Pirola I, Cumetti D, Agosti B, Gandossi E, et al. The predictive value of ultrasound findings in the management of thyroid nodules. QJM. 2007;100(1):29–35.
4. Brito JP, Gionfriddo MR, Al Nofal A, Boehmer KR, Leppin AL, Reading C, et al. The accuracy of thyroid nodule ultrasound to predict thyroid cancer: systematic review and meta-analysis. J Clin Endocrinol Metab. 2014;99(4):1253–63.
5. Remonti LR, Kramer CK, Leitao CB, Pinto LC, Gross JL. Thyroid ultrasound features and risk of carcinoma: a systematic review and meta-analysis of observational studies. Thyroid. 2015;25(5):538–50.
6. Choi SH, Kim EK, Kwak JY, Kim MJ, Son EJ. Interobserver and intraobserver variations in ultrasound assessment of thyroid nodules. Thyroid. 2010;20(2):167–72.
7. Ko SY, Kim EK, Moon HJ, Yoon JH, Kim HY, Kwak JY. Application of thyroid imaging reporting and data system in the ultrasound assessment of thyroid

nodules according to physician experience. Ultrasound Q. 2016;32(2):126–31.
8. Russ G, Royer B, Bigorgne C, Rouxel A, Bienvenu-Perrard M, Leenhardt L. Prospective evaluation of thyroid imaging reporting and data system on 4550 nodules with and without elastography. Eur J Endocrinol. 2013;168(5):649–55.
9. Horvath E, Majlis S, Rossi R, Franco C, Niedmann JP, Castro A, et al. An ultrasonogram reporting system for thyroid nodules stratifying cancer risk for clinical management. J Clin Endocrinol Metab. 2009;94(5): 1748–51.
10. Reading CC, Charboneau JW, Hay ID, Sebo TJ. Sonography of thyroid nodules: a "classic pattern" diagnostic approach. Ultrasound Q. 2005;21(3):157–65.
11. Park JY, Lee HJ, Jang HW, Kim HK, Yi JH, Lee W, et al. A proposal for a thyroid imaging reporting and data system for ultrasound features of thyroid carcinoma. Thyroid. 2009;19(11):1257–64.
12. Kwak JY, Han KH, Yoon JH, Moon HJ, Son EJ, Park SH, et al. Thyroid imaging reporting and data system for US features of nodules: a step in establishing better stratification of cancer risk. Radiology. 2011;260(3):892–9.
13. Kwak JY, Jung I, Baek JH, Baek SM, Choi N, Choi YJ, et al. Image reporting and characterization system for ultrasound features of thyroid nodules: multicentric Korean retrospective study. Korean J Radiol. 2013;14(1):110–7.
14. Russ G. Risk stratification of thyroid nodules on ultrasonography with the French TI-RADS: description and reflections. Ultrasonography. 2016;35(1):25–38.
15. Grant EG, Tessler FN, Hoang JK, Langer JE, Beland MD, Berland LL, et al. Thyroid ultrasound reporting lexicon: white paper of the ACR Thyroid Imaging, Reporting and Data System (TIRADS) Committee. J Am Coll Radiol. 2015;12(12 Pt A):1272–9.
16. Haugen BR, Alexander EK, Bible KC, Doherty GM, Mandel SJ, Nikiforov YE, et al. 2015 American Thyroid Association Management Guidelines for adult patients with thyroid nodules and differentiated thyroid cancer: the American Thyroid Association guidelines task force on thyroid nodules and differentiated thyroid cancer. Thyroid. 2016;26(1):1–133.
17. Yoon JH, Lee HS, Kim EK, Moon HJ, Kwak JY. Malignancy risk stratification of thyroid nodules: comparison between the thyroid imaging reporting and data system and the 2014 American Thyroid Association management guidelines. Radiology. 2016;278(3):917–24.
18. Gharib H, Papini E, Garber JR, Duick DS, Harrell RM, Hegedus L, et al. American Association of Clinical Endocrinologists, American College Of Endocrinology, And Associazione Medici Endocrinologi Medical guidelines for clinical practice for the diagnosis and management of thyroid nodules - 2016 update. Endocr Pract. 2016;22(5):622–39.
19. Rosario PW. Thyroid nodules with atypia or follicular lesions of undetermined significance (Bethesda Category III): importance of ultrasonography and cytological subcategory. Thyroid. 2014;24(7):1115–20.
20. Kim SY, Han KH, Moon HJ, Kwak JY, Chung WY, Kim EK. Thyroid nodules with benign findings at cytologic examination: results of long-term follow-up with US. Radiology. 2014;271(1):272–81.
21. Kim DW, Lee EJ, Lee JH. Role of ultrasound diagnosis in assessing and managing thyroid nodules with inadequate cytology. AJR Am J Roentgenol. 2011;197(5): 1213–9.
22. Moon HJ, Kim EK, Kwak JY. Malignancy risk stratification in thyroid nodules with benign results on cytology: combination of thyroid imaging reporting and data system and Bethesda system. Ann Surg Oncol. 2014;21(6):1898–903.
23. Chng CL, Kurzawinski TR, Beale T. Value of sonographic features in predicting malignancy in thyroid nodules diagnosed as follicular neoplasm on cytology. Clin Endocrinol (Oxf). 2015;83(5):711–6.
24. Moon HJ, Kim EK, Yoon JH, Kwak JY. Malignancy risk stratification in thyroid nodules with nondiagnostic results at cytologic examination: combination of thyroid imaging reporting and data system and the Bethesda System. Radiology. 2015;274(1):287–95.
25. Soelberg KK, Bonnema SJ, Brix TH, Hegedus L. Risk of malignancy in thyroid incidentalomas detected by 18F-fluorodeoxyglucose positron emission tomography: a systematic review. Thyroid. 2012;22(9):918–25.
26. Yoon JH, Cho A, Lee HS, Kim EK, Moon HJ, Kwak JY. Thyroid incidentalomas detected on 18F-fluorodeoxyglucose-positron emission tomography/computed tomography: Thyroid Imaging Reporting and Data System (TIRADS) in the diagnosis and management of patients. Surgery. 2015; 158(5):1314–22.
27. Wei X, Li Y, Zhang S, Gao M. Meta-analysis of thyroid imaging reporting and data system in the ultrasonographic diagnosis of 10,437 thyroid nodules. Head Neck. 2016;38(2):309–15.
28. Davies L, Welch HG. Current thyroid cancer trends in the United States. JAMA Otolaryngol Head Neck Surg. 2014;140(4):317–22.
29. Welch HG, Black WC. Overdiagnosis in cancer. J Natl Cancer Inst. 2010;102(9):605–13.
30. Nikiforov YE, Seethala RR, Tallini G, Baloch ZW, Basolo F, Thompson LD, et al. Nomenclature revision for encapsulated follicular variant of papillary thyroid carcinoma: a paradigm shift to reduce overtreatment of indolent tumors. JAMA Oncol. 2016;2:1023.
31. Kim DS, Kim JH, Na DG, Park SH, Kim E, Chang KH, et al. Sonographic features of follicular variant papillary thyroid carcinomas in comparison with conventional papillary thyroid carcinomas. J Ultrasound Med. 2009;28(12):1685–92.
32. Miyauchi A. Clinical trials of active surveillance of papillary microcarcinoma of the thyroid. World J Surg. 2016;40(3):516–22.

15 Challenges in Pattern Recognition: Navigating Assessment of Thyroid Features and the Subjectivity of Ultrasound Interpretation

Yufei Chen and Sareh Parangi

15.1 Introduction

It is clear that radiologic imaging is becoming increasingly influential in patient care in general. Application of ultrasound to imaging of the thyroid began in the late 1960s and has revolutionized the care of patients with thyroid diseases [1]. It is fair to say that clinicians taking care of patients with thyroid diseases cannot take care of patients without ultrasound. Furthermore, recent advances in ultrasound technologies such as harmonic imaging, spatial compound imaging, contrast studies, three-dimensional reconstruction, and elastography have furthered the field. While ultrasound is often associated with operator dependency, ultimately pattern recognition is the key feature when this technology is used by clinicians. In particular, pattern recognition in radiology is based on recognizing anatomical and physiological appearances on an image and identifying what is normal and how variations from these appearances can represent pathology. This skill requires considerable experience both in the interpretation and acquisition of images. The clinician uses mental extraction of the texture features and then correlates significant texture features with biologic behavior.

Over the last two decades, many studies have evaluated sonographic features as predictors of malignancy. Unfortunately the vast majority of these studies utilize a variety of classification criteria, techniques, and operators, but certain elements of the ultrasound exam have evolved to be considered particularly helpful. Most authors recognized that the use of individual features to predict malignancy was limited due to low sensitivity or specificity of these features alone. Some authors then advocated a change of approach to teach clinicians to recognize specific patterns rather than individual ultrasound features to help separate nodules requiring biopsy from those that might be safely observed [2, 3]. Seven ultrasound components that when combined aid the surgeon in pattern recognition are hypoechogenicity; irregular margins; microcalcifications; anteroposterior to transverse diameter ratio, i.e., "taller than wide" on transverse view; intranodular vascularity; size; and significant growth. Each of these will be separately discussed at later points in this book in detail; here we focus on the challenge, that is, pattern recognition by clinicians performing or evaluating ultrasounds during the routine care of thyroid patients. Familiarity with the

Y. Chen, M.D. (✉)
Department of Surgery, Massachusetts General Hospital, Harvard Medical School,
55 Fruit St, GRB-425, Boston, MA 02114, USA
e-mail: ychen49@partners.org

S. Parangi, M.D.
Department of Surgery, Massachusetts General Hospital, Harvard Medical School, 15 Parkman Street, Suite 460, Boston, MA 02114, USA
e-mail: sparangi@partners.org

M. Milas et al. (eds.), *Advanced Thyroid and Parathyroid Ultrasound*,
DOI 10.1007/978-3-319-44100-9_15

Table 15.1 Summary of 2015 ATA Guidelines for sonographic patterns and their estimated risk of malignancy

Sonographic pattern	US features	Estimated risk of malignancy, %	FNA done for diagnosis size cutoff (largest dimension)
High suspicion	Solid hypoechoic nodule or solid hypoechoic component of a partially cystic nodule with one or more of the following features: irregular margins (infiltrative, microlobulated), microcalcifications, taller-than-wide shape, rim calcifications with small extrusive soft tissue component, evidence of extrathyroidal extension	>70–90	Recommend FNA at ≥1 cm
Intermediate suspicion	Hypoechoic solid thyroid nodule with smooth margins without microcalcifications, ETE, or taller-than-wide shape	10–20	Recommend FNA at ≥1 cm
Low suspicion	Isoechoic or hyperechoic solid nodule or partially cystic nodule with eccentric solid areas, without microcalcification, irregular margin or ETE, or taller-than-wide shape	5–10	Recommend FNA at ≥1.5 cm
Very low suspicion	Spongiform or partially cystic thyroid nodules without any of the sonographic features described in low, intermediate, or high suspicion patterns	<3	Consider FNA at ≥2 cm Observation without FNA is also a reasonable option
Benign	Purely cystic thyroid nodules (no solid component)	<1	No biopsy

Adapted from ATA Guidelines 2015 Table 6 (Ref. [5])

new clinical guidelines and use of algorithms for decision-making on a particular nodule is imperative for practical, safe, and cost-effective care of patients. These guidelines (represented in Table 15.1 and Fig. 15.1) use the best available data from studies of "ultrasound patterns" and size thresholds to help clinical decision-making [4, 5]. Good clinical judgment cannot be replaced by a single sonographic feature or combination of features since ultrasound alone cannot identify all malignancies with a high degree of sensitivity [6].

15.2 Challenge #1: Wide Spectrum of Practitioners Performing Thyroid Ultrasound

Practitioners who perform and interpret thyroid ultrasound range from radiologists to surgeons and endocrinologists. Each of these specialists brings their own background and experience into image interpretation and may perform ultrasound for different reasons. These reasons include diagnosis of thyroid nodules, localization for biopsy, or assessment of characteristics to assist in surgical planning (e.g., proximity to the recurrent laryngeal nerve or malignant involvement of lymph nodes). Furthermore, some practitioners may interpret the images in real time, while others retrospectively view saved cine-images acquired by a technician. This heterogeneity brings with it challenges in the standardized assessment of thyroid nodules. The level of adequacy of training for radiology residents in ultrasound has been addressed in multiple studies. One of the main issues for the radiologist appears to be lack of detailed anatomic knowledge and an overall inability to identify key anatomic landmarks [7].

Most clinicians who use ultrasound in their practices who are not radiologists will learn

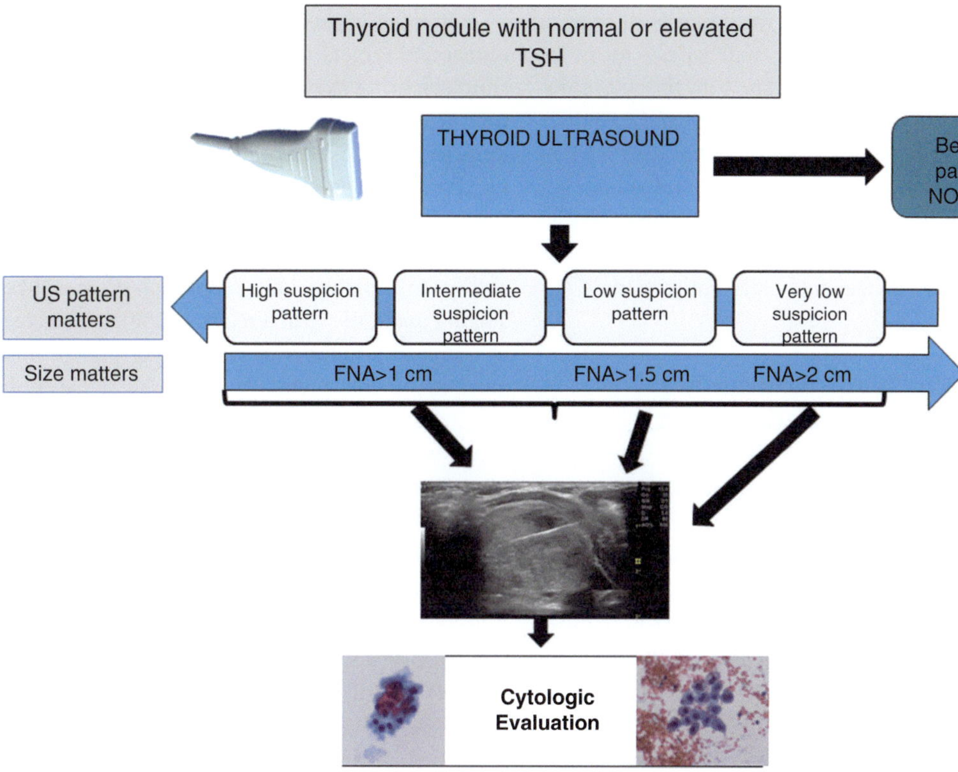

Fig. 15.1 Thyroid nodule with normal or elevated TSH

enough ultrasound skills to be able to provide a careful and systematic assessment of the thyroid and surrounding structures during their daily practice. Precisely because they are not radiologists, they bring unique additional skills that aid in the care of the patient. For the endocrinologist this added value includes knowing the basics of the endocrine diseases that are affecting any particular patient's thyroid, often including a longitudinal relationship with the patient and their long-standing endocrine history as well as laboratory and biomarker values. Surgeons who use ultrasound have the additional benefit of being able to correlate ultrasound findings with intraoperative findings which over time provide an impressive learning tool for correlating pathology, anatomy, and ultrasound images. Of course, the training these clinicians have cannot replace the long and arduous training which a radiologist undergoes, but with adequate time commitments, non-radiologist clinicians can come to recognize the most important patterns in thyroid ultrasound that are commonly seen in their patients.

Unfortunately training of non-radiologist specialists in ultrasound at this time is not an integral process of the training in general surgery or head and neck surgery or medical specialties such as endocrinology. Other residencies such as Obstetrics and Gynecology have successfully integrated ultrasound training into their programs for more than a decade. Efforts to include ultrasound training during surgical residency or fellowship are ongoing. Postgraduate thyroid ultrasound courses are available from multiple organizations in the United States: examples include The American Association of Clinical Endocrinologist, the American College of Surgeons, and the American Academy of Otolaryngology Head and Neck Surgery. Most of these organizations offer 1–2-day courses including didactics and hands-on practice sessions. Furthermore, some of these organizations have created programs with the American Institute of Ultrasound in Medicine to create a voluntary peer review process after which initial accreditation is given enough for a 3-year period.

Clinician performance in the tasks of pattern recognition in ultrasound will surely be influenced by various factors such as fatigue, emotion, reading time, environment, and previous biases. These factors have not been well studied in non-radiologists performing ultrasound, but clinicians should try to minimize fatigue and distractions that will influence their ability to formulate complex images into clear-cut patterns.

15.3 Challenge #2: Training in Pattern Recognition

Practically speaking, basic ultrasound course offerings do not provide an extensive experience in pattern recognition of common thyroid ultrasound findings. While there is no consensus on how many examinations are required to achieve an acceptable level of competency with head and neck ultrasound, several studies focusing on the learning curve in ultrasound examinations have established that approximately 25–50 focused examinations are needed to achieve greater than 90 % concordance with a radiologist interpretation of the same examination [7, 8]. One article recently addressed the issue of observer experience in the evaluation of thyroid malignancy and lymph node metastases. Moon et al. looked at the use of ultrasound by clinicians with less than 2 years of experience versus greater than 7 years of experience in preoperative ultrasound staging in 1421 patients. Preoperative staging ultrasound included an assessment for extrathyroidal extension and ultrasound features of lymph node metastasis, including shape, echogenicity, microcalcifications, cystic change, and vascularity. Their data showed that the two groups differed only in their ability to assess the lateral neck compartment lymph node involvement with the more experienced group showing a 64 % ability to correctly diagnose lateral nodal involvement versus 39 % for the less experienced group [9]. The complexity generated when combining these individual factors into various clinical possibilities requires the practitioner to be well versed in recognizing multiple patterns of pathology, which requires extensive practice and experience.

A number of methods are used to characterize ultrasound targets including pattern recognition, simple scoring systems, and complex classification systems, some of which use mathematical models. Some of these models have been elaborated on in the previous chapter on risk stratification strategies. The technological ability to acquire higher and higher resolution and thus the ability to reliably and reproducibly visualize smaller anatomic structures have come at the cost of increasing number of images per patient that need to be interpreted and mentally analyzed. Pattern recognition training by individuals happens over time and evolves from looking for patterns in a particular nodule to looking at patterns in the entire examination. An example of combining individual features to see the "pattern of a malignant nodule" is shown in Fig. 15.2. An example of combining individual features of an entire thyroid ultrasound to recognize a "pattern of aggressive malignancy" is shown in Fig. 15.3.

In addition, post-ultrasound activities such as analyzing gross and pathologic specimens and comparing them to the ultrasound images will result in dramatically improved clinical judgment over time (see Figs. 15.3 and 15.4, e.g., of how this kind of correlation helps clinicians).

15.4 Challenge #3: Recognizing the Pattern of Benign Nodules

Combining ultrasound features to predict benignity is included in all recent thyroid nodule guidelines since they impart the largest cost saving when applied over large populations [5]. For example, on a group of patients with a prevalence of thyroid cancer set at 10 %, 1000 nodules lacking the future features of hypoechogenicity, taller-than-wide shape, calcifications, and irregular borders would have to be biopsied to detect ten cancers. Pure cysts, small <1 cm colloid-filled cystic nodules, "white knights" (diffuse hyperechoic nodule in the setting of Hashimoto's), and spongiform nodules meet these criteria in multiple studies, and thus most society guidelines report that the chance of malignancy in these nod-

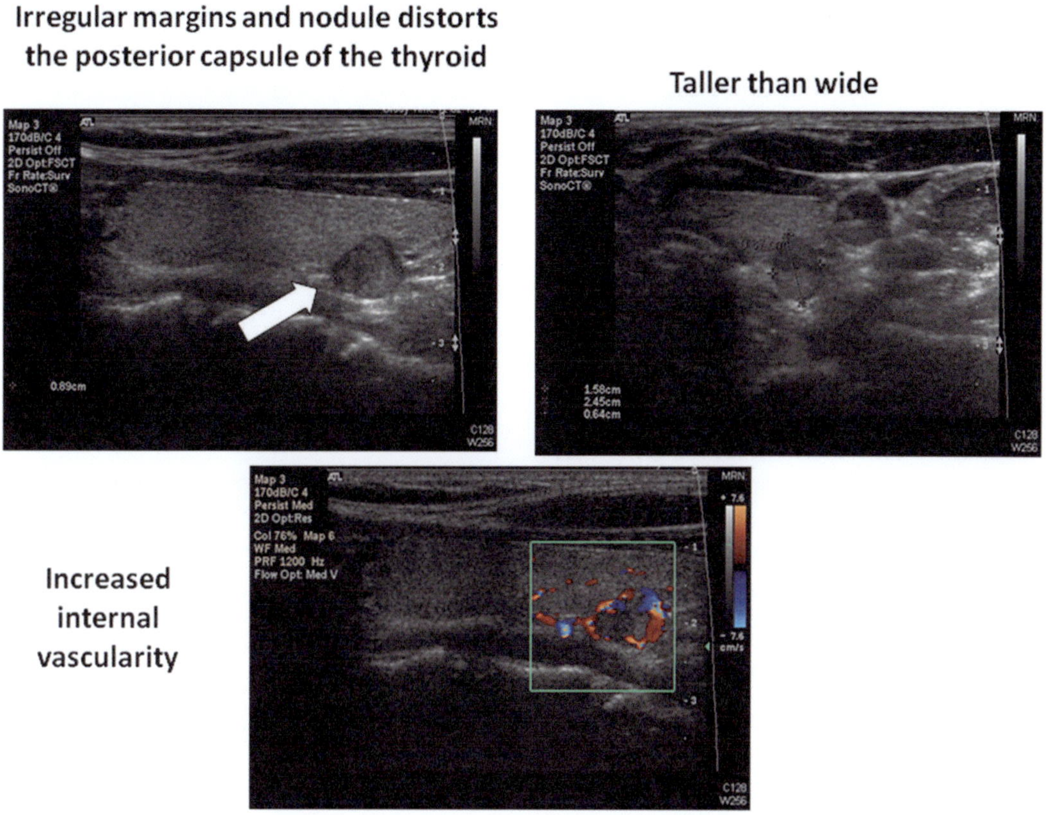

Fig. 15.2 Pattern recognition: combining individual features helps recognize thyroid nodule as malignant

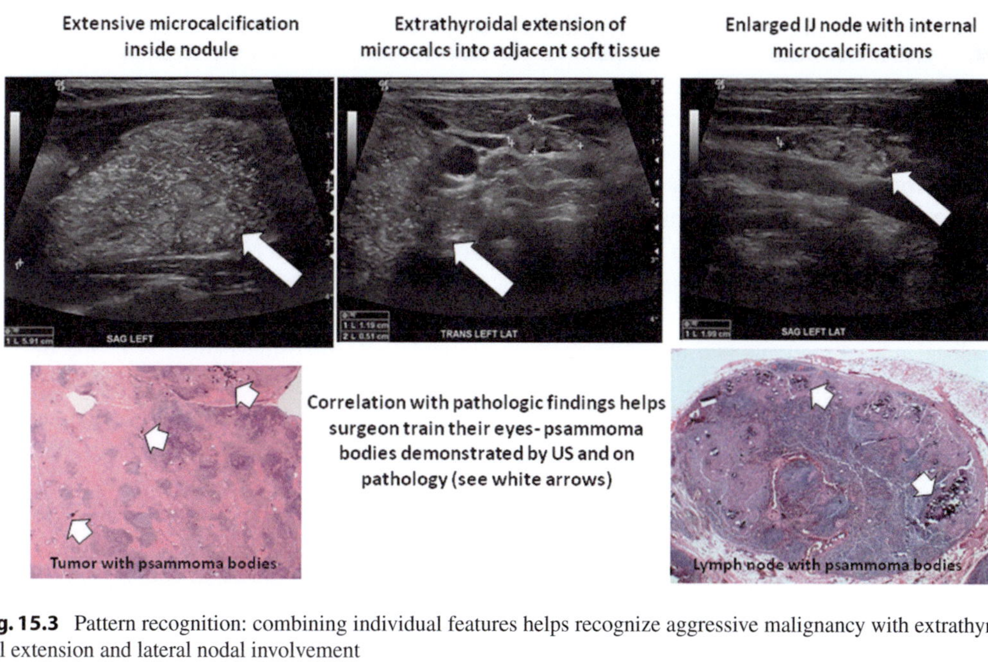

Fig. 15.3 Pattern recognition: combining individual features helps recognize aggressive malignancy with extrathyroidal extension and lateral nodal involvement

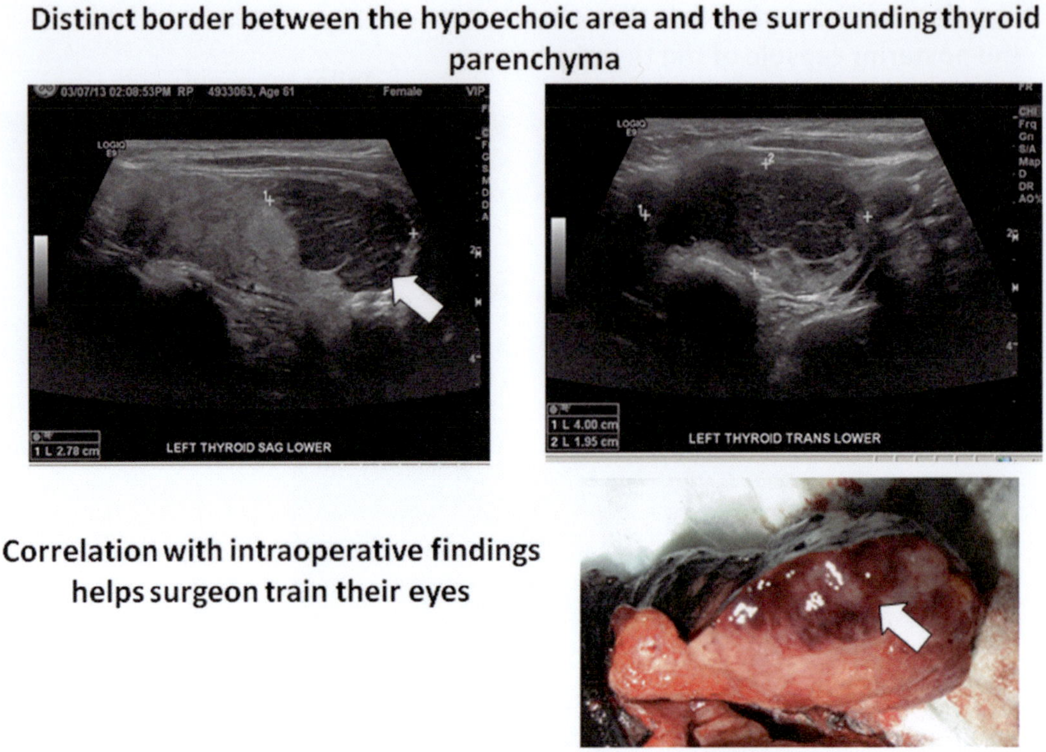

Fig. 15.4 Pattern recognition: comparing individual features helps recognize thyroid nodule as lymphoma

ules is so low that most do not recommend FNA unless there are other factors that drive the need for aspiration [4, 5, 10, 11]. A nodule with diffuse internal cysts described as spongiform (or honeycombed) or an image described as a "puff pastry pattern" with the appearance similar to a many layered flaky puff pastry appears to be characteristic of benign colloid nodules or goiters [2, 3]. When these criteria are applied strictly and with confidence, many FNAs on benign nodules can be avoided. To recognize benign patterns, clinicians must be familiar with the validity of these in their own local referral patterns and assess their own confidence in recognizing these patterns.

15.5 Challenge #4: Pattern Recognition in Inflammatory Conditions

Since 10 % of the US population and an estimated 25 % of women over the age of 65 exhibit antibodies to thyroperoxidase, it is important to be familiar with the altered sonographic patterns in Hashimoto's thyroiditis. Techniques such as sonoelastography have been utilized to help differentiate true nodules from pseudonodules; however, examination of the nodule by visualizing it in multiple planes is likely more reliable. The areas of the thyroid with lymphocytic infiltrate of B cells and cytotoxic T cells show decreased echogenicity, while sound transmission through areas of remaining intact follicles is retained. Generally the degree of hypoechogenicity seen in Hashimoto's is very variable and depends on where the patient is in the disease process and the degree of lymphocytic infiltration. As lymphocytic infiltration progresses, the thyroid echogenicity decreases, approaching that of the surrounding strap muscles and in some cases even exceeding that of the strap muscles.

Sometimes focal lymphocytic thyroiditis areas may be interpreted as sonographically suspicious in the setting of Hashimoto's thyroiditis. When the areas of inflammation are more discrete, the hypoechoic pattern appears more focal, forming localized hypoechoic regions or pseudonodules. These pseudonodules can be small or large, and the larger pseudonodules are often mistaken for true large nodules. Occasionally pseudonodules will be separated by fibrous bands. The hyperechoic bands may be suggestive of peripheral (rim) calcification, but do not produce the characteristic profound posterior shadowing seen in peripheral calcification. A hyperechoic nodule with a background of heterogeneous hypoechogenicity has been termed a "white knight" by Bonavita et al. [3] and is thought to represent a benign regenerative nodule.

The possibility of coexisting malignancy should be considered if an individual region has suspicious features. The sonographic appearance of papillary thyroid cancer (PTC) in Hashimoto's thyroiditis does not differ from PTC found in an otherwise normal thyroid [12–14]. Therefore, the same criteria discussed in the nodule chapter should be applied to the evaluation of nodules detected in Hashimoto's thyroiditis.

There are two typical patterns of thyroid lymphoma that can develop in a gland involved with Hashimoto's thyroiditis. In both cases, a pseudocystic appearance is often seen owing to the excellent transmission of sound and subsequent posterior acoustic enhancement [15]. These two patterns are: (1) A diffuse enlargement and goiter similar to the profoundly hypoechoic pattern. In this case the thyroid parenchyma is almost entirely replaced by lymphocytes. As opposed to discrete germinal centers, the resulting ultrasonographic appearance is homogeneous and profoundly hypoechoic, equal to or darker than adjacent muscle tissue. These diffuse changes may be indistinguishable from the heterogeneous hypoechogenicity commonly seen in Hashimoto's thyroiditis. Therefore, if a diffusely hypoechoic gland exhibits rapid growth, biopsy with flow cytometry should be performed. (2) Nodular lymphoma with distinct borders between the tumor and the surrounding thyroid parenchyma. Therefore, if a hypoechoic nodule with a pseudocystic pattern shows rapid growth in the setting of Hashimoto's, consideration for biopsy with flow cytometry is justified (Fig. 15.4) to rule out lymphoma.

Graves' disease also exhibits lymphoid infiltration, but because the lymphoid cells are in the stroma without direct destruction of the follicles themselves, the ultrasound pattern of the gland shows less heterogeneity than seen in Hashimoto's thyroiditis. Nodules in Graves' disease are often easy to see, and the patterns are not altered from the discussion above. In some cases, Doppler flow may show a decreased pattern of flow in the nodule allowing easy separation from the very hypervascular remainder of the gland [6].

15.6 Challenge #5: Recognizing Anatomic, Structural, and Mental Pitfalls in Pattern Recognition

A number of structures surrounding the thyroid gland may make identification of thyroid nodules difficult. The parathyroid glands lie just deep to the thyroid, and while they are generally not visible, enlarged or calcified parathyroid glands can sometimes be mistaken for abnormal thyroid nodules. In patients with larger necks, the strap muscles, and sometimes the subcutaneous tissues, can significantly attenuate the ultrasound beams, resulting in poor image resolution of the deeper thyroid lesions. This effect can be reduced by increasing transducer pressure on the neck and adjusting the gain and highlights the importance of correct ultrasound technique. Prominent cervical transverse processes, paratracheal air cysts, pharyngoesophageal diverticulum, heavily calcified lymph nodes, and even carotid body tumors can mimic thyroid pathology and lead to misdiagnosis. Recognition of how these structures appear ultrasonographically is essential to help prevent unnecessary biopsies and interventions. Finally, the neck is a highly vascular area, and at times, blood vessels can be mistaken for pathologic lesions. The use of color Doppler and graded compression can help distinguish these blood vessels from true lesions. However, it is important to keep in mind that some pathologic lesions can have marked intrinsic hypervascularity which may confuse the Doppler image.

Image artifacts such as shadowing and enhancement provide useful information, rather than just interfering with creation of a clear image. As experience develops over time, patterns associated with image artifacts will become very helpful to the clinician. One example of an artifact that is helpful is the reverberation artifact known as the "comet tail" which is seen due to the presence of small specks of colloid [16]. Tiny crystals of trapped colloid result in a reverberation of sound waves, and this typical "comet tail appearance" can help differentiate the typically benign densities found in a colloid nodule from highly suspicious microcalcifications. While comet tail artifacts most commonly arise within a benign colloid nodule, they can very rarely be seen in papillary carcinoma as well.

Adding to the subjectivity of ultrasound interpretation is a phenomenon in radiology termed "satisfaction of search," whereby some lesions remain undetected following the detection of other lesions. This underreading of studies leads to false negatives and is particularly true in thyroid ultrasonography where there is often the presence of multiple nodules. A checklist approach ensuring that the whole thyroid gland is inspected is helpful to minimize satisfaction of search errors.

15.7 Challenge #6: Keeping Up with Advancements in the Field of Pattern Recognition

Today, mathematical models are routinely used in radiology and are an essential component of all imaging tools. The hope is that continued fine tuning of these mathematical models will allow software and computer applications to be directly implemented into diagnostic or therapeutic systems. Various methods for automatic detection and investigation of thyroid nodules via ultrasound are currently proposed, and thus far they mostly include computer-aided approaches for nodule delineation. This is particularly important in ultrasound which suffers the most from subjective interpretation. Machine learning is the study of computer algorithms which can learn complex relations or patterns from empirical data provided and make accurate decisions. This is an increasingly complex field with variable components borrowed from artificial intelligence, pattern recognitions, statistics, data mining, and optimization [17]. Some researchers are focusing on discriminating malignancy based on statistical and computation analysis though the challenge remains finding the minimum optimal combination that allows identifying, discriminating, or classifying a particular nodule as malignant. This is due to considerable overlap in the ultrasound features between malignant and benign nodules [18, 19]. Features on high-resolution ultrasound such as microcalcifications, marked hypoechogenicity, absence of broken halo, taller than wide, and irregular margins are very helpful, but interpretative pitfalls remain in many cases. Automated diagnosis support systems are another area of intense research; these systems are meant to ultimately transfer the processing of images from a mental task by a clinician to a computer which might be more cost effective. Most of these computer-aided systems contain a feature extraction step that involves extraction of texture features which are then fed into different algorithms and classifiers [20]. Currently these computer-aided medical systems are currently still viewed as an "aid," and most believe that human decisions are still paramount at this time. However, as algorithms improve, clinicians will have to accept that machine learning will be a critical component of advanced ultrasound software systems and may have clear advantages in analysis of thyroid ultrasound images, thus making it likely to have significantly wider applications in the future.

References

1. Fujimoto Y, Oka A, Omoto R, Hirose M. Ultrasound scanning of the thyroid gland as a new diagnostic approach. Ultrasonics. 1967;5:177–80.
2. Reading CC, Charboneau JW, Hay ID, Sebo TJ. Sonography of thyroid nodules: a "classic pattern" diagnostic approach. Ultrasound Q. 2005;21:157–65.
3. Bonavita JA, Mayo J, Babb J, Bennett G, Oweity T, Macari M, Yee J. Pattern recognition of benign nodules at ultrasound of the thyroid: which nodules can be left alone? AJR Am J Roentgenol. 2009;193:207–13.

4. Gharib H, Papini E, Garber JR, Duick DS, Harrell RM, Hegedus L, Paschke R, Valcavi R, Vitti P, AACE/ACE/AME Task Force on Thyroid Nodules. American Association of Clinical Endocrinologists, American College of Endocrinology, and Associazione Medici Endocrinologi Medical Guidelines for clinical practice for the diagnosis and management of thyroid nodules - 2016 update. Endocr Pract. 2016;22:622–39.
5. Haugen BR, Alexander EK, Bible KC, Doherty GM, Mandel SJ, Nikiforov YE, Pacini F, Randolph GW, Sawka AM, Schlumberger M, Schuff KG, Sherman SI, Sosa JA, Steward DL, Tuttle RM, Wartofsky L. 2015 American Thyroid Association Management Guidelines for adult patients with thyroid nodules and differentiated thyroid cancer: the American Thyroid Association Guidelines Task Force on thyroid nodules and differentiated thyroid cancer. Thyroid. 2016;26:1–133.
6. Baskin HJ, Duick DS, Levine RA. Thyroid ultrasound and ultrasound guided FNA. 3rd ed. New York, NY: Springer; 2013.
7. Hertzberg BS, Kliewer MA, Bowie JD, Carroll BA, DeLong DH, Gray L, Nelson RC. Physician training requirements in sonography: how many cases are needed for competence? AJR Am J Roentgenol. 2000;174:1221–7.
8. Rozycki GS. Surgeon-performed ultrasound: its use in clinical practice. Ann Surg. 1998;228:16–28.
9. Moon HJ, Kim EK, Yoon JH, Kwak JY. Differences in the diagnostic performances of staging US for thyroid malignancy according to experience. Ultrasound Med Biol. 2012;38:568–73.
10. Moon WJ, Jung SL, Lee JH, Na DG, Baek JH, Lee YH, Kim J, Kim HS, Byun JS, Lee DH, Thyroid Study Group, Korean Society of Neuro- and Head and Neck Radiology. Benign and malignant thyroid nodules: US differentiation--multicenter retrospective study. Radiology. 2008;247:762–70.
11. Virmani V, Hammond I. Sonographic patterns of benign thyroid nodules: verification at our institution. AJR Am J Roentgenol. 2011;196:891–5.
12. Anderson L, Middleton WD, Teefey SA, Reading CC, Langer JE, Desser T, Szabunio MM, Hildebolt CF, Mandel SJ, Cronan JJ. Hashimoto thyroiditis: Part 1, sonographic analysis of the nodular form of Hashimoto thyroiditis. AJR Am J Roentgenol. 2010;195:208–15.
13. Anderson L, Middleton WD, Teefey SA, Reading CC, Langer JE, Desser T, Szabunio MM, Mandel SJ, Hildebolt CF, Cronan JJ. Hashimoto thyroiditis: Part 2, sonographic analysis of benign and malignant nodules in patients with diffuse Hashimoto thyroiditis. AJR Am J Roentgenol. 2010;195:216–22.
14. Gul K, Dirikoc A, Kiyak G, Ersoy PE, Ugras NS, Ersoy R, Cakir B. The association between thyroid carcinoma and Hashimoto's thyroiditis: the ultrasonographic and histopathologic characteristics of malignant nodules. Thyroid. 2010;20:873–8.
15. Ota H, Ito Y, Matsuzuka F, Kuma S, Fukata S, Morita S, Kobayashi K, Nakamura Y, Kakudo K, Amino N, Miyauchi A. Usefulness of ultrasonography for diagnosis of malignant lymphoma of the thyroid. Thyroid. 2006;16:983–7.
16. Ahuja A, Chick W, King W, Metreweli C. Clinical significance of the comet-tail artifact in thyroid ultrasound. J Clin Ultrasound. 1996;24:129–33.
17. Wang S, Summers RM. Machine learning and radiology. Med Image Anal. 2012;16:933–51.
18. Savelonas M, Maroulis D, Sangriotis M. A computer-aided system for malignancy risk assessment of nodules in thyroid US images based on boundary features. Comput Methods Programs Biomed. 2009;96:25–32.
19. Bibicu D, Moraru L, Biswas A. Thyroid nodule recognition based on feature selection and pixel classification methods. J Digit Imaging. 2013;26:119–28.
20. Acharya UR, Faust O, Sree SV, Molinari F, Suri JS. ThyroScreen system: high resolution ultrasound thyroid image characterization into benign and malignant classes using novel combination of texture and discrete wavelet transform. Comput Methods Programs Biomed. 2012;107:233–41.

Pattern Recognition: Diffuse Thyroid Disease

16

Mark A. Lupo

16.1 Introduction

Diffuse enlargement of the thyroid gland is a common finding during both physical examination and during ultrasound evaluation. While iodine deficiency is still the most common cause of goiter worldwide, chronic lymphocytic thyroiditis (CLT), also referred to as Hashimoto's thyroiditis, is the most common cause of goiter and hypothyroidism in the United States, most of Europe, and other countries with adequate iodine intake. Table 16.1 lists the most common causes of diffuse thyroid enlargement. Thyroiditis refers to a diverse group of conditions caused by thyroid inflammation. While there is significant overlap in the sonographic findings of these various entities, ultrasound is a very useful tool in evaluating thyroiditis as it provides insight into the etiology and clinical course of the disease process. One easy, although nonspecific, feature of diffuse thyroid enlargement is enlargement of the isthmus to more than 5 mm in the anterior-posterior dimension (Figs. 16.1 and 16.2). Pattern recognition of the various sonographic presentations of autoimmune diffuse thyroid disease is essential in determining if a focal abnormality represents a true nodule which may require fine-needle aspiration biopsy or is simply part of the inflammatory process, often called a pseudonodule. Furthermore, real-time imaging or the use of cine-clips is superior to static imaging in detecting diffuse thyroid disease, especially early in the course of the disease [1] (Fig. 16.3 and Video 16.1).

16.2 Chronic Lymphocytic (Hashimoto's) Thyroiditis (CLT)

Chronic lymphocytic thyroiditis is the most common form of thyroiditis. Approximately 10 % of the US population overall and an estimated 25 % of women over the age of 65 years exhibit antibodies to thyroperoxidase [2]. The presence of thyroid autoantibodies predicts future thyroid dysfunction in patients who are currently euthyroid. The pathologic hallmark of Hashimoto's thyroiditis is lymphocytic infiltration of the gland by B cells and cytotoxic T cells. This results in an overall decrease in parenchymal echogenicity on ultrasound, as the lymphocytic infiltrate allows greater through transmission of sound than the intact thyroid follicles that reflect sound. This hypoechogenicity

Electronic supplementary material: The online version of this chapter (doi:10.1007/978-3-319-44100-9_16) contains supplementary material, which is available to authorized users. Videos can also be accessed at http://link.springer.com/chapter/10.1007/978-3-319-44100-9_16.

M.A. Lupo, M.D., F.A.C.E., E.C.N.U. (✉)
Thyroid & Endocrine Center of Florida,
Florida State University, College of Medicine,
3050 Bee Ridge Road, Sarasota, FL 34239, USA
e-mail: marklupo@thyroidflorida.com

M. Milas et al. (eds.), *Advanced Thyroid and Parathyroid Ultrasound*,
DOI 10.1007/978-3-319-44100-9_16

has been used to predict the presence of autoimmune thyroid disease and the risk of subsequent hypothyroidism. Pederson studied 485 patients with diffuse thyroid hypoechogenicity and 100 normal patients and found that hypoechogenicity had a positive predictive value of autoimmune thyroid disease of 88 % and a negative predictive value of 95 % [3]. Hypoechogenicity of the parenchyma on ultrasound has been shown to have a greater predictive value for development of hypothyroidism than the presence of thyroid autoantibodies [4, 5]. However, in morbidly obese patients, the thyroid may appear more hypoechoic, and this finding is less predictive of autoimmune thyroid disease [6].

Similar to the clinical presentation and the histopathologic findings, the degree of change in echogenicity seen in Hashimoto's thyroiditis is quite variable. Normal thyroid parenchyma has a relatively homogeneous appearance that is significantly brighter (more hyperechoic) than the surrounding strap muscles which are typically markedly hypoechoic. As the lymphocytic infiltration progresses, the echogenicity decreases, approaching that of the surrounding strap muscles and in some cases becoming even more hypoechoic than the strap muscles as shown in Fig. 16.5. In general, the progression and degree of hypoechogenicity are predictive of the severity of hypothyroidism [7].

Table 16.1 Common causes of diffuse thyroid enlargement

Hashimoto's thyroiditis
Graves' disease
Silent thyroiditis
Postpartum thyroiditis
Subacute thyroiditis
Suppurative thyroiditis
Drug-induced thyroiditis
Iodine deficiency

Heterogeneity is another common ultrasonographic feature of autoimmune thyroid disease. A variety of patterns are seen in CLT, reflecting the histopathologic features and the dynamic nature of chronic inflammatory disease (Figs. 16.6 and 16.7). Hallmark pathologic findings include lymphoplasmacytic aggregates with germinal centers, atrophic thyroid follicles, oxyphilic change of the epithelial cells (Hürthle cells), and fibrosis [8]. The patchy nature of these changes produces regional parenchymal distortion that has been described as a pseudonodular appearance. The degree of hypoechogenicity as well as pseudonodular changes in the gland correlates with the titer of thyroperoxidase antibody, but not thyroglobulin antibody [9].

The changes of CLT can be described by seven different patterns or types of appearances [10] and are listed in Table 16.2. These patterns do not necessarily represent a sequential progression. While fibrosis and atrophy are typically later

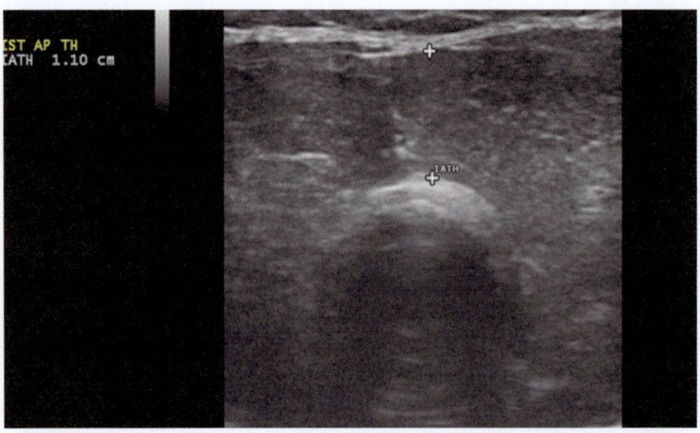

Fig. 16.1 Diffuse thyroid enlargement. Thickened AP dimension of the isthmus (1.1 cm) in this patient with Hashimoto's. Normal AP dimension of the isthmus is typically less than 0.5 cm

events, any of the other patterns can be seen early in the disorder. The inflammation may diffusely involve the thyroid or be geographic in nature.

16.3 Patterns of Heterogeneity Seen in Chronic Lymphocytic Thyroiditis

16.3.1 Pattern 1: Hypoechoic and Heterogeneous

Normal thyroid tissue has an echogenicity that is hyperechoic compared to muscle tissue and is relatively homogeneous (Fig. 16.4). Areas of lymphocytic infiltration of the thyroid are less echogenic than normal thyroid parenchyma. As a result, areas of lymphocytic infiltration appear hypoechoic compared to normal thyroid. The degree of both hypoechogenicity and heterogeneity varies with the distribution and severity of the lymphocytic infiltration creating a spectrum of patterns within this category (Figs. 16.4, 16.5, 16.6, 16.7, and 16.8).

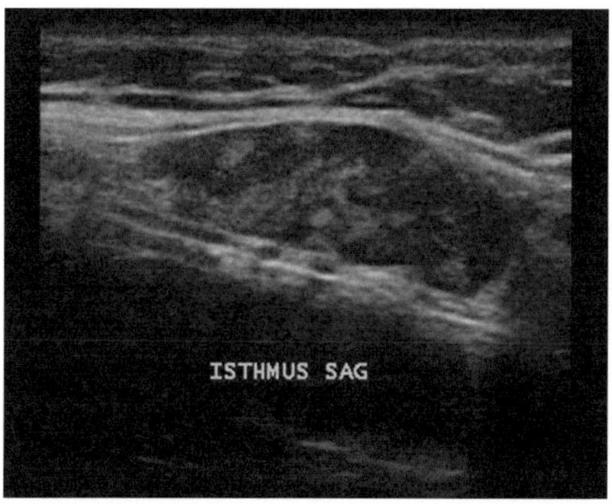

Fig. 16.2 Enlarged isthmus. The isthmus is enlarged on this sagittal view. Note the heterogeneous and hypoechoic echotexture

16.3.2 Pattern 2: Pseudomicronodular

When the areas of inflammation are more discrete, the hypoechoic pattern appears more focal, forming localized hypoechoic regions (pseudonodules) that represent aggregates of lymphocytes (Figs. 16.3, 16.9, and 16.10). The corresponding histopathology includes numerous germinal centers scattered throughout the gland. The hypoechoic pseudomicronodules are subcentimeter in size and often flame shaped and may have a thin hyperechoic rim, representing surrounding fibrosis or an ill-defined margin. This pattern was first described by Yeh in 1996 [36] as characteristic of CLT and should suggest Hashimoto's thyroiditis, rather than a multinodular gland. Pseudonodules are occasionally difficult to differentiate from small, multiple true nodules, especially when few in number and they do not involve the entire gland (Fig. 16.9). If an individual pseudonodule appears different, especially with calcifications or infiltrative margins, the possibility of a coexisting malignancy should be entertained. As the inflammatory process is

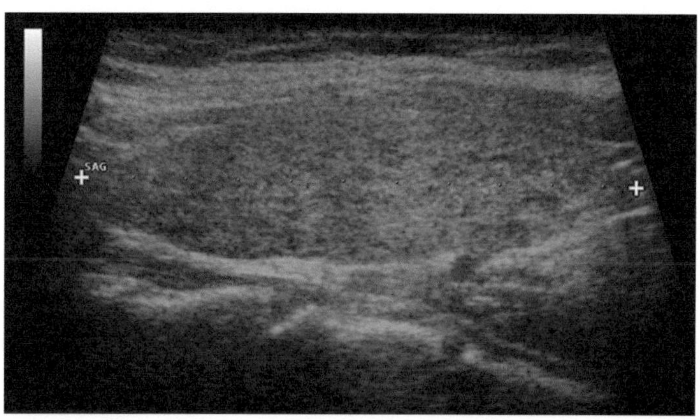

Fig. 16.3 Early changes of chronic lymphocytic thyroiditis. Left lobe sagittal image showing mild heterogeneity and a pseudomicronodular pattern. The pattern is often more easily recognized on real-time imaging

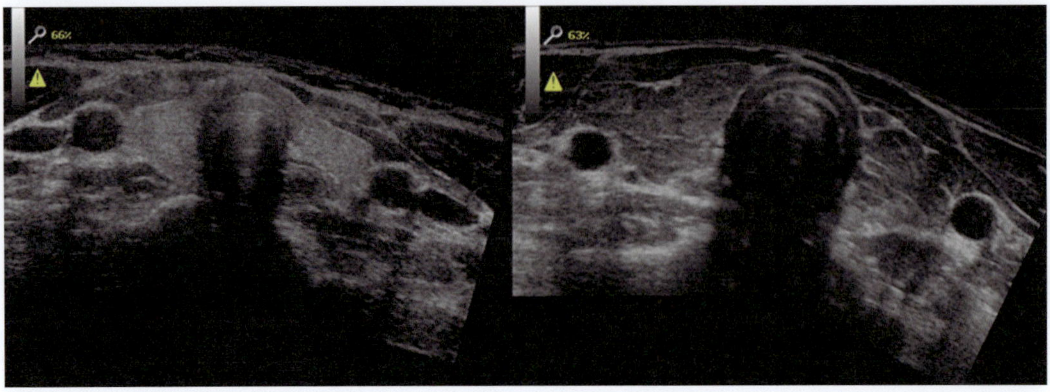

Fig. 16.4 Normal thyroid compared with chronic lymphocytic thyroiditis. Side-by-side panoramic transverse views. *Left panel* demonstrates homogeneous echotexture of a normal thyroid. *Right panel* shows overall hypoechogenicity of the parenchyma, with scatter hypoechoic patchy regions and linear echogenic regions of fibrosis typical of Hashimoto's thyroiditis

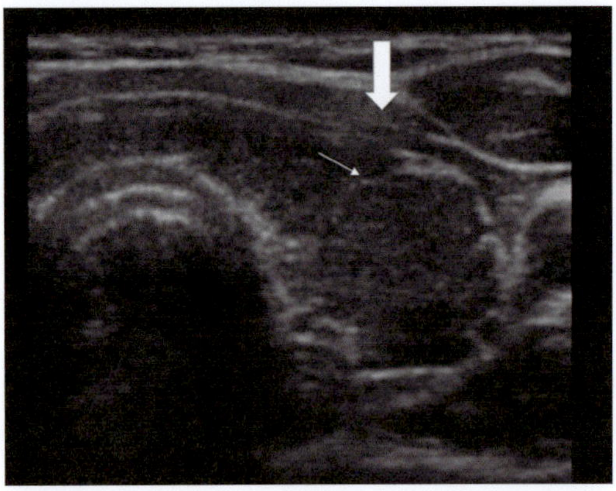

Fig. 16.5 Chronic lymphocytic thyroiditis. Hypoechoic appearance. Transverse image of the left lobe shows decreased parenchyma; echogenicity similar to the surrounding strap muscles (*large arrow*). Early fibrosis appearing as linear echogenic bands (*thin arrow*) is also seen

dynamic, the appearance may vary from study to study, with a change in the number, size, or location of the pseudonodules (Video 16.2).

There are two common subpatterns of pseudomicronodules, which I describe as "Swiss cheese" and "honeycomb." In the former, the areas of inflammation are more discrete and well defined, giving an appearance of numerous well-defined hypoechoic areas (pseudonodules) similar to the holes in Swiss cheese (Fig. 16.10). In contrast to the Swiss cheese pattern in which multiple discrete pseudonodules are seen within the thyroid parenchyma, the "honeycomb" variant is composed of almost confluent small pseudonodules and marked fibrosis with very little parenchyma separating the hypoechoic tissue (Fig. 16.11).

16.3.3 Pattern 3: Pseudomacronodular Pattern

When the areas of inflammation are larger, pseudonodules also appear larger and again are often mistaken for true large nodules (Fig. 16.12). The pseudonodules may appear confluent, with little or no normal intervening thyroid parenchyma. As always, the possibility of coexisting malignancy should be considered if an individual region has suspicious features.

16.3.4 Pattern 4: Profoundly Hypoechoic

This pattern is typically seen with a large, inflamed goiter. The thyroid parenchyma is essentially replaced entirely by lymphocytes, as opposed to discrete germinal centers. The ultrasonographic appearance is relatively homogeneous but profoundly hypoechoic, equal to or darker than adjacent muscle tissue (Fig. 16.13). Importantly, thyroid lymphoma may have a very

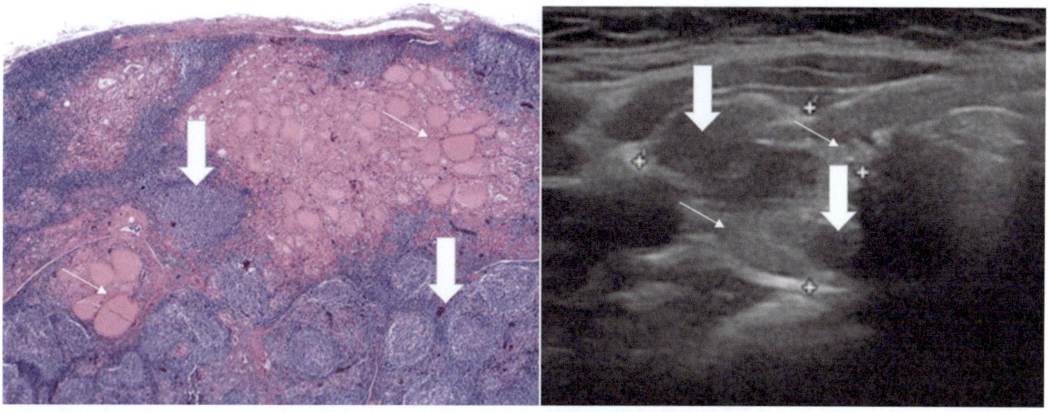

Fig. 16.6 Histologic and sonographic changes of chronic lymphocytic thyroiditis. The histologic appearance (left panel) of Hashimoto's is varied with geographic areas of lymphocytic infiltration (large arrow) amid preserved groups of follicles (thin arrow), similar to the heterogeneity seen on ultrasound (right panel). On sonography, the hypoechoic areas (large arrows) are regions of lymphocytic infiltration, and the echogenic areas (small arrows) are less affected regions and appear as normal echogenic thyroid parenchyma

Table 16.2 Sonographic patterns of Hashimoto's thyroiditis

Hypoechoic and heterogeneous
Pseudomicronodular
Pseudomacronodular
Profoundly hypoechoic
Developing fibrosis
Hyperechoic
Speckled

similar appearance and should be considered in the differential diagnosis, especially if there has been a rapid growth (Video 16.3).

16.3.5 Pattern 5: Developing Fibrosis

Later in the progression of thyroid inflammation, fibrosis develops and appears as hyperechoic linear and curvilinear bands (Figs. 16.14, 16.15, and 16.16). The bands create a pseudonodular appearance by outlining islands of hypoechoic parenchyma with white lines of varying thickness. This appearance of CLT should not be confused with a peri-nodular halo, since a halo surrounding a true nodule is hypoechoic (Fig. 16.12). During real-time imaging in both transverse and longitudinal planes, the band-like nature of the fibrosis can readily be distinguished from underlying nodules. Often these changes are more pronounced in the inferior-posterior aspect of the involved lobe, and a thick band of fibrosis has the appearance of a cleft (Fig. 16.15; Videos 16.4 and 16.5). Often the tubercle of Zuckerkandl becomes prominent in the setting of diffuse thyroid disease and projects from the undersurface of the gland. When the fibrotic bands occur in this portion of the gland, the tubercle can be mistaken for an exophytic nodule (Figs. 16.16 and 16.17 and Video 16.6).

16.3.6 Pattern 6: Hyperechoic and Heterogeneous

When fibrosis is more diffuse, the gland may take on a hyperechoic appearance (Fig. 16.18). This pattern has been observed less frequently, but may be more common later in the course of autoimmune hypothyroidism, associated with the start of goiter regression (Video 16.7).

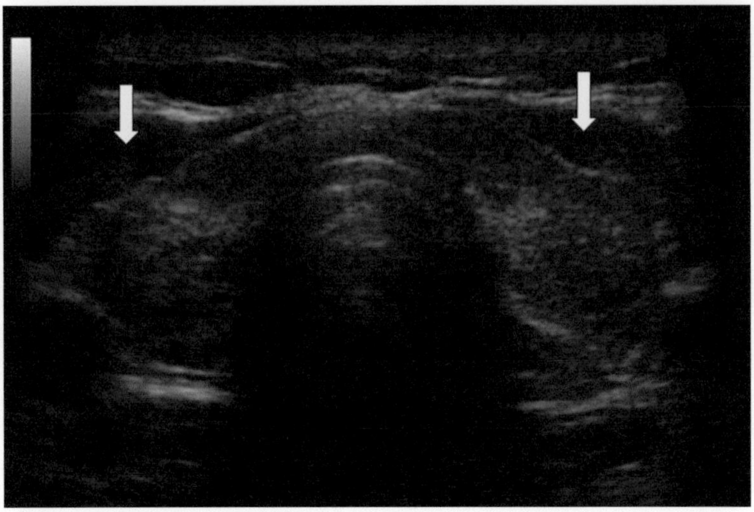

Fig. 16.7 Chronic lymphocytic thyroiditis: mild hypoechogenicity. A transverse image of the thyroid obtained in a patient with early chronic lymphocytic thyroiditis shows mild heterogeneity and hypoechogenicity. Note that strap muscles (arrows) are still more hypoechoic than thyroid parenchyma

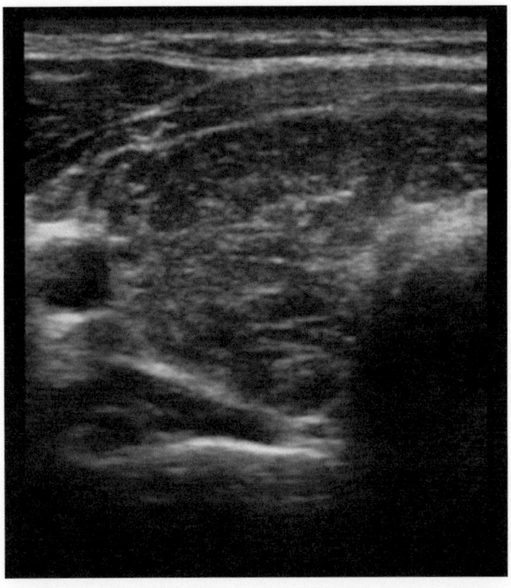

Fig. 16.8 Chronic lymphocytic thyroiditis: moderate hypoechogenicity. Transverse image of the right lobe shows more marked hypoechogenicity and heterogeneity of the parenchyma. The echogenicity of the thyroid is similar to the surrounding muscles

16.3.7 Pattern 7: Speckled

In this very uncommon pattern, numerous punctate non-shadowing echogenic foci are scattered throughout the parenchyma likely due to fibrosis (Figs. 16.19, 16.20, and 16.21, Videos 16.8 and 16.9) With an appearance raising concern for microcalcifications, this pattern usually requires biopsy, to exclude diffuse infiltration by papillary carcinoma. The pattern is very similar to that described for diffuse sclerosing papillary carcinoma which may have a "snowstorm" appearance [11]. The punctate densities do not cast an acoustic shadow and may be similar in origin to the bright linear densities commonly seen in benign colloid nodules [12].

16.4 Thyroid Nodules in Chronic Lymphocytic Thyroiditis

It has been suggested that there is a higher prevalence of papillary thyroid cancer in patients with Hashimoto's thyroiditis [13–16]. Malignant nodules may be camouflaged within the heterogeneity of CLT due to lymphocytic infiltration and fibrosis, making it difficult to identify a discrete potentially suspicious nodule. Careful real-time imaging in two planes along with the aid of Doppler interrogation is required to distinguish a nodule requiring FNA from areas of pseudonodularity (Fig. 16.22).

The sonographic appearance of papillary thyroid cancer in chronic lymphocytic thyroiditis does not differ from PTC found in an otherwise normal thyroid [13, 16, 17]. Therefore, the same

a b

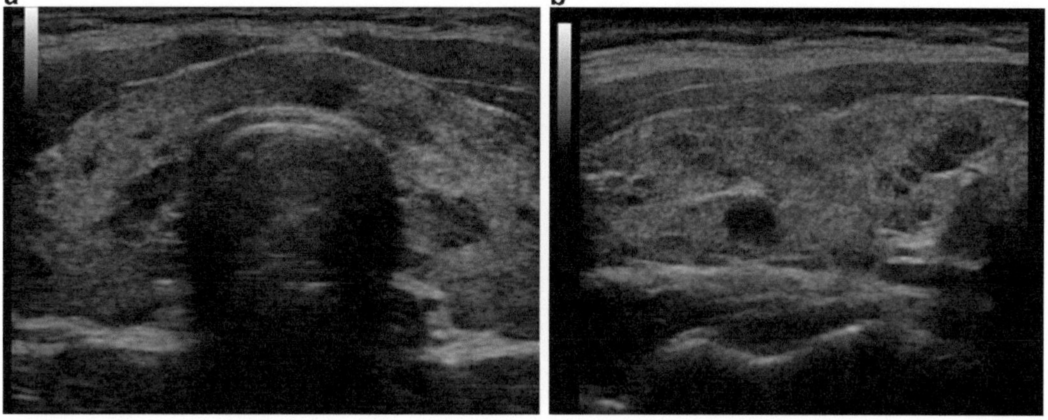

Fig. 16.9 Chronic lymphocytic thyroiditis: pseudomicronodules. Transverse and sagittal views demonstrate multiple subcentimeter hypoechoic areas that represent localized areas of lymphocytic infiltration. The remaining thyroid parenchyma has an isoechoic echotexture

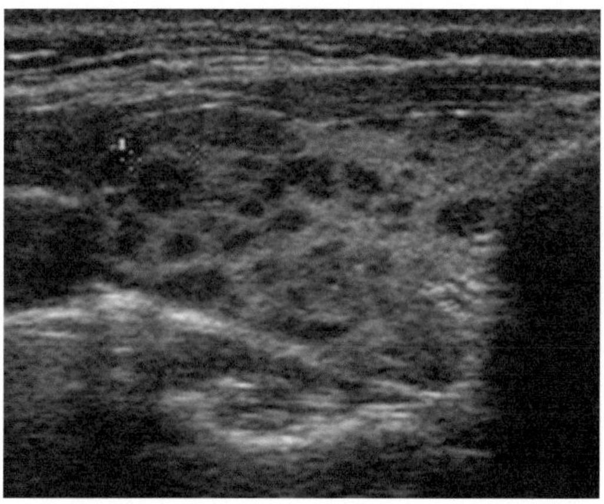

Fig. 16.10 Pseudomicronodules: Swiss cheese pattern. In this pattern the pseudonodules vary in size, have a well-defined border, and replace the much of the normal parenchyma. Reproduced with permission from Springer, Thyroid Ultrasound and Ultrasound-Guided FNA, Editors, Baskin, Duick, and Levine, Chapter 6 pp 99–126

criteria discussed in the thyroid nodule chapter of this text should be applied to evaluation of nodules detected in CLT. There may be a tendency toward denser calcification and less psammomatous calcification in PTC found in Hashimoto's thyroiditis, but any calcification within a nodule should be a cause for potential concern [18]. Additionally, the margins of thyroid cancer are more likely to be irregular or poorly defined when the gland is heterogeneous [19] (Fig. 16.23).

One specific nodular pattern in Hashimoto's is very suggestive of a benign process. A hyperechoic nodule with a background of heterogeneous hypoechogenicity has been termed a "white knight" by Bonavita and colleagues [20] and is thought to represent a benign regenerative nodule (Fig. 16.24). A variant of this pattern is the "giraffe pattern," also described by Bonavita [20] characterized by globular areas of hyperechogenicity surrounded by linear thin areas of hypoechogenicity (Fig. 16.25).

16.5 Lymph Nodes in CLT

Lymph node reactivity and enlargement are almost invariably present in Hashimoto's thyroiditis. These prominent nodes are commonly found in the paratracheal and pretracheal space surrounding the thyroid (Fig. 16.26 and Video 16.10) as well as in surgical levels III and IV of the lateral neck [21] (Fig. 16.27). These lymph nodes may be confluent and have a tendency to appear somewhat rounded. The presence of an echogenic hilum is variable (Fig. 16.28). The prominence and atypical appearance may cause concern in the evaluation for lymph node involvement in patients with both Hashimoto's and thyroid cancer. Any suspicious findings such as calcification, cystic necrosis, or disordered vascularity should prompt

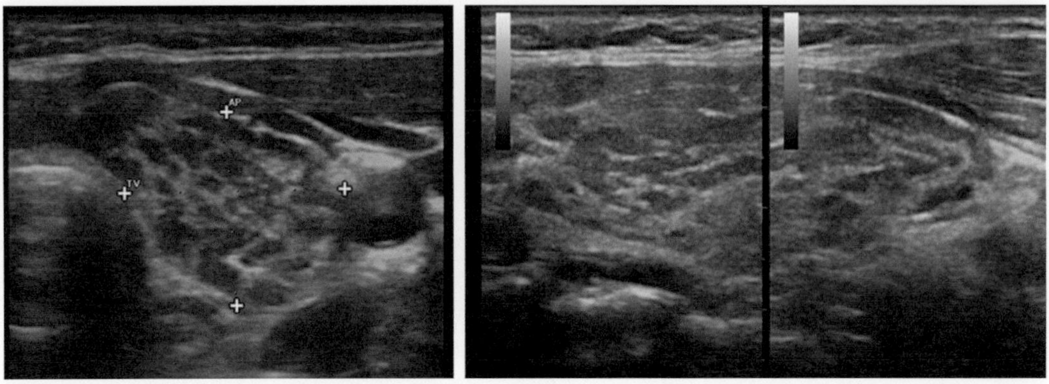

Fig. 16.11 Pseudomicronodules: honeycomb pattern. *Left panel* shows transverse view of the left lobe with overlapping bands of fibrosis outlining hypoechoic regions which could be mistaken for multiple hypoechoic nodules. *Right panel* is the sagittal view which demonstrates the fibrosis and confirms the abnormality as a diffuse process

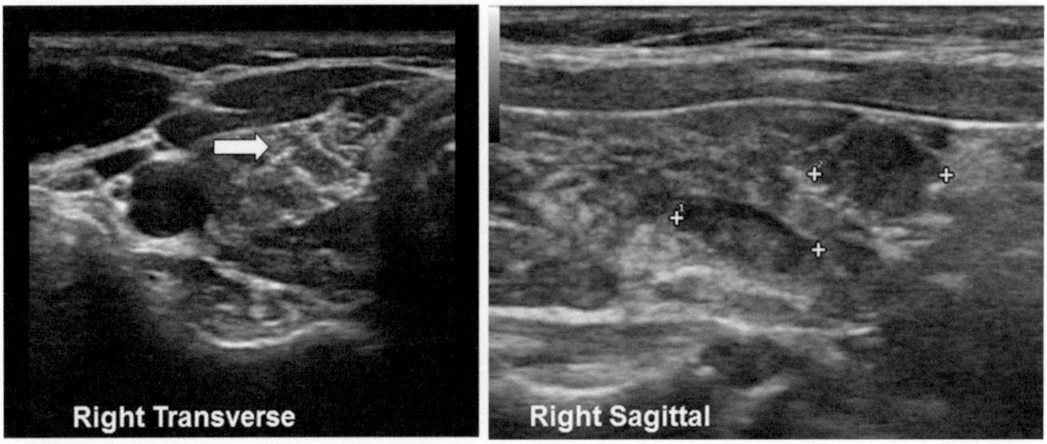

Fig. 16.12 Pseudomacronodules: hyperechoic banding reflecting marked fibrosis (arrow). In sagittal view, hypoechoic pseudonodules (marked by calipers)

FNA evaluation of a lymph node. In addition, lymph nodes at the inferior poles of the thyroid may resemble parathyroid adenomas, making the sonographic evaluation of primary hyperparathyroidism more challenging in patients with chronic lymphocytic thyroiditis (Fig. 16.29).

16.5.1 Atrophic Thyroiditis

Chronic lymphocytic thyroiditis may ultimately result in atrophy of the gland with heterogeneous hypoechogenicity and fibrosis (Fig. 16.30).

16.5.2 Graves' Disease

Histopathologically, Graves' disease exhibits lymphoid infiltration, sometimes with germinal center formation. However the lymphoid cells are strewn in the interfollicular stroma and do not encroach on the follicles themselves. The follicles often show marked epithelial hyperplasia causing the gland to enlarge and become hypoechoic. Fibrosis is unusual unless the disease is long-standing [8] such that the surface of the gland remains smooth, but is often scalloped. Accordingly, on ultrasound there is often less heterogeneity than seen in Hashimoto's thyroiditis. In Graves' disease the decreased echogenicity is due to reduction of colloid to cellular ratio as well as the generalized hypervascularity, but it is not as pronounced as Hashimoto's because the intact and enlarged follicles are reflective of sound waves (Fig. 16.31). In some cases the gland is even hyperechoic.

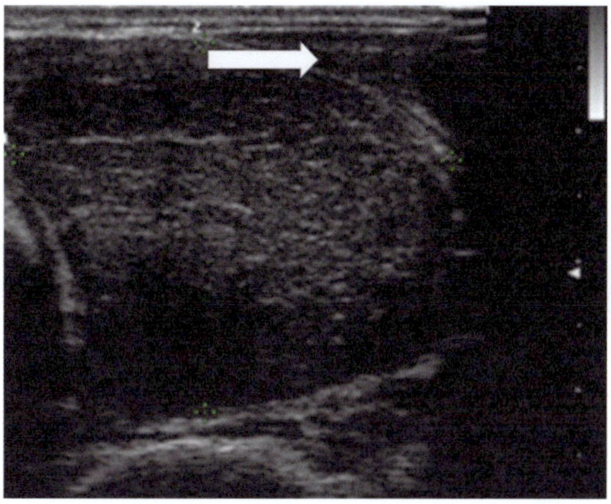

Fig. 16.13 Chronic lymphocytic thyroiditis: profoundly hypoechoic. Transverse image of the left lobe shows marked hypoechogenicity very similar to the strap muscles (arrow). This pattern often seen in clinically swollen thyroid glands. A history of rapid growth should prompt consideration of lymphoma. Reproduced with permission from Springer, Thyroid Ultrasound and Ultrasound-Guided FNA, Editors, Baskin, Duick, and Levine, Chapter 6 pp 99–126

The classic sonographic feature of Graves' disease is intense Doppler flow in the gland referred to as the "thyroid inferno" [22] (Fig. 16.32). Using this observation, some authors have suggested the ability of Doppler flow to distinguish Graves' disease from the thyrotoxicosis due to thyroiditis, with the latter generally showing decreased flow [23, 24]. In this setting, total blood flow may correlate strongly with radioiodine uptake, suggesting it may be a useful technique for patients in whom nuclear studies are contraindicated (pregnancy and breastfeeding) or are not readily available [25]. There is, however, overlap in blood flow patterns between Graves' and thyroiditis so Doppler characteristics alone may not be sufficient to distinguish these two diagnostic entities [26]. While radioiodine uptake remains the gold standard in differentiating Graves' hyperthyroidism from thyrotoxicosis due to thyroiditis [26, 27], when used along with clinical history and laboratory assays of TSH receptor antibodies, ultrasound with Doppler flow may be more cost effective than routine use of nuclear imaging [27] and arguably should be the first line in evaluating a patient with thyrotoxicosis [28–30].

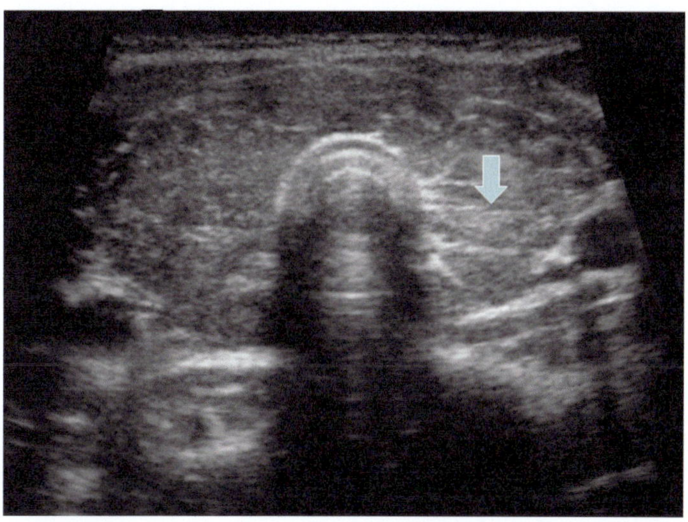

Fig. 16.14 Chronic lymphocytic thyroiditis: developing fibrosis. Developing fibrosis results in hyperechoic bands and echogenic foci without posterior acoustic shadowing. The gland is hypoechoic and the fibrosis appears as subtle white linear echoes of varying lengths (arrow)

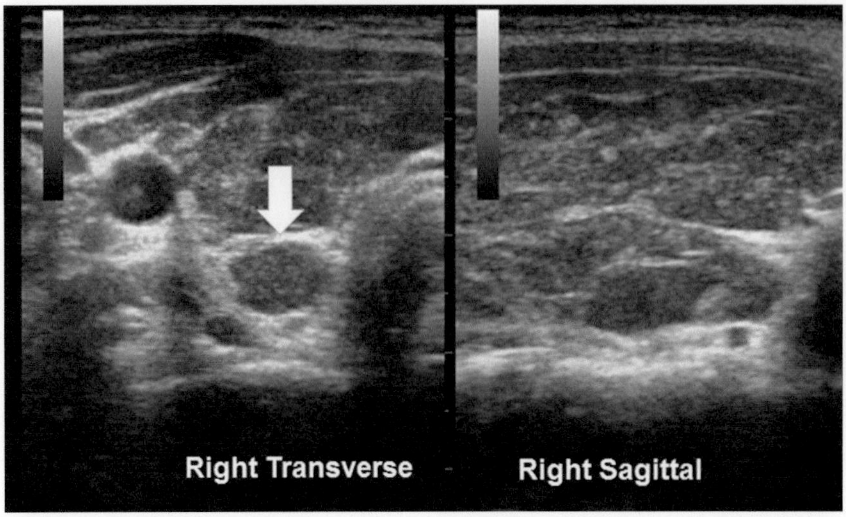

Fig. 16.15 Cleft sign. Thick hyperechoic fibrotic band separates the posterior and anterior components of the lobe in transverse view creating the appearance of a hypoechoic nodule (arrow) outlined by an echogenic circle. The appearance should not be misinterpreted as a nodule with a halo, since halos are hypoechoic. On sagittal view, it is evident that there is no discrete nodule. Reproduced with permission from Springer, Thyroid Ultrasound and Ultrasound-Guided FNA, Editors, Baskin, Duick, and Levine, Chapter 6 pp 99–126

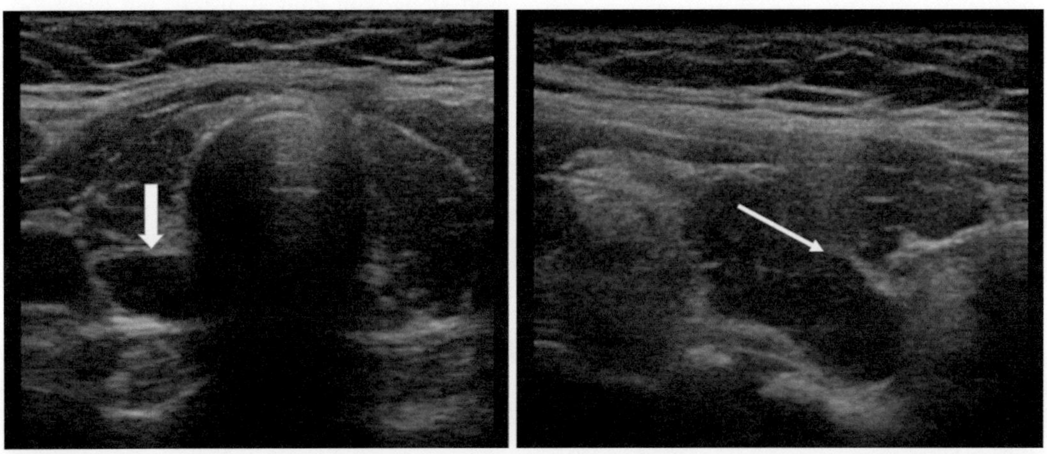

Fig. 16.16 Cleft sign. In transverse view, there appears to be a hypoechoic nodule in the posterior aspect of the right lobe (arrow). In sagittal view, it becomes clear that a band of fibrosis created the appearance of a nodule (thin arrow)

The diagnostic use of blood flow in this way is most appropriate when the TSH is suppressed, as the pattern of "thyroid inferno" can be seen in thyroiditis during the recovery phase when the gland is stimulated by higher levels of thyrotropin. Other authors [31, 32] have used the degree of Doppler flow to determine the dose of antithyroid drug and to predict the long-term outcome in Graves' disease (Fig. 16.33). Demonstration of normal thyroid echotexture and Doppler flow on ultrasound may be more predictive of remission after antithyroid drugs than TSH-R antibody levels [33, 34]. Similar to CLT, the sonographic appearance of papillary

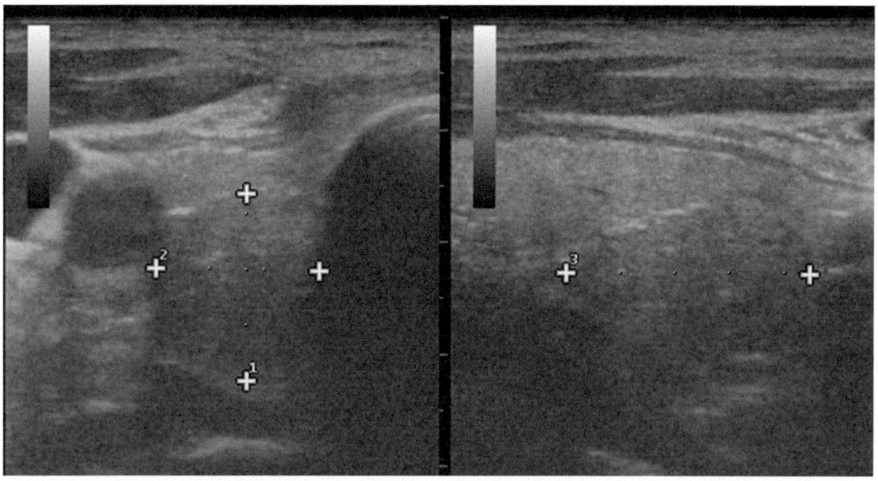

Fig. 16.17 Tubercle of Zuckerkandl. This patient was referred after this "nodule" was incidentally discovered on a chest CT done for cough. Previous core biopsy was interpreted as atypical. Real-time imaging was most consistent with a pseudomacronodule due to a prominent tubercle of Zuckerkandl. TPO antibodies were elevated, and second opinion of the outside biopsy was consistent with Hashimoto's (see also Video 16.6)

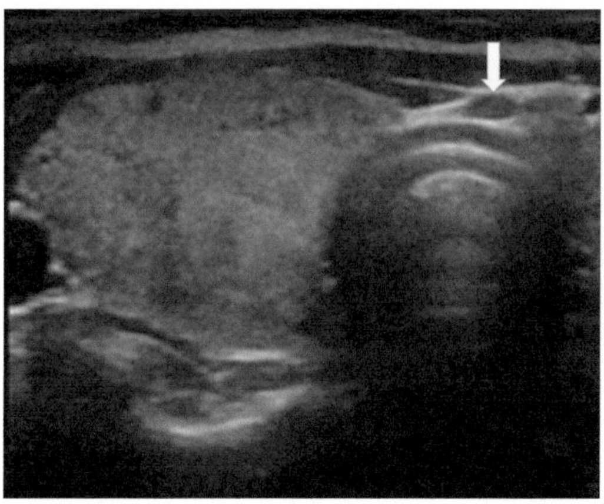

Fig. 16.18 Chronic lymphocytic thyroiditis: hyperechoic and heterogeneous. While the typical pattern in Hashimoto's thyroiditis is hypoechoic, later in the course of the disease, diffuse scarring may predominate over follicles and inflammation resulting in hyperechogenicity. Note the small pretracheal, reactive lymph node (arrow), a frequent finding in autoimmune thyroiditis. Reproduced with permission from Springer, Thyroid Ultrasound and Ultrasound-Guided FNA, Editors, Baskin, Duick, and Levine, Chapter 6 pp 99–126

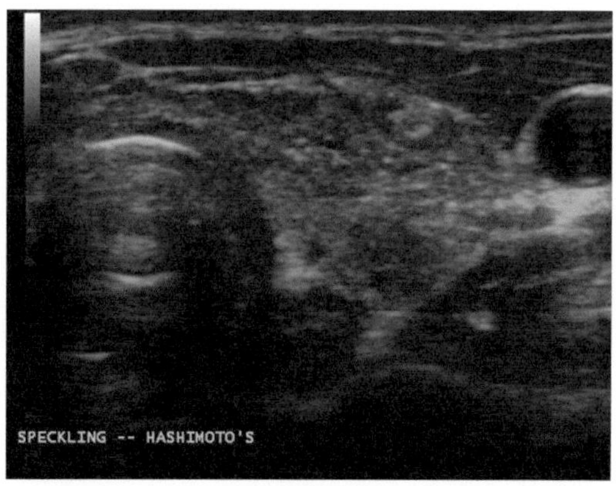

Fig. 16.19 Chronic lymphocytic thyroiditis: speckled pattern. Transverse view, left lobe in patient with Hashimoto's. Note the numerous punctate echogenic foci due to fibrosis. These may mimic microcalcification, and biopsy is often required to confirm the diagnosis

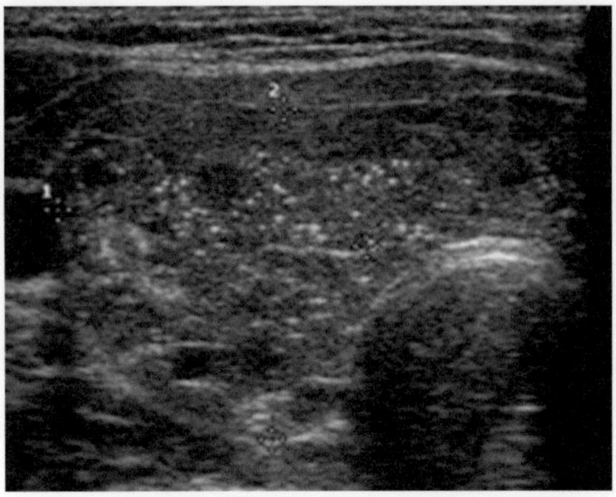

Fig. 16.20 Chronic lymphocytic thyroiditis: speckled pattern. In this very infrequently observed pattern, the gland is enlarged and hypoechoic. Numerous punctate, non-shadowing echogenic foci are present, some with the appearance of "comet tail" artifacts. Biopsy was performed due to the concern that these might represent microcalcifications, but cytology confirmed benign lymphocytic thyroiditis. Reproduced with permission from Springer, Thyroid Ultrasound and Ultrasound-Guided FNA, Editors, Baskin, Duick, and Levine, Chapter 6 pp 99–126

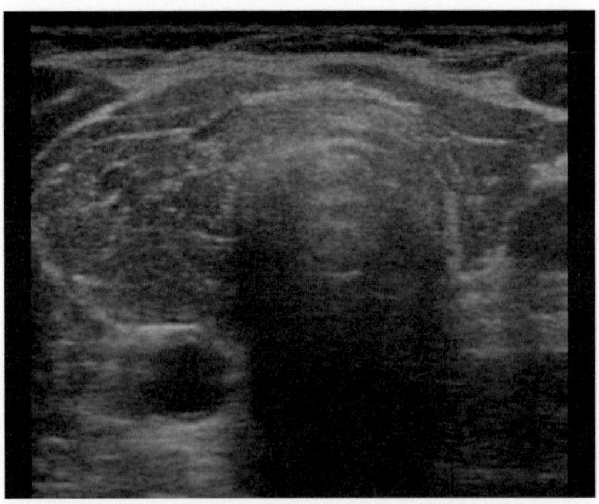

Fig. 16.21 Chronic lymphocytic thyroiditis: speckled and fibrosis. Transverse view of the thyroid showing hypoechogenicity, fibrosis, and slight speckling in the right lobe which is asymmetrically enlarged compared to the left

thyroid cancer in Graves' disease does not differ from PTC found in an otherwise normal thyroid (Fig. 16.34).

16.5.3 Painless Thyroiditis

This category includes both silent thyroiditis and postpartum thyroiditis. Silent thyroiditis is considered to be an autoimmune process and has been referred to subacute lymphocytic thyroiditis as it may be a form of transient Hashimoto's thyroiditis [2]. It occurs primarily in women of 30–50 years of age and tends to have lower levels of thyroid autoantibodies than seen in Hashimoto's thyroiditis. When it presents within 1 year of parturition, it is termed postpartum thyroiditis. Postpartum thyroiditis is seen in up to 10 % of all pregnancies and up to 30 % of type 1 diabetics [2]. The recurrence rate is up to 70 % in subsequent pregnancies. Patients with painless thyroiditis may present either in the thyrotoxic phase (which is usually mild and lasts 1–2 months) or the hypothyroid phase (which is typically transient and lasts up to 4–6 months). The probability of full recovery can be predicted by antibody titers and serial sonographic assessment of echogenicity [35]. Ultrasound evaluation shows hypoechogenicity similar to other forms of autoimmune thyroid disease. The histopathology is similar to Hashimoto's but with relative lack of oncocytic metaplasia, minimal to absent follicular atrophy, and mild to no fibrosis [8]. These differences are reflected in the ultrasound appearance in that hyperechoic fibrotic changes are not seen and the degree of parenchymal hypoechogenicity is not typically profound.

16.5.4 Drug-Induced Thyroiditis

Patients treated with amiodarone, interleukin-2, interferon-alpha, ipilimumab (Fig. 16.35), or tyrosine kinase inhibitors may develop destructive thyroiditis without pain. This relationship should be considered in evaluating patients with diffuse thyroid enlargement that are treated with any of these medications.

16.6 Summary

Diffuse thyroid enlargement may be due to one of several different entities commonly referred to as thyroiditis. Autoimmune thyroid disease is

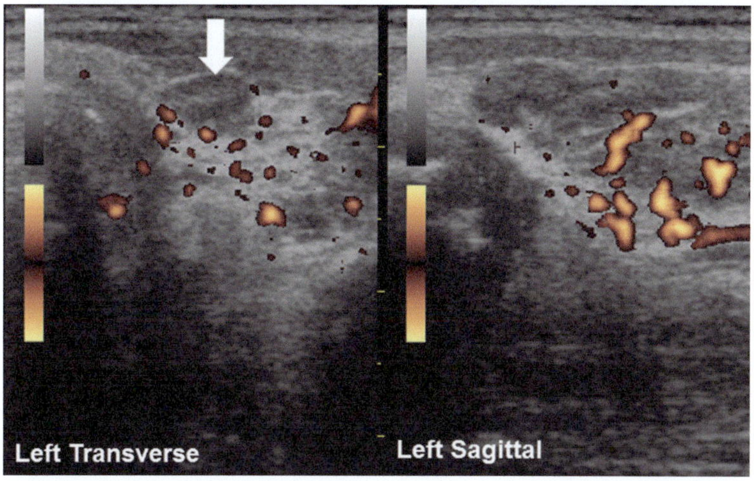

Fig. 16.22 Left superior pseudonodule. In this patient with Hashimoto's, transverse view suggests a discrete hypoechoic nodule (arrow) with possible peripheral blood flow, but in sagittal view, there is no corresponding nodule, and the Doppler pattern of flow is undisturbed. An underlying true nodule would displace the vessels. It is important to image in both planes as this sagittal view confirms the Doppler pattern is that of the background parenchyma and not outlining a nodule

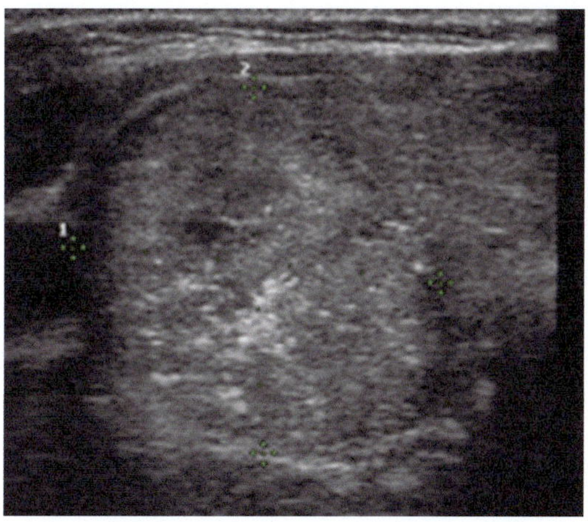

Fig. 16.23 Papillary thyroid cancer in chronic lymphocytic thyroiditis. Transverse image of the right lobe shows a predominantly solid, isoechoic nodule with multiple microcalcifications. FNA biopsy confirmed papillary thyroid cancer in this patient with Hashimoto's. Reproduced with permission from Springer, Thyroid Ultrasound and Ultrasound-Guided FNA, Editors, Baskin, Duick, and Levine, Chapter 6 pp 99–126

by far the most commonly encountered in clinical practice. The sonographic hallmark of thyroid autoimmunity is diffuse hypoechogenicity and heterogeneity, with multiple variants as described. The role of ultrasound is to help confirm diagnosis, to evaluate the size and vascularity of the gland, and to identify any non-palpable nodule which may require FNA biopsy. Familiarity with the wide spectrum of presentation of thyroiditis helps to avoid unnecessary biopsy and avoidable surgery. Real-time imaging of the thyroid and surrounding neck structures can clarify unique situations such as ectopic thyroid (Fig. 16.36 and Video 16.11) or an enlarged pyramidal lobe (Fig. 16.37 and Video 16.12) in patients with diffuse thyroid disease. In the hands of the clinician caring for the patient with thyroiditis, sonography is an efficient and invaluable tool that completes the clinical evaluation of these patients.

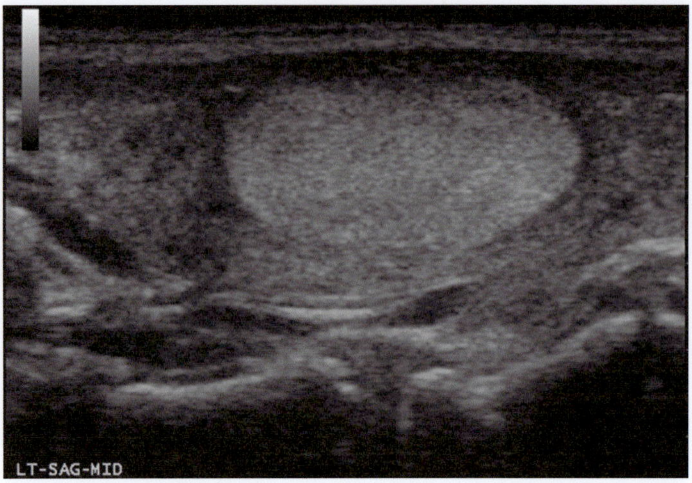

Fig. 16.24 White knight. Transverse image of the left lobe of the thyroid shows a well-marginated, solid hyperechoic nodule occurring in a gland with a background heterogeneous thyroid parenchyma. This type of nodule is invariably benign on biopsy. This appearance has been called a "white knight" and is thought to represent a regenerative nodule in the setting of chronic lymphocytic thyroiditis. Reproduced with permission from Springer, Thyroid Ultrasound and Ultrasound-Guided FNA, Editors, Baskin, Duick, and Levine, Chapter 6 pp 99–126

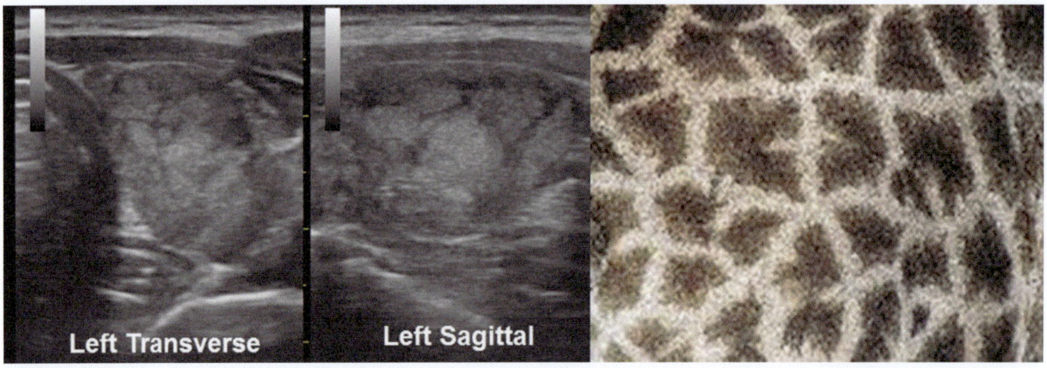

Fig. 16.25 Giraffe pattern in chronic lymphocytic thyroiditis. The sonographic pattern of globular hyperechoic pseudonodules with intervening hypoechoic bands has been termed a giraffe pattern, appearing similar to a photographic negative of a giraffe's hide

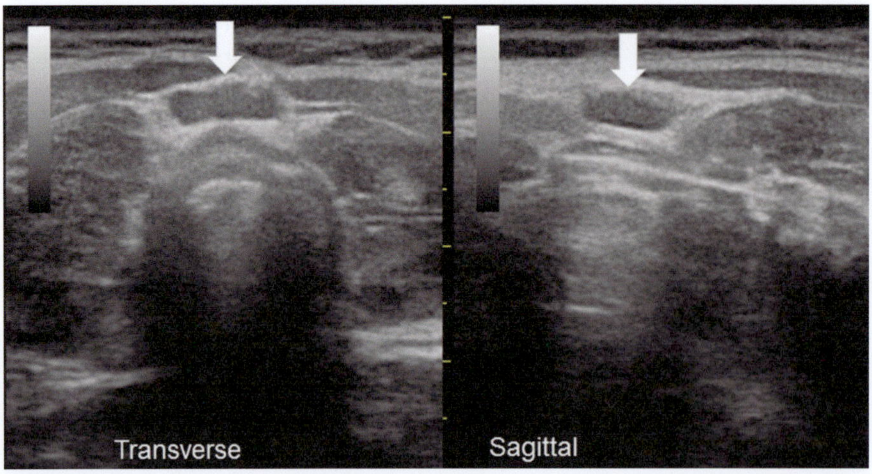

Fig. 16.26 Pre-laryngeal lymph nodes. Anterior to the trachea at the level of the larynx is a hypoechoic lymph node (arrow) that can be easily confused with an isthmus nodule in transverse view, but sagittal view shows this to be superior to the isthmus. This pre-laryngeal node is often referred to as the Delphian node

Fig. 16.27 Lateral lymph nodes. A transverse image of the left neck shows a hypoechoic and heterogeneous left lobe (arrow) in a patient with chronic lymphocytic thyroiditis. Reactive lymph node enlargement is common not only in the paratracheal space but in the lower lateral neck levels of III and IV as seen here marked by *calipers* (*CCA* common carotid artery, *IJV* internal jugular vein)

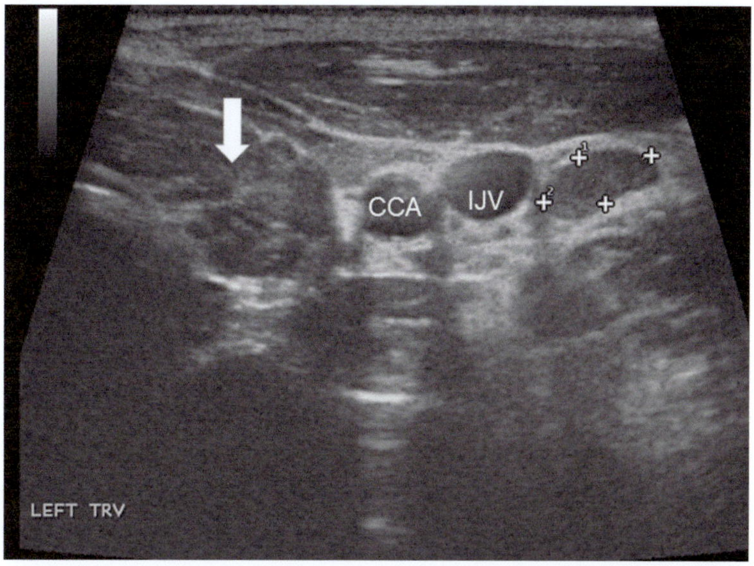

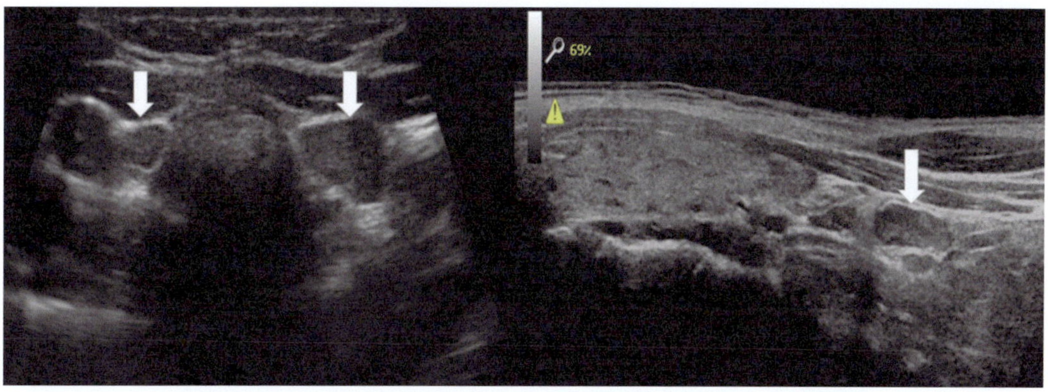

Fig. 16.28 Paratracheal lymph nodes. Transverse view inferior to the thyroid showing left greater than right paratracheal (level VI) lymph nodes in a patient with chronic lymphocytic thyroiditis. *Right panel* shows sagittal view of the left lobe and inferior paratracheal node (arrow)

Fig. 16.29 Lymph nodes (arrows) inferior to the left lobe in a patient with chronic lymphocytic thyroiditis. These can mimic parathyroid adenomas causing potential confusion in patients with primary hyperparathyroidism and Hashimoto's

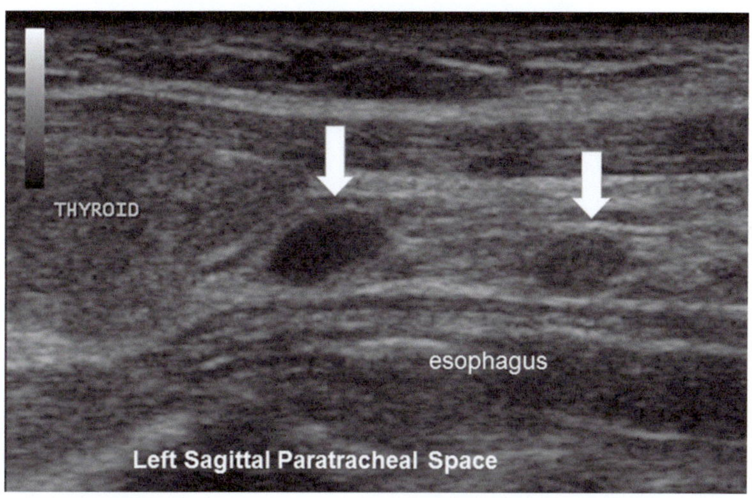

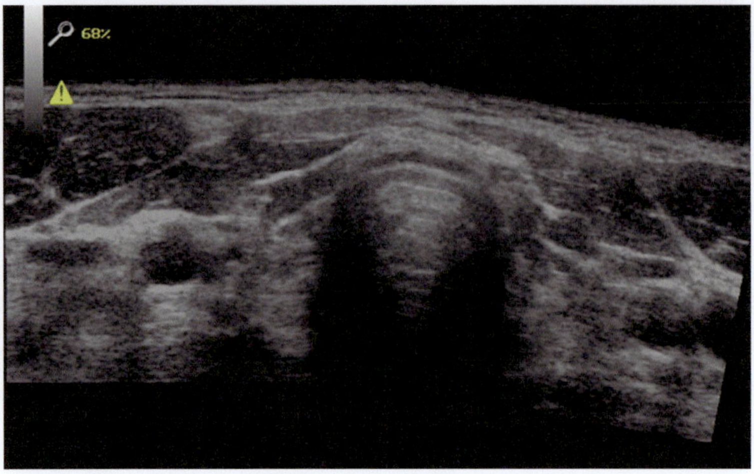

Fig. 16.30 Chronic atrophic thyroiditis. Panoramic view of the neck in a patient with long-standing chronic lymphocytic thyroiditis shows a markedly atrophic and hypoechoic gland. Reproduced with permission from Springer, Thyroid Ultrasound and Ultrasound-Guided FNA, Editors, Baskin, Duick, and Levine, Chapter 6 pp 99–126

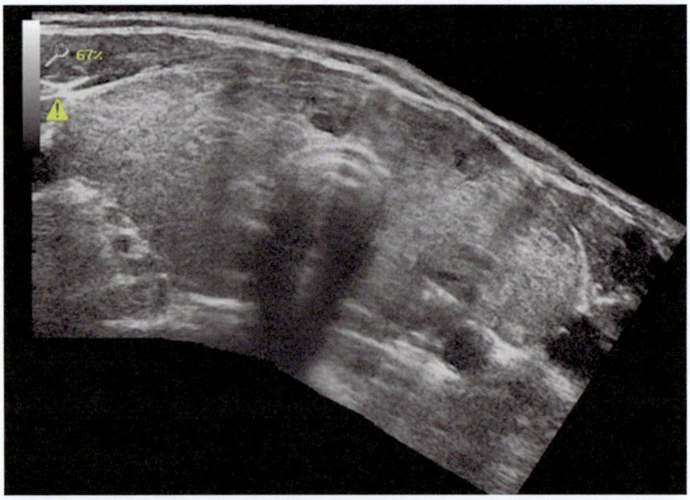

Fig. 16.31 Graves' disease: diffuse enlargement. Virtual panoramic transverse view of the thyroid in a patient with Graves' disease which tends to be more echogenic than Hashimoto's but still demonstrates significant heterogeneity and diffuse enlargement. Reproduced with permission from Springer, Thyroid Ultrasound and Ultrasound-Guided FNA, Editors, Baskin, Duick, and Levine, Chapter 6 pp 99–126

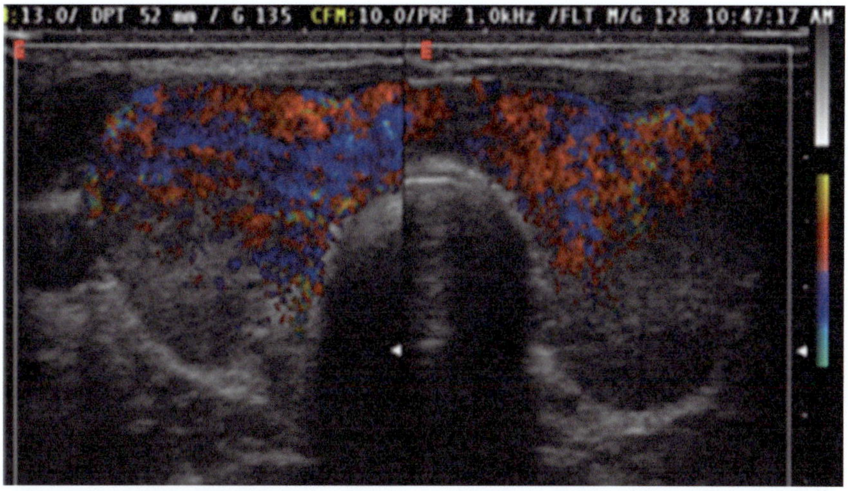

Fig. 16.32 "Thyroid inferno" in Graves' disease. Doppler imaging of this patient with Graves' disease shows intense blood flow. Reproduced with permission from Springer, Thyroid Ultrasound and Ultrasound-Guided FNA, Editors, Baskin, Duick, and Levine, Chapter 6 pp 99–126

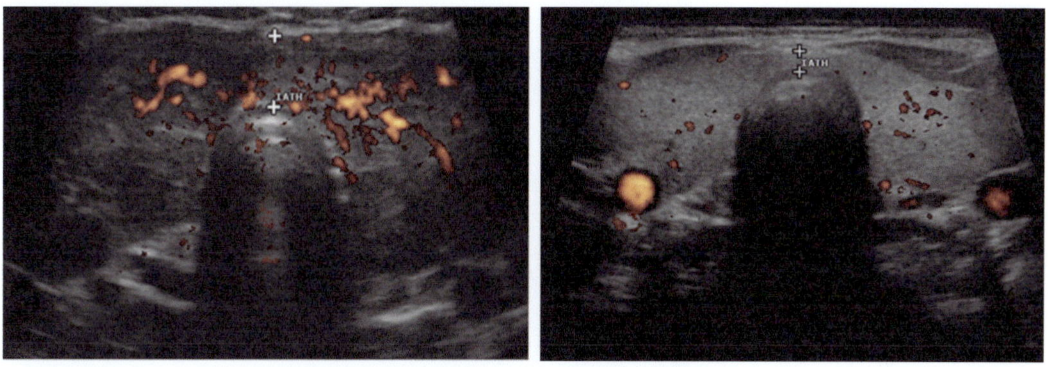

Fig. 16.33 Treated Graves' disease. The *left image* was obtained at the initial presentation of the patient and shows gland enlargement, overall hypoechogenicity, heterogeneity, and moderately increased vascularity. The *right image*, obtained with similar Doppler settings, following 16 months of successful methimazole treatment and normalized TSH-R antibodies shows a normal appearance of the thyroid

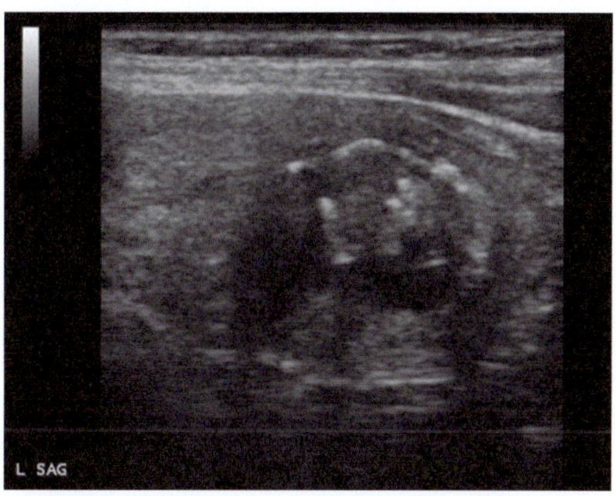

Fig. 16.34 Papillary thyroid cancer in Graves' disease. Sagittal image of the left lobe showing background heterogeneity and a densely calcified nodule which proved to be papillary thyroid cancer on FNA biopsy in this patient with Graves' disease

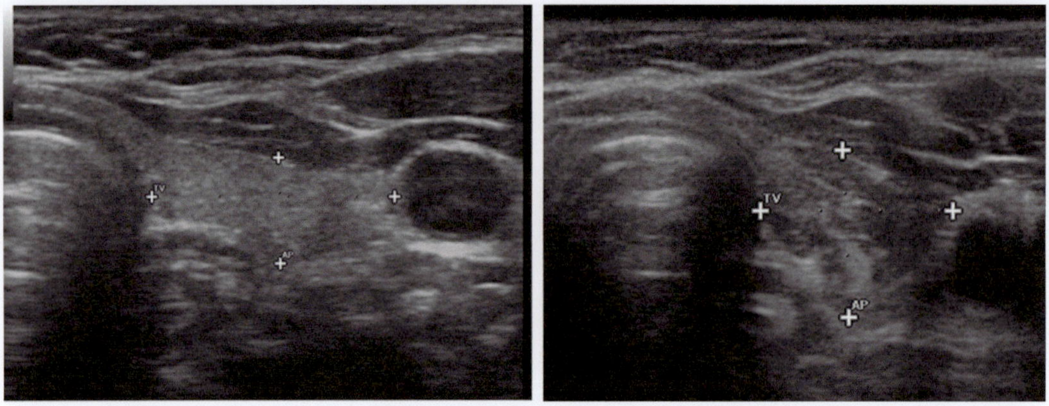

Fig. 16.35 Ipilimumab drug-induced thyroiditis. This patient with metastatic melanoma was initially seen for an incidentally discovered right nodule which was benign. The *left panel* shows the normal left lobe at initial evaluation. Subsequently she was treated with ipilimumab and developed thyroiditis after 4 months with typical sonographic changes of heterogeneity, fibrosis, and hypoechogenicity

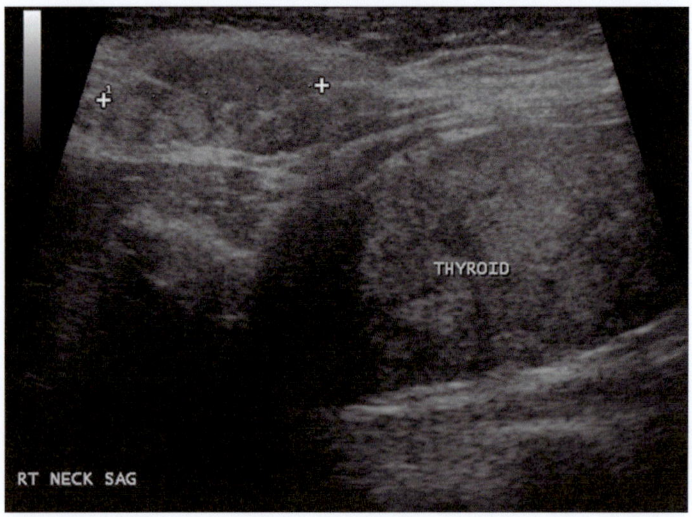

Fig. 16.36 Ectopic Hashimoto's. Patient referred for midline neck mass (calipers) near hyoid thought to be a thyroglossal duct cyst, but ultrasound revealed ectopic thyroid tissue superior to the right lobe, not connected to the thyroid but with same echotexture. FNA biopsy confirmed this to be chronic lymphocytic thyroiditis

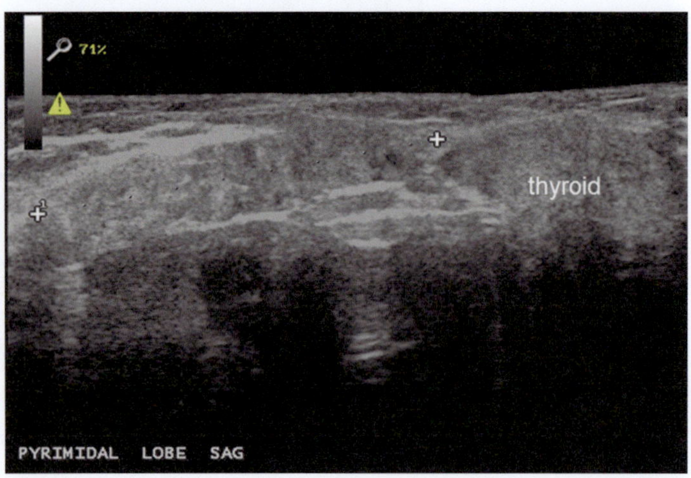

Fig. 16.37 Pyrimidal lobe. This 80-year-old female with long-standing diffuse thyroid enlargement due to Hashimoto's has a prominent pyramidal lobe seen here superior to the thyroid extending to the level of the hyoid bone anterior to the larynx. The *caliper* marks represent a distance of 4.3 cm

References

1. Kim DW. A comparative study of real-time and static ultrasonography diagnoses for the incidental detection of diffuse thyroid disease. Endocr Pract. 2015;21(8):910–6.
2. Pearce E, Farwell A, Braverman L. Current concepts: thyroiditis. N Engl J Med. 2003;384(26):2646–55.
3. Pedersen OM, Aardal NP, Larssen TB, et al. The value of ultrasonography in predicting autoimmune thyroid disease. Thyroid. 2000;10(3):251–9.
4. Raber W, Gessi A, et al. Thyroid ultrasound versus antithyroid peroxidase antibody determination: a cohort study of four hundred fifty-one subjects. Thyroid. 2002;12(8):725–31.
5. Rago T, Chiovato L, Grasso L, et al. Thyroid ultrasonography as a tool for detecting thyroid autoimmune diseases and predicting thyroid dysfunction in apparently healthy subjects. J Endocrinol Invest. 2001;24:763–9.
6. Rotondi M, Cappelli C, Leporati P, et al. A hypoechoic pattern of the thyroid at ultrasound does not indicate autoimmune thyroid diseases in patients with morbid obesity. Eur J Endocrinol. 2010;163(1):105–9.
7. Loy M, Cianchetti ME, Cardia F, et al. Correlation of computerized gray-scale sonographic findings with thyroid function and thyroid autoimmune activity in patients with Hashimoto's thyroiditis. J Clin Ultrasound. 2004;32:136–40.
8. Livolsi VA. The pathology of autoimmune thyroid disease: a review. Thyroid. 1994;4(3):333–9.
9. Williams A, Bieler D, Wieler H, et al. Correlation between sonography and antibody activity in patients with Hashimoto thyroiditis. J Ultrasound Med. 2013;32(11):1979–86.
10. Lupo M, Levine R. Ultrasound of diffuse thyroid enlargement: thyroiditis. In: Baskin J, Duick D, Levine A, editors. Thyroid ultrasound and ultrasound guided FNA. 3rd ed. New York, NY: Springer; 2013.
11. Kim HS, Han BK, Shin JH, et al. Papillary thyroid carcinoma of a diffuse selerosing variant: ultrasonographic monitoring from a normal thyroid gland to mass formation. Korean J Radiol. 2010;11(5):579–82.
12. Beland MD, Kwon L, Delellis RA, Cronin JJ, Grant EG. Nonshadowing echogenic foci in thyroid nodules. Are certain appearances enough to avoid thyroid biopsy? J Ultrasound Med. 2011;30:753–60.
13. Gul K, Dirikoc A, Kiyak G, et al. The association between thyroid carcinoma and Hashimoto's thyroiditis: the ultrasonographic and histopathologic characteristics of malignant nodules. Thyroid. 2010;20:873–8.
14. Fiore E, Rago T, Latrofa F, et al. Hashimoto's thyroiditis is associated with papillary thyroid carcinoma: role of TSH and of treatment with L-thyroxine. Endocr Relat Cancer. 2011;18(4):429–37.
15. Anil C, Goksel S, Gursoy A. Hashimoto's thyroiditis is not associated with increased risk of thyroid cancer in patients with thyroid nodules: a single-center prospective study. Thyroid. 2010;20(6):601–6.
16. Anderson L, Middleton W, et al. Hashimoto thyroiditis: Part 1, Sonographic analysis of the nodular form of hashimoto thyroiditis. AJR Am J Roentgenol. 2010;195:208–15.
17. Anderson L, Middleton W, et al. Hashimoto thyroiditis: Part 2. Sonographic analysis of benign and malignant nodules in patients with diffuse hashimoto thyroiditis. AJR Am J Roentgenol. 2010;195:216–22.
18. Ohmori N, Miyakawa M, Ohmori K, et al. Ultrasonographic findings of papillary thyroid carcinoma with Hashimoto's thyroiditis. Intern Med. 2007;46(9):547–50.
19. Durfee SM, Benson CB, Arthaud DM, et al. Sonographic appearance of thyroid cancer in patients with Hashimoto thyroiditis. J Ultrasound Med. 2015;34(4):697–704.
20. Bonavita JA, Mayo J, Babb J, et al. Pattern recognition of benign nodules at ultrasound of the thyroid: which nodules can be left alone? AJR Am J Roentgenol. 2009;193:207–13.
21. Brancato D, Citarrella R, Richiusa P, et al. Neck lymph nodes in chronic autoimmune thyroiditis: the sonographic pattern. Thyroid. 2013;23(2):173–7.
22. Ralls PW, Mayekawa DS, Lee KP, et al. Color-flow Doppler sonography in Graves disease: "thyroid inferno". AJR Am J Roentgenol. 1988;150(4):781–4.
23. Erdogan MF, Anil C, Cesur M, et al. Color flow Doppler sonography for the etiologic diagnosis of hyperthyroidism. Thyroid. 2007;17:223–8.
24. Kurita S, Sakurai M, Kita Y, et al. Measurement of thyroid blood flow area is useful for diagnosing the cause of Thyrotoxicosis. Thyroid. 2005;15:1249–52.
25. Ota H, Amino N, Morita S, et al. Quantitative measurement of thyroid blood flow for differentiation of painless thyroiditis from Graves' disease. Clin Endocrinol (Oxf). 2007;67:41.
26. Bogazzi F, Vitti P. Could improved ultrasound and power Doppler replace thyroidal radioiodine uptake to assess thyroid disease? Nat Rev Endocrinol. 2008;4:70–1.
27. Bahn RS, Burch HB, Cooper DS, et al. Hyperthyroidism and other causes of thyrotoxicosis: management guidelines of the American Thyroid Association and American Association of Clinical Endocrinologists. Endocr Pract. 2011;17(3):456–520.
28. Cappelli C, Pirola I, de Martino E, et al. The role of imaging in Graves' disease: a cost-effectiveness analysis. Eur J Radiol. 2008;65:99–103.
29. Sipos JA, Kahaly GJ. Imaging of thyrotoxicosis. Am J Med. 2012;125(9):S1–2.
30. Alzahrani AS, Ceresini G, Aldasouqi SA. Role of ultrasonography in the differential diagnosis of thyrotoxicosis: a noninvasive, cost-effective, and widely available but underutilized diagnostic tool. Endocr Pract. 2012;18(4):567–78.
31. Baldini M, Castagnone D, Rivolta R, et al. Thyroid vascularization by color doppler ultrasonography in Graves' disease. Changes related to different phases and to the long-term outcome of the disease. Thyroid. 1997;7(6):823–8.

32. Saleh A, Fürst G, Feldkamp J, et al. Estimation of antithyroid drug dose in Graves' disease: value of quantification of thyroid blood flow with color duplex sonography. Ultrasound Med Biol. 2001;27(8):1137–41.
33. Baldini M, Orsatti A, Bonfanti MT, et al. Relationship between the sonographic appearance of the thyroid and the clinical course and autoimmune activity of Graves' disease. J Clin Ultrasound. 2005;33(8):381–5.
34. Zingrillo M, D'Aloiso L, Ghiggi MR, et al. Thyroid hypoechogenicity after methimazole withdrawal in Graves' disease: a useful index for predicting recurrence? Clin Endocrinol (Oxf). 1996;45(2):201–6.
35. Premawardhana LD, Parkes AB, Ammari F, et al. Postpartum thyroiditis and long-term thyroid status: prognostic influence of TPO antibody and US echogenicity. J Clin Endocrinol Metab. 2000;85:71–5.
36. Yeh H, Futterweit W, Gilbert P. Micronodulation: ultrasonographic sign of Hashimoto thyroiditis. J Ultrasound Med. 1996;15:813–9.

17 Pattern Recognition: Uncommon Clinical Scenarios

Sathya Jyothinagaram and Mira Milas

17.1 Case Vignette 1: Hypoechoic Enlarging Thyroid Mass

A 45-year-old woman presented with a midline neck mass enlarging over a period of 4–6 months. It was soft to palpation, appeared like a midline isthmus nodule with perhaps associated left thyroid fullness, and was located close to the clavicular heads. The patient experienced mild compressive symptoms when swallowing and lying supine. Ten years previously the patient reported having thymectomy for a benign tumor but no old records were available for confirmation. Her TSH was normal. An ultrasound performed during initial consultation revealed a large hypoechoic oval mass (Videos 17.1 and 17.2) centered on the isthmus. Visible portions of the adjacent thyroid lobes appeared normal. Two ultrasound-guided fine-needle aspiration biopsies revealed benign squamous cells and no thyroid follicular cells (Video 17.3). Surgery was advised because of the symptoms, unusual and nondiagnostic cytology, and progressive increase in size. Scrutiny of the ultrasound images more carefully (Fig. 17.1) prior to surgery disclosed that the nodule was actually superficial to the strap muscles (sternothyroid and sternohyoid muscles). This in fact was observed intraoperatively and a benign squamous cell cyst excised and confirmed by cytology (sequence of surgical photos in Fig. 17.2). Neither the midline raphe of the strap muscles nor the thyroid gland required exposure. There was no associated thyroid pathology and no connection between the squamous cyst and any deep anatomical structures (e.g., thymus or paratracheal tissues).

This patient's imaging findings are interesting because they represent a benign superficial cyst mimicking a thyroid nodule, both in exam and ultrasound features. The case also illustrates the need for attentiveness to detail. While it may be instinctive to focus on the main abnormality, especially if it is a large mass, valuable information may come from slowing down the scanning pace to discern nuances such as spatial relationships to surrounding anatomical structures.

Electronic supplementary material: The online version of this chapter (doi:10.1007/978-3-319-44100-9_17) contains supplementary material, which is available to authorized users. Videos can also be accessed at http://link.springer.com/chapter/10.1007/978-3-319-44100-9_17.

S. Jyothinagaram, M.D., F.A.C.E.
Diabetes and Endocrinology Institute, Banner - University Medical Center Phoenix, University of Arizona College of Medicine – Phoenix, Phoenix, AZ, USA
e-mail: sathya.jyothinagaram@bannerhealth.com

M. Milas, M.D., F.A.C.S. (✉)
Department of Surgery and the Endocrinology & Metabolism Institute, University of Arizona College of Medicine - Phoenix, Banner - University Medical Center Phoenix, 1441 North 12th Street 2nd floor, Phoenix, AZ 85006, USA
e-mail: Mira.Milas@bannerhealth.com

M. Milas et al. (eds.), *Advanced Thyroid and Parathyroid Ultrasound*,
DOI 10.1007/978-3-319-44100-9_17

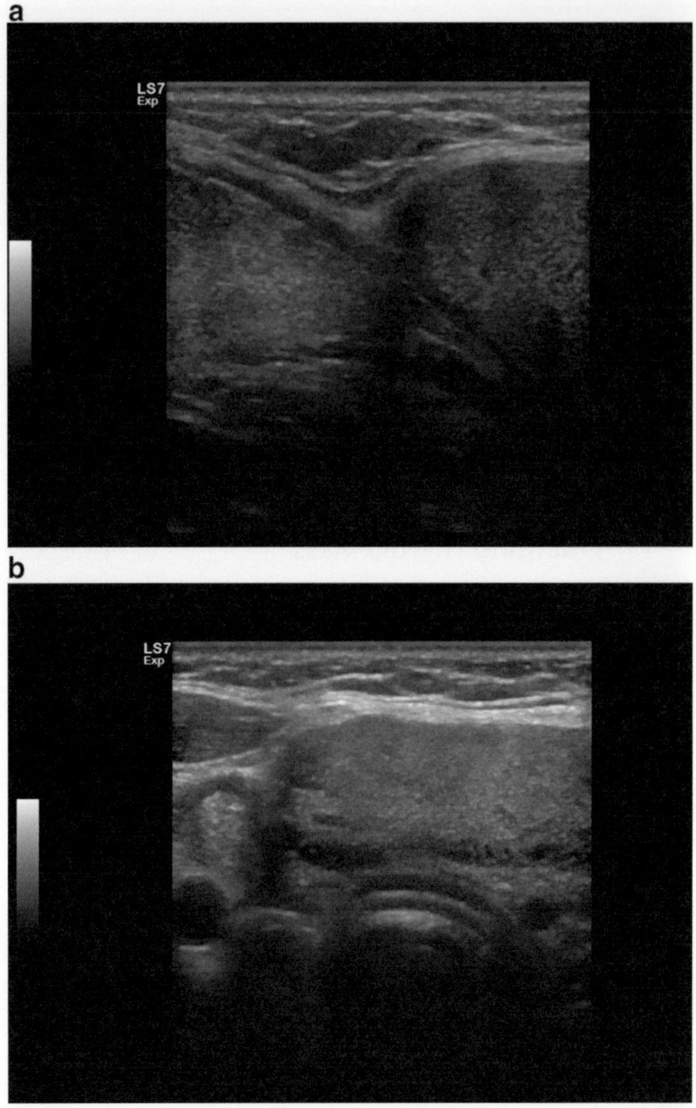

Fig. 17.1 Ultrasound images of squamous cell cyst show it is anterior to the strap muscles (**a**, *right upper corner* of image). In contrast, the normal thyroid is deep to the thin hypoechoic line of the sternothyroid muscle. Both the cyst and the thyroid have the same echogenicity. This relationship is not as evident in the transverse view (**b**) where the nodule appears to arise from the isthmus

17.2 Case Vignette 2: Large Mass with Microcalcifications in the Central Neck

Two years following initial diagnosis and treatment for papillary thyroid cancer (PTC) at age 14, surveillance ultrasound was performed on a 16-year-old boy during routine follow-up visit. The referring physician noticed that the ultrasound report described a previously undetected mass in the central neck with microcalcifications and suspected recurrent PTC. Additional ultrasound imaging during consultation for possible biopsy and/or reoperation clarified that the mass had a different etiology: normal benign thymus. Neither biopsy nor surgery was performed. This case emphasizes that the thymus is a normal component of anatomy in the central neck, particularly in children and young adolescents. In this young population, the thymus typically has

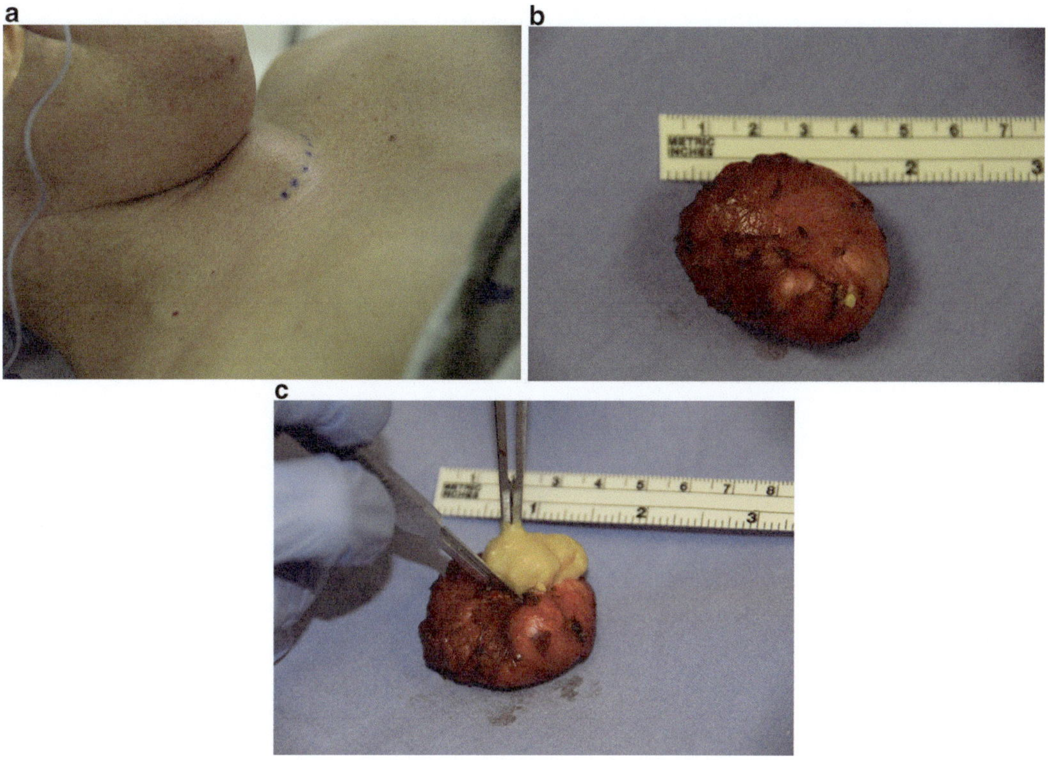

Fig. 17.2 Excised benign squamous cell cyst and contents (**a**–**c**)

scattered hyperechoic foci that mimic microcalcifications (Video 17.4).

17.3 Case Vignette 3: Anaplastic Thyroid Carcinoma

This type of thyroid cancer remains one of the most aggressive, deadly malignancies of any kind. In this 62-year-old man with biopsy-proven anaplastic thyroid cancer, the large left-sided thyroid mass had developed rapidly over the course of 10 days. Normal anatomical structures were displaced laterally, as seen on an early computed tomography (CT) scan (Fig. 17.3). Placement of a tracheostomy tube was necessary for airway security and to allow chemoradiation and palliative care therapies to proceed. While the CT scan demonstrated how compromised and displaced the trachea was, it was impossible to palpate this by exam. Ultrasound played a key role to identify the location of the trachea and guide placement of a tracheostomy (Fig. 17.4).

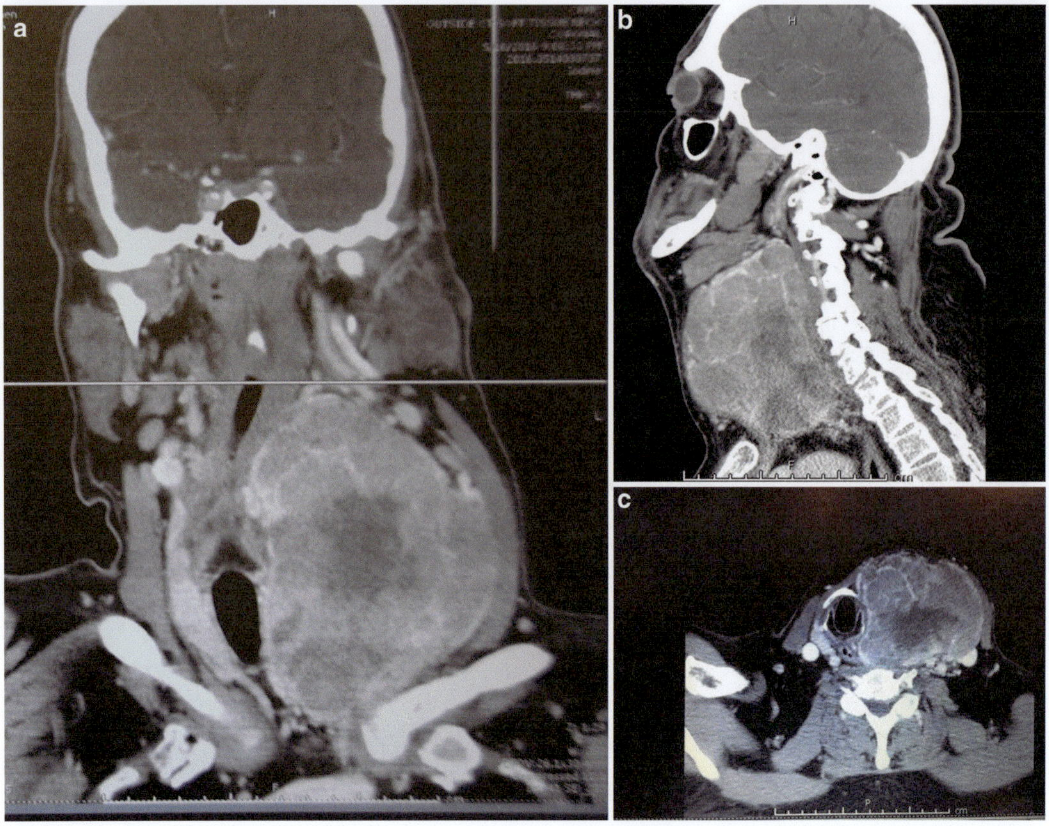

Fig. 17.3 Anaplastic thyroid cancer arising from left thyroid lobe in patient with a prior history of goiter. Computed tomography images are shown in views (**a**)–(**c**)

17.4 Conclusions

Ultrasound appearance of non-endocrine pathologies can imitate the features of thyroid disease [1–5]. Careful study of the ultrasound images, especially in real time during the consultation or via saved cine-clip video files, can identify details that allow a precise direction of evaluation and treatment. The overall pattern of features must be interpreted with awareness of potential biases (e.g., the presence of punctate calcifications is not uniquely associated with malignancy) so as to avoid coming to a premature diagnosis. The versatility of ultrasound is evident in both the office-based and operating room settings, as it can direct appropriate patients to limited surgery, exclude other patients from having unnecessary surgery, and guide interventions to be minimally invasive yet achieve the treatment goals.

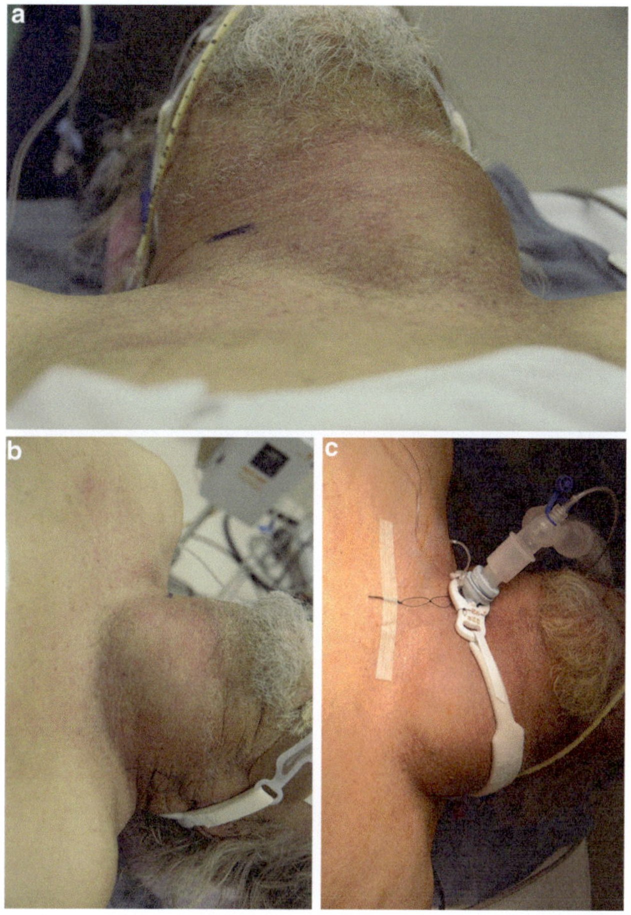

Fig. 17.4 Surgical marking on the skin shows the position of the trachea (**a**, *far right side* of the patient's neck) and the common carotid artery (**b**, *far left side* of the patient's neck, mark in the shape of a *box*). These were identified with ultrasound in surgery to allow placement of tracheostomy (**c**)

References

1. Xie C, Cox P, Taylor N, LaPorte S. Ultrasonography of thyroid nodules: a pictorial review. Insights Imaging. 2016;7(1):77–86.
2. Ginat DT, Butani D, Giampoli EJ, Patel N, Dogra V. Pearls and pitfalls of thyroid nodule sonography and fine-needle aspiration. Ultrasound Q. 2010;26(3):171–8.
3. Bekele W, Gerscovich EO, Naderi S, Bishop J, Gandour-Edwards RF, McGahan JP. Sonography of an epidermoid inclusion cyst of the thyroid gland. J Ultrasound Med. 2012;31(1):128–9.
4. Yildiz AE, Ceyhan K, Sıklar Z, Bilir P, Yağmurlu EA, Berberoğlu M, Fitoz S. Intrathyroidal ectopic thymus in children: retrospective analysis of grayscale and doppler sonographic features. J Ultrasound Med. 2015;34(9):1651–6.
5. Suh HJ, Moon HJ, Kwak JY, Choi JS, Kim EK. Anaplastic thyroid cancer: ultrasonographic findings and the role of ultrasonography-guided fine needle aspiration biopsy. Yonsei Med J. 2013;54(6):1400–6.

18 Pattern Recognition of Benign and Malignant Thyroid Nodules: Ultrasound Characteristics and Ultrasound-Guided Fine Needle Aspiration of Thyroid Nodules

Jason Michael Johnson, Maria K. Gule-Monroe, Michael Kwon, Salmaan Ahmed, Dawid Schlingerhout, Vinodh A. Kumar, Beth S. Edeiken-Monroe, and James M. Debnam

18.1 Introduction

Ultrasound (US) is a practical and reliable imaging modality for assessment of the thyroid. Differentiating malignant from more frequently occurring benign thyroid disease has proved challenging as there may be significant overlap in their clinical presentation and sonographic appearance. High-resolution ultrasound provides a safe and affordable way to identify and characterize diffuse thyroid disease such as thyroiditis and lymphoma, detection of non-palpable masses, diagnosis of palpable masses, staging of known cancer, follow-up evaluation of the thyroid beds after thyroidectomy, and guidance for fine-needle aspiration (FNA).

J.M. Johnson, M.D. • M.K. Gule-Monroe, M.D.
The Department of Diagnostic Radiology, The University of Texas MD Anderson Cancer Center, 1515 Holcombe Blvd., Unit 1482, Houston, TX 77030, USA
e-mail: jjohnson12@mdanderson.org; mgule@mdanderson.org

M. Kwon, M.D., Ph.D. (✉)
Department of Diagnostic Radiology, The University of Texas M. D. Anderson Cancer Center, 1400 Pressler Street, FCT16.5040, Unit 1482, Houston, TX 77030, USA
e-mail: michael.kwon@mdandersong.org

S. Ahmed, M.D.
Department of Diagnostic Radiology, The University of Texas M. D. Anderson Cancer Center, 1400 Pressler Street, Unit 1482, Houston, TX 77030, USA
e-mail: Salmaan.Ahmed@mdanderson.org

D. Schlingerhout, M.D. • J.M. Debnam, M.D.
Section of Neuro Radiology, Department of Diagnostic Radiology, The University of Texas M. D. Anderson Cancer Center, Houston, TX, USA

V.A. Kumar, M.D.
3333 Allen Parkway, Unit 2803, Houston, TX 77019, USA

Department of Diagnostic Radiology, The University of Texas M. D. Anderson Cancer Center, 1400 Pressler Street, Unit 1482, Houston, TX 77030, USA
e-mail: vakumar@mdanderson.org

B.S. Edeiken-Monroe, M.D., F.A.C.R.
Department of Diagnostic Imaging, The University of Texas M. D. Anderson Cancer Center, 1515 Holcombe, Houston, TX 77030, USA

62 East Bend Lane, Houston, TX 77007, USA
e-mail: bedeiken@mdanderson.org

M. Milas et al. (eds.), *Advanced Thyroid and Parathyroid Ultrasound*,
DOI 10.1007/978-3-319-44100-9_18

18.2 Sonographic Evaluation of Thyroid Disease

Ultrasound has high sensitivity but less specificity to distinguish benign from malignant lesions, and diffuse infiltration, in the thyroid. Improvement in US specificity of thyroid disease has been attempted by the employment of contrast agents (1998), harmonic imaging (2001), and elastography (2005) [4, 5]. The experience at MD Anderson Cancer Center (MDACC), in Houston, Texas, is that these systems have not demonstrated the reliability to replace high-frequency B-mode US for the evaluation of benign vs. malignant disease of the thyroid.

Because MDACC is a cancer center, we have had the opportunity to biopsy the thyroid for diffuse disease and well-defined thyroid nodules that would have been followed sonographically rather than biopsy at outlying hospitals. This has afforded the opportunity to have pathology results on diffuse thyroid changes as well as well-defined nodules that were not characteristic of malignancy but did not have a classical benign appearance. Unsuspected medullary cancer, Hurthle cell cancer, metastasis to the thyroid, and lymphoma have been documented. This has led to the conclusion, in our institutional practice, that diffusely infiltrated thyroid glands and thyroid nodules that vary from the classical benign appearance should undergo US-guided biopsy independent of size.

18.3 Sonographic Evaluation of Diffuse Thyroid Disease

Due to the overlap in features, it is difficult to differentiate the etiology of diffuse infiltration of the thyroid. Below are examples of both benign and malignant diffuse thyroid infiltration that required US-guided biopsy for diagnosis.

18.3.1 Case 1: Diffuse Thyroid Disease (Thyroiditis)

Clinical Scenario: A 63-year-old female who presents with painless enlarged thyroid

Imaging Features: Ultrasound. Diffuse enlargement of the right lobe with a heterogeneous echotexture (Fig. 18.1a)

Power Doppler demonstrated increased vascular flow in the thyroid gland (Fig. 18.1b).

Diagnosis of US-Guided FNA/Cytology: (**Right lobe**) **Hashimoto's thyroiditis/lymphocytic thyroiditis**

18.3.2 Case 2: Diffuse Thyroid Disease (Nodular Thyroiditis)

Clinical Scenario: A 56-year-old man with multiple thyroid nodules. US was performed to assess the palpable thyroid nodules.

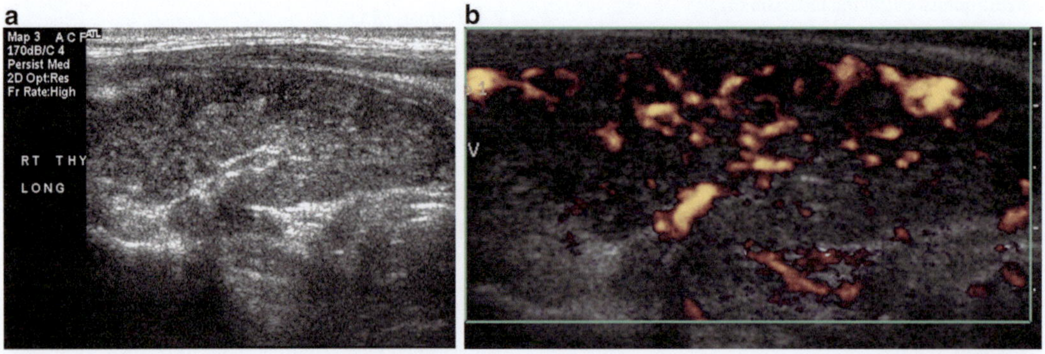

Fig. 18.1 (**a**) **Grayscale US**. Diffusely enlarged right lobe of the thyroid with a heterogeneous echotexture characteristic of thyroiditis. (**b**) **Power Doppler US**. Diffusely enlarged right lobe of the thyroid with a heterogeneous echotexture and increased vascular flow characteristic of thyroiditis

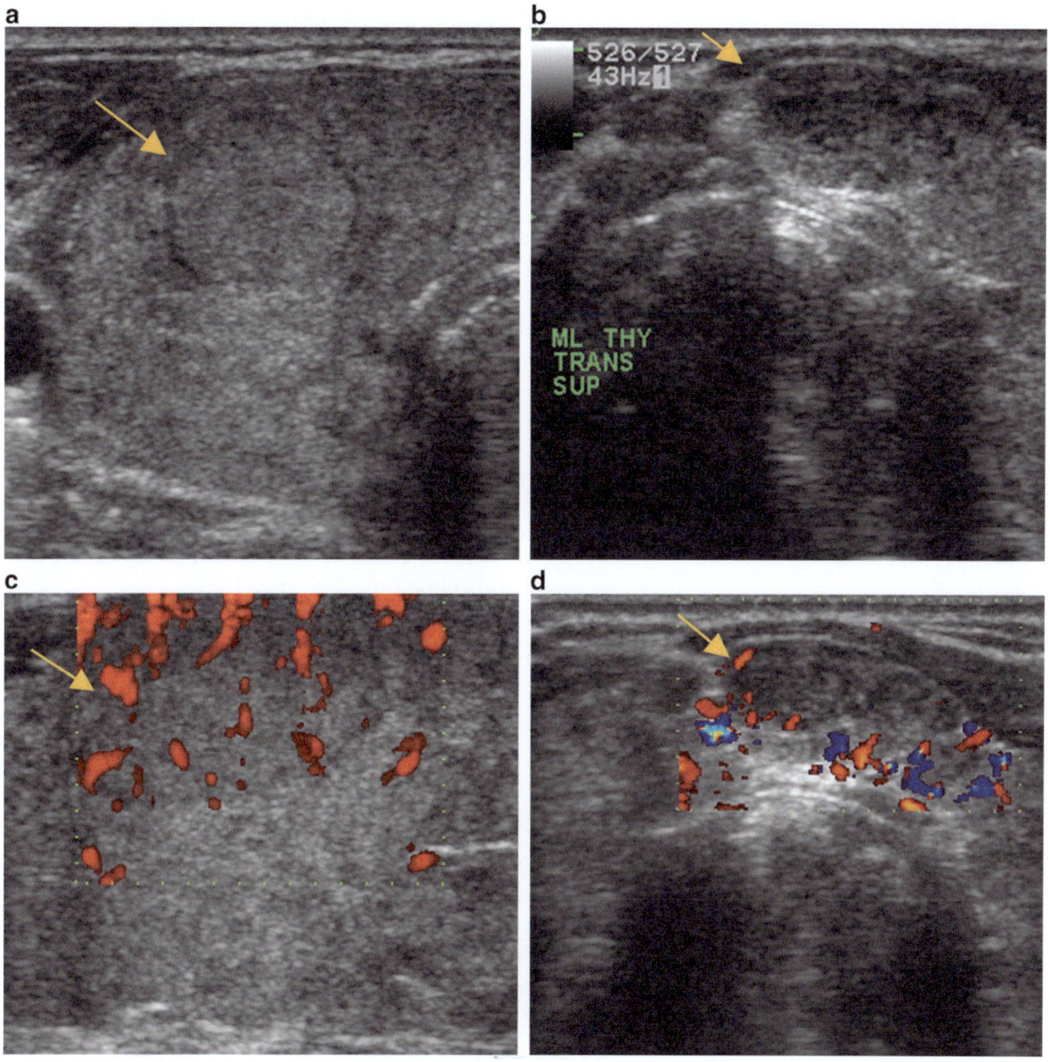

Fig. 18.2 (**a**) **Grayscale US**. Enlarged thyroid gland with what appears to be multiple well-circumscribed nodules in the transverse plane that ultimately proved by US-guided FNA to be pseudo-nodules of thyroiditis (*arrow*). (**b**) **Grayscale US**. Enlarged thyroid gland with what appears to be multiple well-circumscribed nodules in the transverse plane that ultimately proved by US-guided FNA to be pseudo-nodules of thyroiditis (*arrow*). (**c**) **Power Doppler US**. Increased vascular flow demonstrated on power Doppler within suspected multiple thyroid nodules. (**d**) Power Doppler US. Increased vascular flow demonstrated on power Doppler within suspected multiple thyroid nodules that were ultimately found on FNA or cytology to be composed of a polymorphous lymphoid population and Hürthle-like cells consistent with chronic lymphocytic thyroiditis

Imaging Features: Ultrasound. Enlargement of the thyroid gland with what appears to be multiple well-circumscribed nodules in the transverse plane (Fig. 18.2a, b). Increased vascular flow demonstrated on power Doppler within suspected multiple thyroid nodules (Fig. 18.2c, d)

Diagnosis of US-Guided FNA/Cytology: Polymorphous lymphoid population and Hürthle-like cells consistent with chronic lymphocytic thyroiditis documenting that the thyroid contained pseudo-nodules caused by thyroiditis

18.3.3 Case 3: Diffuse Thyroid Disease (Thyroiditis)

Clinical Scenario: A 28-year-old female with familial adenomatous polyposis (FAP). Screening ultrasound examination was performed to exclude an associated thyroid cancer.

Imaging Features: Ultrasound. Non-homogenous thyroid gland in the longitudinal plane with no discrete suspicious nodules present to suggest a thyroid carcinoma (Fig. 18.3a): Power Doppler demonstrates increased vascular flow throughout the thyroid gland (Fig. 18.3b). Benign-appearing lymph nodes are present inferior to the left thyroid lobe which is a characteristic finding of thyroiditis (Fig. 18.3c).

Diagnosis of US-Guided FNA/Cytology: **Biopsy not indicated in this case of well-established thyroiditis based on the US images, even in a patient whose underlying genetic condition (FAP) may predispose to thyroid cancer**

18.3.4 Case 4: Diffuse Thyroid Disease (Thyroiditis vs. Leukemia)

Clinical Scenario: A 31-year-old female who presents with an enlarged, painful thyroid. US was performed to assess the palpable thyromegaly.

Imaging Features: Ultrasound. There is a heterogeneous echotexture of the thyroid gland with a lobulated contour imaged in the longitudinal plane (Fig. 18.4a). Power Doppler. Increased vascular flow throughout the gland (Fig. 18.4b). Computed tomography. Contrast-enhanced CT demonstrates diffuse enlargement of the thyroid gland (Fig. 18.4c).

No suspicious nodes were present in the central compartment or lateral neck.

Diagnosis of US-Guided FNA/Cytology: (**Right thyroid lobe**) **Polymorphous lymphoid infiltrate and rare thyroid follicular epithelium with reactive features, consistent with lymphocytic thyroiditis; immunophenotypic characterization of this aspirate by flow cytometry**

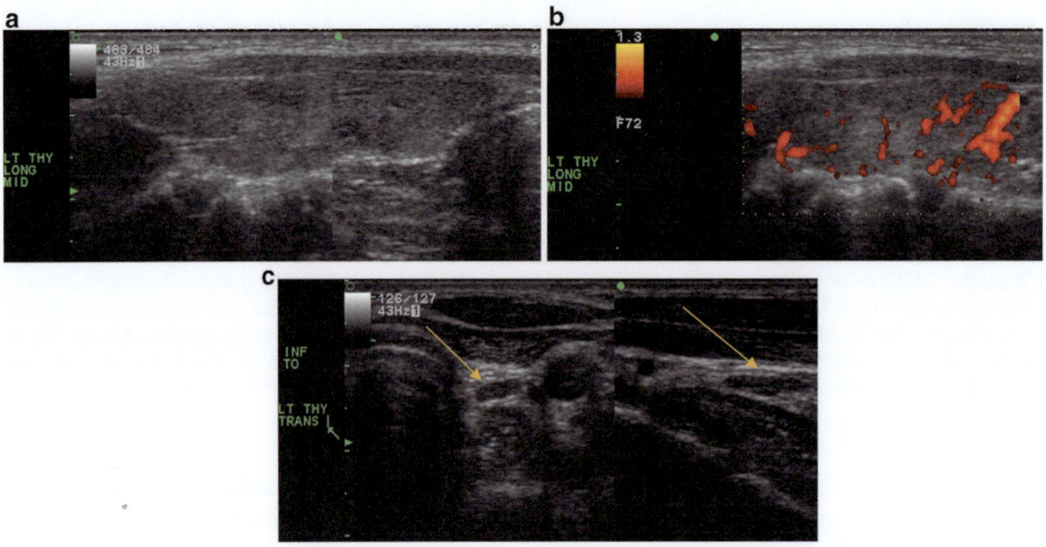

Fig. 18.3 (**a**) **Grayscale US**. Non-homogenous thyroid gland in the longitudinal plane. The appearance is characteristic of thyroiditis with no discrete suspicious nodules to suggest a thyroid carcinoma. (**b**) **Power Doppler US**. Mild increased vascularity of the thyroid gland which combined with the non-homogenous echogenicity is suggestive of thyroiditis. (**c**) **Grayscale US**. Benign-appearing lymph nodes that are present inferior to the left thyroid lobe which combined with the non-homogenous echogenicity are characteristic findings of thyroiditis (*arrow*)

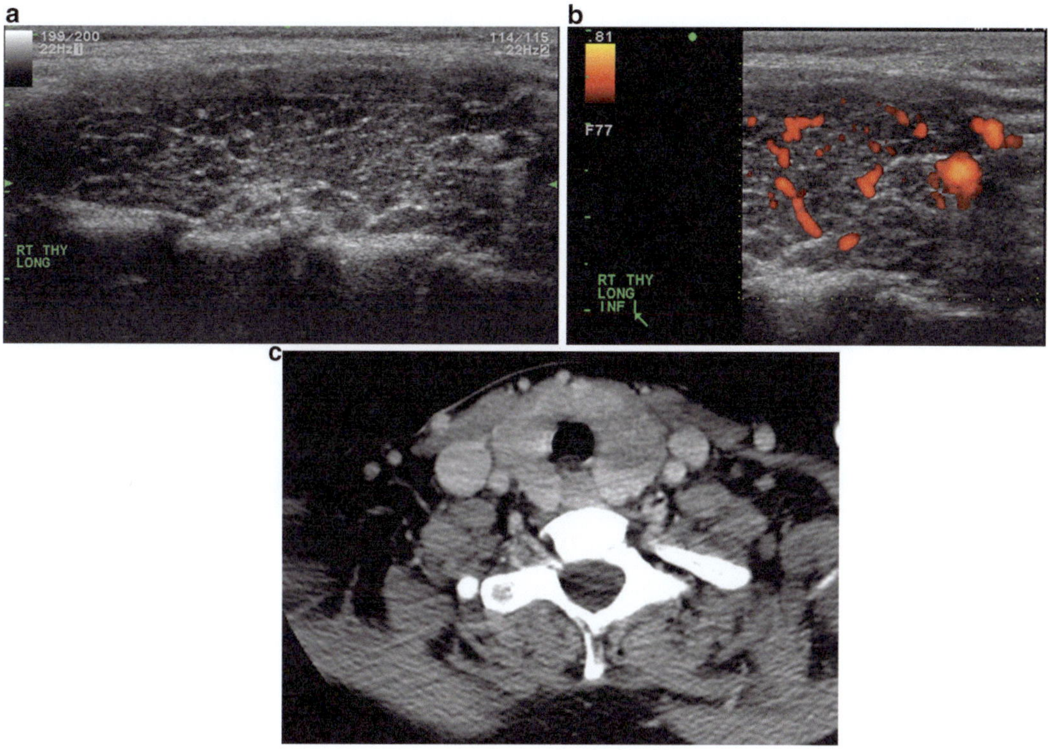

Fig. 18.4 (**a**) **Grayscale US**. There is a heterogeneous echotexture of the thyroid gland with a lobulated contour imaged in the longitudinal plane. (**b**) **Power Doppler US**. Increased vascular flow throughout the thyroid gland. (**c**) **CT**. Contrast-enhanced CT demonstrates diffuse enlargement of the thyroid gland

shows polytypic B cells and unremarkable T and NK cells. There is no immunophenotypic support for a B- or T-cell neoplasm.

Diagnosis of US-Guided FNAs/Cytology: **((A) Right thyroid) Large cell lymphoma**, **((B) Right neck node) large cell lymphoma**

18.3.5 Case 5: Lymphoma

Clinical Scenario: A 63-year-old female with a palpable right neck mass. Ultrasound was performed to assess the mass for thyroid cancer.

Imaging Features: Ultrasound. Diffuse enlargement of the thyroid gland with a heterogeneous echotexture containing multiple nodular components and a lobulated contour seen in the longitudinal plane (Fig. 18.5a). Power Doppler. Increased flow throughout the gland including within one of the nodules (Fig. 18.5b). Contrast-enhanced CT. Diffuse enlargement of the right lobe and a right lateral jugular territory neck node of concern imaged in the transverse plane (Fig. 18.5c)

18.3.6 Case 6: Prostate Cancer

Clinical Scenario: A 67-year-old male who presents with enlarged palpable thyroid. US was performed to assess thyroid and difficulty swallowing.

Imaging Features: Ultrasound. Diffuse enlargement of the left thyroid in the longitudinal plane with multiple punctate hyperechoic foci and no discrete mass (Fig. 18.6a). Power Doppler. Increased vascular flow in the enlarged thyroid gland (Fig. 18.6b). Power Doppler. Increased vascular flow in a suspicious right inferior jugular territory lymph node detected on ultrasound (Fig. 18.6c). Contrast-enhanced CT. Diffuse enlargement of the thyroid gland with a suspicious right inferior neck node (Fig. 18.6d)

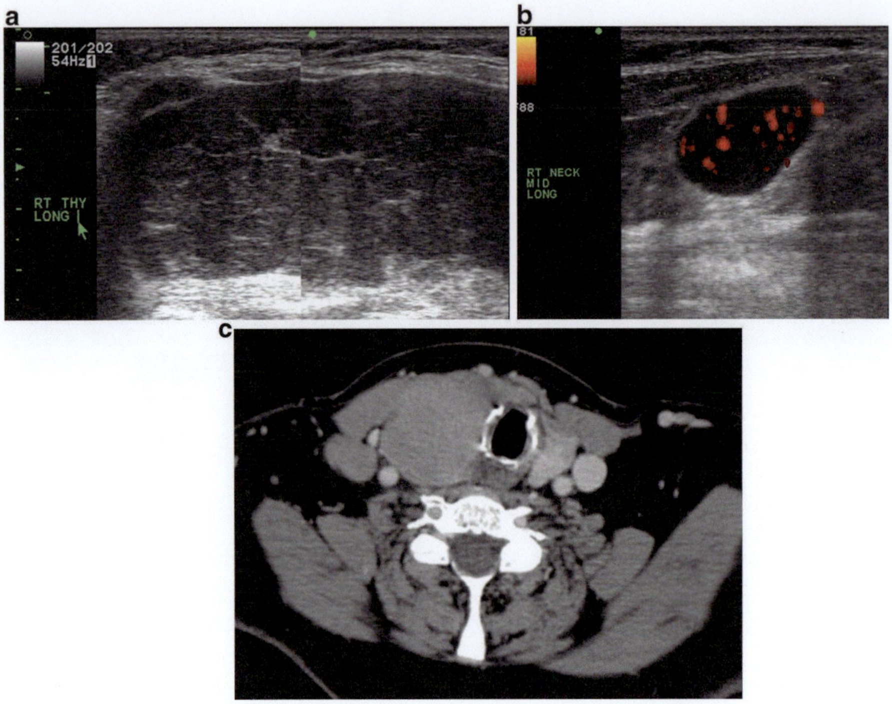

Fig. 18.5 (**a**) **Grayscale US**. Diffuse enlargement of the thyroid gland with a heterogeneous echotexture containing multiple nodules and a lobulated contour seen in the longitudinal plane. (**b**) **Power Doppler US**. Increased flow throughout the thyroid gland including within one of the thyroid nodules. (**c**) **Contrast-enhanced CT**. Diffuse enlargement of the right lobe and a right lateral jugular territory cervical lymph node of concern for malignancy

Diagnosis of US-Guided FNA/Cytology: (**Right thyroid lobe**) **Adenocarcinoma compatible with prostatic primary**

18.3.7 Case 7: Diffuse Papillary Thyroid Carcinoma

Clinical Scenario: A 25-year-old female with the sensation of left neck fullness. Ultrasound was requested to assess for soft tissue mass.

Imaging Features: Ultrasound. Diffuse enlargement of the left thyroid (Fig. 18.7a) with mildly increased vascular flow in the enlarged gland (Fig. 18.7b).

Contrast-enhanced CT. Diffuse enlargement of the thyroid gland (Fig. 18.7c)

Diagnosis of US-Guided FNA/Cytology: ((**A**) **Left thyroid**) **Papillary thyroid carcinoma**

18.4 Sonographic Features of Thyroid Nodules: Benign

Sonographic features that suggest a benign thyroid nodule include a simple thyroid cyst, or complex cyst, with no intranodular calcification or intranodular vascular flow on power Doppler imaging.

18.4.1 Case 8: Thyroid Cyst

Clinical Scenario: A 43-year-old male with multiple palpable thyroid nodules. Ultrasound was requested to assess the palpable thyroid nodules.

Imaging Features: Grayscale ultrasound image of the right thyroid lobe demonstrates a 1.3-cm anechoic thyroid nodule with posterior acoustic

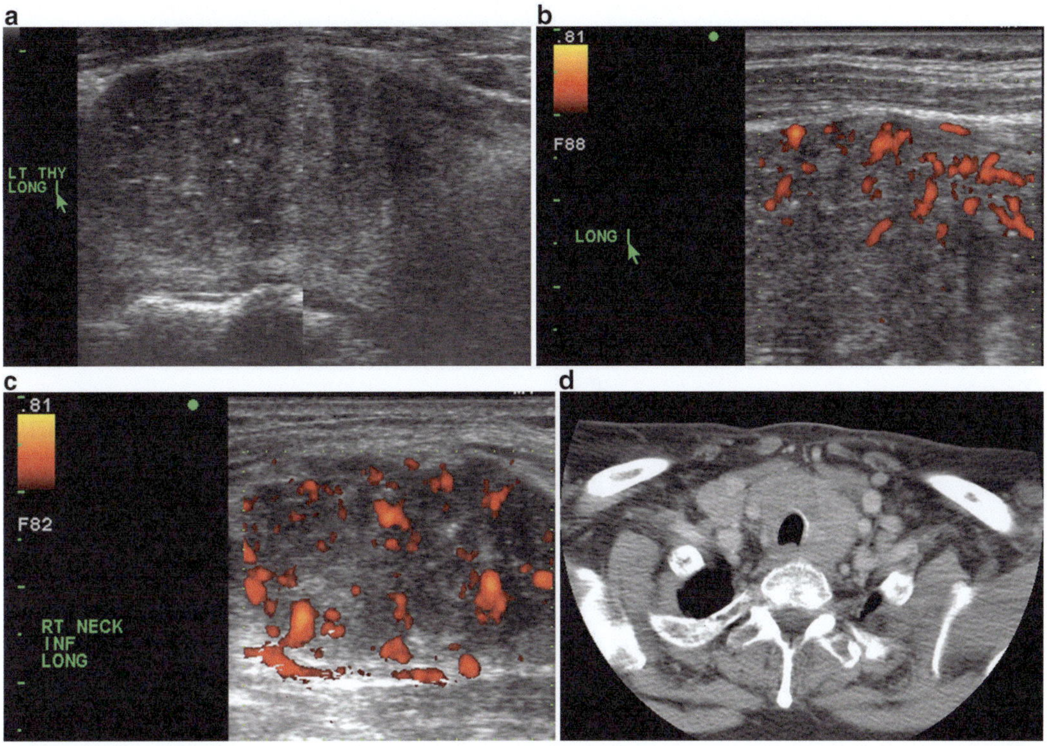

Fig. 18.6 (**a**) **Grayscale US**. Diffuse enlargement of the left thyroid in the longitudinal plane with multiple punctate hyperechoic foci and no discrete mass. (**b**) **Power Doppler US**. Increased vascular flow in the enlarged thyroid gland. (**c**) **Power Doppler US**. Increased disorganized vascular flow in a suspicious right inferior jugular territory lymph node detected on ultrasound. (**d**) **Contrast-enhanced CT**. Diffuse enlargement of the thyroid gland with a suspicious right inferior cervical lymph node

enhancement (Fig. 18.8a). Power Doppler ultrasound image demonstrates no internal vascularity (Fig. 18.8b).

Diagnosis: **Simple thyroid cyst**

18.4.2 Case 9: Crystalline Colloid

Intranodular punctate regions of echogenicity with comet-tail characteristics are indicative of a benign thyroid nodule. These punctuate regions of echogenicity are actually crystalline colloid and must be differentiated from calcifications with acoustic shadowing when assessing the concern for malignancy of a thyroid nodule.

Clinical Scenario: A 54-year-old female with painless enlarged thyroid gland found on routine physical exam. Ultrasound was requested to assess the enlarged palpable thyroid gland.

Imaging Features: Grayscale ultrasound image of the left thyroid gland demonstrates a 1-cm hypoechoic nodule with intranodular echogenic foci demonstrating comet-tail artifact (Fig. 18.9a). Of note is that there is no associated shadowing identified.

Power Doppler ultrasound image of the left thyroid demonstrates the absence of internal vascularity (Fig. 18.9b).

Diagnosis: **Colloid thyroid nodule. Diagnosis was made on the basis of US characteristics**.

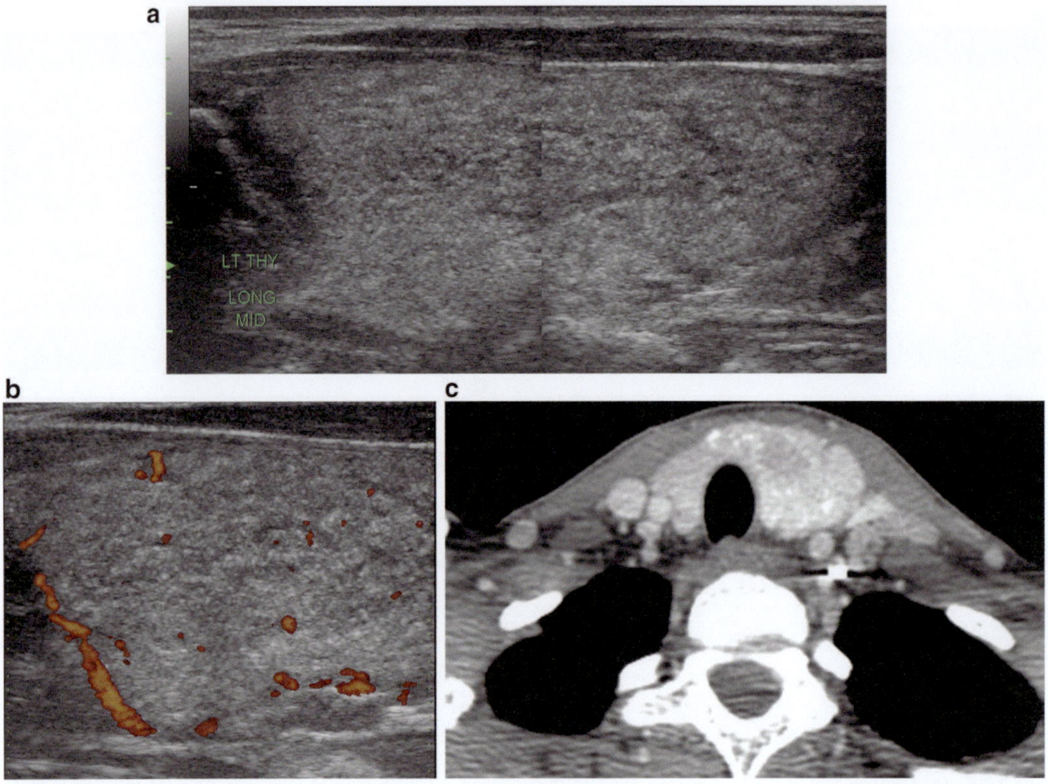

Fig. 18.7 (**a**) **Grayscale US**. Diffuse enlargement of the left thyroid gland. (**b**) **Power Doppler US**. Mildly increased vascular flow in the enlarged thyroid gland. (**c**) Contrast-enhanced CT. Diffuse enlargement of the thyroid gland

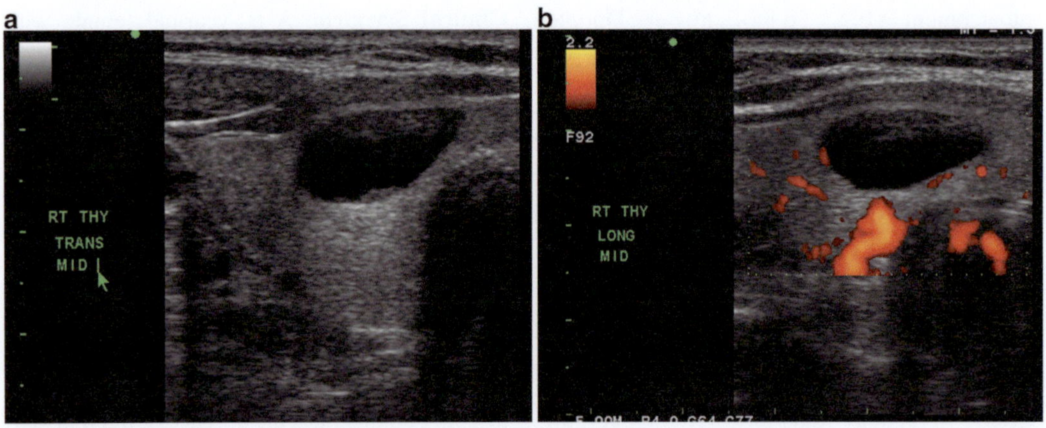

Fig. 18.8 (**a**) Grayscale US image of the right thyroid lobe demonstrates a 1.3-cm anechoic thyroid nodule with posterior acoustic enhancement. (**b**) Power Doppler ultrasound image demonstrates no internal vascularity

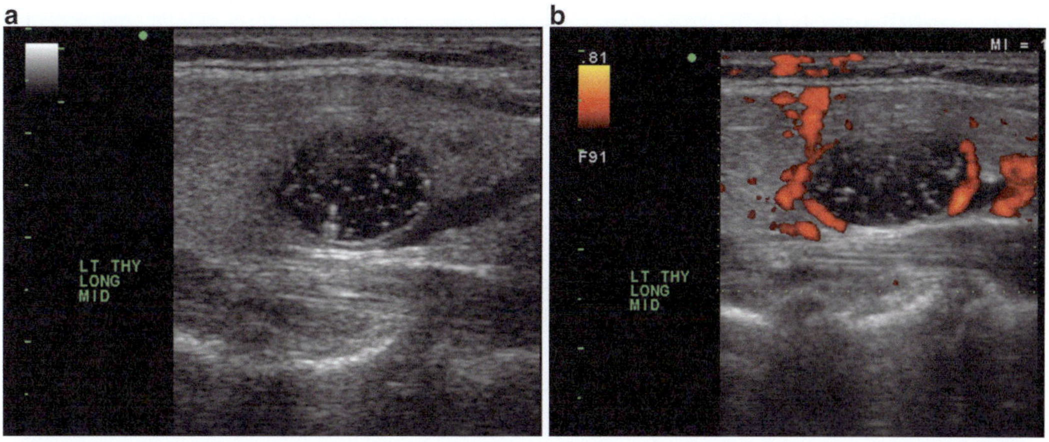

Fig. 18.9 (**a**) Grayscale ultrasound image of the left thyroid gland demonstrates a 1-cm hypoechoic nodule with intranodular echogenic foci demonstrating comet-tail artifact. Of note is that there is no associated shadowing identified. (**b**) Power Doppler ultrasound image of the left thyroid demonstrates absence of internal vascularity

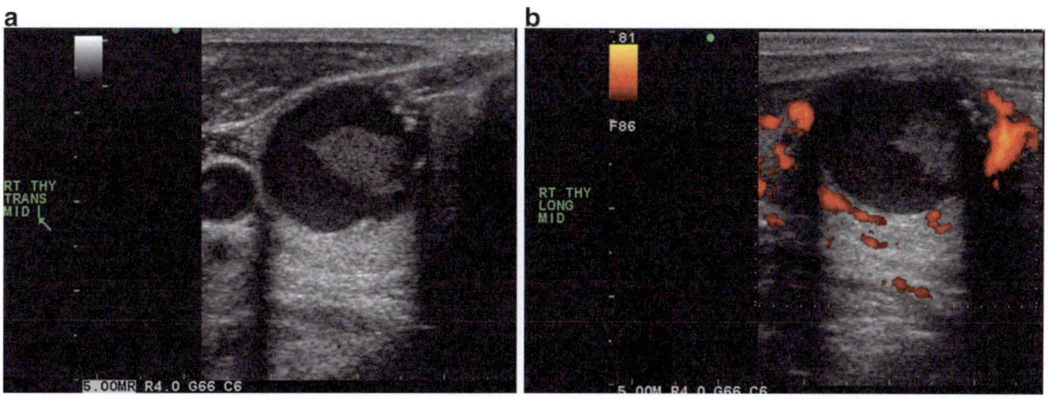

Fig. 18.10 (**a**) Grayscale ultrasound image of the right thyroid lobe demonstrates a 1.6-cm complex solid/cystic thyroid nodule containing layered debris. Note the posterior acoustic enhancement related to the cystic component and presence of edge shadowing. (**b**) Power Doppler US image reveals no internal vascularity of the solid component

18.4.3 Case 10: Complex Avascular Thyroid Nodule

Clinical Scenario: A 49-year-old male with newly diagnosed parotid neoplasm with US of the soft tissues of the neck performed for staging

Imaging Features: Grayscale image of the right thyroid lobe demonstrates a 1.6-cm complex solid and cystic thyroid nodule containing layered debris (Fig. 18.10a). Note the posterior acoustic enhancement related to the cystic component and presence of edge shadowing.

Power Doppler ultrasound image reveals no internal vascularity of the solid component (Fig. 18.10b).

Diagnosis of US-Guided FNA/Cytology: Colloid thyroid nodule

18.5 Sonographic Features of Thyroid Nodules: Malignant

There are several sonographic features traditionally thought to differentiate malignant from benign thyroid nodules. However, we have found that traditional sonographic features of size, halo, and taller-than-wide appearance do not contribute to distinguishing a benign from malignant thyroid nodule.

Malignancy should be suspected in the presence of a hypoechoic or complex thyroid nodule that has intranodular hypervascularity and/or intranodular calcification. Calcifications show the highest accuracy (76 %), specificity (93 %), and positive predictive value (70 %) for malignancy as a single sign; however, there is no single US feature that distinguishes malignant from benign thyroid nodules [6].

In addition to the traditional parameters, there are other features that we have recently added to our concern for a malignant thyroid nodule. Again, we present here our institutional perspective with regard to these parameters. These include:

1. The presence of intranodular calcification and/or power Doppler vascularity independent of the pattern or amount
2. Solitary nodules independent of their appearance
3. A solid or complex isthmus nodule independent of calcification or vascular flow

18.5.1 Case 11: Vascular Complex Thyroid Nodule

Clinical Scenario: A 50-year-old female with CT chest obtained for evaluation for possible pulmonary embolus. Ultrasound was requested to assess the thyroid nodule incidentally found on CT.

Imaging Features: Grayscale image in the transverse (Fig. 18.11a) and longitudinal planes (Fig. 18.11b) of the right thyroid lobe demonstrates a 0.7-cm complex solid and cystic thyroid nodule. The nodule margins also appear irregular.

Power Doppler ultrasound image reveals intranodular vascularity (Fig. 18.11c).

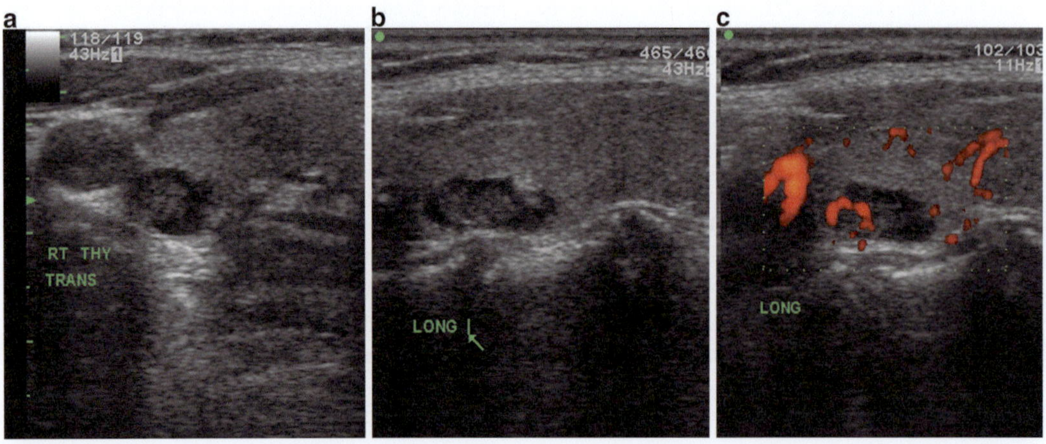

Fig. 18.11 (**a**) Grayscale US image in the transverse plane of the right thyroid lobe demonstrates a 0.7-cm complex solid/cystic thyroid nodule. (**b**) Grayscale US image in the longitudinal plane of the right thyroid lobe demonstrates a 0.7-cm complex solid/cystic thyroid nodule. (**c**) Power Doppler US image reveals intranodular vascularity

Diagnosis of US-Guided FNA/Cytology: Papillary thyroid carcinoma

18.5.2 Case 12: Malignant Thyroid Nodule (Punctate Calcifications)

Clinical Scenario: A 49-year-old female complaining of neck swelling. Ultrasound was requested to assess the patient's concern of neck swelling.

Imaging Features: Grayscale image in the transverse (Fig. 18.12a) and longitudinal (Fig. 18.12b) planes of the right thyroid lobe demonstrates a 0.5-cm solid, isoechoic thyroid nodule subjacent to a thyroid cyst. The smaller nodule has peripheral shadowing calcifications and, thus, was of concern for a papillary thyroid cancer.

Power Doppler reveals internal vascularity of the small thyroid nodule (Fig. 18.12c) which furthers the concern for papillary thyroid cancer.

Diagnosis of US-Guided FNA/Cytology: Papillary thyroid carcinoma

Ultrasound features do not definitively differentiate benign from malignant thyroid nodules as demonstrated in the cases that follow.

18.5.3 Case 13: Colloid Nodule Mimicking Malignant Nodule

Clinical Scenario: A 55-year-old female with incidentally noted thyroid nodule on carotid US

Imaging Features: Grayscale ultrasound images of the right thyroid lobe demonstrate a solitary 1-cm solid nodule containing echogenic punctate calcification with shadowing (Fig. 18.13a).

Power Doppler ultrasound of the same nodule demonstrates internal vascularity which raised the concern for malignancy.

Diagnosis of US-Guided FNA/Cytology: Colloid nodule

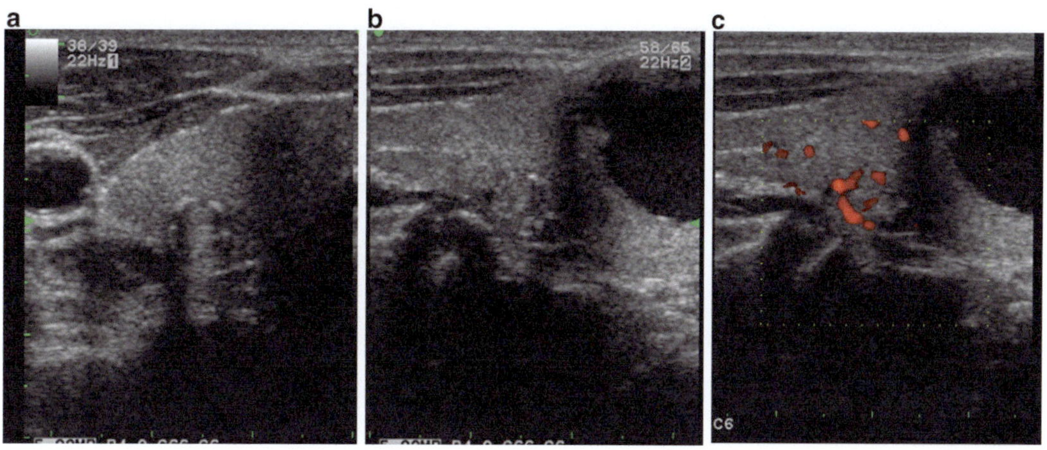

Fig. 18.12 (**a**) Grayscale US image in the transverse plane of the right thyroid lobe demonstrates a 0.5-cm solid, isoechoic thyroid nodule subjacent to a thyroid cyst. The small nodule contains shadowing calcifications and, thus, is of concern for a papillary thyroid cancer. (**b**) Grayscale US image in the longitudinal plane of the right thyroid lobe demonstrates a 0.5-cm solid, isoechoic thyroid nodule subjacent to a thyroid cyst. The small nodule contains shadowing calcifications and, thus, is of concern for a papillary thyroid cancer. (**c**) Power Doppler reveals internal vascularity of the small thyroid nodule which furthers the concern for papillary thyroid cancer

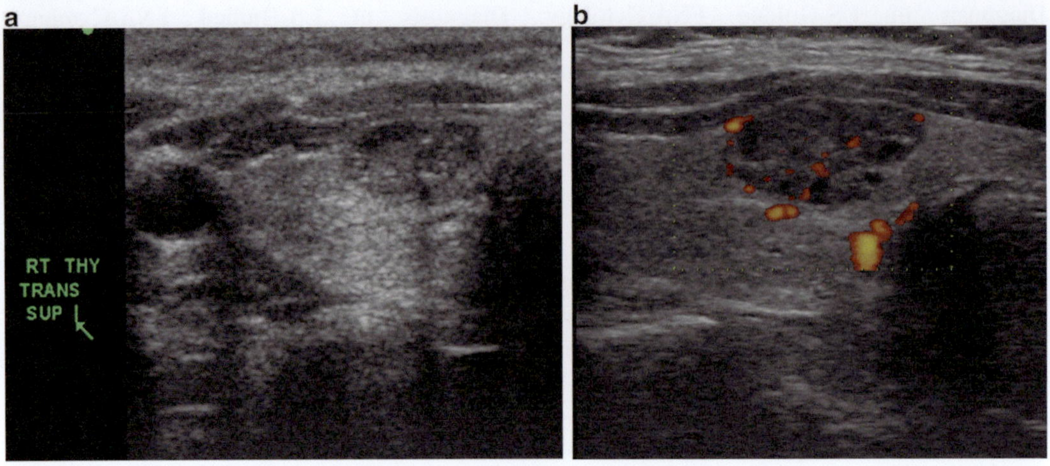

Fig. 18.13 (**a**) Grayscale US images of the right thyroid lobe demonstrate a solitary 1-cm solid nodule containing echogenic punctate calcification with shadowing of concern for malignancy. However, FNA revealed a benign colloid nodule, demonstrating that not all suspicious calcifications lead to the diagnosis of thyroid cancer. (**b**) Power Doppler ultrasound of the 1-cm solid solitary nodule demonstrates internal vascularity that raise the concern for malignancy. However, FNA revealed a benign colloid nodule, demonstrating that not all suspicious calcifications lead to the diagnosis of thyroid cancer

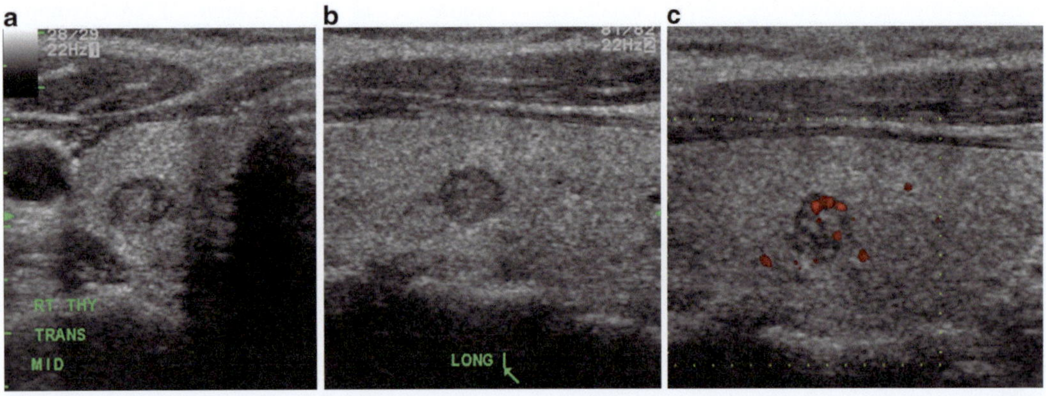

Fig. 18.14 (**a**) Grayscale ultrasound image of the right thyroid gland in the transverse plane demonstrates the presence of a 0.6-cm solitary solid isoechoic to hypoechoic thyroid nodule. No associated calcification is identified. (**b**) Grayscale US image of the right thyroid gland in the longitudinal plane demonstrates the presence of a 0.6-cm solitary solid isoechoic to hypoechoic thyroid nodule. No associated calcification is identified. (**c**) Power Doppler image reveals intranodular vascularity

18.5.4 Case 14: Solitary Nodule Is of Concern Independent of Appearance

Clinical Scenario: A 45-year-old male with malignant melanoma. Ultrasound was performed to assess for metastatic adenopathy.

Imaging Features: Grayscale ultrasound image of the right thyroid gland in the transverse (Fig. 18.14a) and longitudinal planes (Fig. 18.14b) demonstrates the presence of a 0.6-cm solitary solid isoechoic to hypoechoic thyroid nodule. No associated calcification is identified. Power Doppler image reveals internal vascularity (Fig. 18.14c).

The solitary nature of the nodule and the vascular flow were of concern for malignancy.

Diagnosis of US-Guided FNA/Cytology: **Papillary thyroid carcinoma**

18.5.5 Case 15: Malignant Thyroid Nodule Mimicking a Colloid Thyroid Nodule

Clinical Scenario: A 75-year-old female with right thyroid palpable abnormality. Ultrasound was requested to assess the palpable nodule.

Imaging Features: (Fig. 18.15) Power Doppler ultrasound images of the right thyroid lobe demonstrate a 2.3-cm solitary solid nodule with spongiform appearance. No intranodular calcification or vascularity is identified. US-guided FNA was performed based on the solid nature of the nodule.

Diagnosis of US-Guided FNA/Cytology: **Papillary thyroid carcinoma**

18.5.6 Case 16: Malignant Thyroid Nodule Mimicking a Benign Appearance (FDG-Avid, Small Thyroid Nodule)

Clinical Scenario: A 57-year-old female with amyloidosis. FDG-avid thyroid nodule seen on PET/CT as part of workup for the amyloidosis. Ultrasound was requested based on the FDG-avid nodule incidentally found on PET.

Imaging Features: Power Doppler demonstrates a 0.9-cm isoechoic thyroid nodule with no intranodular calcification or vascularity (Fig. 18.16a).

Fused PET/CT axial image at the level of the thyroid gland demonstrates FDG-avid focus in the left thyroid lobe (Fig. 18.16b).

Diagnosis of US-Guided FNA/Cytology: **Papillary thyroid carcinoma**

18.5.7 Case 17: Thyroid Isthmus Nodule

A solid or complex isthmus nodule is of concern for malignancy independent of calcification or vascular flow.

Clinical Scenario: A 37-year-old male with chondrosarcoma of the chest wall found to have calcification in the thyroid on CT chest. Ultrasound was requested to follow up the CT finding.

Ultrasound Features: Grayscale US images of the thyroid isthmus in transverse (Fig. 18.17a) and longitudinal (Fig. 18.17b) planes demonstrate a 0.9-cm ill-defined, solitary nodule in the isthmus containing coarse shadowing calcification.

Diagnosis of US-Guided FNA/Cytology: **Papillary thyroid carcinoma**

18.5.8 Case 18: Isthmus Nodule with Benign Appearance

Clinical Scenario: A 53-year-old woman with breast cancer and an isthmus nodule found incidentally on CT. Ultrasound was requested to assess the isthmus lesion.

Ultrasound Features: Grayscale ultrasound image in transverse plane demonstrates a solid isthmus lesion with scant vascular flow (Fig. 18.18).

Diagnosis: **Follicular neoplasm**

18.6 Ultrasound-Guided FNA of the Thyroid

FNA is a key part of nodule assessment because it is often impossible to predict with sufficient reliability the benign or malignant nature of thyroid disease due to the significant overlap of sonographic features. In the absence of definitive sonographic features of malignant thyroid nodules

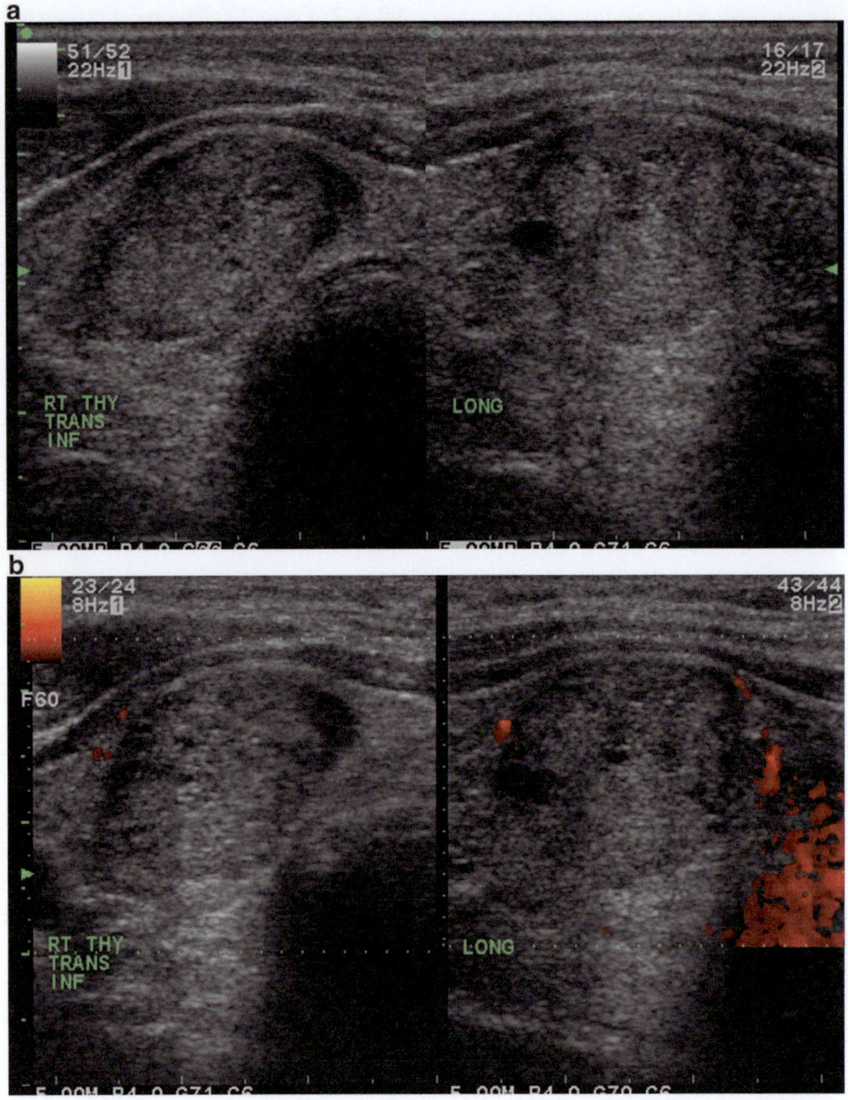

Fig. 18.15 (**a**, **b**) Power Doppler ultrasound images of the right thyroid lobe demonstrate a 2.3-cm solitary solid nodule with a spongiform appearance. No intranodular calcification or vascularity is identified

based on the US images, US-guided FNA has now become the cornerstone in the diagnosis of thyroid cancer or, just as importantly, to confirm the benign nature of a thyroid nodule [7].

US-guided FNA was commonly recommended for nodules >1 cm. It was originally thought that the rate of thyroid malignancy was lower in patients with small incidentally discovered non-palpable thyroid nodules found on MR, CT, or sonography performed for nonthyroid indications. However, the documentation of the potential biological aggressiveness of thyroid nodules <1 cm in size and as small as 0.2 cm, and the higher incidence of associated regional nodal metastasis, indicates that nodules <1 cm should be approached with the same concern for malignancy

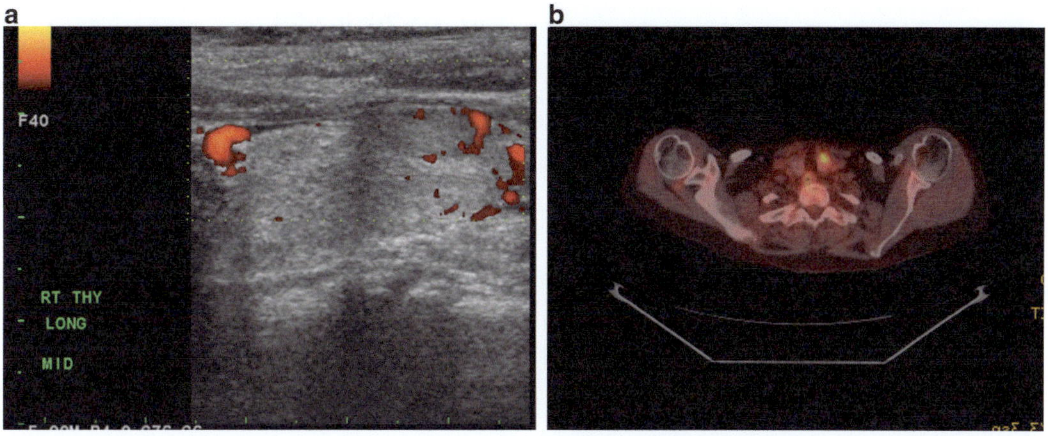

Fig. 18.16 (**a**) Power Doppler US demonstrates a 0.9-cm isoechoic thyroid nodule with no intranodular calcification or vascularity. (**b**) **CT**. Fused PET/CT axial image at the level of the thyroid gland demonstrates an FDG-avid focus in the left thyroid lobe

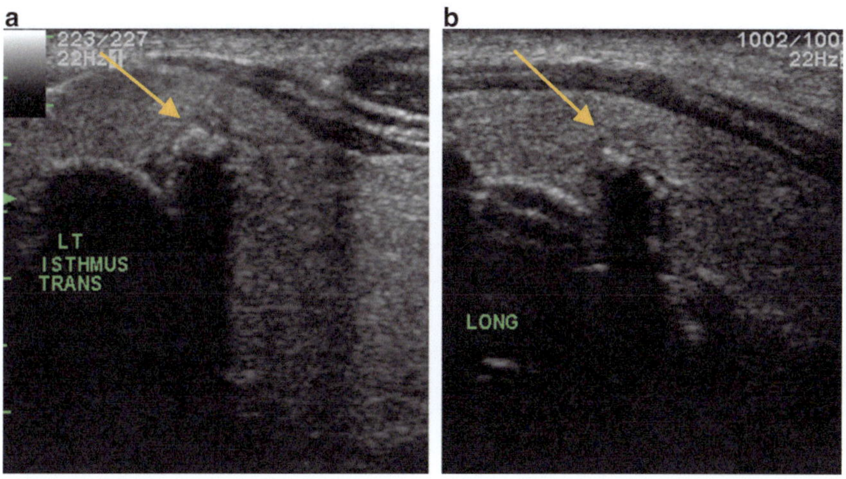

Fig. 18.17 (**a**) Grayscale US images of the thyroid isthmus in the transverse plane demonstrates a 0.9-cm ill-defined, solitary nodule in the isthmus containing coarse shadowing calcification (*arrow*). (**b**) Grayscale US images of the thyroid isthmus in the longitudinal plane demonstrate a 0.9-cm ill-defined, solitary nodule in the isthmus containing coarse shadowing calcification (*arrow*)

as nodules >1 cm in size [8, 9]. Thus, the standard of care for thyroid cancer must now include the detection of <1-cm cancers which implies the capability to perform a US-guided FNA of such minute lesions.

As with other diagnostic tests, the effectiveness of a US-guided FNA is highly dependent on the expertise of the operator performing the procedure and the adequacy of the specimen for interpretation of the cytomorphologic features. At MDACC, US-guided FNA is performed with the freehand technique following preparation of the skin with rubbing alcohol. A 20-gauge needle, attached to a 20-cm^3 syringe, is then inserted under ultrasound guidance, obliquely along the scan plan. The tip of the needle is directed toward, and sonographically confirmed within, the target nodule or lymph node, and aspiration is performed.

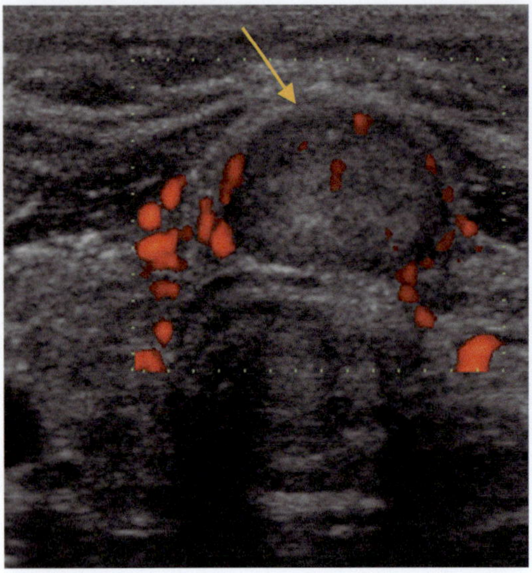

Fig. 18.18 Power Doppler. Ultrasound image in transverse plane demonstrates a solid isthmus lesion with vascular flow (*arrow*)

The needle and tip are readably visible if they are parallel to the transducer. In this manner, there is no need for a specialty needle to improve visibility. A review of 1206 patients at MD Anderson showed a 2 % rate of nondiagnostic specimens and a 1 % rate of false-positive and 2 % rate of false-negative results of US-guided FNA in the diagnosis of thyroid cancer [10].

The high success rate of FNA at MDACC is related in part to the large stiffer needle size used (20 gauge) and a single-pass and vigorous aspiration with a syringe attached to the needle. Complications such as bleeding, infection, and pain are rarely encountered.

Core biopsy of the thyroid is restricted to suspected anaplastic tumors and lymphoma. In suspected lymphoma, core biopsy is performed to obtain tissue for flow cytometry to diagnose small cell lymphoma and in cases where there is concern for transformation of recurrent lymphoma. In documented lymphoma, core biopsy is performed to obtain tissue to assess for treatment options.

18.7 Conclusion

No single sonographic criterion is specific for the benign or malignant nature of thyroid lesions. The combination of different US characteristics (1971) with US-guided fine-needle aspiration (FNA) (1983) and color Doppler (1988) continues to offer a remarkably accurate diagnostic system of evaluation of the thyroid. The combination of sonographic features, color Doppler, and US-guided FNA has a specificity close to 100 % for the characterization of thyroid nodules.

References

1. Solbiati L, Osti V, Cova L, Tonolini M. Ultrasound of thyroid, parathyroid glands and neck lymph nodes. Eur Radiol. 2001;11(12):2411–24.
2. Barraclough BM, Barraclough BH. Ultrasound of the thyroid and parathyroid glands. World J Surg. 2000;24(2):158–65.
3. Baloch ZW, LiVolsi VA. Fine-needle aspiration of thyroid nodules: past, present, and future. Endocr Pract. 2004;10(3):234–41.
4. Holtel MR. Emerging technology in head and neck ultrasonography. Otolaryngol Clin North Am. 2010;43(6):1267–74. doi:10.1016/j.otc.2010.08.003. vii.
5. Sarvazyan A, Hall TJ, Urban MW, Fatemi M, Aglyamov SR, Garra BS. An overview of elastography - an emerging branch of medical imaging. Curr Med Imaging Rev. 2011;7(4):255–82.
6. Kakkos SK, Scopa CD, Chalmoukis AK, et al. Relative risk of cancer in sonographically detected thyroid nodules with calcifications. J Clin Ultrasound. 2000;28:347–52.
7. Yang GC, Liebeskind D, Messina AV. Ultrasound-guided fine-needle aspiration of the thyroid assessed by Ultrafast Papanicolaou stain: data from 1135 biopsies with a two- to six-year follow-up. Thyroid. 2001;11:581–9.
8. Papini E, Guglielmi R, Bianchini A, et al. Risk of malignancy in nonpalpable thyroid nodules: predictive value of ultrasound and color-Doppler features. J Clin Endocrinol Metab. 2002;87:1941–6.
9. Liebeskind A, Sikora AG, Komisar A, Slavit D, Fried K. Rates of malignancy in incidentally discovered thyroid nodules evaluated with sonography and fine-needle aspiration. J Ultrasound Med. 2005;24(5):629–34.
10. Kouvaraki MA, Shapiro SE, Fornage BD, et al. Role of preoperative ultrasonography in the surgical management of patients with thyroid cancer. Surgery. 2003;134:946–55.

Part V

Evaluation of Cervical Lymph Nodes and Thyroid Cancer Metastases

19 Rationale for the Evaluation of Cervical Lymph Nodes in the Setting of Thyroid Cancer

Jennifer A. Sipos

19.1 Introduction

Differentiated thyroid cancer has a strong predilection for metastasis to locoregional lymph nodes. Though the reported frequency of nodal metastases can vary significantly, it is imperative to have an understanding of the impact that these findings can have on the clinical course of an individual patient. This chapter will discuss the bearing that malignant lymph nodes have on the surgical approach, the recurrence risk, and the decision to utilize adjunctive therapy. Additionally, it will outline the role of postoperative surveillance ultrasonography in thyroid cancer patients. Finally, the limitations of sonographic imaging of the neck will be discussed. The sonographic appearance of nodal metastases will be discussed in detail in the following chapter.

J.A. Sipos, M.D. (✉)
Division of Endocrinology, Diabetes and Metabolism, The Ohio State University Wexner Medical Center, 1581 Dodd Dr, Columbus, OH 43210, USA
e-mail: Jennifer.Sipos@osumc.edu

19.2 Preoperative Identification of Metastatic Lymph Nodes

Ultrasonography of the neck is a critical instrument in the arsenal of those treating patients with thyroid cancer. Identification of abnormal lymph nodes on ultrasound examination of the neck not only changes the likelihood of malignancy in any given thyroid nodule in that patient [1], but it also changes the surgical management [2]. In fact, one retrospective study found that the preoperative US of the neck changed the surgical approach in 40 % of patients [2]. Similarly, another study found that performing a US of the neck prior to initial surgery for thyroid cancer reduced the number of repeat surgeries by 39 % [3]. For this reason, a survey of the cervical lymph nodes with ultrasound should be performed in all patients suspected of having a thyroid nodule [1].

19.2.1 Frequency of Lymph Node Metastases

The incidence of nodal metastases in papillary thyroid cancer is highly variable in the literature, with rates reported as high as 90 % on polymerase chain reaction amplification of thyroglobulin (Tg) measurement [4]. With less stringent criteria for malignant diagnosis, however, the rates of nodal involvement are lower, though the majority

M. Milas et al. (eds.), *Advanced Thyroid and Parathyroid Ultrasound*, DOI 10.1007/978-3-319-44100-9_19

of patients with papillary thyroid cancer probably have diseased nodes [3, 5–8]. The likelihood of nodal metastases in the individual patient is dependent on several demographic factors and tumor features. Tumor size correlates with risk of metastatic spread; larger lesions are more likely to exhibit nodal involvement [9]. Additionally, multifocal [10] and poorly differentiated tumors [11] are more often associated with lymphatic spread. The frequency of nodal metastases also varies with histologic subtype, papillary and Hurthle cell cancers having a higher predilection than follicular carcinomas [12]. Patient factors are also important in predicting the likelihood of nodal disease; men [13] and children [14] more often have locoregional metastases. The extent of surgical dissection and thoroughness of the pathologist also increases the nodal yield [15].

It is well recognized that the central compartment is difficult to examine sonographically with an intact thyroid; up to 50 % of malignant nodes are missed preoperatively [16]. Prophylactic central compartment dissection in patients with tumors less than 1 cm reveals that over 50 % have lymph node metastases [17]. With such a high rate of nodal disease and relative insensitivity of preoperative imaging, it begs the question of the legitimacy for prophylactic central neck dissection [17–22].

The potential benefit of a prophylactic surgery is that more diseased nodes are successfully identified and removed. The recognition of nodal involvement may also change the management of patients. In fact, one study found that prophylactic central neck dissection upstaged nearly 30 % of patients to stage III disease, which resulted in higher doses of radioactive iodine [7]. Importantly, however, there was no significant difference in postoperative serum Tg levels in those patients who had the central neck dissection compared to those who did not undergo the more extensive surgery [7].

A valid argument against prophylactic neck dissections relates to the complication rates. Numerous studies have determined that a central neck dissection increases the risk of permanent hypoparathyroidism and recurrent laryngeal nerve paralysis compared to thyroidectomy alone [23, 24]. In addition, a recent study reported no difference in recurrence rates after prophylactic neck dissection in patients with and without pathologically malignant central neck lymph nodes when the preoperative ultrasound performed by an expert operator did not identify suspicious lymph nodes, indicating that small volume central neck disease likely has negligible effects on recurrence [19]. Others counter-argue that reoperation for nodal involvement identified after thyroidectomy is also associated with a high risk of complications [15] and an initial prophylactic surgery is therefore the preferable approach [24]. With little hope for a prospective, randomized controlled trial to settle the debate [25], arguments for and against the role of prophylactic central neck dissections will likely persist. Current recommendations from the American Thyroid Association (ATA) indicate that a prophylactic central compartment dissection may be considered in patients with papillary thyroid cancer when the primary tumor is more advanced or in the presence of lateral neck node involvement [1].

The sonographic identification of lateral lymph node involvement is more sensitive than the central neck, though prophylactic surgeries have also revealed that up to 39 % of nodes may be missed by ultrasonography alone [17]. Indeed, a recent meta-analysis revealed that 57.5 % of patients had nodal metastases on prophylactic dissections of the lateral neck, while only 12.8 % had disease that was identified on preoperative imaging [26]. However, prophylactic dissection of the lateral neck is not recommended [1]. Similar to the central neck, removal of sonographically normal nodes, even if subsequently found to be pathologically positive, does not improve recurrence-free survival [18, 19].

19.2.2 Clinical Impact of Lymph Node Metastases

Any discussion of indications for prophylactic nodal dissection should be tempered by the clinical impact of the identification of nodal disease. There has been ongoing debate about the significance of lymph node involvement and its influence on patient prognosis. An early report published four decades ago reported better outcomes in patients with nodal diseases [27], but a second study shortly thereafter suggested that the presence of nodal disease was associated with a higher risk of recurrence and death [28]. Deliberation ensued. Some studies found adverse effects on survival but not on structural recurrence [29, 30]. Others upheld the findings of increased mortality with nodal disease [31, 32]. A larger study showed that survival is only worse with lymph node metastases in those patients over the age of 45 years [33]. More recent studies evaluating recurrence risk suggest that removal of microscopic malignant nodes identified only on prophylactic neck dissection does not impact disease-free survival [18, 19].

With the high frequency of nodal metastases and the seemingly conflicting data on prognosis, their true impact was unclear, posing a potential barrier to the successful management of patients. The ATA therefore created a task force to address the prognostic significance of nodal metastases from papillary thyroid cancer after a careful analysis of the literature [8]. The conclusion from this study indicates that not all nodal disease is equivalent; some metastatic nodes have a worse prognosis than others (see Table 19.1). Those lymph nodes that are identified preoperatively as abnormal by palpation or with ultrasound or those malignant nodes visually identified intraoperatively are termed clinical node positive (cN1). These clinically apparent nodes are associated with a risk of recurrence approaching 20 % [18, 19, 34–38]. In contrast, those patients with either a few nodes with microscopic malignant involvement (<2 mm) or pathologic malignant nodes that are clinically or sonographically normal pre- or intraoperatively are considered clinically node negative (cN0) [8, 18, 19, 38]. The median likelihood of recurrent disease in cN0 patients is between 2 and 4 % [8]. Additionally, the number of nodes involved with disease factors into the risk; when greater than five metastatic nodes are identified, the median risk of recurrence increases to 19 %, even with microscopic metastases [8, 39, 40]. Moreover, the size of the metastatic deposit impacts recurrence risk. Foci less than 2 mm have a very low likelihood of recurrence [8], whereas a metastatic node measuring over 3 cm has a very high associated risk [40]. Likewise, extranodal extension is associated with a 24 % risk of recurrent disease [8, 39, 41]. It is therefore very important for the clinician to consider the size and number of nodal metastases when establishing an individual patient's risk of recurrent disease and determining the need for adjunctive therapy. Further, the preoperative ultrasound appearance of the nodal metastases impacts patient outcomes [18, 19, 34–38].

Table 19.1 Risk of recurrent disease based on characteristics of lymph node metastases

Characteristic	Median recurrence risk (%)	Range (%)	References
Clinical N0	2	0–9	[5, 38, 42]
<5 metastatic nodes	4	3–8	[5, 39, 40]
>5 metastatic nodes	19	7–21	[39, 40]
Clinical N1	22	10–42	[18, 19, 34–38]
Clinical N1 with extranodal extension	24	15–32	[39, 41]

Clinical N0 signifies lymph nodes that appear normal on ultrasound evaluation and are microscopic metastases. Clinical N1 nodes are those that are identified by palpation or sonographically prior to surgery or appear abnormal intraoperatively. Modified from Randolph et al. [8]

19.3 Postoperative Surveillance

19.3.1 Risk of Recurrent Disease

The term recurrent disease is often used interchangeably with persistent disease, though the two entities are distinct [43]. A recurrence is defined as the appearance of tumor in a patient previously thought to have no evidence of disease [43]. Persistent disease is that which is identified prior to a patient being labeled as having no evidence of disease [43]. Historically, thyroid cancer has a high rate of recurrent disease, up to 30 %, at 40 years of follow-up [44]. This data, however, is derived from utilization of historically more insensitive means for detecting residual disease, including palpation of the neck and diagnostic whole-body scans [44]. Palpation examination may miss nearly 40% of nodal disease subsequently detected with sonography [2, 3]. Furthermore, diagnostic whole-body scans fail to identify many metastatic lesions now recognizable with serum Tg measurement and US examination of the neck [45]. Therefore, the majority of "recurrences" identified by Mazzaferri et al. [44] more likely represented persistent disease that was unable to be distinguished with the imperfect modes of detection available at the time. Moreover, the recurrent disease probably took many years of growth to come to clinical detection. With improved preoperative sonographic detection of metastatic disease, modern patients are undergoing more extensive initial surgeries [46]. And, with very sensitive means of detection of residual thyroid tissue, once a patient is labeled as being free of disease, it seems unlikely that the rates of recurrence with long-term follow-up will remain as high as 30%. More recent short-term estimates of recurrence rates are very low, though long-term follow-up with the current imaging modalities and ultrasensitive Tg measurements remains unavailable [6, 47–49].

The majority of recurrences in patients with papillary thyroid cancer involve locoregional lymph nodes. Sonography of the neck is a critical tool for detection of these metastases as diagnostic whole-body scanning and palpation are very insensitive [2, 3, 45]. For this reason, sonography of the neck is an indispensable component of the long-term follow-up in patients with papillary thyroid cancer. The optimal timing of the initial postoperative ultrasound examination and the subsequent need for repeat examinations is dependent on the initial risk of recurrence [1]. This stratification system is outlined in the sections below. The ultrasound examination is thus an important component of the determination that a patient has been rendered free of disease [1].

Tumor recurrence rates escalate with increasing tumor size; in one study those tumors less than 1 cm had a 10-year recurrence risk of 4.6%, and the risk increased incrementally to 24.8% in those larger than 8 cm [50]. Additional factors impacting recurrence include tumor histology, patient age, extent of nodal involvement, and possibly BRAF mutation status [1]. Variable rates of recurrence risk across studies may also stem from the vigor with which one searches for residual disease. The contemporary definition of biochemical cure should include both imaging and biochemical parameters, however. The current criteria for disease-free status from the ATA, now termed an "excellent response to therapy," include no clinical or imaging evidence of tumor and a serum Tg level during TSH suppression of <0.2 ng/mL or after stimulation of <1 ng/mL in the absence of interfering antibodies [1]. The frequency for performance of neck sonography in patients with differentiated thyroid cancer should be adapted to that individual's risk of structural recurrence. Therefore it is important for clinicians to understand the benefits and limitations of staging systems to predict recurrence.

19.3.2 Staging Systems

The tumor, node, and metastasis (TNM) system proposed by the American Joint Committee on Cancer (AJCC) is the most widely used staging system for thyroid cancer and is designed to predict risk of mortality [51]. Other staging systems, including European Organisation for Research and Treatment of Cancer (EORTC) [52], Age, Metastasis, Extent of disease, Size (AMES) [53], and Metastasis, Age at presentation, Completeness of surgical resection, Invasion (extrathyroidal), Size (MACIS) [54], were created to capture additional clinicopathologic factors that impact survival such as patient age or tumor invasiveness. Numerous studies have demonstrated that the TNM and MACIS systems offer the most reliable estimates of mortality [55, 56]. These systems have significant shortcomings, however. One major limitation is that no single staging system adequately captures all tumor and patient features that impact prognosis. Consequently, the ability of any of these staging systems to accurately predict death from thyroid cancer in the individual patient is limited [55, 56]. The clinician should be aware of these limitations when discussing the tumor stage with a patient, regardless of the system employed.

Fortunately, prediction of mortality is typically a secondary concern for most patients with differentiated thyroid cancer; the risk for recurrence is more probable and consequently of more immediate interest. Because the TNM system does not accurately differentiate the risk of recurrence among the vast majority of patients who are either stage 1 or stage 2, the ATA developed a three-tiered classification of tumors based upon surgical pathology features [1]. Differentiated thyroid cancers are categorized as low, intermediate, or high risk for structural recurrence based on various tumor features that are obtained on surgical pathology. Small, intrathyroidal tumors with minimal nodal involvement are at low risk for recurrence, between 1 and 8 % [1]. Intrathyroidal tumors less than 4 cm with vascular invasion, clinically evident nodal disease, greater than five nodal metastases, or BRAF mutation have an intermediate risk of recurrence, between 10 and 30 % [1]. Papillary cancers larger than 4 cm with BRAF mutations or gross extrathyroidal extension, tumors with nodal disease measuring >3 cm or extranodal extension, and follicular carcinomas with extensive vascular invasion are deemed high risk with a recurrence rate between 40 and 50 % [1]. This stratification system not only aids the clinician in determining the need for additional therapy but also helps to guide the initial timing and intensity of surveillance and the level of TSH suppression in the first 12–18 months postoperatively [1].

19.3.3 Initial Ultrasound Surveillance

Active surveillance for recurrent disease initially combines measurement of serum thyroglobulin and ultrasound of the neck [1]. At a minimum, ultrasound of the neck should be performed at 6–12 months after surgery for papillary thyroid cancer and then periodically thereafter, depending on the patient's risk for recurrence and thyroglobulin status [1]. The central and lateral cervical nodal compartments should be interrogated by an experienced sonographer utilizing a high-frequency probe (≥10 MHz) [1].

19.3.4 Long-Term Ultrasound Surveillance

It is important to recognize that the risk of recurrence may change over time depending on the clinical course of the disease and the response to therapy [1]. A dynamic stratification system has been proposed to assess the response to treatment and hence modify the initial structural recurrence risk estimation [57, 58]. This system may be used at each visit to reassess an individual's likelihood of recurrent disease; the information is then incorporated into the surveillance strategy and guides the extent of TSH suppression and other treatment decisions, the most common of which is frequency of neck sonography [1, 57]. The system has been retrospectively validated in two studies [57, 58].

Response to therapy is divided into one of four groups: excellent, biochemical incomplete, structural incomplete, and indeterminate [1]. An excellent response to therapy is typified by a lack of clinical, biochemical, or structural evidence of disease. Initially low- and intermediate-risk patients who achieve this status have a very low risk of recurrence, between 1 and 4 %. In contrast, high-risk patients to reach this benchmark have a risk of recurrence of 14 % [57]. A biochemical incomplete response is marked by an abnormal thyroglobulin value (suppressed serum Tg between 1 and 10 ng/ml or stimulated Tg >10 ng/ml) or rising anti-Tg antibody level in the absence of visible disease [57]. During follow-up, approximately 30 % of these patients will be reclassified as having no evidence of disease, 20 % will achieve disease-free status after additional therapy, and 20 % will develop structural disease during follow-up [57]. Those with persistent visible disease are classified as structural incomplete response to therapy [57]. The majority of these patients, 50–85 %, will have persistent disease despite additional therapy. Finally, an indeterminate response to therapy is denoted by nonspecific structural findings that cannot be confidently viewed as malignant or benign, a low-level detectable suppressed Tg (greater than the low limit of normal for the assay but less than 1 ng/ml), a stimulated Tg <10 ng/ml, or declining anti-Tg antibody levels [57]. During follow-up, 15–20 % of these patients will have structural disease identified, and 80–85 % will have stable or resolving clinical findings [57].

The response to therapy stratification is used to guide the clinician in long-term follow-up and management decisions, including the intervals for US surveillance. In patients with an excellent response to therapy, a reduction in the intensity and frequency of follow-up is appropriate [1]. In fact, low-risk patients with no detectable disease can be followed primarily with clinical examination and serum Tg measurement while on levothyroxine replacement therapy [1]. Because initially high-risk patients that achieve an excellent response to therapy may have a higher risk of recurrence, a more intensive follow-up strategy may be appropriate, with yearly follow-up and periodic US examinations for the first 5 years after achieving disease-free status. Patients with a biochemical incomplete response to therapy may require additional imaging if the Tg or Tg-antibody titer is rising [1]. If a structural incomplete response is seen, continued imaging with US is appropriate for determination of rate of growth and potentially the development of new lesions [1]. Those patients with an indeterminate response to therapy and nonspecific findings on US may require serial sonographic imaging to identify changing features or growth [1].

19.4 Observation of Small Nodal Disease

Sonography is very sensitive for identifying minimal residual thyroid tissue and nodal metastases as small as 2–3 mm in diameter. These tiny foci may be very difficult to identify intraoperatively, however. And the clinical impact of this minimal residual disease is questionable [1]. Nearly half of the "suspicious" US findings that are aspirated are ultimately deemed to be benign [59–61]. Additionally, several studies have demonstrated that the majority of suspicious lesions in the postoperative neck do not demonstrate significant growth [62–64]. Though the percentage of lesions that exhibited growth was variable in the studies, it remained low, between 9 and 20 %, even with long-term follow-up (3.5–14 years) [62–64]. The studies consistently found that the variable which best predicted the growth of a lesion was the largest lesional diameter; bigger masses were more likely to grow [62, 64]. Even among the minority of malignant lesions that demonstrated enlargement, the rate of growth was typically slow, with a 1.3 mm/year increase [64]. Fortunately, when the structurally progressing lesion was ultimately resected, there was no evidence of local invasion or distant metastases [63, 64]. Taken together, these data point to the conclusion that with careful sonographic follow-up including serial measurement of Tg, observation rather than surgical removal may be warranted in properly selected patients with minimal residual disease [1, 43]. Alternatively, those sonographically suspicious lesions measuring greater than 8–10 mm in smallest diameter may be considered for fine-needle aspiration with cytology and thyroglobulin measurement in the needle washout fluid and, ultimately, removal [1]. Suspicious lesions that are smaller than 8–10 mm also may be considered for intervention if there is growth or if the node threatens vital structures [1].

19.5 Limitations of Ultrasound Imaging for Cervical Lymph Nodes

Clinicians should be cognizant of the limitations of neck sonography. First, sound waves cannot penetrate air, bone, or cartilage. Consequently, nodes posterior to the trachea may be difficult to identify. Second, the depth of a structure may exceed the limits of high-resolution sonography. As a result, the superior mediastinal and deep level IV lymph nodes may be difficult to see, particularly in patients with a large body habitus. Third, artifacts from normal anatomic structures may also obscure visualization of nodal metastases. For example, isoechoic nodes that lie posterior to a large vessel may be difficult to delineate.

The posterior acoustic enhancement associated with the sound waves traveling through the vessel may disguise an isoechoic metastatic node.

Computerized tomography may therefore improve the sensitivity of identifying disease in the retropharyngeal space and the superior mediastinum [65] and may be a useful adjunct to ultrasonography in preoperative planning [1]. Indeed, the combination of CT and US was found to have increased sensitivity to either modality alone for the identification of nodal disease in the central compartment [66].

Extrathyroidal extension may be seen in up to 15 % of patients with papillary thyroid cancer, with the severity ranging from microscopic invasion to gross extension of the tumor into the surrounding vital structures and soft tissues [67]. Though gross extrathyroidal extension may be identified on ultrasonography [68], invasion into the trachea or esophagus cannot be assessed sonographically. CT offers improved visualization of the integrity of these structures [66, 69]. Knowledge of the extent of tumor invasion could significantly impact the surgical approach [70].

Another limitation of sonography includes the identification of lesions and structures not related to the cancer but which may be confused with a recurrence. These include suture granulomata, neuromas, parathyroid adenomas, thymic tissue, and metastases from other primary tumors, to name a few [71, 72]. The distinction between benign and malignant nodes may also be confusing, particularly with plump reactive nodes in which the characteristic hilar stripe cannot be readily identified. These often may be seen in level II, as repeated microtrauma in the mouth chronically stimulates the node and causes resultant hypertrophy [71, 72]. The distinction between suspicious and malignant lymph nodes is discussed in greater detail in Chap. 20.

19.6 Summary

Ultrasound plays an important role in the diagnosis and surveillance of patients with thyroid cancer. Preoperative US of the neck is a critical component of the surgical planning; identification of metastatic nodes changes the operative approach. Sonography also helps identify recurrent disease in the neck in the postoperative patient; all patients should have a surveillance US 6–12 months after surgery. The importance of the ultrasound examination in the management of thyroid cancer patients is further established in that it is a central component of the definition of freedom from disease. The necessity of, and interval for, subsequent imaging is based on the response to therapy. Though sonography is pivotal to the evaluation and surveillance of thyroid cancer, there are important limitations to its use. The clinician should not only have expertise in the distinction of those metastatic foci of disease but also have a facile understanding of the mimics of thyroid cancer recurrence. Furthermore, when suspicion is high for the presence of persistence or recurrence in the absence of a sonographic suspect lesion, other imaging modalities may be necessary to examine the regions of the neck that are not adequately visualized sonographically.

References

1. Haugen BR, et al. 2015 American Thyroid Association Management Guidelines for adult patients with thyroid nodules and differentiated thyroid cancer: the American Thyroid Association Guidelines Task Force on thyroid nodules and differentiated thyroid cancer. Thyroid. 2016;26(1):1–133.
2. Stulak JM, et al. Value of preoperative ultrasonography in the surgical management of initial and reoperative papillary thyroid cancer. Arch Surg. 2006;141(5):489–94. discussion 494-6.
3. Kouvaraki MA, et al. Role of preoperative ultrasonography in the surgical management of patients with thyroid cancer. Surgery. 2003;134(6):946–54. discussion 954-5.
4. Arturi F, et al. Early diagnosis by genetic analysis of differentiated thyroid cancer metastases in small lymph nodes. J Clin Endocrinol Metab. 1997;82(5):1638–41.
5. Bardet S, et al. Macroscopic lymph-node involvement and neck dissection predict lymph-node recurrence in papillary thyroid carcinoma. Eur J Endocrinol. 2008;158(4):551–60.
6. Grant CS, et al. Risks and adequacy of an optimized surgical approach to the primary surgical management of papillary thyroid carcinoma treated during 1999-2006. World J Surg. 2010;34(6):1239–46.

7. Hughes DT, et al. Influence of prophylactic central lymph node dissection on postoperative thyroglobulin levels and radioiodine treatment in papillary thyroid cancer. Surgery. 2010;148(6):1100–6. discussion 1006-7.
8. Randolph G, et al.; ATA Surgical Affairs Committee's Taskforce on Thyroid Cancer Nodal Surgery. The prognostic significance of nodal metastases from papillary thyroid carcinoma can be stratified based on the size and number of metastatic lymph nodes, as well as the presence of extranodal extension. Thyroid, 2012; 22: 1144.
9. Machens A, Holzhausen HJ, Dralle H. The prognostic value of primary tumor size in papillary and follicular thyroid carcinoma. Cancer. 2005;103(11):2269–73.
10. Carcangiu ML, et al. Papillary carcinoma of the thyroid. A clinicopathologic study of 241 cases treated at the University of Florence, Italy. Cancer. 1985;55(4):805–28.
11. Sugitani I, et al. Prospective outcomes of selective lymph node dissection for papillary thyroid carcinoma based on preoperative ultrasonography. World J Surg. 2008;32(11):2494–502.
12. Grebe SK, Hay ID. Follicular thyroid cancer. Endocrinol Metab Clin North Am. 1995;24(4):761–801.
13. Choi YJ, et al. Clinical and imaging assessment of cervical lymph node metastasis in papillary thyroid carcinomas. World J Surg. 2010;34(7):1494–9.
14. Frankenthaler RA, et al. Lymph node metastasis from papillary-follicular thyroid carcinoma in young patients. Am J Surg. 1990;160(4):341–3.
15. Clark OH. Thyroid cancer and lymph node metastases. J Surg Oncol. 2011;103(6):615–8.
16. Shimamoto K, et al. Preoperative staging of thyroid papillary carcinoma with ultrasonography. Eur J Radiol. 1998;29(1):4–10.
17. Ito Y, et al. An observation trial without surgical treatment in patients with papillary microcarcinoma of the thyroid. Thyroid. 2003;13(4):381–7.
18. Ito Y, et al. Preoperative ultrasonographic examination for lymph node metastasis: usefulness when designing lymph node dissection for papillary microcarcinoma of the thyroid. World J Surg. 2004;28(5):498–501.
19. Moreno MA, et al. In papillary thyroid cancer, preoperative central neck ultrasound detects only macroscopic surgical disease, but negative findings predict excellent long-term regional control and survival. Thyroid. 2012;22(4):347–55.
20. American Thyroid Association Guidelines Taskforce on Thyroid, N., et al. Revised American Thyroid Association management guidelines for patients with thyroid nodules and differentiated thyroid cancer. Thyroid. 2009;19(11):1167–214.
21. Bonnet S, et al. Prophylactic lymph node dissection for papillary thyroid cancer less than 2 cm: implications for radioiodine treatment. J Clin Endocrinol Metab. 2009;94(4):1162–7.
22. Henry JF, et al. Morbidity of prophylactic lymph node dissection in the central neck area in patients with papillary thyroid carcinoma. Langenbecks Arch Surg. 1998;383(2):167–9.
23. Cheah WK, et al. Complications of neck dissection for thyroid cancer. World J Surg. 2002;26(8):1013–6.
24. White ML, Gauger PG, Doherty GM. Central lymph node dissection in differentiated thyroid cancer. World J Surg. 2007;31(5):895–904.
25. Carling T, et al. American Thyroid Association design and feasibility of a prospective randomized controlled trial of prophylactic central lymph node dissection for papillary thyroid carcinoma. Thyroid. 2012;22(3):237–44.
26. Mulla MG, et al. Lateral cervical lymph node metastases in papillary thyroid cancer: a systematic review of imaging-guided and prophylactic removal of the lateral compartment. Clin Endocrinol (Oxf). 2012;77(1):126–31.
27. Cady B, et al. Changing clinical, pathologic, therapeutic, and survival patterns in differentiated thyroid carcinoma. Ann Surg. 1976;184(5):541–53.
28. Harwood J, Clark OH, Dunphy JE. Significance of lymph node metastasis in differentiated thyroid cancer. Am J Surg. 1978;136(1):107–12.
29. Hay ID, et al. Papillary thyroid microcarcinoma: a study of 535 cases observed in a 50-year period. Surgery. 1992;112(6):1139–46. discussion 1146-7.
30. Spires JR, et al. Metastatic papillary carcinoma of the thyroid: the significance of extranodal extension. Head Neck. 1989;11(3):242–6.
31. Mazzaferri EL, Young RL. Papillary thyroid carcinoma: a 10 year follow-up report of the impact of therapy in 576 patients. Am J Med. 1981;70(3):511–8.
32. Scheumann GF, et al. Prognostic significance and surgical management of locoregional lymph node metastases in papillary thyroid cancer. World J Surg. 1994;18(4):559–67. discussion 567-8.
33. Zaydfudim V, et al. The impact of lymph node involvement on survival in patients with papillary and follicular thyroid carcinoma. Surgery. 2008;144(6): 1070–7. discussion 1077-8.
34. Ito Y, et al. Prognosis of patients with papillary thyroid carcinoma having clinically apparent metastasis to the lateral compartment. Endocr J. 2009;56(6):759–66.
35. Ito Y, et al. Clinical significance of lymph node metastasis of thyroid papillary carcinoma located in one lobe. World J Surg. 2006;30(10):1821–8.
36. Ito Y, et al. Ultrasonographically and anatomopathologically detectable node metastases in the lateral compartment as indicators of worse relapse-free survival in patients with papillary thyroid carcinoma. World J Surg. 2005;29(7):917–20.
37. Wada N, et al. Lymph node metastasis from 259 papillary thyroid microcarcinomas: frequency, pattern of occurrence and recurrence, and optimal strategy for neck dissection. Ann Surg. 2003;237(3):399–407.
38. Wada N, et al. Clinical outcomes in older or younger patients with papillary thyroid carcinoma: impact of

lymphadenopathy and patient age. Eur J Surg Oncol. 2008;34(2):202–7.
39. Leboulleux S, et al. Prognostic factors for persistent or recurrent disease of papillary thyroid carcinoma with neck lymph node metastases and/or tumor extension beyond the thyroid capsule at initial diagnosis. J Clin Endocrinol Metab. 2005;90(10):5723–9.
40. Sugitani I, et al. A novel classification system for patients with PTC: addition of the new variables of large (3 cm or greater) nodal metastases and reclassification during the follow-up period. Surgery. 2004;135(2):139–48.
41. Yamashita H, et al. Extracapsular invasion of lymph node metastasis. A good indicator of disease recurrence and poor prognosis in patients with thyroid microcarcinoma. Cancer. 1999;86(5):842–9.
42. Cranshaw IM, Carnaille B. Micrometastases in thyroid cancer. An important finding? Surg Oncol. 2008;17(3):253–8.
43. Tufano RP, et al. Management of recurrent/persistent nodal disease in patients with differentiated thyroid cancer: a critical review of the risks and benefits of surgical intervention versus active surveillance. Thyroid. 2015;25(1):15–27.
44. Mazzaferri EL, Jhiang SM. Long-term impact of initial surgical and medical therapy on papillary and follicular thyroid cancer. Am J Med. 1994;97(5):418–28.
45. Pacini F, et al. Recombinant human thyrotropin-stimulated serum thyroglobulin combined with neck ultrasonography has the highest sensitivity in monitoring differentiated thyroid carcinoma. J Clin Endocrinol Metab. 2003;88(8):3668–73.
46. Hay ID, et al. Papillary thyroid carcinoma managed at the Mayo Clinic during six decades (1940-1999): temporal trends in initial therapy and long-term outcome in 2444 consecutively treated patients. World J Surg. 2002;26(8):879–85.
47. Giordano D, et al. Treatment and prognostic factors of papillary thyroid microcarcinoma. Clin Otolaryngol. 2010;35(2):118–24.
48. Jonklaas J, et al. Outcomes of patients with differentiated thyroid carcinoma following initial therapy. Thyroid. 2006;16(12):1229–42.
49. Toniato A, et al. Papillary thyroid carcinoma: factors influencing recurrence and survival. Ann Surg Oncol. 2008;15(5):1518–22.
50. Bilimoria KY, et al. Extent of surgery affects survival for papillary thyroid cancer. Ann Surg. 2007;246(3): 375–81. discussion 381-4.
51. Edge SB, Byrd D, Compton CC, Fritz AG, Greene FL, Trotti A. Thyroid cancer staging. In: Byrd D, Edge SB, Compton CC, Fritz AG, Greene FL, Trotti A, editors. AJCC cancer staging manual. New York, NY: Springer; 2010. p. 59–64.
52. Byar DP, et al. A prognostic index for thyroid carcinoma. A study of the E.O.R.T.C. Thyroid Cancer Cooperative Group. Eur J Cancer. 1979;15(8):1033–41.
53. Cady B, Rossi R. An expanded view of risk-group definition in differentiated thyroid carcinoma. Surgery. 1988;104(6):947–53.
54. Hay ID, et al. Predicting outcome in papillary thyroid carcinoma: development of a reliable prognostic scoring system in a cohort of 1779 patients surgically treated at one institution during 1940 through 1989. Surgery. 1993;114(6):1050–7. discussion 1057-8.
55. Brierley JD, et al. A comparison of different staging systems predictability of patient outcome. Thyroid carcinoma as an example. Cancer. 1997;79(12): 2414–23.
56. Sherman SI, et al. Prospective multicenter study of thyroiscarcinoma treatment: initial analysis of staging and outcome. National Thyroid Cancer Treatment Cooperative Study Registry Group. Cancer. 1998;83(5):1012–21.
57. Tuttle RM, et al. Estimating risk of recurrence in differentiated thyroid cancer after total thyroidectomy and radioactive iodine remnant ablation: using response to therapy variables to modify the initial risk estimates predicted by the new American Thyroid Association staging system. Thyroid. 2010;20(12): 1341–9.
58. Castagna MG, et al. Delayed risk stratification, to include the response to initial treatment (surgery and radioiodine ablation), has better outcome predictivity in differentiated thyroid cancer patients. Eur J Endocrinol. 2011;165(3):441–6.
59. Baloch ZW, et al. Utility of Thyroglobulin measurement in fine-needle aspiration biopsy specimens of lymph nodes in the diagnosis of recurrent thyroid carcinoma. Cytojournal. 2008;5:1.
60. Boi F, et al. The diagnostic value for differentiated thyroid carcinoma metastases of thyroglobulin (Tg) measurement in washout fluid from fine-needle aspiration biopsy of neck lymph nodes is maintained in the presence of circulating anti-Tg antibodies. J Clin Endocrinol Metab. 2006;91(4):1364–9.
61. Snozek CL, et al. Serum thyroglobulin, high-resolution ultrasound, and lymph node thyroglobulin in diagnosis of differentiated thyroid carcinoma nodal metastases. J Clin Endocrinol Metab. 2007;92(11):4278–81.
62. Choudhary C, et al. Evaluation of thyroid bed nodules on ultrasonography after total thyroidectomy: risk for loco-regional recurrence of thyroid cancer. Eur Thyroid J. 2015;4(2):106–14.
63. Robenshtok E, et al. Suspicious cervical lymph nodes detected after thyroidectomy for papillary thyroid cancer usually remain stable over years in properly selected patients. J Clin Endocrinol Metab. 2012;97(8):2706–13.
64. Rondeau G, et al. Ultrasonographically detected small thyroid bed nodules identified after total thyroidectomy for differentiated thyroid cancer seldom show clinically significant structural progression. Thyroid. 2011;21(8):845–53.
65. Ahn JE, et al. Diagnostic accuracy of CT and ultrasonography for evaluating metastatic cervical lymph nodes in patients with thyroid cancer. World J Surg. 2008;32(7):1552–8.
66. Lesnik D, et al. Papillary thyroid carcinoma nodal surgery directed by a preoperative radiographic map

utilizing CT scan and ultrasound in all primary and reoperative patients. Head Neck. 2014;36(2):191–202.
67. Andersen PE, et al. Differentiated carcinoma of the thyroid with extrathyroidal extension. Am J Surg. 1995;170(5):467–70.
68. Kamaya A, et al. Sonographic detection of extracapsular extension in papillary thyroid cancer. J Ultrasound Med. 2015;34(12):2225–30.
69. Kim E, et al. Preoperative diagnosis of cervical metastatic lymph nodes in papillary thyroid carcinoma: comparison of ultrasound, computed tomography, and combined ultrasound with computed tomography. Thyroid. 2008;18(4):411–8.
70. Yeh MW, et al. American Thyroid Association statement on preoperative imaging for thyroid cancer surgery. Thyroid. 2015;25(1):3–14.
71. Kobaly K, Mandel SJ, Langer JE. Clinical review: thyroid cancer mimics on surveillance neck sonography. J Clin Endocrinol Metab. 2015;100(2):371–5.
72. Sipos JA. Advances in ultrasound for the diagnosis and management of thyroid cancer. Thyroid. 2009;19(12):1363–72.

20 Normal Cervical Lymph Node Appearance and Anatomic Landmarks in Neck Ultrasound

Lisa A. Orloff and Maisie L. Shindo

20.1 Introduction

Lymph nodes involved in metastatic thyroid cancer can be classified into central neck and lateral neck subsets. These regions are defined by normal anatomic landmarks in the neck, which separate lymph node clusters into six levels or compartments (Fig. 20.1) [1]. The central neck contains the thyroid gland itself, and its immediate lymphatic basin (level VI) consists of paratracheal, pretracheal, and prelaryngeal nodes [2]. Boundaries of the level VI compartment are the hyoid bone superiorly, carotid arteries bilaterally, innominate artery inferiorly, and prevertebral fascia posteriorly (Fig. 20.2). The lateral neck lymph nodes (compartments I–V) are grouped into the following:

Electronic supplementary material: The online version of this chapter (doi:10.1007/978-3-319-44100-9_20) contains supplementary material, which is available to authorized users. Videos can also be accessed at http://link.springer.com/chapter/10.1007/978-3-319-44100-9_20.

L.A. Orloff, M.D., F.A.C.S., F.A.C.E. (✉)
Director of Endocrine Head & Neck Surgery, Professor of Otolaryngology - Head & Neck Surgery, Thyroid & Parathyroid Surgery, Stanford University School of Medicine and Stanford Cancer Center, 875 Blake Wilbur Drive, CC-2225, Stanford, CA 94305, USA
e-mail: lorloff@stanford.edu

M.L. Shindo (✉)
Director of Thyroid & Parathyroid Center, Director of Head & Neck Endocrine Surgery, Department of Otolaryngology, Oregon Health & Science University, Portland, OR, USA
e-mail: shindom@ohsu.edu

20.2 Level I: Submandibular

This group is very rarely involved in thyroid cancer. It consists of lymph nodes within the boundaries of the anterior and posterior bellies of the digastric muscles, the stylohyoid muscle, and the body of the mandible. Lymph nodes in this compartment are at greatest risk for harboring metastases from oral cavity, anterior nasal cavity, midface soft tissue, and submandibular gland malignancies. Inflammatory lymphadenopathy is also very common in level I, related to benign dental and oral cavity processes. Of note, the submandibular glands are located in level I, and these salivary glands are not infrequently affected by radioactive iodine therapy (Fig. 20.3).

20.3 Level II: Upper Jugular

This group is comprised of lymph nodes located around the upper third of the internal jugular vein. Its boundaries are the skull base superiorly, inferior border of the hyoid bone inferiorly, lateral border of the sternohyoid and stylohyoid muscles anteromedially, and the posterior border of the sternocleidomastoid

M. Milas et al. (eds.), *Advanced Thyroid and Parathyroid Ultrasound*,
DOI 10.1007/978-3-319-44100-9_20

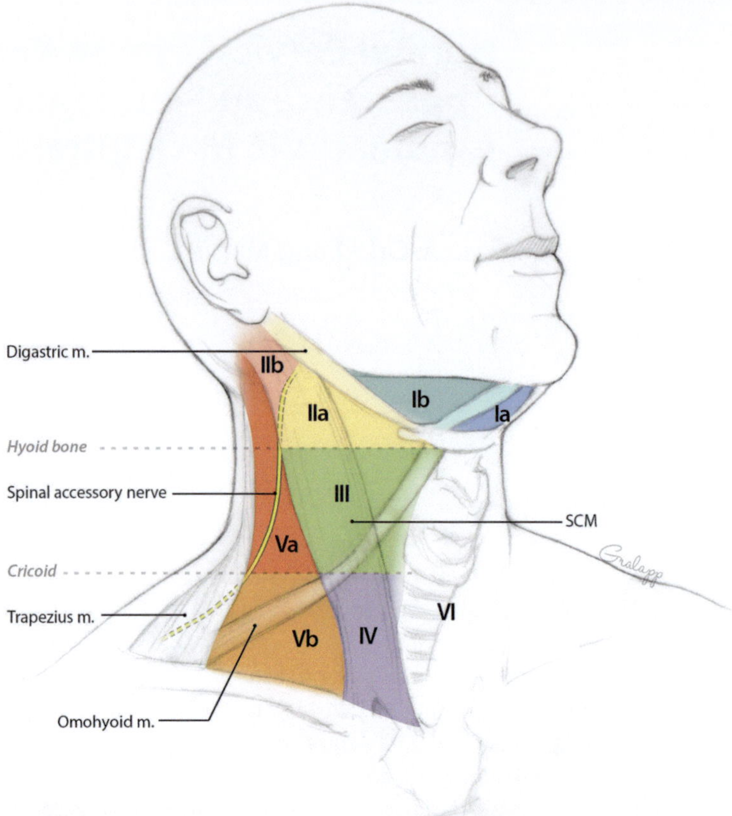

Fig. 20.1 Levels I–VI of the neck (and level VII, superior mediastinum)

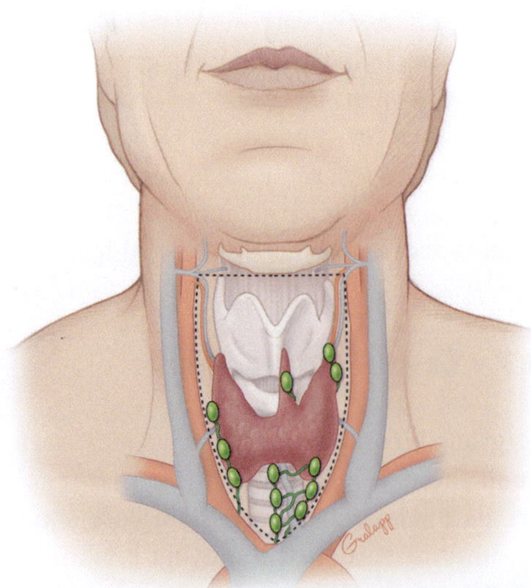

Fig. 20.2 Level VI, anterior view

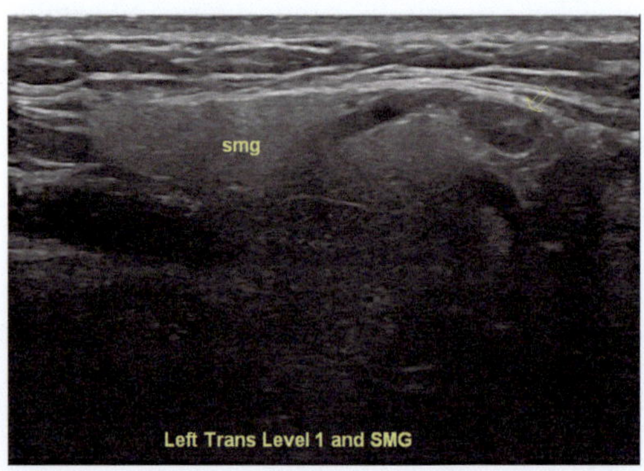

Fig. 20.3 Level I lymph node (*arrow*) with adjacent submandibular gland

muscle posterolaterally. The spinal accessory nerve is within this compartment and subdivides this compartment into IIA which are nodes located anterior (medial) to the nerve and IIB which are nodes located posterior to the nerve. Level II nodes are at risk for harboring metastases from cancers arising from the oral cavity, nasal cavity, nasopharynx, oropharynx, thyroid, hypopharynx, larynx, and parotid gland (Fig. 20.4, Video 20.1).

20.4 Level III: Middle Jugular

This group consists of lymph nodes located around the middle third of the internal jugular vein. Its boundaries are the hyoid bone superiorly, cricoid cartilage inferiorly, lateral border of the sternohyoid muscle anteromedially, and posterior border of the sternocleidomastoid muscle posterolaterally. These nodes are at greatest risk for harboring metastases from cancers arising from the thyroid, oral cavity, nasopharynx, oropharynx, hypopharynx, and larynx (Fig. 20.5, Video 20.2).

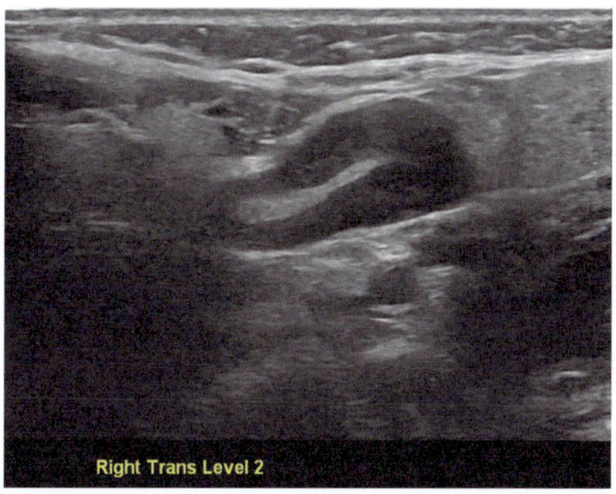

Fig. 20.4 Benign level II lymph node (right transverse view)

20.5 Level IV: Lower Jugular

This group consists of lymph nodes located around the lower third of the internal jugular vein. Its boundaries are the cricoid cartilage superiorly, clavicle inferiorly, lateral border of the sternohyoid muscle anteromedially, and posterior border of the sternocleidomastoid muscle posteriorly. These nodes are at greatest risk for harboring metastases from cancers arising from the thyroid, hypopharynx, cervical esophagus, and larynx (Fig. 20.6).

20.6 Level V: Posterior Triangle

This group is comprised predominantly of the lymph nodes located along the lower half of the spinal accessory nerve and the transverse cervical artery, along with the supraclavicular nodes. The superior boundary is the apex formed by a convergence of the sternocleidomastoid and the trapezius muscles, the inferior boundary is the clavicle, the anterior boundary is the posterior border of the sternocleidomastoid muscle, and the posterior boundary is the anterior border of the trapezius muscle. Sublevel VA is separated from sublevel VB by a horizontal plane marking the inferior border of the arch of the cricoid cartilage. Sublevel VA includes the spinal accessory nodes, and sublevel VB includes the nodes fol-

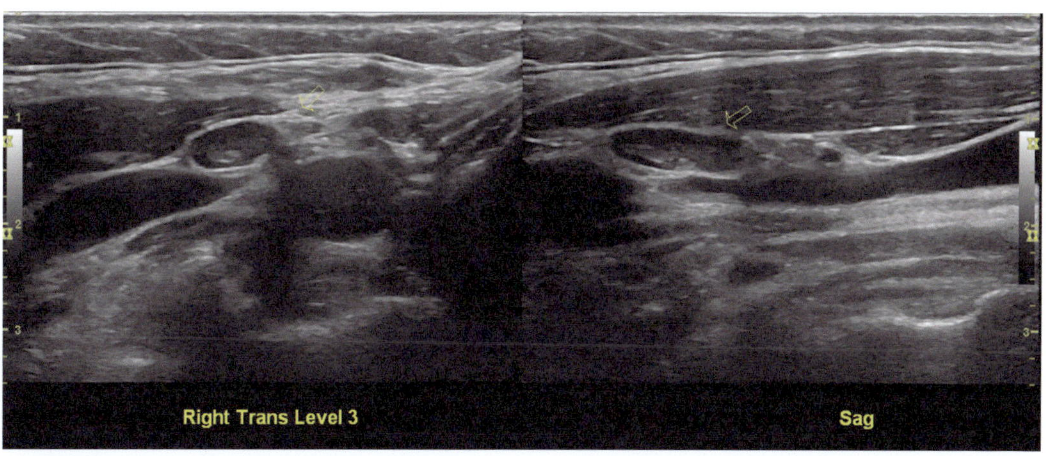

Fig. 20.5 Right level III benign lymph node, transverse and sagittal views

lowing the transverse cervical vessels and the supraclavicular nodes. Level V nodes are at greatest risk for harboring metastases from cancers arising from the thyroid, nasopharynx, and oropharynx (Fig. 20.7).

In practice, some of the landmarks noted above are not easily visible by ultrasound during scanning of the neck. Therefore, a surrogate landmark for the boundary between levels I and II is the posterior border of the submandibular gland; an alternative landmark for the boundary between levels II and III is the carotid bifurcation and between levels III and IV is the omohyoid muscle as it crosses over the internal jugular vein from superomedial to inferolateral. It is important to be aware of variations in usage of landmarks by different examiners and through different imaging modalities (ultrasound vs. cross-sectional), as well as variations in individual patient anatomy, so that imaging can be properly correlated with pathology, treatment planning, and outcomes.

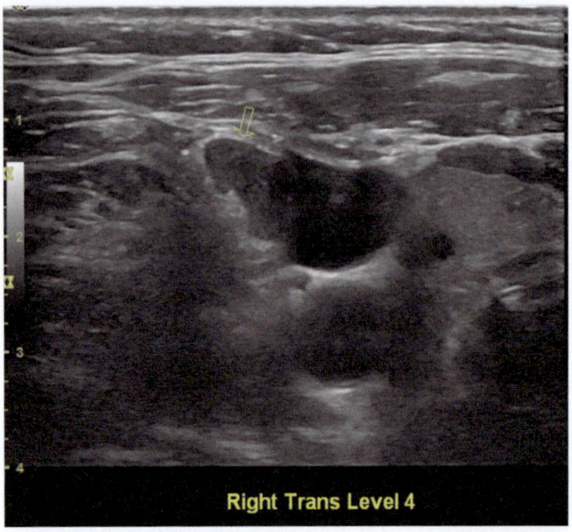

Fig. 20.6 Right transverse level IV, somewhat amorphous but benign lymph node

20.7 Level VI: Central Neck

As noted above, this compartment is bounded inferiorly by the innominate artery. However, the ability to visualize this lower limit is quite variable depending on patient body habitus, ability to extend the neck, and position of the larynx relative to the sternum. In some patients, it is not possible to visualize soft tissue structures, including lymph nodes, more inferior than the sternal notch. At the other extreme, there are some patients whose superior mediastinal structures (level VII) can be visualized even inferior to the innominate artery (Fig. 20.8 and Video 20.3).

20.8 Scanning Lymph Nodes

A 7.5-MHz linear transducer is the minimum requirement for ultrasonography of neck lymph nodes. A higher-frequency transducer (>10 MHz) allows better resolution of the lymph node archi-

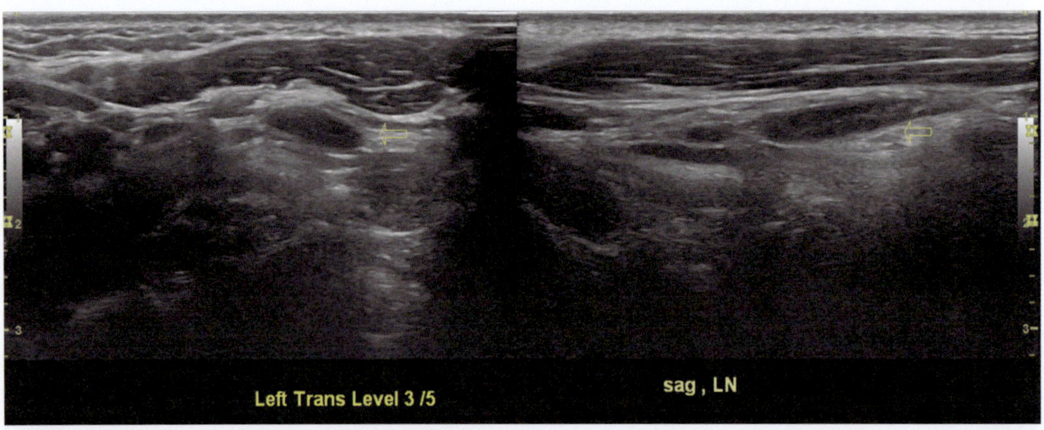

Fig. 20.7 Benign lymph node at junction of levels III and V, left transverse and sagittal views. Note flattened shape and absence of visible hilum despite benign nature

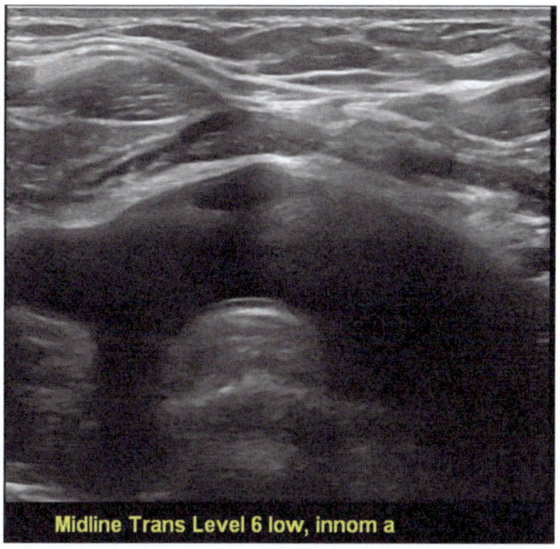

Fig. 20.8 Level VI inferior limit at innominate artery

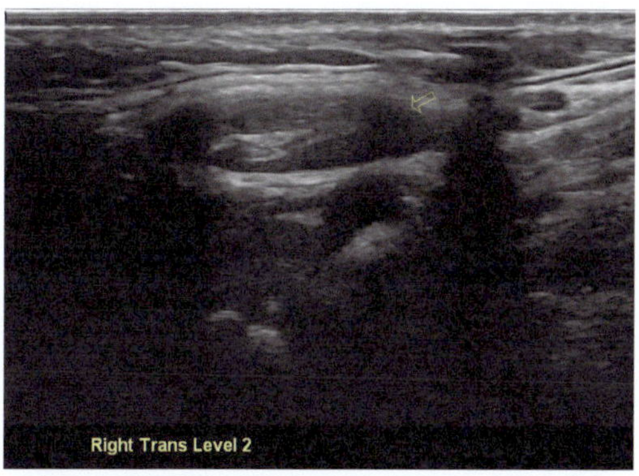

Fig. 20.9 Benign level II lymph node, oval in shape, visible hilum

tecture. Ultrasound can help differentiate benign nodes from those that are suspicious for malignancy. The next chapter (Chap. 21) discusses malignant lymph nodes in greater detail. To distinguish benign from malignant lymph nodes, the shape of the lymph node provides a useful starting point. Normal or reactive nodes (Fig. 20.9) are usually oval or fusiform, whereas malignant nodes tend to be round. A short to long axis ratio greater than 0.5 indicates a rounded and suspicious lymph node. Although rounded lymph nodes are more likely to be malignant, one must be cautious in using this rule with submandibular and parotid nodes, since nodes in these regions are frequently round even when benign (Fig. 20.10). Size of lymph nodes alone cannot be used for identifying malignant nodes, particularly since level II nodes tend to be quite large (Fig. 20.11). However, in a patient with a known malignancy, the serial change in nodal size is useful. Enlarging lymph nodes on serial examinations are highly suspicious for metastases. The medullary sinuses in the lymph node act as multiple acoustic interfaces and reflect the ultrasound waves, producing an echogenic structure know as echogenic hilum or hilus (Fig. 20.12). Fatty deposition makes the hilum more visible on ultrasound. Malignant nodes frequently lack an echogenic hilum. The presence of an echogenic hilum is suggestive of a benign node but is not absolute since nodes with small malignant deposits that have not completely replaced the

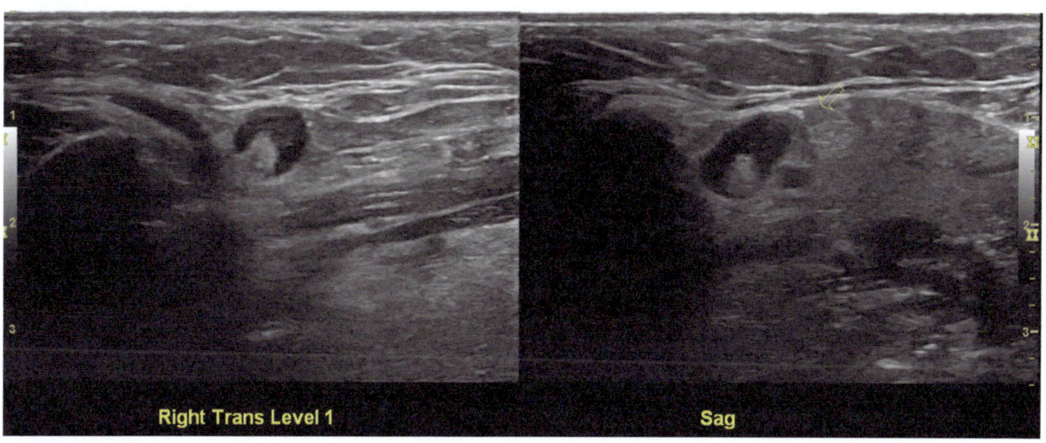

Fig. 20.10 Right level I benign lymph node, transverse and sagittal views. Note somewhat rounded shape. Visible hilum

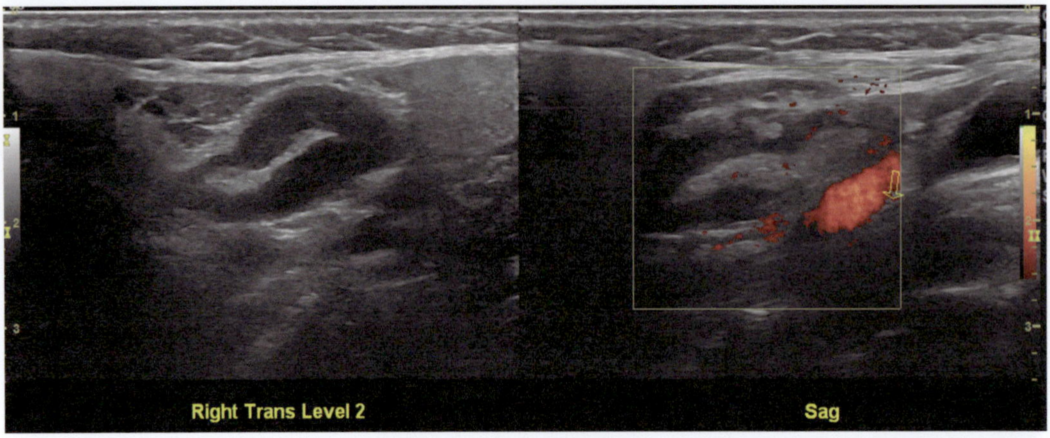

Fig. 20.11 Large right level II benign lymph node, transverse and sagittal (with power Doppler) views

Fig. 20.12 Left level II benign lymph node with visible hilum, transverse view

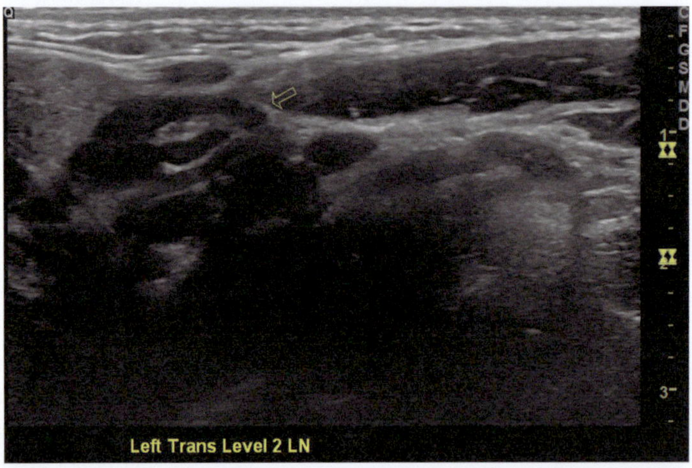

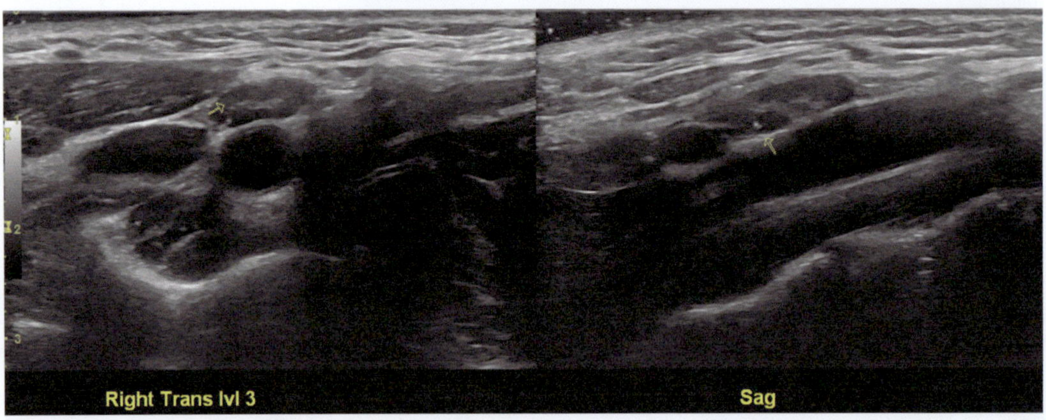

Fig. 20.13 Benign-appearing right level III lymph node except for tiny microcalcification (*arrow*)

lymph node may preserve the echogenic hilum (Fig. 20.13 and Video 20.4). Color and power Doppler are invaluable to help differentiate benign-appearing nodes from those that are suspicious for malignancy. Normal lymph nodes only exhibit vascularity along the echogenic hilum [Video 20.5].

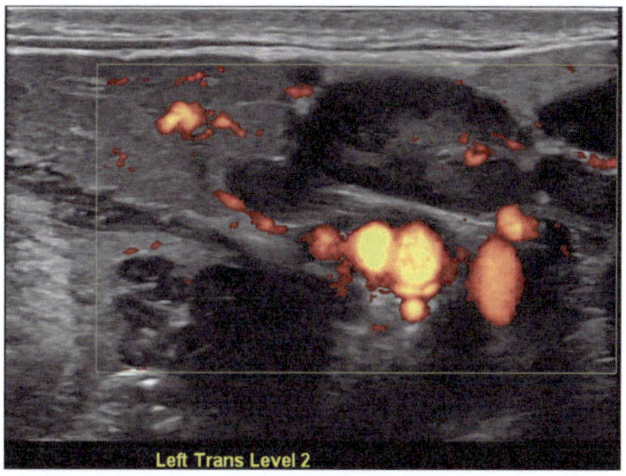

Fig. 20.14 Reactive lymphadenitis in level II; note somewhat diffuse hilar flow on power Doppler

Acute reactive lymphadenitis may exhibit increased vascularity with branching of the hilar vessels, but the flow is still within the core of the lymph node (Fig. 20.14). Increased vascularity around the periphery or throughout the lymph node cortex is suspicious for malignancy (Fig. 20.15). The increased peripheral vascularity in malignant lymph nodes is related to tumor angiogenesis. Other findings suspicious for thyroid malignancy are irregular lymph node borders, presence of calcifications, and cystic and/or hyperechoic soft tissue component within the node (Fig. 20.16a, b). More examples are shown in the next chapter.

In order to ensure that pathology is not missed in the performance of a neck ultrasound exam, it

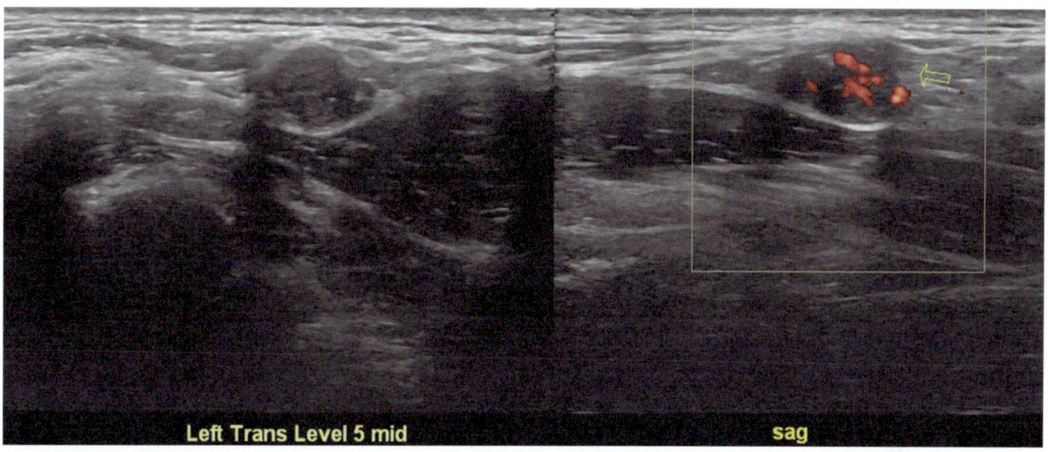

Fig. 20.15 Left transverse (B-mode) and sagittal (power Doppler) views of level V lymph node with metastatic papillary thyroid carcinoma

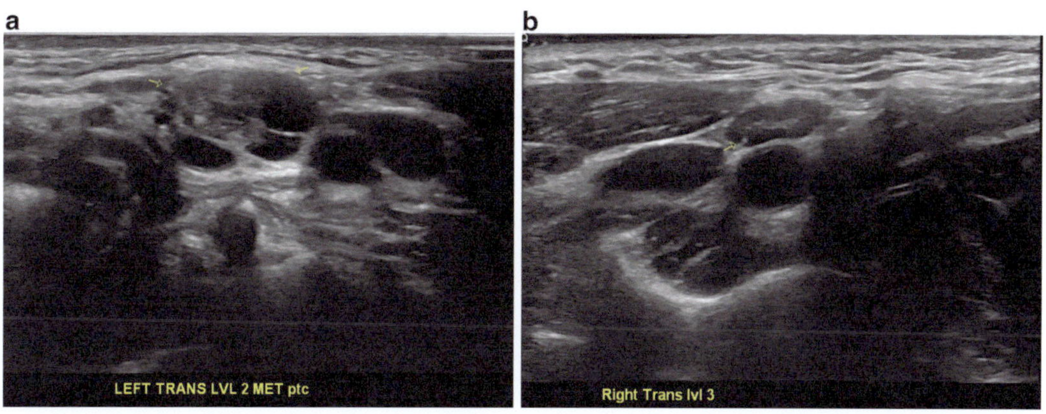

Fig. 20.16 (**a**) Metastatic papillary carcinoma. Left level II lymph node, transverse view. (**b**) Metastatic papillary carcinoma. Right level III, transverse view, *arrow* points to microcalcification in otherwise benign-appearing lymph node

is important to be systematic in scanning [3]. The sequence of exam is less important than the consistency by a given examiner and the conscious effort to include all six levels of the neck. Most scanning is performed in the transverse plane, sweeping superiorly and inferiorly, with corroboration of findings and completion of measurements by rotating to a sagittal (longitudinal) plane. Doppler is typically applied to discrete structures after B-mode (grayscale) ultrasound has delineated specific areas of interest. Level VI is typically examined in combination with the thyroid gland (if present) or as a starting point after thyroidectomy, and the lateral neck compartments are then scanned sequentially. Annotation of images and an effort to commit findings to specific compartments in the neck will greatly enhance communication of findings, and ultimately management of disease, by collaborating specialists.

References

1. Robbins KT, Clayman G, Levine PA, Medina J, Sessions R, Shaha A, Som P, Wolf GT, Committee for Head and Neck Surgery and Oncology, American Academy of Otolaryngology – Head and Neck Surgery. Neck dissection classification update. Arch Otolaryngol Head Neck Surg. 2002;128(7):751–8.
2. Carty SE, Cooper DS, Doherty GM, Duh QY, Kloos RT, Mandel SJ, Randolph GW, Stack Jr BC, Steward DL, Terris DJ, Thompson GB, Tufano RP, Tuttle RM, Udelsman R, The American Thyroid Association Surgery Working Group. Consensus statement on the terminology and classification of central neck dissection for thyroid cancer. Thyroid. 2009;19(11):1153–8.
3. Yeh MW, Bauer AJ, Bernet VA, Ferris RL, Loevner LA, Mandel SJ, Orloff LA, Randolph GW, Steward DL. American Thyroid Association Statement on preoperative imaging for thyroid cancer surgery. Thyroid. 2015;25(1):3–14.

21 Sonographic Appearance of Abnormal Cervical Lymph Nodes in the Preoperative and Reoperative/"Empty" Neck: A Surgeon's Perspective

Marlon A. Guerrero

21.1 Introduction

Thyroid cancer has a propensity for cervical lymph node metastasis. Metastasis to the cervical lymph nodes may develop early during initial presentation or may present during surveillance as recurrence. Lymph node metastases arise as either macro-metastasis, which is clinically or radiographically apparent, or micro-metastasis, which is identified within seemingly benign-appearing lymph nodes on pathologic examination. Macro-metastasis is clinically important because morphologic changes in the cervical lymph nodes can be detected radiographically preoperatively and ultimately alter operative management [1, 2].

Cervical lymph node metastases may arise in any type of thyroid cancer, but with varying frequency. Of the five types of thyroid cancer, papillary thyroid cancer is the most common accounting for nearly 90 % of all cases, followed by follicular thyroid cancer (5 %); Hürthle cell cancer, now termed oncocytic follicular cancer (2 %); medullary thyroid cancer (1.7 %); and anaplastic thyroid cancer (0.8 %) [3]. Papillary, follicular, and Hürthle cell carcinomas are grouped together and termed well-differentiated thyroid cancer. Lymph node metastases may be found in up to 50 % of people initially diagnosed with well-differentiated thyroid cancer [4, 5]. In papillary thyroid cancer, clinically apparent lymph node metastases occur in up to 36 % of adults and 80 % of children during initial presentation [6]. Cervical lymph node metastases are found in 5–17 % of follicular thyroid cancers [6, 7], 25 % of Hürthle cell carcinomas [7], and up to 75 % of medullary thyroid cancers [8]. Anaplastic thyroid cancer is fatal and aggressive cancer that presents with lymph node metastasis in 38 % of patients [9].

The importance of thorough perioperative sonographic evaluation of the neck cannot be stressed enough. Sonographic evaluation of cervical lymph nodes is important in all patients with known thyroid cancer or suspicious thyroid nodules [10]. Performing routine preoperative ultrasound lymph node mapping has been shown to alter the operative management in 20 % of those undergoing initial surgery [1] and 68 % undergoing reoperative surgery for recurrence [2]. Cervical ultrasound is an extremely useful tool in detecting cervical lymph node metastasis with a sensitivity of 70 % and specificity of 98 % in patients with thyroid cancer [11].

Electronic supplementary material: The online version of this chapter (doi:10.1007/978-3-319-44100-9_21) contains supplementary material, which is available to authorized users. Videos can also be accessed at http://link.springer.com/chapter/10.1007/978-3-319-44100-9_21.

M.A. Guerrero, M.D., F.A.C.S. (✉)
Department of Surgery, Banner - University Medical Center, Tucson Campus, University of Arizona, 1501 N. Campbell Avenue, Tucson, AZ 85724, USA
e-mail: mguerrero@surgery.arizona.edu

M. Milas et al. (eds.), *Advanced Thyroid and Parathyroid Ultrasound*,
DOI 10.1007/978-3-319-44100-9_21

21.2 Ultrasound Technique and Reporting

Sonographic evaluation of cervical lymph nodes necessitates a standard method of imaging and reporting. A common language in reporting is essential for communication and for proper therapeutic planning. Cervical lymph nodes are grouped into seven levels according to anatomical distribution as proposed by Robbins et al. in 2008 [12]. The borders of each level are as follows:

Level 1: Mandible, hyoid bone, anterior belly of the digastric muscle, and posterior border of the submandibular gland.
Levels 2–4 are bordered medially by the medial border of the carotid artery and laterally by the posterior border of the sternocleidomastoid muscle. The cephalad to caudad borders are:
Level 2: Skull base and angle of the mandible to the inferior border of the hyoid bone
Level 3: Inferior border of the hyoid bone to the inferior border of the cricoid cartilage
Level 4: Inferior border of cricoid cartilage to the clavicle
Level 5: Posterior border to the sternocleidomastoid muscle to the anterior border of the trapezius muscle from the convergence of the sternocleidomastoid and trapezius muscles down to the clavicle. Level 5 is divided in half at the level of the cricoid cartilage, with 5a being cephalad and 5b being caudad.
Level 6: Medial border of the carotid arteries from the hyoid bone to the suprasternal notch.
Level 7: Upper mediastinum (sternal notch to the innominate vessels).

Cervical lymph nodes are also categorized according to the compartments of the neck. The neck is divided into central and lateral compartments. This nomenclature is utilized for imaging and operative descriptions.

The central neck compartment encompasses cervical lymph node levels 6 and 7. This compartment is bordered by the carotid arteries laterally, trachea medially, hyoid bone superiorly, innominate vessels inferiorly, and paraspinous muscles posteriorly. The central neck also incorporates the prelaryngeal (Delphian) and pretracheal lymph nodes. The prelaryngeal lymph nodes are located anterior to the trachea between the hyoid bone and superior border of the isthmus. The pretracheal lymph nodes are found anterior to the trachea from the inferior border to the isthmus down to the innominate vessels.

The lateral compartment is made up of levels 2 through 5 and is bordered by the medial border to the carotid artery medially, the trapezius muscle laterally, angle of the mandible superiorly, clavicle inferiorly, and paraspinous and scalene muscles posteriorly.

Reporting of lymph nodes should comprise the following information:

1. Location: the level of the neck
2. Measurement (in three dimensions): length × width × height (anterior-posterior)
3. Fatty hilum: presence or absence
4. Vascularity pattern
5. Echogenicity
6. Composition (cystic degeneration, calcifications, uniformity)

21.3 Normal Morphology

Detailed description of normal-appearing lymph nodes is detailed in Chap. 23. Briefly, normal- or benign-appearing cervical lymph nodes have a distinct morphologic appearance. Benign lymph nodes are elliptical and small (Fig. 21.1a). However, even when benign lymph nodes enlarge (Fig. 21.1b), they usually maintain an elongated shape in which the length and width of the node are longer than the height (or anterior-posterior dimension). The echogenicity of benign lymph nodes is uniform and hypoechoic with a fatty hilum (hyperechoic streak) running centrally through the node. However, benign or reactive lymph nodes may present without a hyperechoic hilum [13].

21.4 Abnormal Cervical Lymph Nodes

Metastatic disease to the cervical lymph nodes is common in thyroid cancer. The pattern of spread tends to follow a specific course in

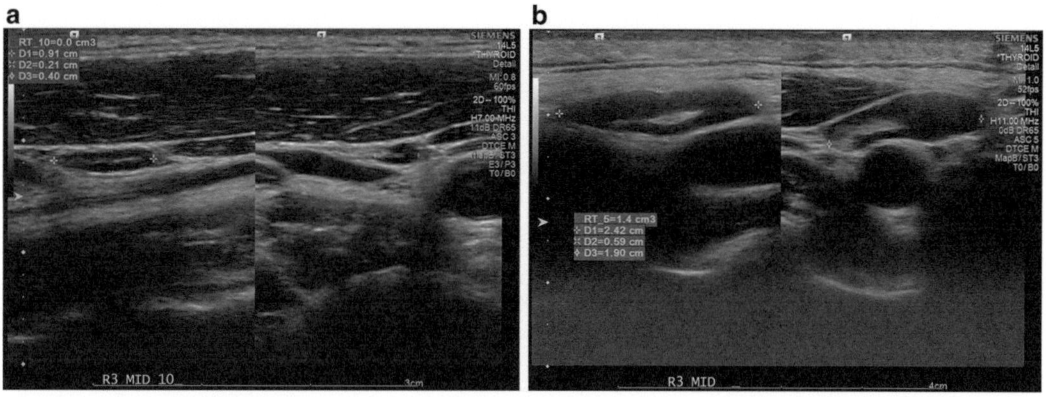

Fig. 21.1 Normal lymph nodes. Note that both small (**a**) and large (**b**) lymph nodes are hypoechoic and maintain an elongated shape with a hyperechoic fatty hilum coursing centrally

which the central compartment is typically affected first, followed by the lateral comportment. The proximity of the central lymph nodes to the thyroid gland makes these lymph nodes more susceptible to local spread. However, visualization of these lymph nodes is often difficult during initial presentation due to the presence of the thyroid parenchyma anteriorly. Level 6 and 7 lymph nodes are commonly involved first, followed by levels 3 and 4. Levels 2 and 5 are less commonly involved, but may still harbor metastasis; metastasis to level 1 is very rare [14, 15]. The lower third of the neck (low jugular, midline low neck, and supraclavicular neck regions) is affected in 66.5 % and the middle third in 20.4 % of patients with metastatic thyroid cancer. Only 13 % of patients had metastasis to the upper third of the neck [15]. In evaluating level-specific metastasis in the lateral compartment, levels 3 and 4 harbor 71 % and 79 %, respectively, of the lymph node metastasis [16]. Therefore, identification of metastasis in any lateral neck lymph node during initial evaluation suggests involvement in the central neck. Understanding this pattern of spread is essential to proper operative management. For instance, positive lateral neck metastasis would necessitate a lateral neck dissection in combination with a central neck dissection.

21.5 Ultrasound Abnormalities

Abnormal lymph nodes consistently show deviation from normal morphologic patterns. However, ultrasound is limited in that there is no single sonographic finding or criterion that is diagnostic of malignancy. Specificity and sensitivity for malignancy vary according to individual features. A study evaluating the sonographic criteria for malignancy found that loss of the fatty hyperechoic hilum had the highest sensitivity (100 %), but the lowest specificity (29 %) in predicting malignancy. On the contrary, cystic appearance and hyperechoic punctuations had the highest specificity (100 %), but low sensitivities (11 % and 46 %, respectively) [14]. The importance in analyzing sonographic images is recognizing that deviation from the typical lymph node morphology should prompt further evaluation. Sonographic findings suggestive of malignancy are as follows:

21.5.1 Shape

Shape of cervical lymph nodes can be utilized to differentiate malignant from benign cervical lymph nodes. The classic elliptical form of benign

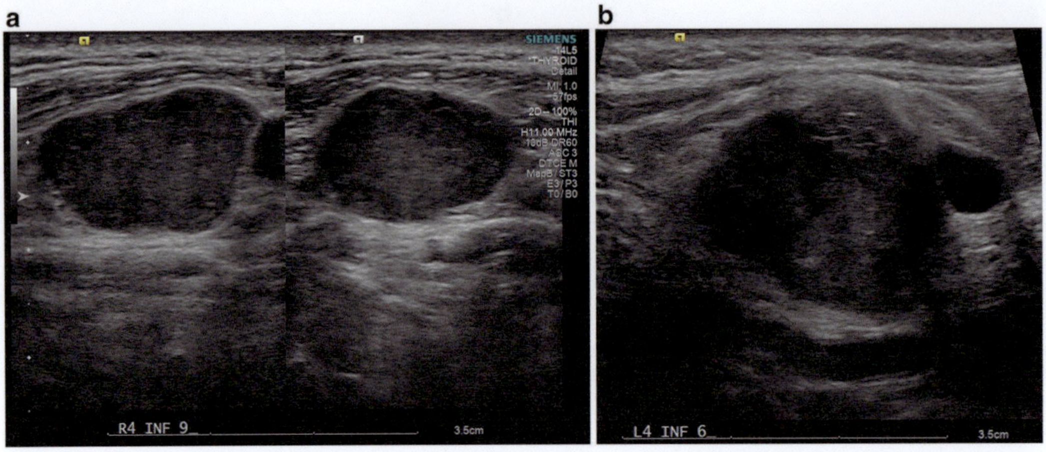

Fig. 21.2 Metastatic lymph nodes. (**a**) Lateral lymph node (level 4) with loss of elliptical shape, fatty hilum. Also note the irregular margins and heterogeneous echogenic pattern. (**b**) Level 4 lymph node with round appearance, irregular margins, heterogeneous solid echogenic pattern, and microcalcifications

lymph nodes is lost in malignant lymph nodes, and the shape becomes more rounded. Malignant lymph nodes also tend to develop an irregular contour and lose the smooth margin seen in benign lymph nodes (Fig. 21.2a). A round shape has been reported in 80 % of malignant lymph nodes, but in only 30 % of benign lymph nodes [17]. Shape of lymph nodes may be determined on transverse view with measurement of the width (transverse dimension) and height (anteroposterior dimension). Malignant lymph nodes are suspected when the height of the lymph node is equal to or greater than the width causing a more rounded appearance. A round shape is present when the ratio of the lymph node's shortest to longest dimension is >0.5 [16, 17]. 80 % of malignant and only 30 % of benign lymph nodes have a ratio greater than 0.5, with a sensitivity and specificity of 80 and 71 %, respectfully [17]. A more specific assessment was proposed in which the largest and smallest dimensions are utilized to calculate the longitudinal/transverse ratio. A ratio of >2 defines an oval lymph node and a ratio of <2 defines a round lymph node [15]. Utilizing the longitudinal/transverse ratio of 2, 88 % of benign lymph nodes have a ratio of 2 or greater, while 66 % of malignant lymph nodes have a ratio of less than 2 [15]. Nonetheless, round shape is only 70 % specific and 37 % sensitive for identifying malignant lymph nodes [10, 14].

21.5.2 Echogenic Pattern

Echogenicity is another sonographic finding that can be utilized to stratify the risk of metastatic cervical lymph nodes in patients with thyroid cancer. Hypoechoic lymph nodes, especially with a hyperechoic fatty hilum, are typically benign. In contrast, hyperechogenicity is more commonly associated with malignant lymph nodes. It has been demonstrated that 86 % of malignant lymph nodes are hyperechoic as opposed to only 4.5 % of benign lymph nodes [17]. Hyperechogenicity alone is a strong indicator of malignancy. Hyperechogenicity, with the loss of the fatty hilum, on ultrasound has a predictive value of 96 %, negative predictive value of 84 %, and accuracy of 90 % in identifying malignant lymph nodes in patients with thyroid cancer [17].

In addition to a hyperechogenicity, a heterogeneous solid ultrasound appearance also identifies a malignant lymph node. Benign lymph nodes exhibit a homogenous hypoechoic appearance on sonogram (Fig. 21.1). Malignant lymph nodes, on the other hand, may have a heterogeneous appearance with mixed hypo- and hyperechoic patterns (Fig. 21.2b). Hyperechogenicity and heterogeneity are also found in the solid component of cystic lymph nodes that harbor metastasis (Fig. 21.3). A recent study introducing a predic-

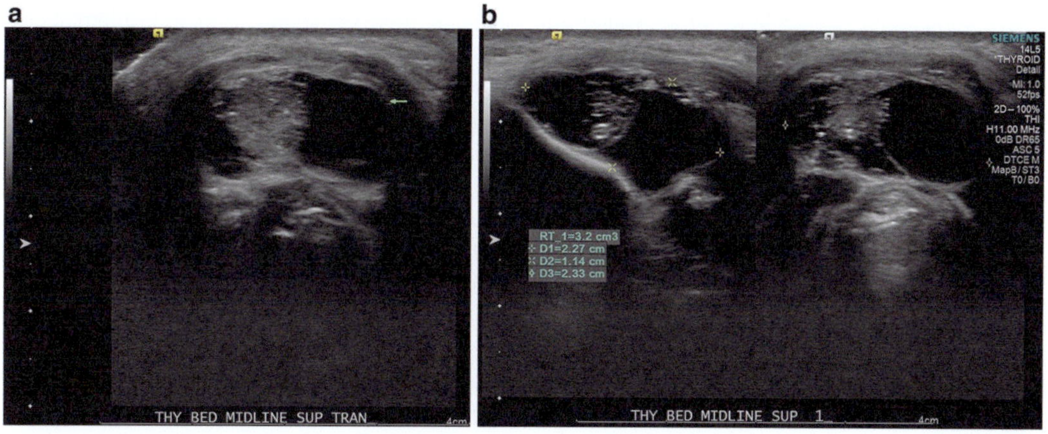

Fig. 21.3 Cystic degeneration of malignant lymph nodes. Note that the cystic lymph node may be associated with a (**a**) dense or (**b**) sparse central component. (**a**) Cystic lymph node with a dense, hyperechoic, central solid component with hyperechoic spots. (**b**) Cystic lymph node with sparse solid component. The solid component has irregular margins and hyperechoic spots

tive model utilizing sonogram demonstrated that the existence of microcalcifications in the presence of a heterogeneous echogenic pattern was the best predictor of malignancy in cervical lymph nodes [18].

21.5.3 Size

Size in itself is not definitive for the diagnosis of malignancy. However, size may affect the malignant potential of lymph nodes. Metastatic lymph nodes in general tend to be larger than benign lymph nodes. When a minimum axial diameter was set at 6 mm, metastases were found in 93 % of lymph nodes, while only 17 % were benign [17]. The malignant potential significantly increases when lymph nodes are larger than 2 cm. Approximately 22 % of malignant lymph nodes are between 2 and 3 cm, compared to 12 % of benign lymph nodes. One study reported that 14 % of malignant lymph nodules were larger than 3 cm (Fig. 21.2), but only 1 % of benign lymph nodes reached this size cutoff. No difference existed in differentiating malignant risk in lymph nodes smaller than 1 cm, while lymph nodes measuring between 1 and 2 cm were more likely to be benign [15].

21.5.4 Cystic Degeneration

Lymph nodes, whether benign or malignant, are frequently solid. Earlier studies showed that over 80 % of metastatic lymph nodes were homogenous [13] and solid. Less often, malignancy may lead to cellular degeneration resulting in cystic formation within a lymph node. Cystic lymph nodes may also be found in benign diseases such as tuberculosis lymphadenitis, branchial cysts, and lymphoceles [10, 14]. In one study, cystic lymph nodes were found in approximately 20 % of thyroid cancer patients with malignant lymph nodes, and no benign lymph nodes exhibited cystic change [15]. However, others have shown that cystic degeneration may occur in up to 70 % of patients with papillary thyroid cancer [19, 20]. Most cystic lymph nodes are from papillary thyroid cancer (93 %); however, poorly differentiated thyroid cancer (3 %) and papillary serous carcinoma of the ovary (3 %) may also present with cystic degeneration [21]. Although identification of a cystic component has a specificity of 100 %, this finding is limited by a low sensitivity (10–34 %) [10].

Sonographic appearance of cystic lymph nodes varies. Generally, cystic lymph nodes lose the elliptical shape of a benign lymph node. The cystic component is anechoic under sonogram evaluation and may encompass a small single focus and multiple cystic areas or completely replace the lymph node [20]. The solid component is iso- to hyperechoic and may be dense or sparse relative to the cystic portion. Sonographic features of the solid component parallel findings typical of non-cystic malignant lymph nodes. Irregular margins, heterogeneity, microcalcifications, and increased vascularity are typical findings within the solid portion of cystic lymph nodes (Fig. 21.3).

21.5.5 Microcalcifications

Microcalcifications are classic finding in malignant thyroid nodules and lymph nodes of thyroid cancer patients, most commonly with well-differentiated thyroid cancer. Microcalcifications may be found in nearly 70 % of metastatic lymph nodes in patients with thyroid cancer [13, 15]. Though commonly associated with papillary thyroid cancer, microcalcifications may also occur in medullary thyroid cancer [22]. Identification of microcalcifications within a lymph node has a specificity of 100 %, but only 46 % sensitivity for malignancy [14]. A recent study showed that microcalcifications in the presence of a heterogeneous echo pattern were predictive of malignancy [18].

On ultrasound, microcalcifications appear as hyperechoic bright spots or reflectors (Fig. 21.4). As opposed to macrocalcifications found in thyroid nodules, microcalcifications do not refract the ultrasound waves. Therefore, the posterior acoustic shadow typical of macro-

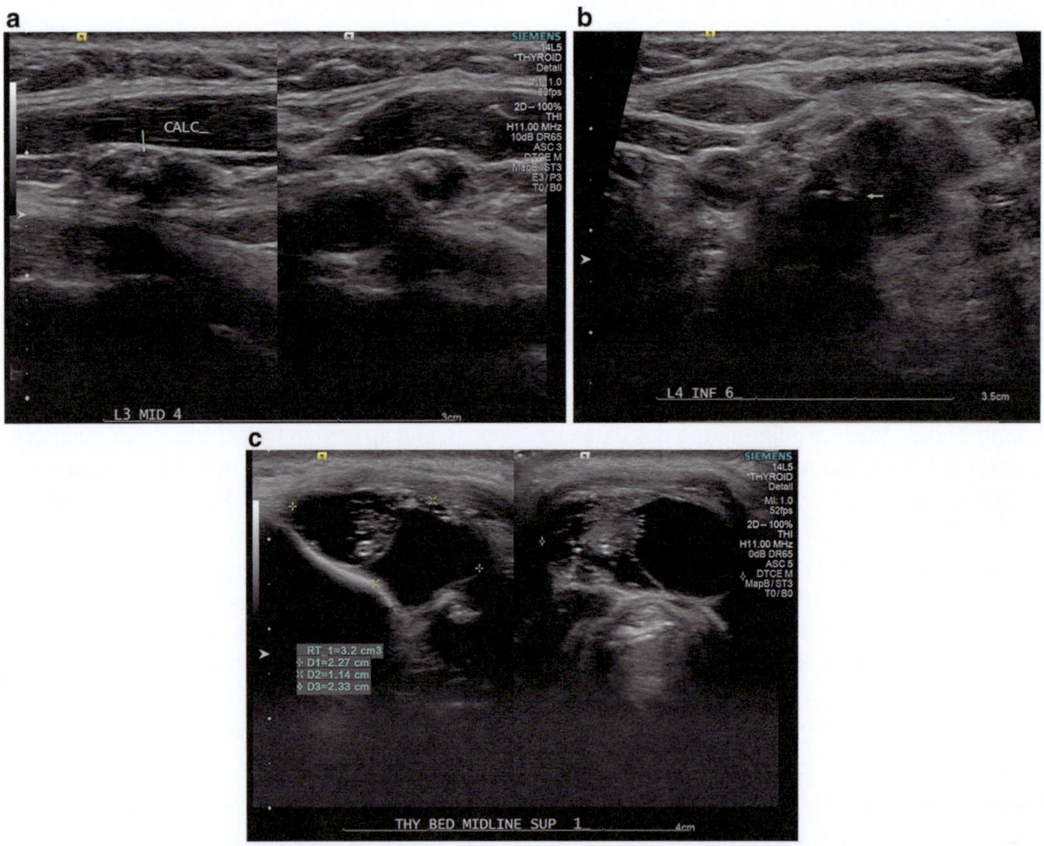

Fig. 21.4 Metastatic lymph nodes depicting varying patterns of microcalcifications. (**a**) Level 3 lymph node with aggregate of calcifications. (**b**) Heterogeneous lymph node with irregular margins and microcalcifications (*arrow*). (**c**) Metastatic lymph node with cystic degeneration and small punctate microcalcifications within the solid component

calcifications is not visible with microcalcifications. Microcalcifications may be found in homogenous lymph nodes or within the solid component of partially cystic lymph nodes.

21.5.6 Vascularity

Increased vascularity within a tumor is commonly associated with malignancy. This is an important factor in evaluating cervical lymph nodes. Yet, benign factors (inflammation and infection) may also affect vascularity in cervical lymph nodes. Therefore, increased vascularity cannot be used as a single diagnostic criterion for malignancy. However, taking other ultrasound features into account, peripheral vascularity is one of the best factors for assessing malignant potential with a specificity of 82 % and sensitivity of 86 % for lymph node metastasis [14]. Other studies have shown a broader range with specificity of 57–93 % and sensitivity of 40–86 % [10].

Patterns of vascularity within metastatic lymph nodes vary. Peripheral enhancement is the principal vascular pattern that has been associated with thyroid cancer metastasis (Fig. 21.5) [10, 14, 17]. Peripheral vascularity may also be apparent within the solid component of a cystic lymph node. Other lymph nodes may harbor a diffuse pattern of increased vascularity throughout the lymph node, including central and prominent peripheral vascular flow. The solid component of cystic lymph nodes may also show diffuse vascular flow. On the other hand, vascularity is not exclusive of malignancy as some metastatic lymph nodes may present with little or no vascularity on Doppler.

21.6 The Technique of Preoperative and Surveillance Ultrasound

There are a few key aspects to review about the strategy of performing ultrasound for the purpose of detecting cervical lymph node metastases. These aspects are offered here as a systematic listing and then supplemented with a photo of the lateral neck with an incision and ultrasound cine-clips demonstrating lymph nodes confirmed by cytology or histology to be thyroid cancer metastases (Fig. 21.6, Videos 21.1, 21.2, 21.3, 21.4, 21.5, 21.6, 21.7, 21.8, 21.9, 21.10, 21.11, 21.12, 21.13, 21.14, 21.15, 21.16, 21.17, 21.18, 21.19, 21.20, 21.21, 21.22, 21.23, 21.24, 21.25, 21.26, 21.27, 21.28, 21.29, 21.30, and 21.31).

1. The most significant aspect is to ensure that this ultrasound actually gets performed. As simple and basic as this seems, the fact remains that preoperative ultrasound for lymph node mapping is often omitted prior to the initial surgery or that it is assumed that lymph nodes are normal because no mention of abnormal lymph nodes is made in the ultrasound report. It is a joint responsibility of treating physicians to ensure, by communication, that this ultrasound is performed and that the expected information is available before surgery. During the surveillance period postoperatively, since again a number of physicians may share in the care of the patient, communication and attentiveness to accomplishing the ultrasound are of paramount importance.
2. Methodical conduct of lymph node mapping is exceptionally helpful. There is no standard technique or sequence in which this is accomplished or advocated by professional associations. The key is to perform it in the same way each time and in each patient and to include all of the cervical lymph node levels described above. A practical admonition is to inform even the patients to expect a comprehensive evaluation of cervical lymph nodes; if the patients do not feel the ultrasound probe covering their entire neck, then as advocates of their own medical care, they should make that known to their physicians who can request another, properly thorough ultrasound exam. The transducer probe and ultrasound gel should cover the following regions thoroughly (Fig. 21.6): level of the angle of the mandible/mastoid process (superiorly) all the way down to the clavicle (inferiorly), the posterior neck to the trapezius muscle (laterally), and all of the central neck (medially).

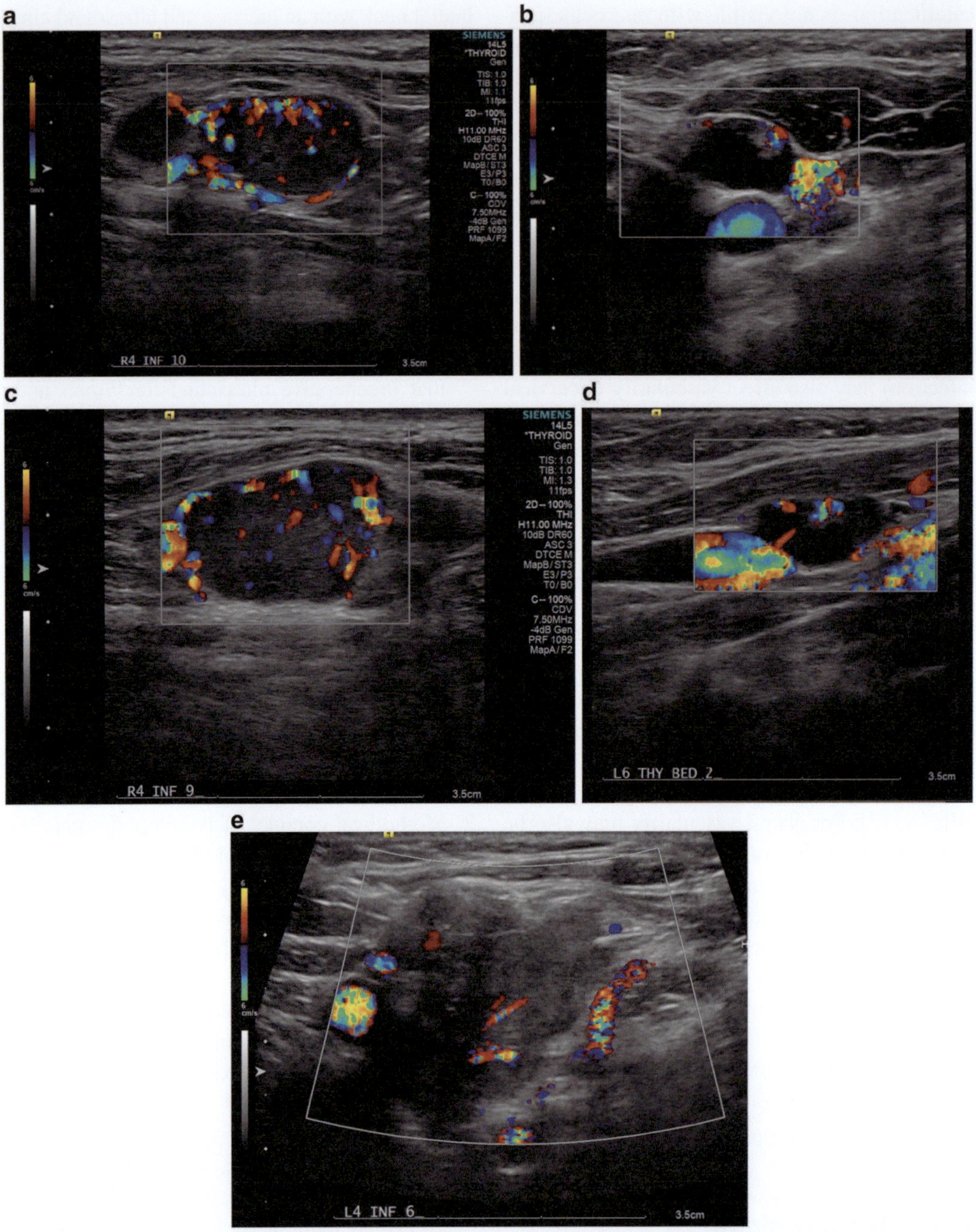

Fig. 21.5 Vascular patterns in malignant lymph nodes. (**a**) Metastatic lymph node with increased peripheral vascularity. (**b**) Peripheral vascularity within the solid component of a metastatic lymph node with cystic degeneration. (**c**) Metastatic lymph node with diffusely increased vascularity, both centrally and peripherally. (**d**) Cystic lymph node with increased vascularity of the solid component. (**e**) Metastatic lymph node with irregular margins, heterogeneous echotexture, and minimal vascularity

One method is to start by examination of the central neck (level 6) because that is where the thyroid is or was located. In transverse orientation, the transducer remains centered on the trachea while acquiring images from the sternal notch up to the thyroid cartilage. The

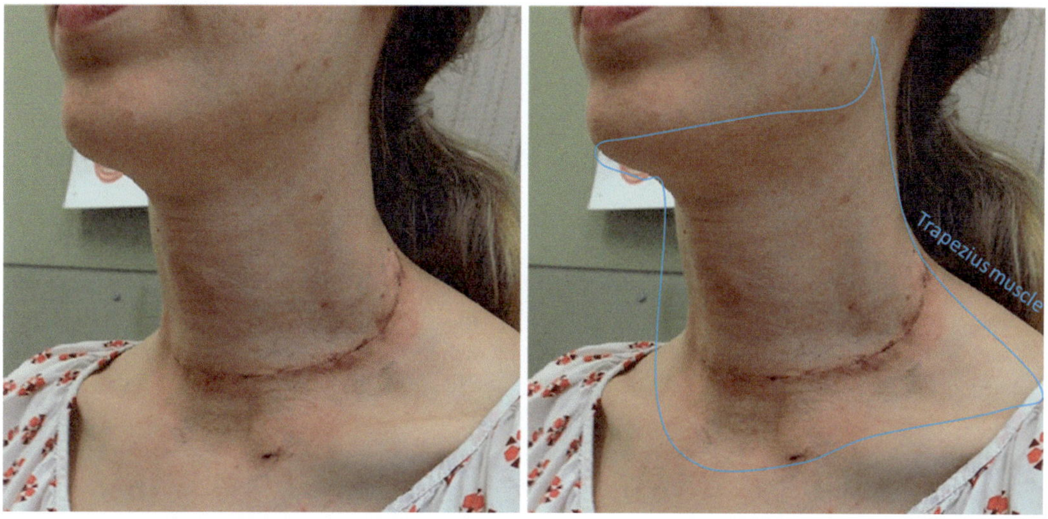

Fig. 21.6 Area of the neck that requires imaging by ultrasound, essentially from the chin and the mandible to the hairline and to the clavicle and all in the central neck. The incision used here was required to access the all regions of the neck for a comprehensive cervical lymph node clearance of metastatic papillary thyroid cancer. Refer also to Videos 21.1, 21.2, 21.3, 21.4, 21.5, 21.6, 21.7, 21.8, 21.9, 21.10, 21.11, 21.12, 21.13, 21.14, 21.15, 21.16, 21.17, 21.18, 21.19, 21.20, 21.21, 21.22, 21.23, 21.24, 21.25, 21.26, 21.27, 21.28, 21.29, and 21.30

paratracheal areas are inspected for presence of abnormal lymph nodes. The transducer can then be positioned over the right and left thyroid bed spaces, and pressure altered, so as to elicit further any abnormalities, particularly those that may be deeply positioned. The space is then examined in longitudinal views. Returning to a transverse transducer probe orientation, the flanking zones are examined: level 7 (superior mediastinum) and level 1 (submental triangle). While lymph node metastases in these zones are not very common, they are also not rare, especially in level 7, where they may represent an extension of inferior level 6 nodes, Thus, the ultrasound probe and gel should cover the area from the chin to the chest, and the probe angles deeply into the mediastinum until even the aortic arch can be seen in some patients. To accomplish this, the patient really has to be in gentle neck hyperextension, supported by a soft pillow below the shoulders, and asked to turn their chin to the side to expose the lateral neck surface. Patients who have cervical spine issues or arthritis or are limited from other discomfort can avoid the extension, but more attentiveness needs to be given to each zone when the ultrasound probe is applied.

Laterally, the neck cannot be examined in just a single motion of the ultrasound probe, but it takes several "painting" motions of the ultrasound probe, held in transverse orientation, to cover the territory of levels 2, 3, 4, and 5. Starting at the clavicle (level 4), the probe can proceed superiorly until it can go no further, limited by the mandible (level 2). The probe can then be moved ever so slightly laterally, still in transverse orientation, to scan back down to the clavicle, and this is repeated again in the superior-inferior axis until the trapezius muscle is reached ("painting"). The sternocleidomastoid muscle (SCM) serves as the "roof" of the lateral neck space for levels 2–4. Therefore, when the SCM is displaced so only a small portion of it is visible on the edge of the ultrasound, the posterior neck (level 5) is in focus. This area is a broad, vague stretch of gray-scale background with few discreet anatomical structures. A notable exception is the brachial plexus at the border with the clavicle (Video 21.30). The goal of imaging in level 5 is to detect round hypoechoic densities that stand out from the usually monotonous gray-scale background.

Remember that the benefit of clinician-performed ultrasound is real-time imaging. Any of the regions can be scrutinized with isolated focus again. The probe can be oriented in any direction to capture a lymph node along its longest axis or to determine how it appears in different views. Symmetry in appearance of structures from the left compared to the right neck supports a benign pattern. For example, lymph nodes adjacent to the submandibular gland can be as large as 2–3 cm but maintain normal architecture and appear the same on the right and left sides of the neck. This symmetry may help avoid their misdiagnosis as thyroid cancer metastases. Furthermore in the lateral neck, the transverse processes of the cervical spine should not be mistaken for calcified masses—these are normal structures and several processes can be visible and tracked in a superior to inferior direction (Video 21.31).

3. Ultrasound of the "empty neck," after a patient has had thyroid surgery and even lymph node dissection surgery, benefits from repetition to gain mastery. The anatomical relationships in the central neck are different as the carotid artery moves closer to the trachea. Videos 21.5, 21.6, and 21.9 provide some examples for consideration.
4. Earlier chapters in this textbook have elaborated on the use of color Doppler settings and the interpretation of patterns of vascularity. In examining lymph nodes, the gain setting of the color Doppler mode can be increased to detect chaotic or disorganized vascularity that may not be apparent at lower gain intensity. However, the best strategy is to remain flexible in adjusting both overall B-mode and color Doppler gain settings as the exam is being performed. This allows the image appearance to be optimized in relationship to the adjacent carotid artery and jugular vein or the high submandibular region (level 2) which can hide lymph nodes unless the sonographer scrutinizes the area carefully. At the angle of the mandible, especially several limitations to ultrasound exist. The probe cannot move beyond the mandibular bone: thus a smaller or small fingerprint/curvilinear probe may be helpful if available. The area is markedly hypoechoic because of density of normal hypoechoic structures (blood vessels, larynx, retropharyngeal space), and these may obscure adjacent or deep lymph nodes, which are also hypoechoic. If these areas are not imaged to the desired degree of satisfaction or confidence, and lymphadenopathy is suspected, a CT scan with IV contrast is exceptionally helpful.
5. The Thyroid Cancer Care Collaborative (TCCC) provides a methodical way to record the findings of cervical lymph node ultrasound (https://www.thyroidccc.org/) and offers guidelines, based on the American Thyroid Association, with points of consideration for optimal management of patients with initial or persistent/recurrent lymph node metastases [23].

21.7 Conclusion

Preoperative and surveillance ultrasound evaluation of the cervical lymph nodes is fundamental in the management of thyroid cancer. Though no specific criterion exists to diagnose metastatic disease, sonographic findings that deviate from benign lymph node morphology help stratify the risk of malignancy and prompt further diagnostic work-up.

References

1. O'Connell K, Yen TW, Quiroz F, Evans DB, Wang TS. The utility of routine preoperative cervical ultrasonography in patients undergoing thyroidectomy for differentiated thyroid cancer. Surgery. 2013;154(4):697–701. discussion 701-3.
2. Kouvaraki MA, Shapiro SE, Fornage BD, Edeiken-Monro BS, Sherman SI, Vassilopoulou-Sellin R, Lee JE, Evans DB. Role of preoperative ultrasonography in the surgical management of patients with thyroid cancer. Surgery. 2003;134:946–54.
3. Howlader N, Noone AM, Krapcho M, Garshell J, Miller D, Altekruse SF, Kosary CL, Yu M, Ruhl J,

Tatalovich Z, Mariotto A, Lewis DR, Chen HS, Feuer EJ, Cronin KA (eds). SEER Cancer Statistics Review, 1975-2012, National Cancer Institute. Bethesda, MD, http://seer.cancer.gov/csr/1975_2012/, based on November 2014 SEER data submission, posted to the SEER web site, April 2015.
4. Chow SM, Law SC, Chan JK, Au SK, Yau S, Lau WH. Papillary microcarcinoma of the thyroid-Prognostic significance of lymph node metastasis and multifocality. Cancer. 2003;98:31–40.
5. Grebe SK, Hay ID. Thyroid cancer nodal metastases: biologic significance and therapeutic considerations. Surg Oncol Clin N Am. 1996;5:43–63.
6. Mazzaferri EL. Management of a solitary thyroid nodule. N Engl J Med. 1993;328:553–9.
7. Soh EY, Clark OH. Surgical considerations and approach to thyroid cancer. Endocrinol Metab Clin North Am. 1996;25:115–39.
8. Quayle FJ, Moley JF. Medullary thyroid carcinoma: management of lymph node metastases. Curr Treat Options Oncol. 2005;6(4):347–54.
9. Kebebew E, Greenspan FS, Clark OH, Woeber KA, McMillan A. Anaplastic thyroid carcinoma. Treatment outcome and prognostic factors. Cancer. 2005;103(7):1330–5.
10. Haugen BR, Alexander EK, Bible KC, Doherty GM, Mandel SJ, Nikiforov YE, Pacini F, Randolph GW, Sawka AM, Schlumberger M, Schuff KG, Sherman SI, Sosa JA, Steward DL, Tuttle RM, Wartofsky L. 2015 American Thyroid Association Management Guidelines for adult patients with thyroid nodules and differentiated thyroid cancer: the American Thyroid Association Guidelines Task Force on thyroid nodules and differentiated thyroid cancer. Thyroid. 2016;26(1):1–133.
11. Wu LM, Gu HY, Qu XH, et al. The accuracy of ultrasonography in the preoperative diagnosis of cervical lymph node metastasis in patients with papillary thyroid carcinoma: a meta-analysis. Eur J Radiol. 2012;81:1798–805.
12. Robbins KT, Shaha AR, Medina JE, Califano JA, Wolf GT, Ferlito A, Som PM, Day TA, Committee for Neck Dissection Classification, American Head and Neck Society. Consensus statement on the classification and terminology of neck dissection. Arch Otolaryngol Head Neck Surg. 2008;134(5):536–8.
13. Ahuja AT, Chow L, Chick W, King W, Metreweli C. Metastatic cervical nodes in papillary carcinoma of the thyroid: ultrasound and histological correlation. Clin Radiol. 1995;50:229–31.
14. Leboulleux S, Girard E, Rose M, Travagli JP, Sabbah N, Caillou B, Hartl DM, Lassau N, Baudin E, Schlumberger M. Ultrasound criteria of malignancy for cervical lymph nodes in patients followed up for differentiated thyroid cancer. J Clin Endocrinol Metab. 2007;92:3590–4.
15. Kuna SK, Bracic I, Tesic V, Kuna K, Herceg GH, Dodig D. Ultrasonographic differentiation of benign from malignant neck lymphadenopathy in thyroid cancer. J Ultrasound Med. 2006;25:1531–7.
16. Roh JL, Park JY, Kim JM, Song CJ. Use of preoperative ultrasonography as guidance for neck dissection in patients with papillary thyroid carcinoma. J Surg Oncol. 2009;99(1):28–31.
17. Rosário PW, de Faria S, Bicalho L, Alves MF, Borges MA, Purisch S, Padrão EL, Rezende LL, Barroso AL. Ultrasonographic differentiation between metastatic and benign lymph nodes in patients with papillary thyroid carcinoma. J Ultrasound Med. 2005;24:1385–9.
18. Patel NU, McKinney K, Kreidler SM, Bieker TM, Russ P, Roberts K, Glueck DH, Albuja-Cruz M, Klopper J, Haugen BR. Ultrasound-based clinical prediction rule model for detecting papillary thyroid cancer in cervical lymph nodes: a pilot study. J Clin Ultrasound. 2016;44:143.
19. Sohn YM, Kwak JY, Kim EK, Moon HJ, Kim SJ, Kim MJ. Diagnostic approach for evaluation of lymph node metastasis from thyroid cancer using ultrasound and fine- needle aspiration biopsy. AJR Am J Roentgenol. 2010;194:38.
20. Kessler A, Rappaport Y, Blank A, Marmor S, Weiss J, Graif M. Cystic appearance of cervical lymph nodes is characteristic of metastatic papillary thyroid carcinoma. J Clin Ultrasound. 2003;31(1):21–5.
21. Landry CS, Grubbs EG, Busaidy NL, Monroe BJ, Staerkel GA, Perrier ND, Edeiken-Monroe BS. Cystic lymph nodes in the lateral neck as indicators of metastatic papillary thyroid cancer. Endocr Pract. 2011;17(2):240–4.
22. Gorman B, Charboneau JW, James EM, Reading CC, Wold LE, Grant CS, Gharib H, Hay ID. Medullary thyroid carcinoma: role of high resolution US. Radiology. 1987;162:147–50.
23. Urken ML, Milas M, Randolph GW, Tufano R, Bergman D, Bernet V, Brett EM, Brierley JD, Cobin R, Doherty G, Klopper J, Lee S, Machac J, Mechanick JI, Orloff LA, Ross D, Smallridge RC, Terris DJ, Clain JB, Tuttle M. Management of recurrent and persistent metastatic lymph nodes in well-differentiated thyroid cancer: a multifactorial decision-making guide for the Thyroid Cancer Care Collaborative. Head Neck. 2015;37(4):605–14.

22 Ultrasound Characteristics and Ultrasound-Guided Fine-Needle Aspiration of Lymph Nodes in the Cervical Soft Tissues: A Radiology Perspective

Maria K. Gule-Monroe, Michael Kwon, Komal B. Shah, Jason Michael Johnson, Thinh Vu, and Beth S. Edeiken-Monroe

22.1 Introduction

Characterization of a lymph node as benign or malignant in the soft tissues of the neck in patients with head and neck cancers can be challenging even for the most experienced radiologist. In the past decade, ultrasound (US) and US-guided fine-needle aspiration (FNA) have become the methods of choice for early and preoperative diagnosis of cervical adenopathy [1]. In this chapter, we discuss the technique of US imaging of cervical lymph nodes, radiographic findings that portend early and also well-established metastatic lateral cervical adenopathy, assessment for HPV, and the preoperative documentation of metastatic adenopathy by US-guided FNA.

22.2 Technique: Routine US Evaluation of Cervical Lymph Nodes

Routine sonographic evaluation of the soft tissues of the neck includes imaging in the anterior and posterior jugular territories from the supraclavicular regions to the superior neck and the submandibular and submental regions. The parotid glands are included in patients with lymphoma, melanoma, and where there is concern for a parotid tumor on alternate imaging modalities. Retropharyngeal lymph nodes, well seen on CT, cannot be assessed by routine ultrasound. Sonographic evaluation of retropharyngeal lymph nodes requires the transoral approach. Centrally, lymph nodes are evaluated in the pre-

M.K. Gule-Monroe, M.D. • M. Kwon, M.D., Ph.D.
K.B. Shah, M.D. • J.M. Johnson, M.D. • T. Vu, M.D.
The Department of Diagnostic Radiology,
The University of Texas MD Anderson Cancer Center,
1515 Holcombe Blvd., Unit 1482, Houston,
TX 77030, USA
e-mail: mgule@mdanderson.org; michael.kwon@mdandersong.org; komal.Shah@mdanderson.org; jjohnson12@mdanderson.org; thinh.Vu@mdanderson.org

B.S. Edeiken-Monroe, M.D., F.A.C.R. (✉)
The Department of Diagnostic Imaging,
The University of Texas MD Anderson Cancer Center,
1515 Holcombe, Unit 1350, Houston, TX 77030, USA
e-mail: bedeiken@mdanderson.org

M. Milas et al. (eds.), *Advanced Thyroid and Parathyroid Ultrasound*,
DOI 10.1007/978-3-319-44100-9_22

tracheal, pre-laryngeal, and suprasternal regions. The thyroid obscures paratracheal lymph nodes along with other lymph nodes posterior to the thyroid gland.

The metastatic spread of head and neck cancers is usually to the ipsilateral cervical lymph nodes; however, contralateral metastasis may occur. Thus, at The MD Anderson Cancer Center (MDACC) in Houston, Texas, US of the soft tissues of the neck always includes evaluation of the lymph nodes in the bilateral jugular territories. In this manner, US detection of metastic adenopathy has altered the staging and treatment of head and neck cancers allowing complete treatment/resection of disease and minimizing local-regional recurrence.

22.2.1 Case 1: Sonographic Evaluation of Benign Cervical Lymph Nodes in the Lower and Mid-Jugular Territories

Lymph nodes are evaluated in both the longitudinal and transverse planes. Benign cervical lymph nodes in the lower and mid-jugular territories have an almond or oval shape with a central echogenic hilum, hypoechoic cortex, and organized vascular flow.

Clinical Scenario: PET/CT suggested an FDG avid left jugular territory lymph node in a 46-year-old male with a biopsy proven Hurthle cell carcinoma in the left lobe of the thyroid. Ultrasound was requested to evaluate the FDG avid left jugular territory lymph node.

Imaging Features: Ultrasound. Benign appearing oval lymph node in the longitudinal (Fig. 22.1a) and transverse (Fig. 22.1b) planes with a central echogenic hilum. The central hilum is composed of the lymphatics, artery, and vein. The normal course of the vein within the central hilum is demonstrated as linear in the transverse (Fig. 22.1c, d) and longitudinal (Fig. 22.1e) planes.

Diagnosis: **Benign appearing 0.7-cm oval lymph node in the soft tissues of the left mid-jugular territory. No biopsy was performed due to the benign appearance of the node in both the longitudinal and transverse planes. In this patient, the echogenic central hilum is normal.**

22.2.2 Case 2: The Importance of Assessing for Symmetry of Cervical Lymph Nodes in the Superior Jugular Territories to Assess for Benign or Metastatic Involvement

Interestingly, the benign lymph nodes in the superior jugular territories vary in appearance compared to the benign lymph nodes in the mid- and lower jugular territories. Left and right lymph nodes in the superior jugular territories should be compared on side-by-side images to assess symmetry. Asymmetry suggests metastatic involvement.

Clinical Scenario: A 51-year-old female with a 3-year history of bilateral papillary thyroid cancer who presents with a palpable right superior neck lymph node which by patient history has been enlarging. US was requested to assess the palpable lymph node.

Imaging Features: Ultrasound. On initial US evaluation, the 1.3-cm right superior neck lymph node (Fig. 22.2a) was thought to potentially be metastatic with loss of central hilum. There was no vascular flow or calcification. US-guided biopsy was considered.

Comparison with the contralateral 1.4-cm left superior neck node (Fig. 22.2b) revealed a symmetrical appearance suggesting that the lymph nodes were either both benign or bilateral metastatic adenopathy.

US-guided FNA was considered based on concern for absent hilum and prominent rounded lymph nodes which may have been caused by bilateral metastasis.

Diagnosis: **US-guided biopsy was performed on the right and left superior neck lymph nodes. The FNAs revealed benign nodes with no malignant cells. In this case, the symmetry of the superior neck nodes was within normal limits.**

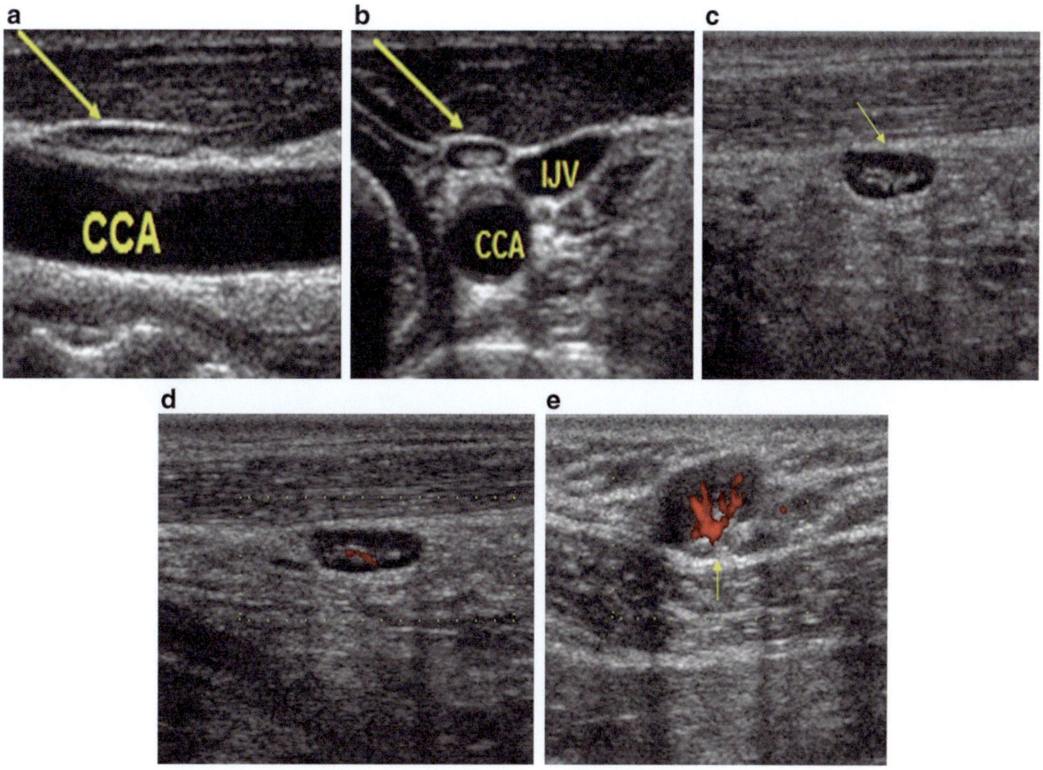

Fig. 22.1 (**a**) Gray-scale US. Benign appearing oval 1-cm lymph node, in the longitudinal plane, with a normal central echogenic hilum (*arrow*). (**b**) Gray-scale US. Benign appearing oval 1-cm lymph node, in the transverse plane, with normal echogenic hilum (*arrow*). (**c**) Gray-scale US. Benign 0.8-cm lymph node in the longitudinal plane demonstrating the linear hypoechoic course of the vessels through the central echogenic hilum. (**d**) Power Doppler. US demonstration of the linear course of the vein within the central hilum of a 0.8-cm benign lymph node imaged in the longitudinal plane. (**e**) Power Doppler US demonstration of the organized course of the vein within the central hilum of a 0.8-cm lymph node imaged in the transverse plane

22.2.3 Case 3: The Importance of Assessing for Symmetry of Cervical Lymph Nodes in the Superior Jugular Territories to Assess for Metastatic Involvement

Ultrasound imaging of the soft tissues of the neck should include a two-on-one image of the right and left superior neck lymph nodes for comparison. Symmetry may assist in defining the benign appearance of the superior neck nodes in a specific patient.

Clinical Scenario: A 47-year-old male with right thyroid follicular variant of papillary cancer and palpable lymph nodes in the right and left superior neck. US was requested to assess the palpable superior neck lymph nodes.

Imaging Features: Right superior neck palpable 1.4-cm lymph node (Fig. 22.3a) created concern for an enlarged metastatic lymph node until comparison of 1.5-cm palpable left superior neck lymph node (Fig. 22.3b). The asymmetry suggests that the left superior neck lymph node is the metastatic node.

Diagnosis: **US-guided FNA of the right and left superior neck lymph nodes revealed that the 1.4-cm right superior neck palpable lymph node was benign and the left 1.5-cm palpable lymph node was metastatic papillary carcinoma.**

We have found that traditional criteria of size greater than 0.5 cm, shape of taller than wide,

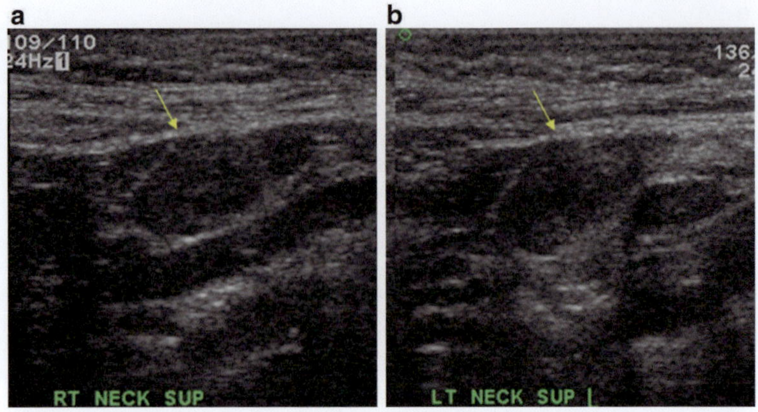

Fig. 22.2 (**a**) Gray-scale US. 1.3-cm right superior neck lymph node, imaged in the longitudinal plane, with absent central hilum initially of concern for a metastatic lymph node (*arrow*). (**b**) Gray-scale US. Contralateral 1.4-cm left superior neck lymph node, imaged in the longitudinal plane, with a symmetrical appearance suggesting benign symmetrical lymph nodes in the superior jugular territories (*arrow*)

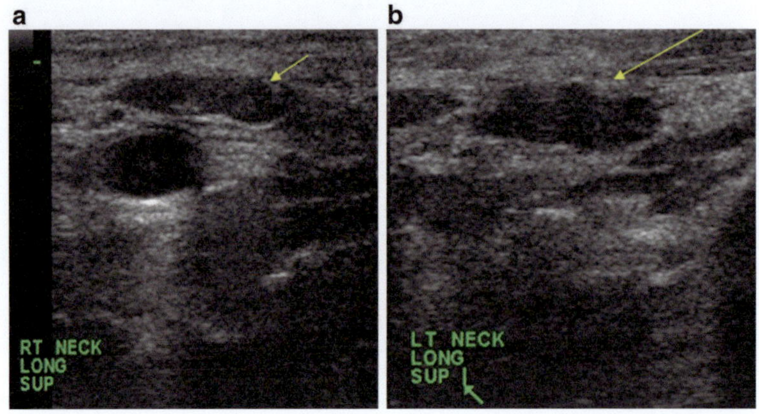

Fig. 22.3 (**a**) Gray-scale US. Palpable right superior neck 1.4-cm lymph node was of concern for an enlarged metastatic lymph node (*arrow*). (**b**) Gray-scale US. Comparison of contralateral 1.5-cm palpable asymmetric left superior neck lymph node with asymmetry suggesting a metastatic lymph node (*arrow*)

and irregular borders are not powerful indicators of malignancy. Although no single sonographic feature is pathognomonic for a metastatic lymph node, certain features should raise suspicion of a malignant lymph node. The combination of several features may be even more suggestive of metastatic adenopathy. These features include a full or rounded shape, disrupted or displaced hilum, disorganized vascularity, calcifications, cystic change, bulging of a component of the lymph node, and the presence of intranodal punctate regions of increased echogenicity. Of importance is that ultrasound characteristics are sensitive but not disease specific for a metastatic lymph node. Thus, US-guided FNA should be performed on lymph nodes of concern to establish the diagnosis.

22.2.4 Clinical Case 4: Distorted Hilum in a Metastatic Lymph Node

Metastatic involvement of a lymph node may present as distortion of the normal echogenic central hilum.

Clinical Scenario: A 46-year-old female with 0.9-cm right papillary thyroid carcinoma and 1.1-cm right mid-neck node.

Imaging Features: Abnormal right mid-neck lymph node with displaced hilum in the longitudinal (Fig. 22.4a) and transverse (Fig. 22.4b) planes.

Diagnosis: **US-guided FNA (Fig. 22.4c) revealed metastatic PTC**.

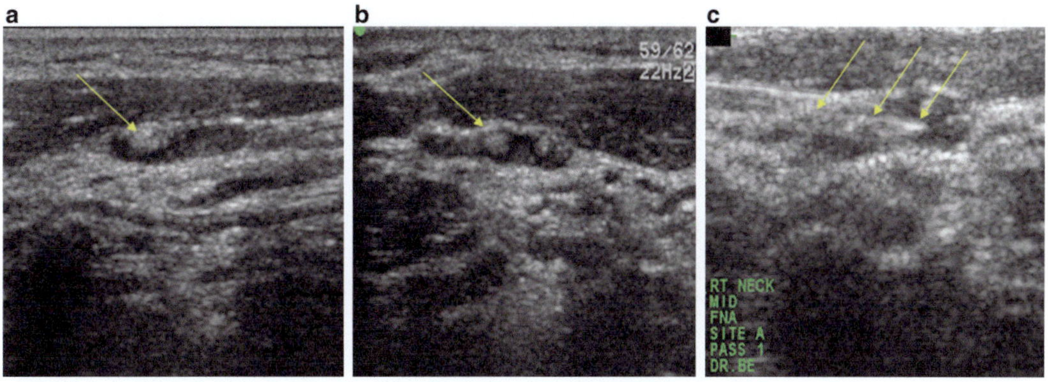

Fig. 22.4 (**a**) Gray-scale US. Abnormal-appearing 1.1-cm right mid-neck lymph node, in the longitudinal plane, with a displaced hilum causing concern for metastasis (*arrow*). (**b**) Gray-scale US. Abnormal-appearing 1.1-cm right mid-neck lymph node, in the transverse plane, with a displaced hilum causing concern for metastasis (*arrow*). (**c**) Gray-scale US. US-guided FNA of the right mid-neck lymph node with the biopsy needle tip within the lymph node (*arrows*)

22.2.5 Case 5: Absent Hilum in a Metastatic Lymph Node

The hilum may be absent in a metastatic lymph node due to infiltration of metastasis.

Clinical Scenario: A 72-year-old male with a 3-year history of 0.6-cm right PTC and a new palpable left mid-neck lymph node. Ultrasound was requested to assess the jugular territory lymph nodes.

Imaging Features: Abnormal 0.5-cm left inferior neck lymph node (Fig. 22.5a) and 1.2-cm palpable left mid-neck lymph node (Fig. 22.5b) in the transverse planes with hilum absent in both lymph nodes.

Diagnosis: **US-guided FNA revealed anaplastic transformation of PTC in the left and right jugular territories**.

22.2.6 Case 6: Disorganized Vascular Flow in a Metastatic Lymph Node

Vascular flow normally transverses the central echogenic hilum in a linear configuration. Metastatic infiltration of a lymph node may cause disorganization of the vascular flow.

Clinical Scenario: A 40-year-old female a with 2-year history of 2.5-cm right PTC and currently with a palpable right inferior jugular territory lymph node.

Imaging Features: Abnormal 0.8-cm right inferior neck lymph node, in the longitudinal plane, with disorganized vascular flow (Fig. 22.6a) and a 2.5-cm right superior jugular territory lymph node in the longitudinal plane with normal central hilar vascular flow for comparison (Fig. 22.6b).

Diagnosis: **US-guided FNA revealed papillary thyroid cancer**.

22.2.7 Case 7: Calcification in Metastatic Lymph Nodes

Metastatic infiltration of the lymph node may cause calcification which may present with varied appearances that include punctate regions of increased echogenicity to coarse calcifications.

Clinical Scenarios: The following are five patients with metastatic lymph nodes of concern for metastasis based on the presence of calcifications. US-guided FNA documented metastatic adenopathy in each patient.

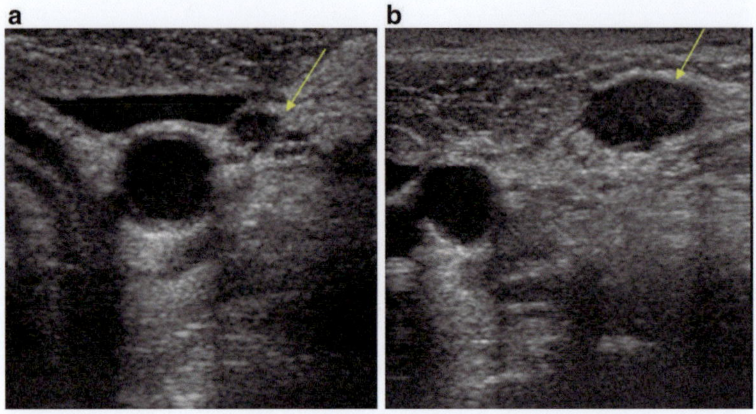

Fig. 22.5 (**a**) Gray-scale US. Abnormal 0.5-cm left inferior neck lymph node, in the transverse plane, with absent hilum causing concern for a metastatic lymph node (*arrow*). (**b**) Gray-scale US. Abnormal 1.2-cm left inferior neck lymph node, in the transverse plane, with absent hilum causing concern for a metastatic lymph node (*arrow*)

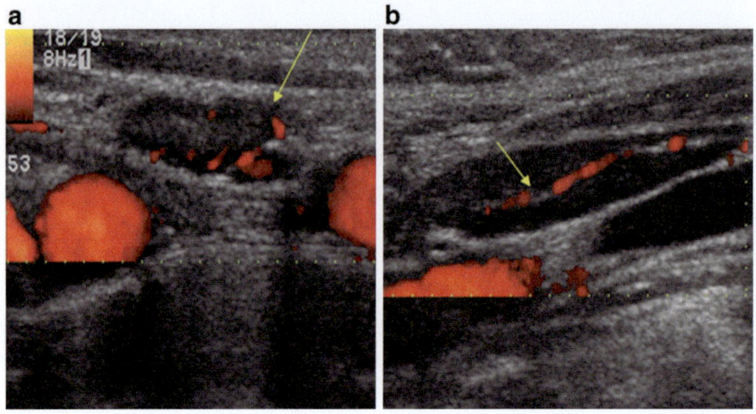

Fig. 22.6 (**a**) Power Doppler US. Abnormal 0.8-cm right inferior neck lymph node, in the longitudinal plane, with disorganized vascular flow causing concern for metastatic adenopathy. (**b**) Power Doppler US. Comparison of superior jugular territory lymph node in the longitudinal plane with normal central hilar vascular flow

Imaging Features: Abnormal jugular territory lymph nodes with calcifications.

Diagnosis: **US-guided FNA documented papillary ca in a 1-cm node in the right mid-jugular territory in the longitudinal plane with shadowing punctate calcification (Fig. 22.7a) and disorganized vascular flow on power Doppler (Fig. 22.7b).**

Diagnosis: **US-guided FNA documented papillary ca in a 0.8-cm node in the right inferior jugular territory in the transverse (Fig. 22.7c) and longitudinal (Fig. 22.7d) planes with a single shadowing punctate calcification.**

Diagnosis: **US-guided FNA documented papillary ca in a 0.6-cm node in the right mid-jugular territory in the longitudinal plane (Fig 22.7e) with a multiple punctate calcifications with no shadowing or abnormal vascular flow on power Doppler.**

Diagnosis: **(Fig 22.7f) US-guided FNA documented medullary cancer in a 1-cm node in the right inferior jugular territory in the longitudinal plane with coarse calcifications with shadowing.**

Diagnosis: **Patient with papillary cancer and suspected metastatic adenopathy with punctate calcification in a 1.4-cm lymph node in the right supraclavicular jugular territory in the transverse (Fig 22.7g) plane. US-guided FNA and core biopsy documented unsuspected and previously undiagnosed Hodgkin's disease. This case once again demonstrates that ultrasound is an imaging modality that is sensitive but not specific.**

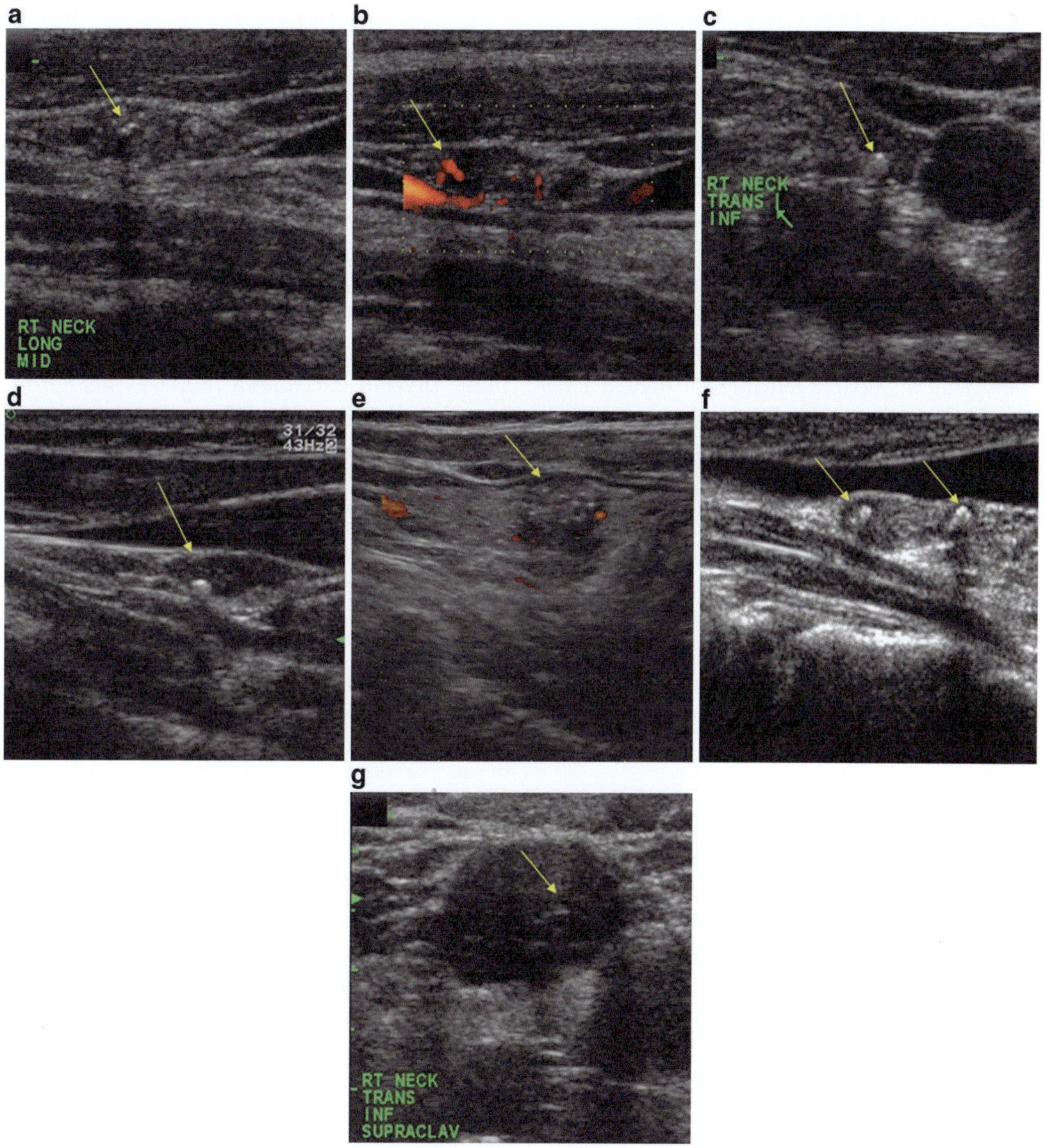

Fig. 22.7 (**a**) Gray-scale US. Abnormal 1-cm lymph node in the right mid-jugular territory, in the longitudinal plane, with shadowing punctate calcification raising the concern for metastatic adenopathy. (**b**) Power Doppler US. Abnormal 1-cm lymph node in the right mid-jugular territory, in the longitudinal plane, with disorganized vascular flow raising the concern for metastatic adenopathy. (**c**) Gray-scale US. 0.8-cm jugular territory lymph node, in the transverse plane, with a single shadowing punctate calcification causing concern for metastatic adenopathy (*arrow*). (**d**) Gray-scale US. 0.8-cm jugular territory lymph node, in the longitudinal plane, with a single shadowing punctate calcification causing concern for metastatic adenopathy (*arrow*). (**e**) Power Doppler US. A 0.6-cm lymph node in the right mid-jugular territory, in the longitudinal plane, with multiple punctate calcifications raising the concern for metastatic adenopathy even in the absence of shadowing or abnormal vascular flow (*arrow*). (**f**) Gray-scale US. A 1-cm lymph node with coarse shadowing calcifications, in the longitudinal plane, in the right inferior jugular territory documented by US-guided FNA as medullary cancer (*arrow*). (**g**) Gray-scale US. A 1.4-cm right supraclavicular lymph node, in the transverse plane, with punctate calcifications documented by US-guided FNA and core biopsy as unsuspected and previously undiagnosed Hodgkin's disease in a patient with simultaneous papillary cancer (*arrow*)

22.2.8 Case 8: Metastatic Lymph Nodes with Cystic Change

Metastatic infiltration of lymph nodes in thyroid cancer may cause complete or partial cystic change. In these lymph nodes, it may be difficult to document metastasis emphasizing the importance of sending the aspirate for a thyroglobulin count in addition to cytological evaluation.

Clinical Scenario: A 40-year-old female with a 2-year history of 2.5-cm right PTC and currently with a palpable left inferior jugular territory lymph node evaluated by ultrasound.

Imaging Features: Abnormal 1.3-cm left inferior neck lymph node, in the longitudinal (Fig. 22.8a) and transverse (Fig. 22.8b) planes with a solid and cystic component and a small calcification. On power Doppler, abnormal vascular flow was demonstrated in the solid component of the abnormal lymph nodes (Fig. 22.8c).

Diagnosis: **US-guided FNA revealed papillary thyroid cancer with an elevated thyroglobulin (Tg)**.

NOTE: **On cytology, FNA of nodes with cystic change may initially appear cytologically as nondiagnostic because the cellularity may wash off of the slides. The Tg may be necessary to confirm metastasis** [2].

22.2.9 Case 9: Diagnosis of Early Metastatic Lymph Node Involvement

Diagnosis of early metastatic infiltration of lymph nodes is critical for preoperative planning. One ultrasound finding that raises the concern for metastatic adenopathy is the presence of one or several punctate regions of increased echogenicity. These may occur with no associated shadowing or vascular disorganization. They may also be seen in benign lymph nodes.

Clinical Scenario: A 40-year-old female with a newly diagnosed papillary thyroid carcinoma in the right thyroid and isthmus and to a lesser extent the left thyroid. Ultrasound was requested to assess for adenopathy.

Imaging Features: CT was negative for left jugular territory adenopathy. There were no PET FDG avid nodes in the left jugular territory. On ultrasound, there is a 1.3-cm lymph node in the left mid-jugular territory with a single punctate region of increased echogenicity with no shadowing and no abnormal vascular flow (Fig. 22.9a).

Diagnosis: **US-guided FNA revealed papillary thyroid cancer in the left mid-jugular territory and for comparison is a lymph node that also was of concern in a patient with papillary thyroid carcinoma that was benign on US-guided FNA (Fig. 22.9b)**. **The punctate regions of echogenicity in the lymph nodes raise concern for metastatic infiltration but are also seen occasionally in benign lymph nodes. US-guided FNA is required to document the status of the lymph node**.

22.2.10 Case 10: Diagnosis of Early Metastatic Lymph Node Involvement

An additional ultrasound finding that raises the concern for early metastatic adenopathy is bulging of a portion of the lymph node even in the absence of other findings that may be of concern for metastasis.

Clinical Scenario: A 43-year-old male with a diagnosed Hurthle cell carcinoma of the right thyroid 8 years previous with ultrasound performed for routine follow-up.

Imaging Features: Abnormal 1.7 × 0.7 × 0.3-cm lymph node in the longitudinal plane in the right mid-jugular territory with a bulge in the medial portion (Fig 22.10).

Diagnosis: **US-guided FNA of the right mid-jugular territory lymph node revealed Hurthle cell carcinoma**.

22.2.11 Case 11: Do Not Touch Me Cervical Soft Tissue Nodules and Lymph Nodes

Nodules within the soft tissues of the neck may include lesions other than lymph nodes. These

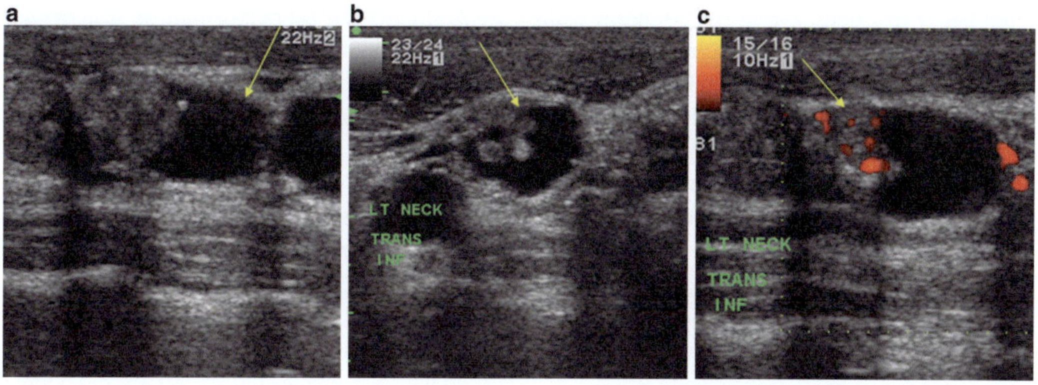

Fig. 22.8 (**a**) Gray-scale US. A 1.3-cm left inferior jugular territory lymph node, in the longitudinal plane, with complex solid and cystic components and a small calcification causing concern for a metastatic adenopathy. (**b**) Gray-scale US. A 1.3-cm left inferior jugular territory lymph node, in the transverse plane, with complex solid and cystic components and a small calcification causing concern for metastatic adenopathy. (**c**) Power Doppler US. Abnormal disorganized vascular flow in the solid component of the 1.3-cm left inferior jugular territory lymph node raising concern for metastatic adenopathy

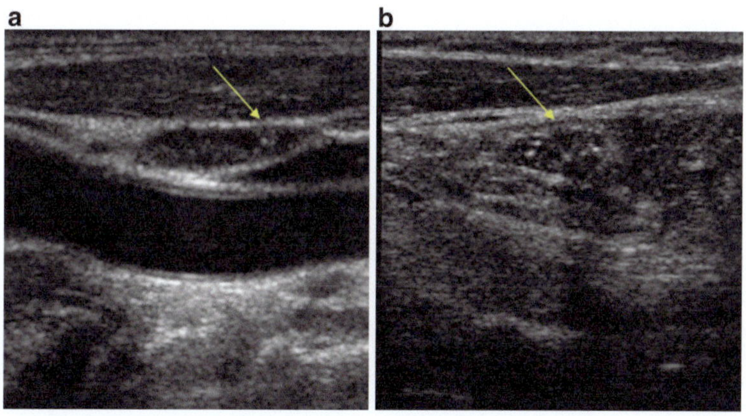

Fig. 22.9 (**a**) Gray-scale US. A 1.3-cm lymph node in the left mid-jugular territory with a punctate region of increased echogenicity causing concern for metastatic adenopathy even in the absence of shadowing and abnormal vascular flow (*arrow*). (**b**) Doppler US. Comparison of lymph nodes. Lymph node in the left mid-jugular territory, in the longitudinal plane, with multiple punctate regions of increased echogenicity causing concern for metastatic adenopathy. US-guided FNA of a different node in the left inferior neck had revealed a benign lymph node (*arrow*)

should be considered in the decision-making process to perform a US-guided fine-needle aspiration.

Clinical Scenario: A 13-year-old male was diagnosed with right medullary thyroid carcinoma 3 years ago. On initial diagnosis, there was metastasis to the right jugular territory extending from the inferior soft tissues of the neck to the superior jugular territory. The patient underwent total thyroidectomy and right neck dissection at that time. The patient now presents with a palpable mass in the right mid-jugular territory.

Imaging Features: In the lateral compartment of the right mid neck, there is a new heterogeneous (Fig. 22.11a) vascular nodule (Fig. 22.11b) measuring 2.2×0.6×0.4 cm. The remaining lymph nodes along the jugular territories in the lateral compartment of the neck are unremarkable.

Diagnosis: **The palpable lesion was exquisitely tender on palpation and with pressure**

from the transducer. When the 20-gauge aspiration needle entered the lesion (Fig. 22.11c), the patient experiences a feeling of electric shock transverse from the mid-jugular territory to the submandibular region with pain characteristic of a neuroma. Even with vigorous aspiration, no sample could be obtained. FNA should not be performed on a neuroma which can be diagnosed by characteristic pain but is difficult to distinguish by US imaging from a lymph node.

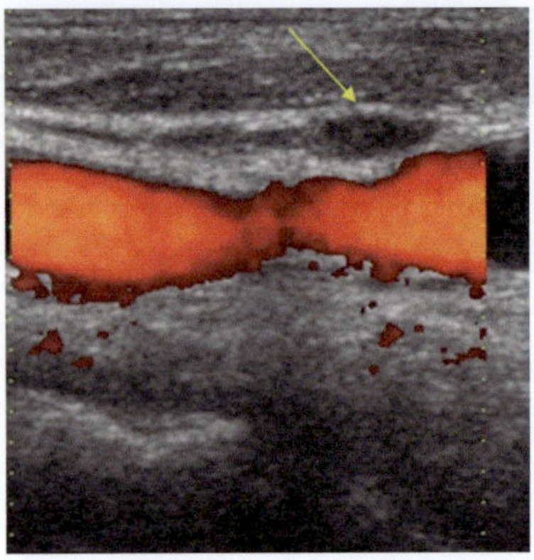

Fig. 22.10 Power Doppler US. Abnormal 1.7 × 0.7 × 0.3-cm lymph node, in the longitudinal plane, in the right mid-jugular territory with a bulge in the medial portion creating concern for metastasis (*arrow*)

22.2.12 Case 12: Do Not Touch Me Cervical Soft Tissue Nodules and Lymph Nodes

Clinical Scenario: A 56-year-old female diagnosed with a palpable solitary left thyroid nodule suspicious for papillary thyroid carcinoma. Ultrasound was performed to assess for metastatic adenopathy.

Imaging Features: Ultrasound. In addition to the solitary thyroid nodule, there is a 1.3-cm nodule superior jugular territory in the bifurcation of the carotid artery and jugular vein (Fig. 22.12a) demonstrated on vascular ultrasound (Fig. 22.12b).

CT: Findings. There is an avidly enhancing mass in the left carotid space located at the carotid bifurcation extending superiorly. It splays the left internal and external carotid arteries and

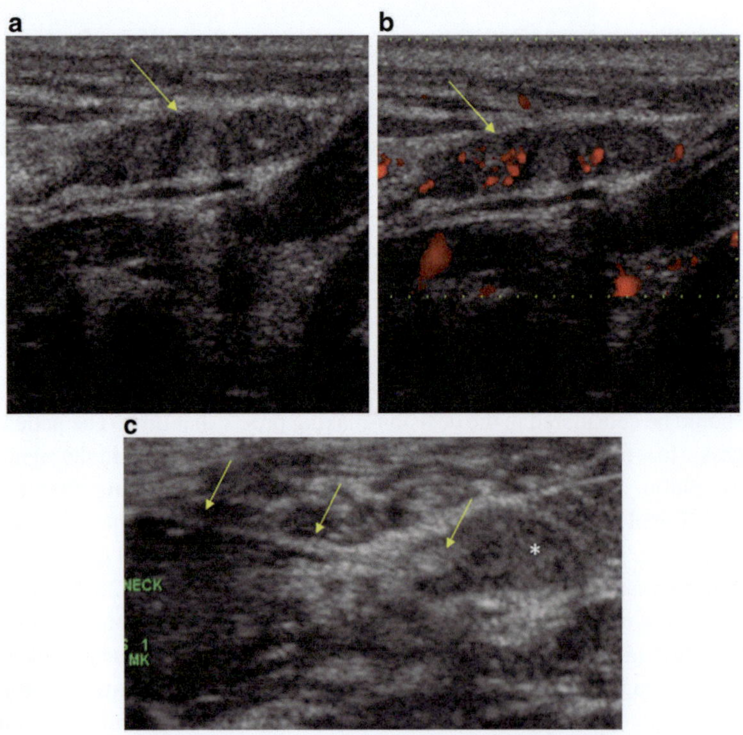

Fig. 22.11 (**a**) Gray-scale US. A 2.2 × 0.6 × 0.4-cm new heterogeneous palpable nodule/node in the right mid-jugular territory exquisitely tender on palpation and of concern for a metastatic lymph node. (**b**) Power Doppler US. Right mid-jugular territory suspected lymph node with disorganized vascular flow raising concern for metastatic adenopathy. (**c**) Gray-scale US. US-guided FNA with needle tip (*arrows*) within the suspected lymph node (*) just prior to aborting the biopsy due to exquisite pain feeling like an electric shock radiating to the submandibular region

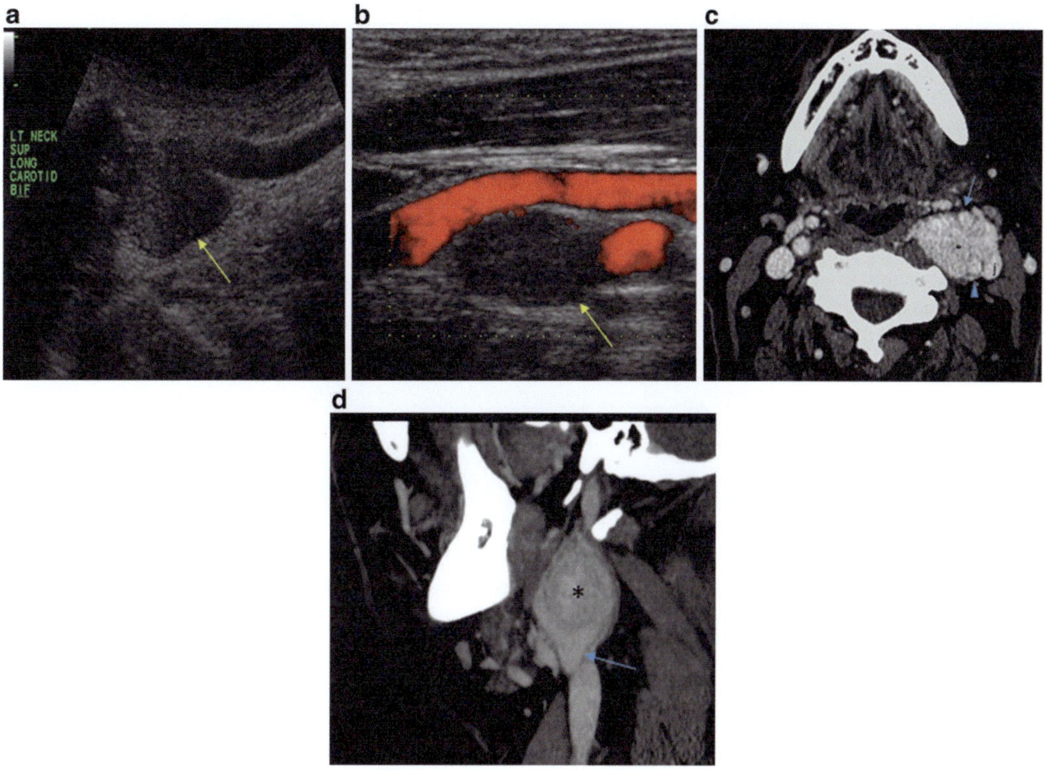

Fig. 22.12 (**a**) Gray-scale US. A 1.3-cm carotid body tumor in the superior jugular territory located in the bifurcation of the carotid artery and jugular vein imaged in the longitudinal plane. (**b**) Location of the carotid body tumor in the bifurcation of the carotid artery and jugular vein demonstrated on power Doppler ultrasound imaged in the longitudinal plane. (**c**) Axial contrast-enhanced CT shows the avidly enhancing carotid body tumor (*) partially splaying the internal carotid artery (*arrowhead*) and external carotid artery (*arrow*). Mass effect is seen on the left internal jugular vein (j). (**d**) Sagittal reconstruction of contrast-enhanced CT demonstrating the avidly enhancing carotid body tumor in the left carotid space located at the carotid bifurcation (*arrow*)

enhances similarly to that of the arteries. It extends medially abutting the left pharyngeal wall and extends laterally distorting the left internal jugular vein.

Diagnosis: **No US-guided FNA should be performed on this carotid body tumor. Diagnosis of a carotid body tumor may be suggested by its precarious location alone. Furthermore, correlation to other available clinical information such as hypertension, history of paragangliomas, and appearance of the mass on other imaging modalities such as CT can help determine that FNA would be inadvisable.**

Clinical Scenario 13: A 63-year-old female with ultrasound performed to assess for adenopathy after detection of a papillary carcinoma in the isthmus.

Imaging Features: Ultrasound. There are mildly vascular nodules at the bilateral carotid bifurcations, in the superior soft tissues of the neck, presumably representing carotid body paragangliomas (Fig. 22.13a), demonstrated on vascular ultrasound (Fig. 22.13b).

Diagnosis: **No US-guided FNA was performed on the bilateral carotid body paragangliomas at the bifurcation of the left jugular vein and carotid artery due to their vascular composition and characteristic imaging appearance.**

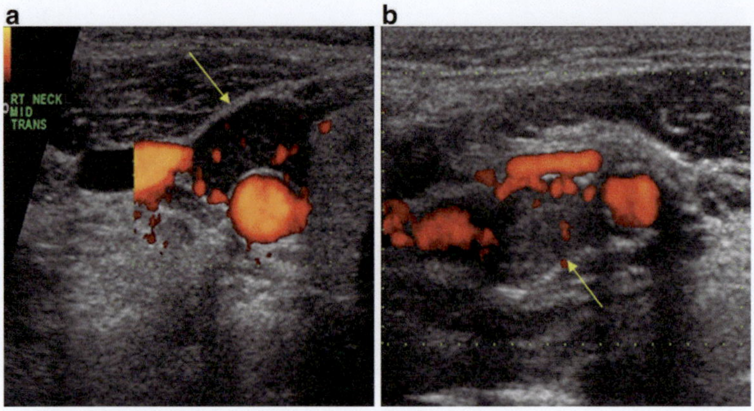

Fig. 22.13 (**a**) Power Doppler US. Mildly vascular 1.2-cm right carotid body paraganglioma at the carotid bifurcation in the superior soft tissues of the right neck imaged in the transverse plane. (**b**) Power Doppler US. Mildly vascular 1.4-cm left carotid body paraganglioma at the carotid bifurcation in the superior soft tissues of the left neck imaged in the transverse plane

22.3 Ultrasound-Guided FNA of Lymph Nodes

While some lymph nodes have an appearance highly suggestive of metastatic lymph nodes, the ultrasound appearance of abnormal nodes is not specific. In the absence of definitive sonographic features of malignant lymph nodes based on the US images, US-guided FNA has now become the cornerstone to confirm the benign or malignance nature of a lymph node [3].

At MDACC, US-guided FNA is performed with the free-hand technique following preparation of the skin with rubbing alcohol. Approximately 2 cc of Xylocaine is injected through a 25-gauge needle along the planned scan plane to the edge of the targeted lymph node. A 20-gauge needle attached to a 20-cc syringe is then inserted under ultrasound guidance, parallel to the transducer and obliquely along the scan plane. The tip of the needle is directed toward, and sonographically confirmed within, the targeted nodule and aspiration is performed.

The high success rate of US-guided FNA at MDACC is related in part to the needle size (20 gauge), constant visualization of the needle tip within the targeted lymph node, and vigorous aspiration. The 20-gauge 1.5-in. hypodermic needle is stiffer than the commonly employed 25-gauge or 27-gauge needles. This stiffer needle allows accurate guidance into calcified, deep, fibrotic, small, or mobile lymph nodes. The 20-gauge needle also facilitates placement of the needle tip and aspiration within the suspicious portion of the lymph node, a luxury not readily afforded with a smaller gauge needle or with FNA performed without imaging guidance. Complications such as bleeding, infection, and pain are rarely encountered.

The larger size of a 20-gauge needle allows aspiration of abundant material for cytologic review minimizing the number of passes required to obtain sufficient aspirate for diagnosis. In 97 % of the patients, a single biopsy pass yields sufficient aspirate for a diagnosis with a 98 % accuracy.

22.4 Conclusion

Ultrasound is sensitive but not specific due to the overlap of benign and malignant sonographic features. Sonographic features, either independent or in combination, raise the suspicion for malignancy, but remain insufficient to be reliable in the definitive diagnosis of malignancy. Ultrasound-guided FNA can document the malignant nature of a lymph node and is as critical in the documentation of the benign nature of a node.

References

1. Tseng FY, Hsiao YL, Chang TC. Cytologic features of metastatic papillary thyroid carcinoma in cervical lymph nodes. Acta Cytol. 2002;46(6):1043–8.
2. Cignarelli M, Ambrosi A, Marino A, Lamacchia O, Campo M, Picca G, Giorgino F. Diagnostic utility of

thyroglobulin detection in fine-needle aspiration of cervical cystic metastatic lymph nodes from papillary thyroid cancer with negative cytology. Thyroid. 2003;13(12):1163–7.

3. Boland GW, Lee MJ, Mueller PR, Mayo-Smith W, Dawson SL, Simeone JF. Efficacy of sonographically guided biopsy of thyroid masses and cervical lymph nodes. AJR Am J Roentgenol. 1993;161(5):1053–6.

Ultrasound Characteristics of Non-endocrine Cervical Pathology

23

Caitlin P. McMullen, Daniel Rocke, Jean-François Cléroux, Sangeet Ghai, and Jeremy L. Freeman

23.1 Introduction

Ultrasound for the head and neck may have its greatest utility for evaluating the thyroid and parathyroid glands, but it is also an extremely useful tool for evaluating other neck pathology. Combined with physical exam, ultrasound can help narrow the differential diagnosis, as well as guide and increase the diagnostic yield of fine needle aspiration biopsies.

23.2 Congenital Lesions

Congenital neck lesions are most commonly seen in a pediatric population, but they can be seen in the adult population as well. The location of the lesion is key in differentiating the type and treatment for these lesions. Midline congenital neck masses include thyroglossal duct cysts, dermoid cysts, epidermoid cysts, and teratomas. A lateral congenital neck mass is most commonly a branchial cleft cyst.

Electronic supplementary material: The online version of this chapter (doi:10.1007/978-3-319-44100-9_23) contains supplementary material, which is available to authorized users. Videos can also be accessed at http://link.springer.com/chapter/10.1007/978-3-319-44100-9_23.

C.P. McMullen, M.D. (✉)
770 Bay Street, Suite 2504, Toronto, ON, Canada, M5G0A6

Department of Otolaryngology - Head and Neck Surgery, Mount Sinai Hospital, University of Toronto, 600 University Avenue, Rm 401, Toronto, ON, Canada, M5G1X5
e-mail: caitlinmcmullen@gmail.com

D. Rocke, M.D., J.D.
Department of Surgery, Division of Head and Neck Surgery & Communication Sciences, Duke University Medical Center, DUMC Box 3805, Durham, NC 27710, USA
e-mail: daniel.rocke@dm.duke.edu

J.-F. Cléroux, M.D., F.R.C.P.C.
33 Charles St E, #1611, Toronto, ON, Canada, M4Y 0A2

Jt Department of Medical Imaging, University Health Network – Mt Sinai Hospital – Women's College Hospital, University of Toronto, 1PMB-283, 585 University Avenue, Toronto, ON, Canada, M5G 2N2
e-mail: jf.cleroux@hotmail.com

S. Ghai, M.D., F.R.C.R.
Jt Department of Medical Imaging, University Health Network – Mt Sinai Hospital – Women's College Hospital, University of Toronto, 1PMB-283, 585 University Avenue, Toronto, ON, Canada, M5G 2N2
e-mail: sangeet.ghai@uhn.ca

J.L. Freeman, M.D., F.R.C.S., F.A.C.S.
Department of Otolaryngology - Head and Neck Surgery, Mount Sinai Hospital, University of Toronto, 600 University Avenue, Rm 401, Toronto, ON, Canada, M5G1X5
e-mail: JFreeman@mtsinai.on.ca

M. Milas et al. (eds.), *Advanced Thyroid and Parathyroid Ultrasound*, DOI 10.1007/978-3-319-44100-9_23

23.2.1 Thyroglossal Duct Cysts

Thyroglossal duct cysts are remnants of the thyroglossal duct, which the thyroid anlage traverses during its descent from the foramen cecum to the inferior neck beginning in the third week of gestation. Approximately half of these cysts are found in close proximity to the hyoid bone, but they can be located anywhere from the foramen cecum to the pyramidal lobe of the thyroid gland [1, 2]. These cysts are classically anechoic or hypoechoic with a thin cyst wall and posterior enhancement [Video 23.1; Fig. 23.1]. This classic appearance is seen in less than half of cases, however, and there is often a homogeneous or heterogeneous hypoechoic appearance. They are located deep to or within the strap muscles and may have internal septations [1, 3–7]. Often hypoechoic debris is present within the cyst, and air-fluid levels can be seen [Fig. 23.2] [1, 2, 6]. The cyst's relation to the hyoid bone should be examined, and it should be noted whether a fistula or sinus tract is present [2]. Ultrasound is also useful to rule out an ectopic thyroid. Occasionally thyroid cancer can arise from a thyroglossal duct cyst, and suspicious ultrasound findings such as a solid component or microcalcifications can direct the surgeon accordingly [5].

23.2.2 Dermoid and Epidermoid Cysts and Teratomas

Dermoid and epidermoid cysts and teratomas are classified as dysontogenetic cysts. Dermoid and epidermoid cysts are found in the floor of mouth region and are thought to develop from trapped tissue in embryonic fusion planes. Dermoid cysts are typically found in the second and third decade of life and are midline in nature. The less common epidermoid cysts tend to be found during infancy, but are also found in the suprahyoid midline [1].

Ultrasound can be useful for evaluating these lesions if they are superficial in nature. Deeper cysts are better evaluated with a contrasted CT scan [1]. Superficial dermoid cysts that are evaluable with ultrasound will typically be hypoechoic and thin walled, but can have a heterogeneous appearance due to hair, sebum, or fluid within the lesion [2, 4, 6, 7]. Coalescent fat and calcifications within a dermoid cyst give rise to what is known as a "pseudosolid" or "sac-of-marbles" appearance, and this is nearly pathognomonic for this lesion [1, 7]. Epidermoid cysts tend to be more homogeneous in appearance due to the lack of dermal appendages [1]. Calcification with visible blood flow is characteristics of a teratoma [2, 8].

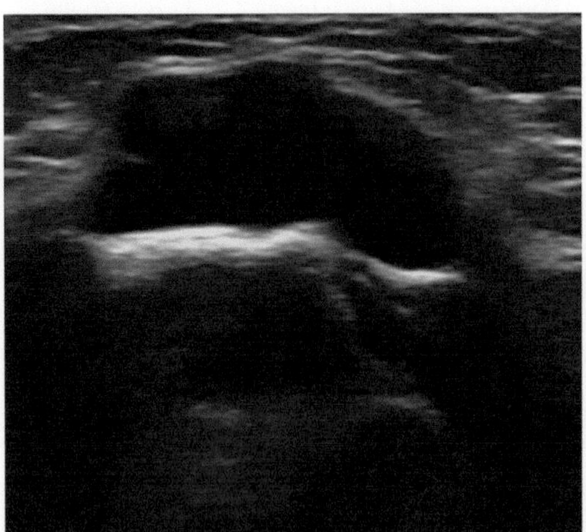

Fig. 23.1 Ultrasound of a midline suprahyoid lobulated cyst, measuring 2 cm, consistent with a thyroglossal duct cyst

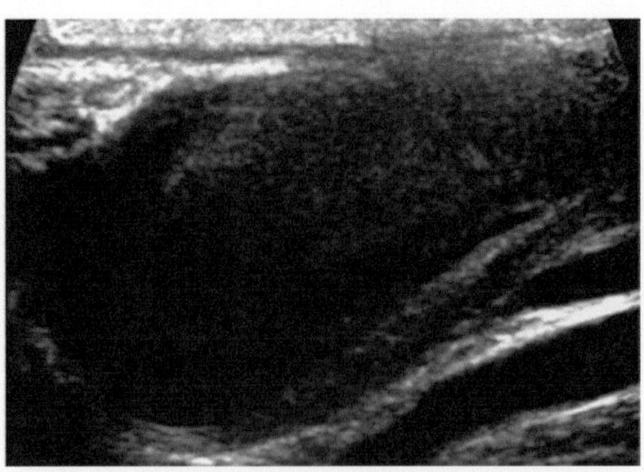

Fig. 23.2 A young man presented with recurrent episodes of infection in this complicated right paramidline infrahyoid thyroglossal duct cyst with internal debris, measuring 2.4 cm

23.2.3 Branchial Cleft Abnormalities

Branchial cleft abnormalities include cysts, which are most common, fistulas, and sinuses [2]. The vast majority of branchial cleft abnormalities are from the second branchial arch and are found near the carotid bifurcation [Fig. 23.3]. Those found in the parotid region are more likely from the first arch [1, 2]. Third-arch lesions are most commonly found in the posterior cervical space, while fourth-arch abnormalities are typically adjacent to the left lobe of the thyroid [1]. It is important to perform a careful evaluation for a sinus tract, as this can aide in the operative management of these lesions [2].

Regardless of location, these lesions are hypoechoic or anechoic, thin walled, and compressible [Fig. 23.4]. One can occasionally see sedimentation levels within the fluid, thick cyst walls, or septations, but this is not typical [1, 2, 7, 9]. More frequently these lesions show fine echogenic regions that are secondary to cholesterol crystals or debris [2]. Infected branchial cleft lesions can have thickened cyst walls, internal echogenic foci, and associated reactive lymphadenopathy [Video 23.2] [1, 2].

23.3 Neoplastic Lesions

Neoplastic lesions in the head and neck are more commonly seen in an adult population. Ultrasound can provide immediate information to the clinician about exact location and can narrow the differential diagnosis.

23.3.1 Benign Neoplastic Lesions

23.3.1.1 Lipoma

Lipomas in the head and neck are relatively common lesions and are typically easily diagnosed by clinical history and physical examination alone. Occasionally these can be located deeper within the neck, and ultrasound may be a useful adjunct in these cases. Lipomas are typically located superficially in the subcutaneous tissues, and their appearance can vary based on the amounts of fat and fibrous tissue that are present. Lipomas are well-circumscribed lesions that are ovoid and have a characteristic striated appearance [Fig. 23.5]. Some describe a hypoechoic appearance to lipomas, but they are more frequently isoechoic or hyperechoic [2, 10]. There is no to minimal internal blood flow seen, and liposarcoma should be considered lesions that appear to be lipomas with internal blood flow [10].

23.3.1.2 Paraganglioma

Paragangliomas in the head and neck are more typically evaluated with other imaging modalities, but ultrasound can be useful in establishing

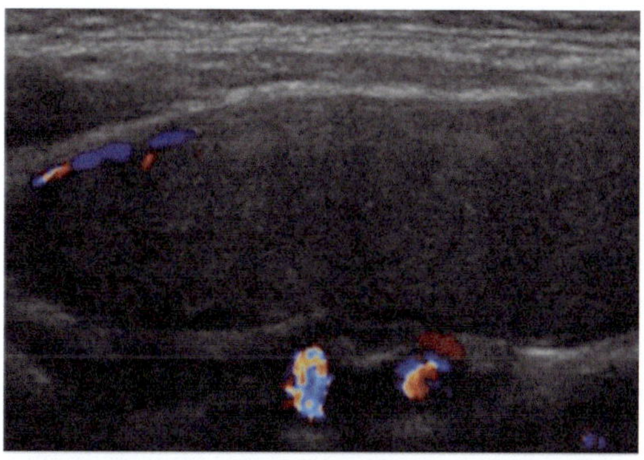

Fig. 23.3 Ultrasound of a large, well-defined avascular mass, suggestive of a branchial cleft cyst type II

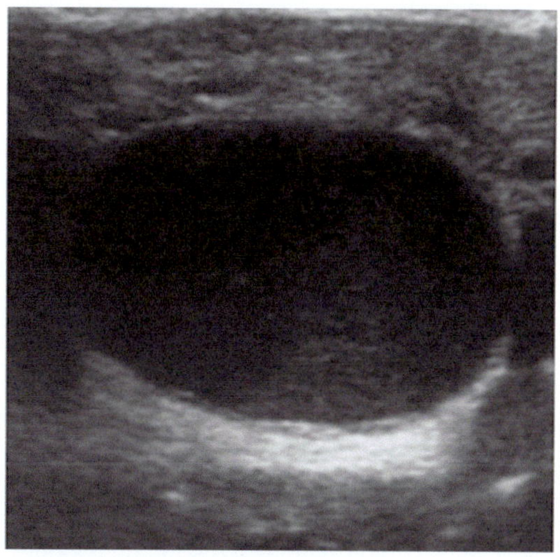

Fig. 23.4 The ultrasound appearance of a fluid-filled cyst with posterior enhancement

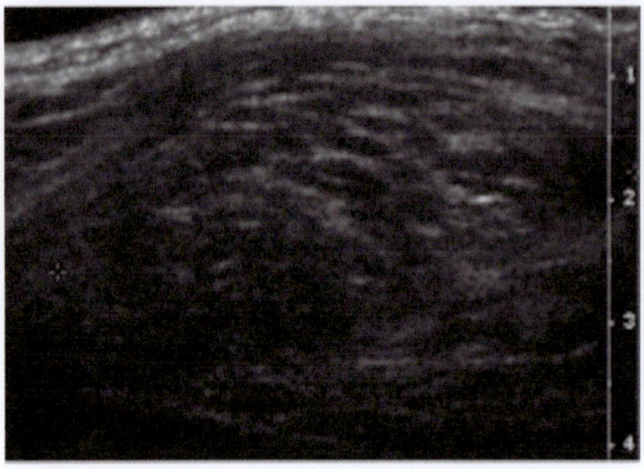

Fig. 23.5 A young man presented with a palpable soft right supraclavicular mass. Ultrasound demonstrated a 4.8 cm ovoid isoechoic heterogeneous mass with no vascularity, consistent with a lipoma

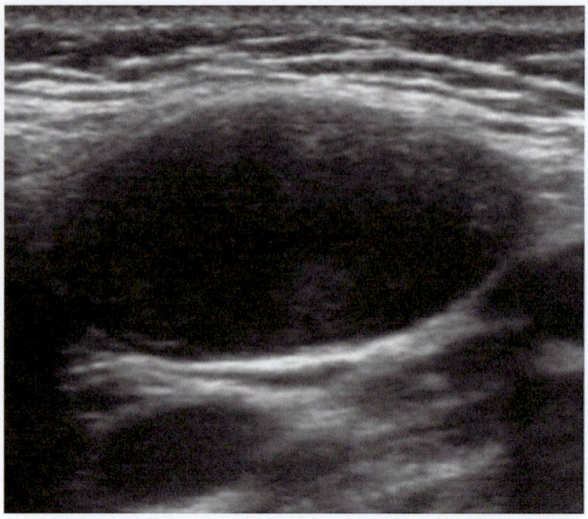

Fig. 23.6 This level III neck mass along the carotid sheath was proven to be a schwannoma along the vagus nerve

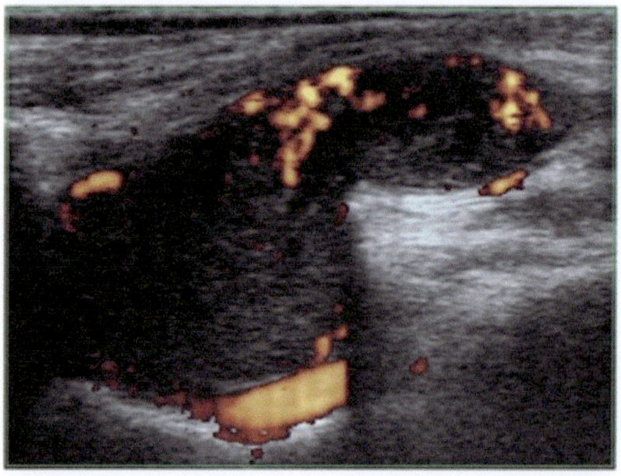

Fig. 23.7 In a patient with history of neurofibromatosis type 2, ultrasound demonstrated a large, lobulated, hypoechoic, vascular mass with a dumbbell appearance. The deep component is located within an enlarged vertebral foramen, consistent with a neurofibroma

this as a diagnosis in a new patient with a neck mass. Ultrasound can also be used to monitor for recurrence of carotid body tumors. Paragangliomas are solid, hypoechoic masses that are highly vascular on Doppler imaging. Carotid body paragangliomas splay the internal and external carotid arteries. Due to overlying bony anatomy, glomus jugulare tumors cannot usually be evaluated with ultrasound [2, 10].

23.3.1.3 Schwannoma and Neurofibroma

Neurogenic tumors, including schwannomas and neurofibromas, are hypoechoic, often vascular masses that can sometimes be seen in continuity with a peripheral nerve on ultrasound exam [Figs. 23.6 and 23.7]. In those that can be visualized relative to their nerve of origin, the surgeon can see schwannomas based more marginally relative to the nerve [Video 23.3]. Neurofibromas, on the other hand, originate more centrally. These lesions are most often located in the posterior triangle of the neck and are fusiform with smooth margins [2, 10].

23.3.1.4 Hemangioma

Hemangiomas are vascular lesions that are usually diagnosed early in life [Video 23.4]. Not surprisingly, they demonstrate vascularity on Doppler imaging [Fig. 23.8]. In lower-flow lesions, the power Doppler setting may be useful. When the vascular spaces are small, these lesions can be hyperechoic. Larger spaces are hypoechoic. The compressibility of the lesion as well as the vascularity can help distinguish this from other lesions, and sometimes a feeding vessel can be identified as well [2, 10]. Calcifications may also be present.

23.3.1.5 Lymphangioma

Like hemangiomas, lymphangiomas are diagnosed early in life in most cases. Lymphangiomas will have a complex and multiloculated appearance and are compressible on ultrasound

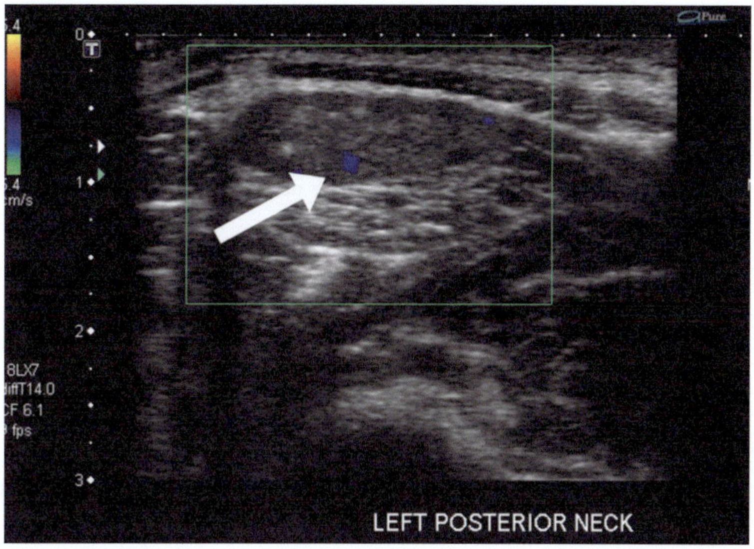

Fig. 23.8 Ultrasound imaging using color Doppler of a patient with Klippel-Trenaunay syndrome demonstrating flow within the lesion. Speckled calcification can also be visualized

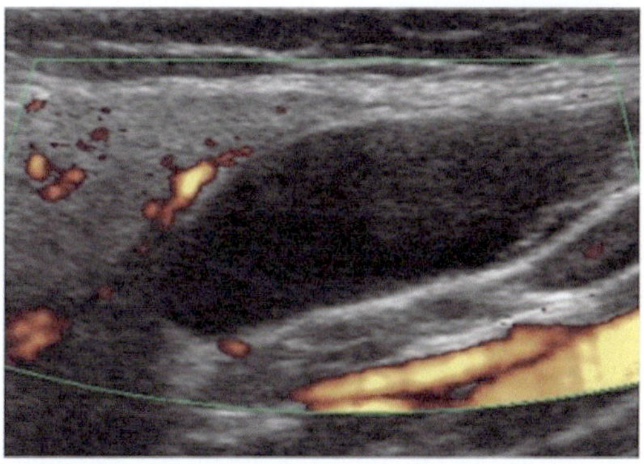

Fig. 23.9 Ultrasound of a soft, multiseptated, avascular, complex cystic lesion with internal debris next to the submandibular gland, in keeping with a lymphangioma

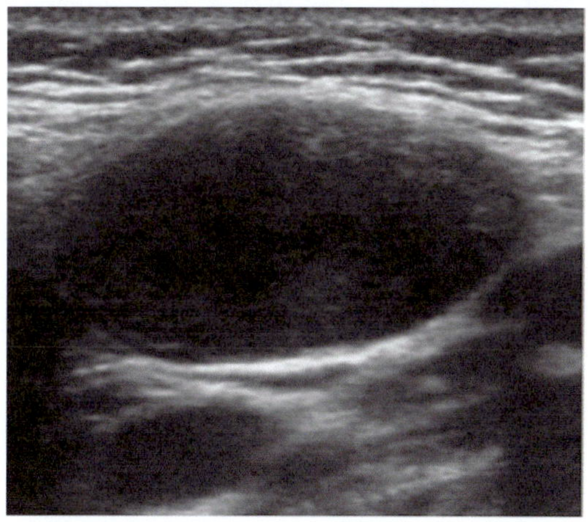

Fig. 23.10 A patient with a history of B-cell lymphoma in remission presented with a palpable right neck mass. Ultrasound shows an enlarged, homogeneous, hypoechoic adenopathy with loss of the fatty hilum in level III. Biopsy revealed lymphoma recurrence

[Fig. 23.9]. Hyperechoic areas may also be seen and these are due to clustered lymphatic channels. The lack of vascularity on Doppler imaging helps to distinguish the lymphangioma from a hemangioma [2, 7, 10].

23.3.2 Malignant Neoplastic Lesions

23.3.2.1 Lymphoma

Lymphomatous lymph nodes can be difficult to distinguish sonographically from reactive lymph nodes and nodes in inflammatory diseases like sarcoidosis. They are hypoechoic in nature, rounded or oval in shape, and have smooth margins [Fig. 23.10]. Necrosis and extranodal extension are uncommon. Doppler imaging can show hilar vascularity, similar to reactive nodes, or a mix of hilar and peripheral vascularity [2, 11].

23.3.2.2 Non-thyroid Metastatic Lesions

Squamous cell carcinoma is the most common metastatic lesion found in the neck, but other metastatic lesions can be seen, especially in the supraclavicular region [2]. As with other entities mentioned above, ultrasound may not be the imaging modality of choice in staging and initial treatment due to its inability to image areas like the retropharyngeal lymph node basin. It does, however, offer a useful adjunct both in the initial diagnostic setting and for follow-up.

As in thyroid lymph node metastases, non-thyroid metastases have a rounded appearance with a loss of the fatty hilum. There is often a heterogeneous internal appearance due to necrosis. The border of involved nodes can be indistinct, and there can be evidence of invasion of adjacent structures. Doppler assessment can show a disorganized vascular pattern [2, 12, 13].

23.4 Reactive Lymph Nodes

The differential diagnosis of cervical lymphadenopathy is quite extensive. The ultrasonographer must be able to distinguish reactive or benign lymph nodes from those that are pathologic so the patient may avoid unnecessary invasive testing and distress. Fortunately, there are characteristic ultrasound features of benign and pathologic lymph nodes that can assist in making the diagnosis.

Reactive and normal lymph nodes, both benign, share many of the same ultrasound features. Pathologic lymph nodes tend to appear rounded, and reactive nodes are oval in shape [14]. The oval shape for reactive nodes is defined as a short axis/long axis ratio of <0.5 [15]. Benign lymph nodes are typically anechoic or hypoechoic. The most characteristic finding of benign or reactive lymph nodes is a bright fatty hilum containing a vascular strip. This finding has a 90 % accuracy in diagnosing a benign lymph node [16]. Benign lymph nodes typically maintain a sharp border, while malignant or otherwise pathologic nodes may infiltrate into surrounding structures [15].

The vascular flow pattern may also assist in determining the nature of the node. Peripheral vascularity is generally suggestive of a pathologic process [17]. With color flow Doppler, the hilum of a reactive or normal node demonstrates a vascular pattern, with the surrounding nodal structure relatively avascular [14, 17]. Reactive nodes will also lack many of the features characteristic of certain malignancies: heterogeneous echogenicity, calcifications, cystic spaces, or intranodal necrosis [16].

23.5 Sarcoidosis

Sarcoidosis is a systemic disease process whose etiology is not definitively known. A systemic inflammatory response, perhaps a reaction to an as-of-yet unknown antigen, results in the formation of noncaseating granulomas, usually involving the hilar mediastinal lymph nodes. The diagnosis must be made by histopathologic analysis of tissue specimens. Most patients present with pulmonary symptoms; however, the head and neck soft tissues are affected in 10–15 % of cases, with approximately 50 % of these patients displaying cervical lymphadenopathy [18].

Sonographic features of sarcoidosis within the cervical nodes and salivary glands are relatively nonspecific, and definitive diagnosis is made with tissue analysis. Lymph nodes involved with sarcoidosis are hypoechoic and lose the vascular hilum. They are frequently large and palpable. The lateral, supraclavicular, and posterior neck compartments are typically involved, and findings may be bilateral and asymmetric. Cervical nodes in sarcoidosis usually occur in a cluster and display a rounded shape, rather than the typical ovoid shape of benign reactive lymph nodes [Fig. 23.11] [19]. These nodes do not display extracapsular extension or infiltrate into surrounding tissues. Large nodes are hypoechoic/anechoic and may display a "punctate echo structure" with small hyperechoic areas within the node [20].

Sarcoidosis also may involve the salivary glands. Ultrasound of these areas in sarcoidosis patients may demonstrate intraparotid nodal enlargement, as well as variable echogenicity and mixed involvement of the gland [21, 22]. The parenchyma of the gland may appear heterogeneous and may display multiple septae. Small hypoechoic nodules may be present throughout the parenchyma. Upon color flow Doppler imaging of these hypoechoic areas, they may appear hypervascular [21].

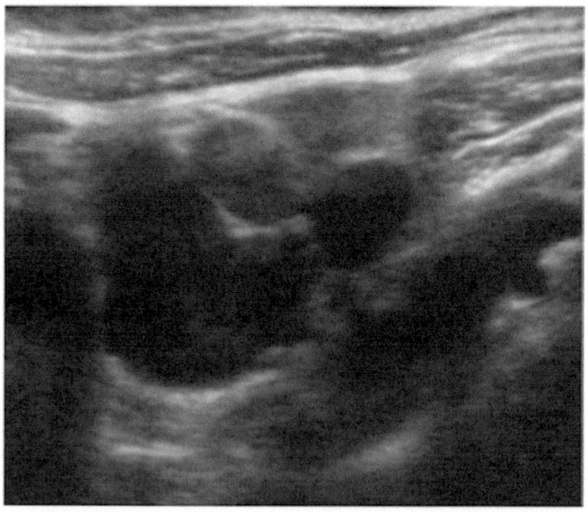

Fig. 23.11 A patient with history of sarcoidosis presented with bilateral enlarged, asymmetric cervical/supraclavicular suspicious lymph nodes, which were hypoechoic with a loss of the fatty hilum. Biopsy was consistent with sarcoidosis

Heerfordt syndrome, the classic presentation of parotitis, facial nerve paralysis, and uveitis caused by sarcoidosis, is a rare entity, occurring in 6 % or less of patients with the disease [23]. With this syndrome, ultrasound may reveal diffuse enlargement of the parotid glands with multiple hypoechogenic nodules. These hypoechoic areas correlate clinically with granuloma formation within the glands [20]. Duplex ultrasound of the involved parotid demonstrates hypervascularity [24].

Ultrasound-guided biopsy of mediastinal nodes in sarcoidosis has been described as a useful method of diagnosis, with a diagnostic yield >93 % [25, 26]. Tissue specimens display the characteristic noncaseating epithelioid cell granuloma. Within the neck, ultrasound-guided fine needle aspiration biopsy has been reported for sarcoidosis involving supraclavicular nodes [27], but there is limited evidence of its use within the neck for the indication of sarcoidosis.

23.6 Ranula

Ranula is a mucocele formed by the obstruction of the sublingual ducts and a subsequent collection of salivary fluid. Physical exam of the patient may reveal a soft fullness in the floor of mouth or a neck mass. Many individuals presenting with a ranula are young adults or pediatric patients, and consequently radiation-free ultrasound is an ideal method for initial assessment and diagnosis. Treatment is surgical and involves removal of the ranula with removal of the offending sublingual gland and/or marsupialization.

Ultrasound findings of the ranula are characteristic. Findings include a homogeneous, hypoechoic, compressible, unilocular cyst with well-defined borders and a thin cyst wall [28, 29]. The sublingual gland and mylohyoid muscle are visualized adjacent to the lesion. Occasionally there may be protinaceous intralesional debris. A "plunging ranula" is defined by the cystic lesion descending beyond the posterior aspect of the mylohyoid muscle and into the neck into the submandibular space, resulting in the presence of a soft, nontender, neck mass. The mylohyoid defect through which the ranula descends may be visualized with high-resolution ultrasound [29]. Ultrasound has been advocated for monitoring these patients for recurrence postoperatively as a noninvasive, low-cost, and radiation-free imaging modality [28].

23.7 Laryngocele

Laryngoceles are rare air-filled laryngeal lesions that form as an acquired dilation of the laryngeal ventricle and communicate with the lumen. These dilations typically form from increased glottic pressure and may be bilateral. Laryngeal tumors potentially causing supraglottic obstruction should be ruled out. Laryngoceles may be internal or external (also called a combined laryngocele), as defined by whether or not they herniate through the thyrohyoid membrane. External laryngoceles may present as a soft, compressible neck mass. Mucous or serous material may fill the lesion.

Ultrasound is highly diagnostic for fluid-filled laryngoceles, in particular due to its anatomic relationships. Ultrasound for the external laryngocele reveals an anechoic mass lateral to

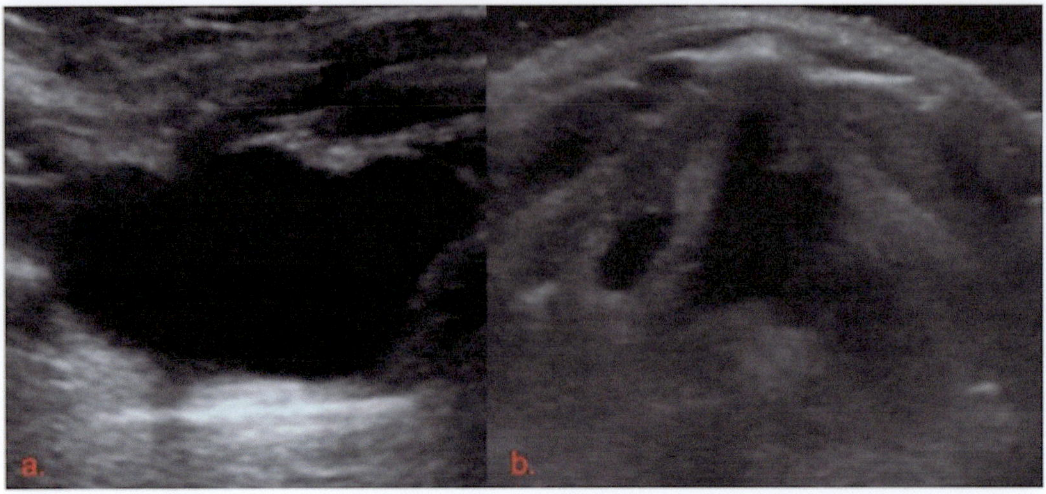

Fig. 23.12 Ultrasound of a lobulated cystic lesion, located deep to the left thyrohyoid membrane in the paralaryngeal space consistent with a fluid-filled internal laryngocele (**a**). Transverse midline view showing the lesion beneath the thyrohyoid membrane (**b**)

the larynx at the level of the thyrohyoid membrane [Fig. 23.12]. Borders are well defined and non-infiltrative. Internal laryngoceles have a characteristic appearance as anechoic, rounded structures contained within the thyroid cartilage [30].

Air-filled, pressure-related laryngoceles may be difficult to visualize without active patient participation. A closed-mouth and nasopharynx forced expiration may create dilation of the laryngocele. Ultrasound of this lesion will demonstrate a bright linear echo adjacent to the thyroid cartilage with shadowing and reverberation effect due to the air content. Real-time ultrasound will show a gradual decrease in size of the sac [31].

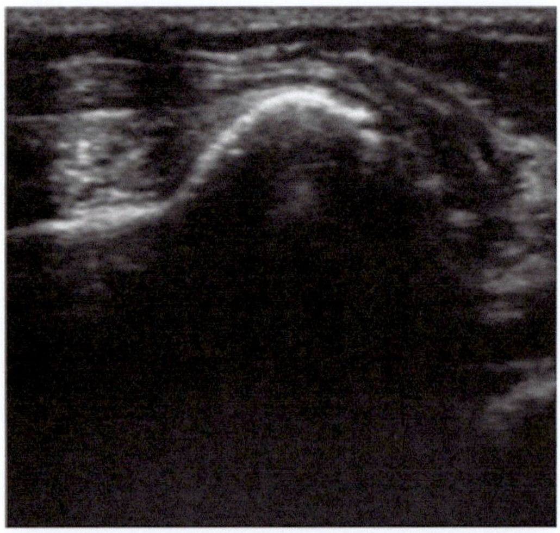

Fig. 23.13 Ultrasound demonstrating a transverse process of a cervical vertebra in a thin patient. The bony structure creates a markedly hyperechoic line with strong posterior shadowing

23.8 Transverse Processes of Cervical Spine

Ultrasound beams do not penetrate bone well; therefore, boney structures appear anechoic with a posterior acoustic shadow and a bright hyperechoic rim [Fig. 23.13]. The cervical spine can be visualized with routine neck ultrasound, especially within the posterior triangle. All human vertebrae possess lateral elongated bony protuberances bilaterally called transverse processes. The transverse processes of the upper six cervical vertebrae contain a foramen through which the vertebral artery, vertebral vein, and sympathetic plexus travel. The transverse process of C1 is the most superficial and prominent bony landmark. The transverse processes can be visualized on posterior triangle cervical ultrasound and should not be mistaken for pathology.

23.9 Salivary Gland Pathology

The differential diagnosis of a mass presenting in the salivary glands is broad: benign, malignant, autoimmune, inflammatory, infectious, and others. Histology is essential to obtain a definitive diagnosis. The majority of tumors—whether benign or malignant—appears in the superficial lobe of the parotid but may occasionally present in the deep lobe or enter the parapharyngeal space. Tumors of the submandibular and sublingual salivary glands are more likely to be malignant. Comprehensive history and physical exam of the patient are indispensible, but ultrasound is a useful adjunct for patient evaluation. Ultrasound-guided fine needle biopsy of salivary gland masses is frequently used to suggest the diagnosis and guide surgical planning.

The structure of salivary glands is complex, but the normal glandular tissue itself is typically homogeneous on ultrasound [Fig. 23.14]. Within a normal gland, well-defined, tubular anechoic ductal structures may be visualized. Lymph nodes may also be present in the parotid with their characteristic appearance. The ultrasound findings of common parotid pathologies are discussed in this section [Table 23.1].

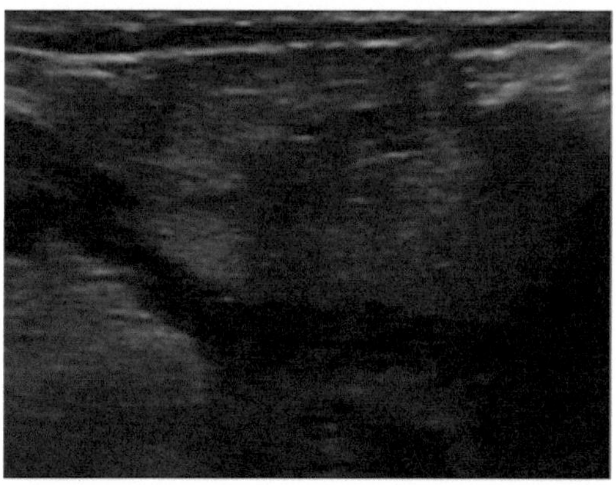

Fig. 23.14 Normal ultrasound appearance of the left submandibular gland

23.10 Benign Tumors

The most common benign tumors of the salivary glands are pleomorphic adenoma and Warthin's tumors. The most common parotid tumor is the pleomorphic adenoma [32]. This lesion is most often located in the superficial lobe of the parotid. Ultrasound demonstrates homogeneously hypoechoic, rounded lesions that are regular in appearance with well-defined borders [Video 23.5; Fig. 23.15] [33]. The tumor capsule may be visualized as a thin, hyperechoic line around the mass [34]. Pleomorphic adenomas are also frequently lobulated and do not typically have cystic components [35]. Though generally benign tumors are relatively hypovascular, a peripheral vascularization pattern may be seen with Doppler mode [22, 34]. Occasionally, calcifications may be visualized as brightly hyperechoic areas within the mass [36]. Bright posterior enhancement, a brightly hyperechoic area posterior to a hypoechoic or anechoic structure, is often seen with this benign lesion [Fig. 23.16] [34, 36]. Recurrent pleomorphic adenoma in a postoperative surgical bed may be multicentric and nodular.

Warthin's tumor, also known as papillary cystadenoma lymphomatosum, is the second most common benign parotid tumor. These tumors usually occur in older, male smokers and can occur bilaterally. These benign tumors are round or ovoid with well-defined, regular borders and low vascularity with Doppler imaging [37]. They are hypoechoic with more heterogeneous echotexture than the pleomorphic adenoma. Anechoic cystic areas with thin septae may be

Table 23.1 Ultrasound characteristics of various salivary gland pathology

	Echogenecity	Heterogeneity	Shape	Vascularity
Pleomorphic adenoma	Hypoechoic	Homogeneous	Lobular	Peripheral
Warthin tumor	Hypoechoic	Heterogeneous	Round or ovoid	Hypovascular
Salivary malignancy	Hypoechoic	Heterogeneous	Irregular	Hypervascular
Sjogren's	Mixed	Heterogeneous	Diffuse	Hypervascular

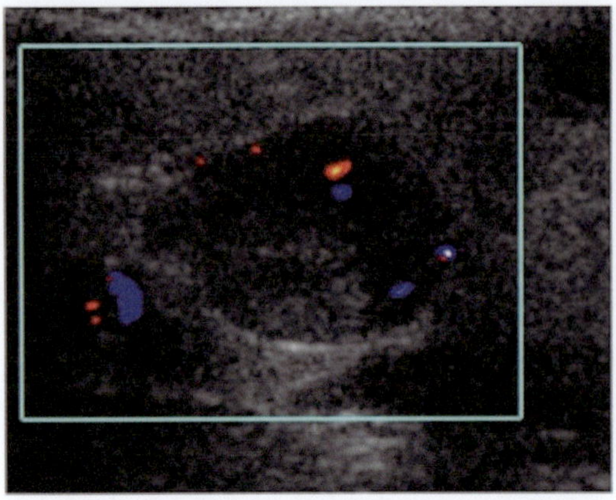

Fig. 23.15 Ultrasound of a parotid mass shows a round, well-defined, hypoechoic, solid lesion with vascularity, in keeping with a pleomorphic adenoma

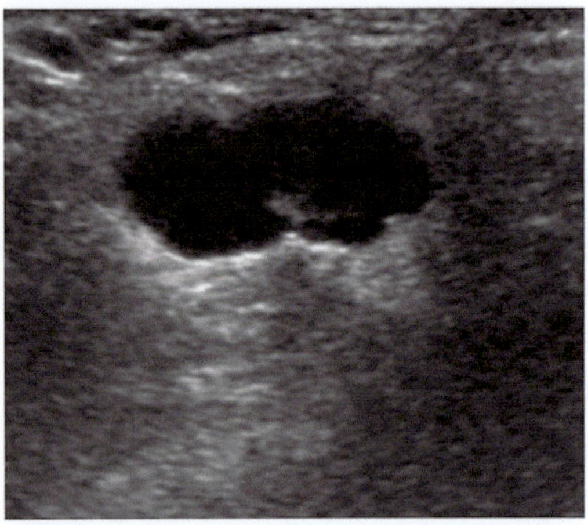

Fig. 23.16 Ultrasound of a pleomorphic adenoma, a lobulated, well-defined, markedly hypoechoic structure with characteristic posterior enhancement within the parotid gland

visualized. Multiple cystic areas within the mass upon ultrasound are a sensitive finding for Warthin tumors [Fig. 23.17] [37]. Posterior acoustic enhancement does occur with Warthin tumors, but this is seen much less frequently than with pleomorphic adenoma [36].

23.11 Malignant Tumors

Lesions presenting the submandibular gland are more likely to be malignant than those presenting in the parotid glands. Small and low-grade tumors

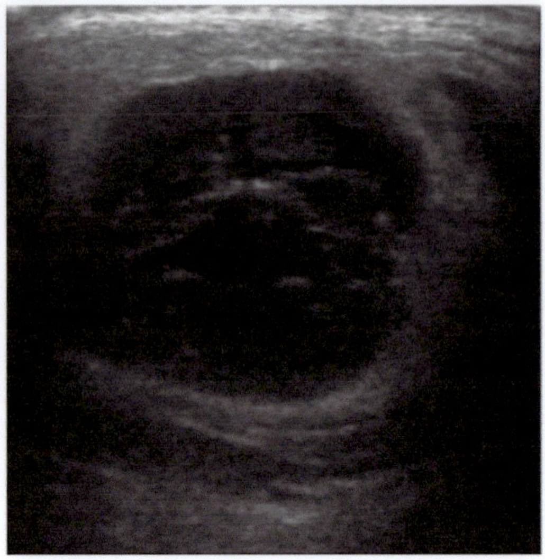

Fig. 23.17 A mass within the left parotid gland, with small cystic components, consistent with a Warthin's tumor

may have an ultrasonographic appearance similar to a benign mass lesion. Larger malignant tumors may have poorly defined edges with infiltrative borders. Nodal basins associated with the salivary lesion should be thoroughly assessed with physical exam and imaging. Ultrasound is helpful for rapid initial assessment, but it is not highly sensitive or specific in the diagnosis of malignant salivary tumors [38]. If there is high suspicion of a malignant process, cross-sectional imaging such as MRI may be necessary to delineate the extent of disease.

Mucoepidermoid carcinoma is the most common malignant tumor of the salivary glands and may be low, intermediate, or high grade [32]. These lesions are hypoechoic and may contain anechoic areas of necrosis. Small and low-grade lesions may have regular, well-defined borders and appear similar to a benign salivary mass. High-grade tumors infiltrate into the surrounding parenchyma, which can be visualized on ultrasound as a poorly defined border and heterogeneous echotexture [33, 36].

Adenoid cystic carcinoma is the most common malignancy of the submandibular glands. This tumor is aggressive but tends to present insidiously and has a predilection for perineural invasion. Distant metastases may present many years after initial diagnosis. Unfortunately, the characteristic perineural invasion cannot be visualized with ultrasound. As with other malignant salivary pathologies, adenoid cystic tumors may be hypervascular and can have poorly defined borders when high grade [22].

23.12 Inflammatory and Other Diseases

Acute infectious sialoadenitis typically presents with a painful, swollen mass in the parotid or submandibular area. History and physical, demonstrating acute painful swelling of the salivary gland with purulent drainage from the duct, are usually adequate for diagnosis. Ultrasound can be a useful adjunct, especially to rule out abscess formation. The gland itself may appear enlarged and heterogeneous, with multiple hypoechoic and anechoic areas [Fig. 23.18]. Hyperechoic obstructing stones may be visualized with a proximal, anechoic dilated duct [39]. Abscesses, in severe cases, demonstrate anechoic liquefied areas with echoic debris [40].

Sialolithiasis, frequently a cause of acute sialoadenitis, is more common in the submandibular glands than the parotid glands. Within the submandibular gland, most stones are calcified and can be visualized well with various imaging modalities [Fig. 23.19]. Ultrasound has a high specificity and positive predictive value for sialolithiasis: 95 % and 94 %, respectively [41]. Small calculi <3 mm in size may be missed with ultrasound, and false positives may occur in the presence of ductal stenosis with fibrosis [41]. Stones appear as an echogenic mass with posterior shadowing, though stones <2 mm may not display this artifact [2]. Salivation may be stimulated in order to further dilate the ducts and more distinctly visualize the location of an obstructing stone.

Chronic inflammation and infection of the salivary glands can result in eventual atrophy of the glands. Causes include chronic ductal obstruction by stone or fibrosis, recurrent infections, granulomatous disease, and systemic autoimmune processes. Findings of chronic sialoadenitis generally include heterogeneous glandular tissue, ductal strictures, and ectasias. Punctate or nodular hypoechoic areas are intermixed with hyperechoic areas of fibrosis [Fig. 23.20]. Adenopathy within the parotid gland may be encountered [33].

Autoimmune processes, such as Sjogren's syndrome, may demonstrate ultrasound findings similar to chronic sialoadenitis. Sjogren's syn-

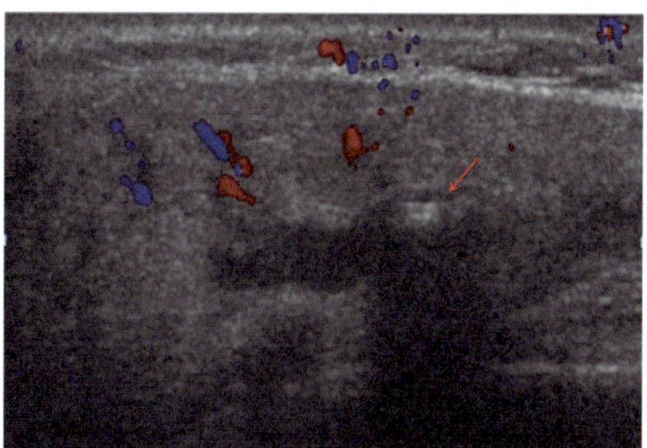

Fig. 23.18 A patient presented with swelling, erythema, and pain in the right parotid area. Ultrasound shows a mildly hypoechoic, heterogeneous, and hypervascular right parotid gland. One small stone is seen in a dilated canal inside the gland (*arrow*), in keeping with acute calculous sialadenitis

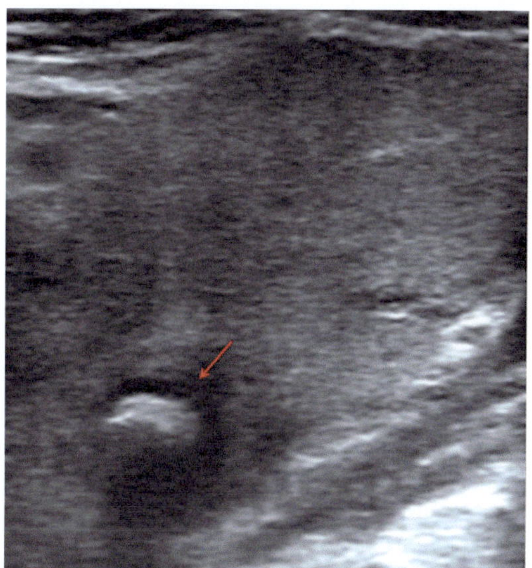

Fig. 23.19 Ultrasound demonstrating acute calculous sialadenitis of the submandibular gland. A 1.1 cm stone is seen in the proximal Wharton's canal

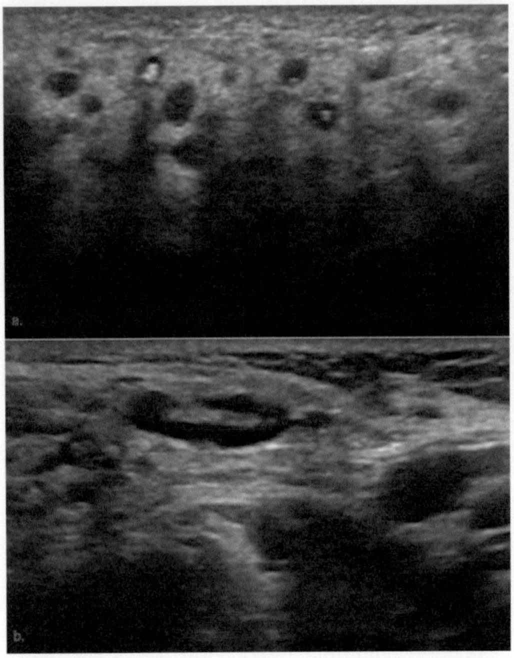

Fig. 23.20 Ultrasound appearance of chronic sialoadenitis, demonstrating symmetric, heterogeneous changes of both parotid glands, with multiple tiny cystic spaces and microcalcifications (**a**). Reactive lymph nodes are also noted (**b**)

drome results in cystic glandular changes and characteristic sialectasis and may even appear as a solid mass lesion on ultrasound [42]. Glands tend to be diffusely hypervascular [22] with hypoechogenic nodules within the gland as the disease advances. Eventually, the gland atrophies. Patients with Sjogren's syndrome are at high risk for the development of intraparotid lymphoma, and intraparotid adenopathy in this setting should be viewed with suspicion.

23.13 Conclusion

Ultrasound affords a low-cost, radiation-free imaging modality that is highly useful in the assessment of various head and neck pathologies, both benign and malignant. Knowledge of the characteristic appearance of normal anatomy and various pathologies is essential for the sonographer who may encounter unexpected findings upon routine ultrasound.

References

1. Gaddikeri S, Vattoth S, Gaddikeri RS, Stuart R, Harrison K, Young D, et al. Congenital cystic neck masses: embryology and imaging appearances, with clinicopathological correlation. Curr Probl Diagn Radiol. 2014;43(2):55–67.
2. Gritzmann N, Hollerweger A, Macheiner P, Rettenbacher T. Sonography of soft tissue masses of the neck. J Clin Ultrasound. 2002;30(6):356–73.
3. Hong HS, Lee EH, Jeong SH, Park J, Lee H. Ultrasonography of various thyroid diseases in children and adolescents: a pictorial essay. Korean J Radiol. 2015;16(2):419–29.
4. Oyewumi M, Inarejos E, Greer ML, Hassouneh B, Campisi P, Forte V, et al. Ultrasound to differentiate thyroglossal duct cysts and dermoid cysts in children. Laryngoscope. 2015;125(4):998–1003.
5. Chou J, Walters A, Hage R, Zurada A, Michalak M, Tubbs RS, et al. Thyroglossal duct cysts: anatomy, embryology and treatment. Surg Radiol Anat. 2013;35(10):875–81.
6. Sidell DR, Shapiro NL. Diagnostic accuracy of ultrasonography for midline neck masses in children. Otolaryngol Head Neck Surg. 2011;144(3):431–4.
7. Ibrahim M, Hammoud K, Maheshwari M, Pandya A. Congenital cystic lesions of the head and neck. Neuroimaging Clin N Am. 2011;21(3):621–39. viii.
8. Rahbar R, Vogel A, Myers LB, Bulich LA, Wilkins-Haug L, Benson CB, et al. Fetal surgery in otolaryngology: a new era in the diagnosis and management of fetal airway obstruction because of advances in prenatal imaging. Arch Otolaryngol Head Neck Surg. 2005;131(5):393–8.
9. Valentino M, Quiligotti C, Carone L. Branchial cleft cyst. J Ultrasound. 2013;16(1):17–20.
10. DiDomenico P, Middleton W. Sonographic evaluation of palpable superficial masses. Radiol Clin North Am. 2014;52(6):1295–305.
11. Averill LW, Acikgoz G, Miller RE, Kandula VV, Epelman M. Update on pediatric leukemia and lymphoma imaging. Semin Ultrasound CT MR. 2013;34(6):578–99.
12. Ashraf M, Biswas J, Jha J, Nayak S, Singh V, Majumdar S, et al. Clinical utility and prospective comparison of ultrasonography and computed tomography imaging in staging of neck metastases in head and neck squamous cell cancer in an Indian setup. Int J Clin Oncol. 2011;16(6):686–93.
13. Shetty D, Jayade BV, Joshi SK, Gopalkrishnan K. Accuracy of palpation, ultrasonography, and computed tomography in the evaluation of metastatic cervical lymph nodes in head and neck cancer. Indian J Dent. 2015;6(3):121–4.
14. Dragoni F, Cartoni C, Pescarmona E, Chiarotti F, Puopolo M, Orsi E, et al. The role of high resolution pulsed and color Doppler ultrasound in the differential diagnosis of benign and malignant lymphadenopathy: results of multivariate analysis. Cancer. 1999;85(11):2485–90.

15. Ying M, Ahuja A, Metreweli C. Diagnostic accuracy of sonographic criteria for evaluation of cervical lymphadenopathy. J Ultrasound Med. 1998;17(7):437–45.
16. Rosario PW, de Faria S, Bicalho L, Alves MF, Borges MA, Purisch S, et al. Ultrasonographic differentiation between metastatic and benign lymph nodes in patients with papillary thyroid carcinoma. J Ultrasound Med. 2005;24(10):1385–9.
17. Ahuja A, Ying M. Sonography of neck lymph nodes. Part II: abnormal lymph nodes. Clin Radiol. 2003; 58(5):359–66.
18. Dash GI, Kimmelman CP. Head and neck manifestations of sarcoidosis. Laryngoscope. 1988;98(1):50–3.
19. Garwood S, Judson MA, Silvestri G, Hoda R, Fraig M, Doelken P. Endobronchial ultrasound for the diagnosis of pulmonary sarcoidosis. Chest. 2007;132(4): 1298–304.
20. Koischwitz D, Gritzmann N. Ultrasound of the neck. Radiol Clin North Am. 2000;38(5):1029–45.
21. Teymoortash A, Werner JA. Parotid gland involvement in sarcoidosis: sonographic features. J Clin Ultrasound. 2009;37(9):507–10.
22. Martinoli C, Derchi LE, Solbiati L, Rizzatto G, Silvestri E, Giannoni M. Color Doppler sonography of salivary glands. AJR Am J Roentgenol. 1994;163(4):933–41.
23. James DG, Sharma OP. Parotid gland sarcoidosis. Sarcoidosis Vasc Diffuse Lung Dis. 2000;17(1):27–32.
24. Fischer T, Filimonow S, Petersein J, Zimmer C, Beyersdorff D, Guski H. Diagnosis of Heerfordt's syndrome by state-of-the-art ultrasound in combination with parotid biopsy: a case report. Eur Radiol. 2002;12(1):134–7.
25. Oki M, Saka H, Kitagawa C, Kogure Y, Murata N, Ichihara S, et al. Prospective study of endobronchial ultrasound-guided transbronchial needle aspiration of lymph nodes versus transbronchial lung biopsy of lung tissue for diagnosis of sarcoidosis. J Thorac Cardiovasc Surg. 2012;143(6):1324–9.
26. Wong M, Yasufuku K, Nakajima T, Herth FJ, Sekine Y, Shibuya K, et al. Endobronchial ultrasound: new insight for the diagnosis of sarcoidosis. Eur Respir J. 2007;29(6):1182–6.
27. Lohela P, Tikkakoski T, Strengell L, Mikkola S, Koskinen S, Suramo I. Ultrasound-guided fine-needle aspiration cytology of non-palpable supraclavicular lymph nodes in sarcoidosis. Acta Radiol. 1996;37(6):896–9.
28. Sigismund PE, Bozzato A, Schumann M, Koch M, Iro H, Zenk J. Management of ranula: 9 years' clinical experience in pediatric and adult patients. J Oral Maxillofac Surg. 2013;71(3):538–44.
29. Jain P, Jain R, Morton RP, Ahmad Z. Plunging ranulas: high-resolution ultrasound for diagnosis and surgical management. Eur Radiol. 2010;20(6):1442–9.
30. Baatenburg de Jong RJ, Rongen RJ, Lameris JS, Knegt P, Verwoerd CD. Ultrasound in the diagnosis of laryngoceles. ORL J Otorhinolaryngol Relat Spec. 1993;55(5):290–3.
31. Conkbayir I, Keyik B, Hekimoglu K, Cifci E, Yanik B. Trumpet maneuver in the sonographic diagnosis of an external laryngocele. J Clin Ultrasound. 2010;38(1):56–8.
32. Spiro RH. Salivary neoplasms: overview of a 35-year experience with 2,807 patients. Head Neck Surg. 1986;8(3):177–84.
33. Katz P, Hartl DM, Guerre A. Clinical ultrasound of the salivary glands. Otolaryngol Clin North Am. 2009;42(6):973–1000. Table of Contents.
34. Fodor D, Pop S, Maniu A, Cosgaria M. Gray scale and Doppler ultrasonography of the benign tumors of parotid gland (pleomorphic adenoma and Warthin's tumor) Pictorial essay. Med Ultrason. 2010;12(3):238–44.
35. Yuan WH, Hsu HC, Chou YH, Hsueh HC, Tseng TK, Tiu CM. Gray-scale and color Doppler ultrasonographic features of pleomorphic adenoma and Warthin's tumor in major salivary glands. Clin Imaging. 2009;33(5):348–53.
36. Shimizu M, Ussmuller J, Hartwein J, Donath K. A comparative study of sonographic and histopathologic findings of tumorous lesions in the parotid gland. Oral Surg Oral Med Oral Pathol Oral Radiol Endod. 1999;88(6):723–37.
37. Kim J, Kim EK, Park CS, Choi YS, Kim YH, Choi EC. Characteristic sonographic findings of Warthin's tumor in the parotid gland. J Clin Ultrasound. 2004;32(2):78–81.
38. Wu S, Liu G, Chen R, Guan Y. Role of ultrasound in the assessment of benignity and malignancy of parotid masses. Dentomaxillofac Radiol. 2012;41(2):131–5.
39. Ching AS, Ahuja AT, King AD, Tse GM, Metreweli C. Comparison of the sonographic features of acalculous and calculous submandibular sialadenitis. J Clin Ultrasound. 2001;29(6):332–8.
40. Nusem-Horowitz S, Wolf M, Coret A, Kronenberg J. Acute suppurative parotitis and parotid abscess in children. Int J Pediatr Otorhinolaryngol. 1995; 32(2):123–7.
41. Terraz S, Poletti PA, Dulguerov P, Dfouni N, Becker CD, Marchal F, et al. How reliable is sonography in the assessment of sialolithiasis? AJR Am J Roentgenol. 2013;201(1):W104–9.
42. Bradus RJ, Hybarger P, Gooding GA. Parotid gland: US findings in Sjogren syndrome. Work in progress. Radiology. 1988;169(3):749–51.

Part VI

Parathyroid Ultrasound: Anatomy and Fundamental Features

24 Ultrasound and FNA in Parathyroid Disease: Fundamentals of Appearance and Evaluation of Abnormal Parathyroid Glands

Devaprabu Abraham

24.1 Introduction

Neck ultrasonography has become an integral part of most endocrine practice for the evaluation of parathyroid adenoma or enlarged parathyroid glands, prior to surgical intervention. It is also the most cost and time-effective study for the evaluation of coexistent thyroid disease in subjects who undergo parathyroid surgery. Ultrasonograms facilitate parathyroid biopsy and alcohol ablation to be performed in select patients in the office.

24.2 Historical Perspectives

Parathyroid glands are one of the last organs to be identified in humans. The first description of parathyroid glands was in 1852 by Sir Richard Owens in the first recorded dissection of an Indian rhinoceros [1]. Subsequently, Ivor Sandstrom described it in humans when he was a medical student in Stockholm, Sweden [2]. The first parathyroid surgery was performed in 1925 by Dr. Felix Mandl in Vienna, on a tram car conductor named Albert Gahn. The first parathyroidectomy in the USA was by EJ Lewis, at Cook County Hospital in Chicago [3]. The need for multiple surgeries was observed in the case of Captain Charles Martell, who was operated for the seventh time for parathyroid adenoma removal [4]. In the 1990s Tc^{99}-Sestamibi (MIBI) was utilized as an isotope of choice for the evaluation of mitochondria rich tissue, such as the heart. It was observed during cardiac studies that parathyroid adenomas also trap this isotope, which stimulated the concept of presurgical localization prior to minimally invasive surgeries [5]. Ultrasound evaluation for parathyroid glands was largely considered not effective due to lack of understanding of imaging phenotype and operator inexperience. Over the years, ultrasound evaluation for parathyroid localization has become the mainstay in the USA and in Europe. This is partly due to easy availability of equipment and mostly as a result of understanding of the US appearance of enlarged parathyroid glands and adenomas. The lack of ionizing radiation enables easy procurement and maintenance of US equipment in physicians and surgeons offices.

Electronic supplementary material: The online version of this chapter (doi:10.1007/978-3-319-44100-9_24) contains supplementary material, which is available to authorized users. Videos can also be accessed at http://link.springer.com/chapter/10.1007/978-3-319-44100-9_24.

D. Abraham, M.D. (✉)
Department of Medicine, University of Utah,
615 Arapeen Drive Suite 100, Salt Lake City, UT
84108, USA
e-mail: dev.abraham@hsc.utah.edu

M. Milas et al. (eds.), *Advanced Thyroid and Parathyroid Ultrasound*,
DOI 10.1007/978-3-319-44100-9_24

24.3 Surgical Anatomy and Embryologic Development of Parathyroid Glands

Normal parathyroid glands are approximately 5×4×2 mm in size, length, width, and depth respectively, and weigh 20–40 mg [6]. There is considerable variation in the size and weight of the "normal" glands. The size variation was astutely observed by Ivor Sandstrom, who reported this observation in his landmark monograph in 1877 [2]. The glands have a distinct anatomic vascular supply from the thyroid gland and encased in a thin fibrous capsule. The location of parathyroid glands is quite variable. The superior glands are typically located posterior to the thyroid lobes and the inferior glands are located along its posterior and caudal aspect [7–10]. Due to the small size of the parathyroid glands and the presence of physiologic central compartment lymph nodes that are indistinguishable from parathyroid glands, it is generally considered not possible to visualize physiologic, nonenlarged, and normal parathyroid glands with ultrasound. Therefore, it is also not possible to identify the total number of parathyroid glands present in an individual. In one postmortem study, where such information has typically been obtained, four glands were visualized in greater than 90 % of subjects, three glands in 5 %, and five glands in 4 % [9]. The superior parathyroid glands originate in the fourth branchial arch and the inferior parathyroid glands originate from the third branchial arch. Due to the close developmental relationship of the inferior parathyroid glands to the thymus gland, they can be located within the thymus, at the thoracic inlet, or within the mediastinum. The typical location of superior parathyroid glands is extra-thyroidal and about the mid-portion of the posterior margin of the thyroid gland. The vast majority of superior parathyroid glands are within a few millimeters at the junction of inferior thyroid artery and recurrent laryngeal nerve. An inferiorly displaced superior thyroid gland is still located posterior (deep) to the inferior thyroid artery and recurrent laryngeal nerve. The inferior parathyroid glands are often located posterior to the lower third of the thyroid gland or within a few centimeters of the caudal pole of the thyroid gland, but their plane is anterior to the recurrent laryngeal nerve. The superior pair holds their anatomical relationship to the thyroid gland more constantly. A mal-positioned superior parathyroid gland is often displaced posteriorly within the tracheoesophageal groove or into the retropharyngeal space. The inferior parathyroid glands are often located variable in location posteriorly and caudally to the thyroid lobes and into the mediastinum. They can be located within the thymus gland and can also be as inferior in location as the aortic arch. Intrathyroidal parathyroid glands are quite uncommon. The superior pair is more likely to be intrathyroidal within the posterior thyroid capsule, perhaps due to the embryological co-development with the C-cells of the thyroid gland, from the fourth branchial pouch. The typical location within the thyroid lobes is subcapsular location and can often be visualized through the posterior capsule of the thyroid.

24.4 Epidemiology of Primary Hyperparathyroidism

The dominant clinical phenotype of PHPT in the USA is asymptomatic hypercalcemia, invariably identified fortuitously in patients undergoing yearly physical examination. The apparent increase in the incidence of PHPT was correlated to the wide availability and use of multichannel laboratory testing since the 1970s [11]. In the Kaiser Permanente study involving 3.5 million people, the incidence of primary hyperparathyroidism varied from 34 to 124 per 100,000 person years. The incidence increases with advancing age and was highest among African Americans followed by Caucasians, with rates for Asians and Hispanics lowest among the ethnicities. Women are affected threefold more frequently than men [12]. Along with the increase in the diagnosis of patients with PHPT, the surgical case volume increased an astounding 177 % in a statewide health planning study from California between 1999 and 2008 [13].

Endorgan dysfunctions include chronic renal disease, stone formation, and bone loss. The vast majority of patients with bone disease are asymptomatic and diagnosed using screening DXA. The lumbar spine BMD is relatively conserved and there is preferential site specific loss of cortical bone site such as the distal third of the radius. The trabecular skeleton in primary hyperparathyroidism is relatively spared; therefore, three site assessments with DXA that includes forearm should be performed in these subjects. Successful parathyroid gland surgery is associated with increase in bone density most rapid at the lumbar spine and hip followed by the distal radius. Therapies such as bisphosphonates and estrogens are also effective. Cinacalcet reduces the elevated serum calcium levels without improvement in bone density. Therefore, surgery appears to be the most definitive treatment for primary hyperparathyroidism [13, 14]. Percutaneous ethanol ablation in selected cases is also effective. These patients are either of advancing age, or have high intra or postoperative risks or those patients who have failed multiple surgeries. The most recent multidisciplinary workshop on asymptomatic primary hyperparathyroidism addressed these themes in 2014 to the current state of knowledge [14].

In the past 10 years, there has been emerging appreciation of eucalcemic primary hyperparathyroidism, often identified during evaluation for fatigue or nonspecific symptoms. Early surgical treatment of normocalcemic patients with isolated elevation or upper end of parathyroid hormone (PTH) levels is controversial [14]. Since surgery is the only definitive treatment to halt the progression of end organ damage due to PHPT, if renal or bone disease remains unexplained or progressive, surgery appears justified. Therefore, normo-alcemic PHPT patients should be evaluated for end organ dysfunction and the most conservative approach would be that they are carefully followed until more information regarding management policies becomes available.

24.5 Imaging Features of Parathyroid Adenomas, Atypical Adenomas and Parathyroid Carcinomas

The size of a parathyroid adenoma is critical for visualization during ultrasonography. Normal, non-enlarged parathyroid glands cannot be visualized reliably with US equipment available at the present time. In eucalcemic, subclinical PHPT patients, it is entirely possible to have a solitary small adenoma and yet elude detection by the USA, even when they are located in the typical sites. Therefore, ultrasound evaluation should not be used as a diagnostic study in any suspected patients with PHPT, including those who have normal or mildly elevated calcium level with elevation of PTH. The characteristic ultrasound appearances of an adenoma are the following:

1. Extrathyroidal and posterior in location to the thyroid lobes
2. The presence of an echogenic line separating the thyroid gland from the adenoma
3. Indentation sign—this can be seen either with superior or inferior adenomas that are abutting the posterior capsule of the thyroid
4. Enlarged parathyroids are uniformly hypoechoic in texture
5. Demonstration of a distinct and independent feeding vessel during color Doppler interrogation (See Video 24.1, references [15–17]).

Parathyroid adenomas present in variable sizes and shapes. They conform to the anatomic pressures of surrounding structures and “meld” into facial planes almost seamlessly. Due to the gradual growth within the facial planes, the can be surprisingly mobile in relation to the neighboring structures. Therefore, they can move or be displaced by excessive pressure with US transducers, swallowing or by asking the patient to make a Valsalva maneuver. Similarly, they can also be better visualized by any of the above maneuvers. Asking the patient to rotate their head in different directions, swallowing, coughing, and staining (Valsalva) should be a part of real-time US evaluation.

Patient positioning is critical for the success of parathyroid localization. Placing one or two pillows under the shoulder for neck extension, and supporting of the neck and vertex with rolled towels, can enable optimal visualization of the superior mediastinal structures. Lower frequency settings (10 mHz or lower) should be chosen for visualization of deeper structures in the neck. Tissue harmonics settings, if available, can also improve visualization of enlarged parathyroid glands. The region below the hyoid bone to the visualized portions of superior mediastinum and trapezius muscles bilaterally should be systematically studied. Particular attention should be devoted to the posterior and the caudal aspect of the thyroid lobes. Also, careful visualization of the thyroid gland and surgical levels of the neck can identify incidental thyroid abnormalities, which is a unique advantage of US compared to MIBI imaging.

24.6 Location of Parathyroid Adenomas

The majority of superior adenomas, up to 70 %, are located posterior to the mid portion of the thyroid lobes. The inferior glands are more variable in their location, but nearly 80 % of the lower glands are still located either just posterior to the lower portion of the thyroid gland or immediately caudal to the lower pole of the thyroid lobes. Less than 10 % of the glands can be located in close approximation to or embedded within the thymus gland. The most difficult to visualize of adenomas by the USA is the posteriorly displaced upper adenomas. These glands can be partially or entirely retropharyngeal, mobile, or can be flattened along the TE grooves. In one large autopsy series from Athens, Greece, which involved examination of 942 cadavers, 5 % had supernumerary glands, 2 % had three glands, 8.5 % were ectopic within the neck, 0.2 % intra-thyroidal, and 6 % were within the mediastinum [18]. The reported frequency of ectopic parathyroid glands following surgical intervention is quite variable, ranging from 5 to 20 %, most likely due to lack of universal definition for what constitutes ectopic locations. For example, in one series involving secondary hyperparathyroidism patients with renal failure reported 39 % frequency of ectopic glands [19]. Figures 24.1, 24.2, 24.3, 24.4, 24.5, 24.6, 24.7, and 24.8 illustrate these principles and the typical appearance of abnormal parathyroid glands on ultrasound.

Parathyroid carcinomas differ in their clinical presentation compared to parathyroid adenomas, rather than by consistent US image findings. Parathyroid carcinoma should be suspected in patients who present with sudden and considerable calcium and PTH elevation. Parathyroid carcinomas can also be palpable. Even very large benign adenomas are not palpable due to their soft consistency. Parathyroid carcinomas or atypical adenomas are usually large, with our without calcific or cystic change (Fig. 24.7). Additionally, irregular margins and lack of distinct planes between the thyroid and an enlarged parathyroid gland should prompt consideration of parathyroid carcinoma.

24.7 Fine Needle Aspiration (FNA) of Parathyroid Glands or Adenomas

FNA can be performed in clinically benign appearing parathyroid tumors for confirmation prior to surgery or percutaneous ethanol injection [20, 21]. Needle tracking of malignant tumor following FNA can occur. Therefore, FNA is best avoided in suspected cases of atypical adenomas or parathyroid carcinomas. It is also best avoided at all during the initial evaluation of primary parathyroid disease. One helpful application of parathyroid FNA is to confirm a suspected lesion as parathyroid tissue in preparation for reoperative parathyroid surgery, especially when other imaging remains ambiguous or the clinical scenario is unusual.

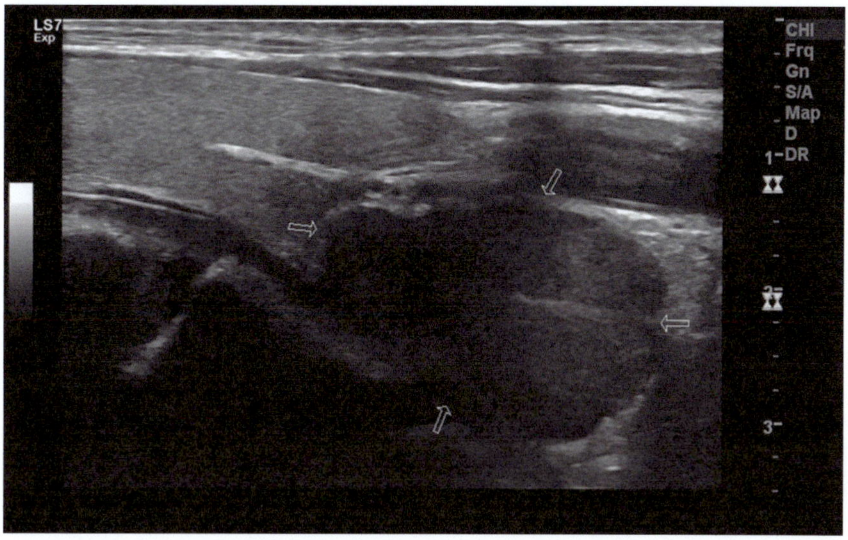

Fig. 24.1 Large inferior adenoma

Fig. 24.2 Trans-upper PA

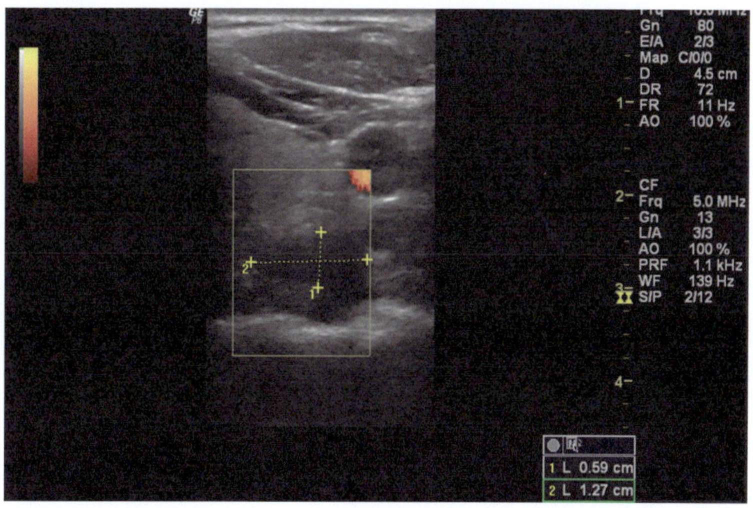

24.8 Procedure of Parathyroid FNA

Parathyroid FNA is performed in the standard manner as one would for FNA of thyroid nodules with few differences. The use of smaller gauge needles causes less trauma and fibrosis of parathyroid adenomas and does not make subsequent surgical removal difficult [22, 23]. Parathyroid FNA can be performed using 25 or 27 G needles with or without local anesthesia. Jabbing technique is best avoided, particularly of smaller lesions to avoid multiple anterior or posterior capsular punctures. Rotation technique with aspiration is sufficient in most occasions. Blood and aspirate materials can be allowed into the hub of the needle. Parathyroid lesions yield a "bloody tap," whereas a "dry-tap" is often encountered in the inadvertent sampling of a central compartment lymph-node.

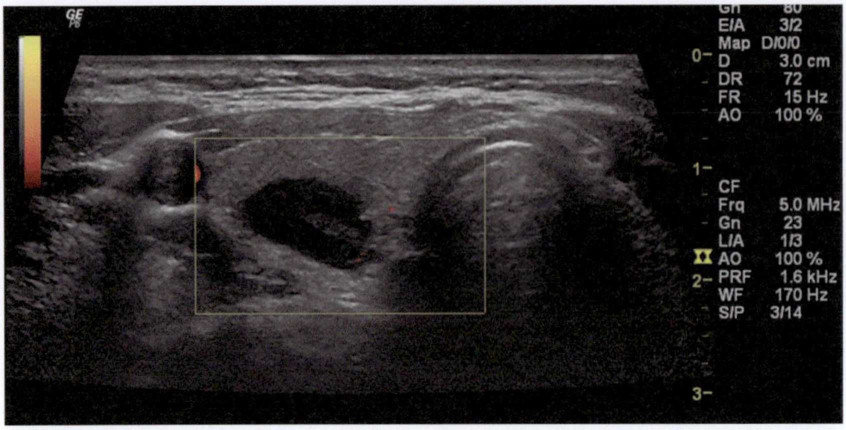

Fig. 24.3 Intrathyroidal adenoma. Note lack of echogenic line

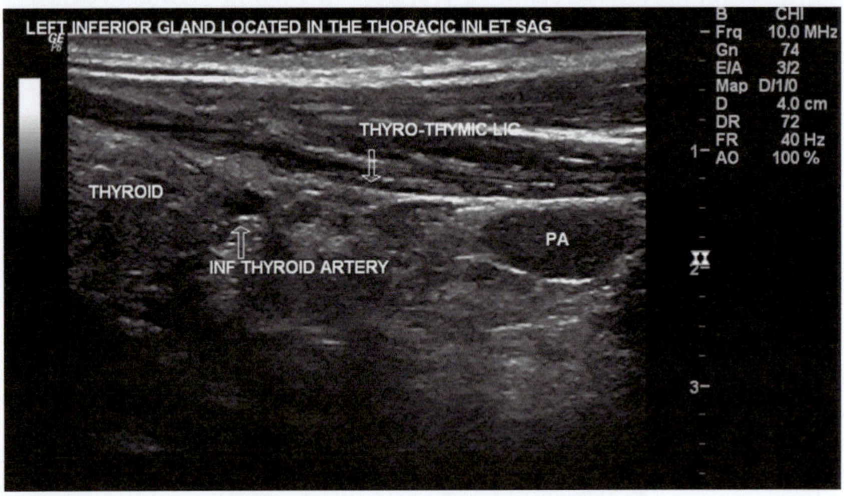

Fig. 24.4 Mediastinal thymic lesion SAG

24.9 A Protocol for Specimen Processing, Handling, and Smear Preparation of Parathyroid FNA (See Fig. 24.9)

Following completion of the biopsy of the suspected abnormal parathyroid gland, one or two direct smears are made with the material. The reminder of the specimen is washed from the syringe with 2 cm^3 of saline and spun in a red top tube (contains no EDTA) for 5 min. The clear or often blood tinged supernatant is separated and submitted for PTH measurement. The specimen should be kept cold or ideally frozen prior to transportation to the laboratory. The cell pellet is saved and refrigerated as a duplicate specimen. In the unfortunate event of lost or mishandled specimen, the pellet can be resuspended in 2 cm^3 of saline and re-spun to yield a second specimen. This technique can avoid unnecessary second FNA on patients. The slides are saved until the PTH FNA washout results are available. If the levels are low, then the slides along with the saved cell pellet should be submitted for cytological analysis. If the PTH FNA washout levels are elevated, then there is no need to submit the smears for cytological analysis. If the PTH levels are low, cytological analysis of the specimen

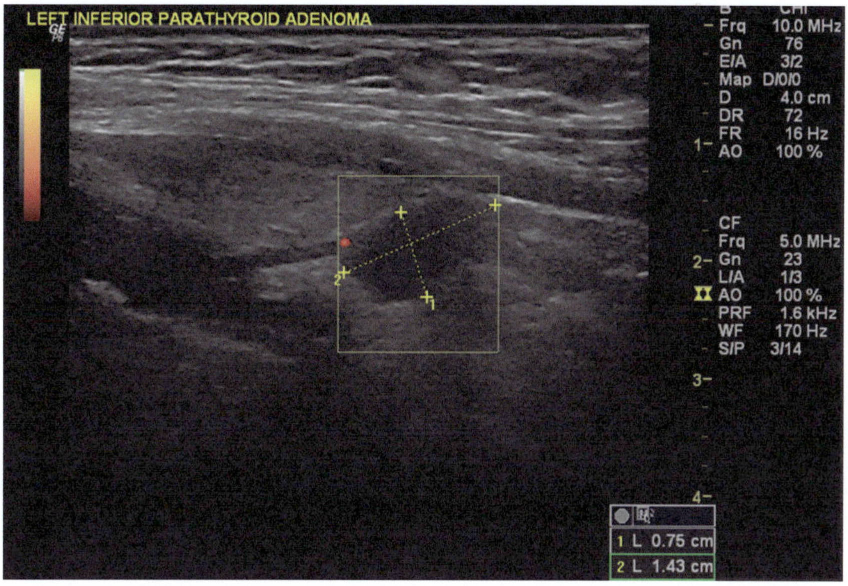

Fig. 24.5 Inferior PA sagittal view

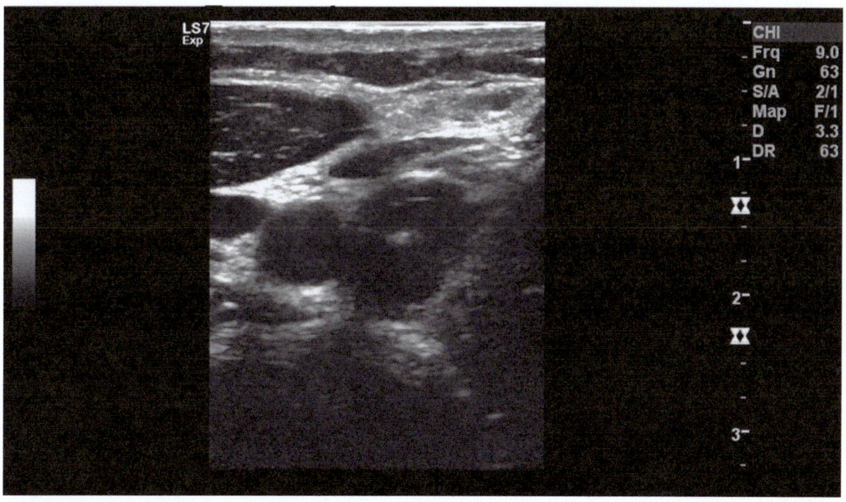

Fig. 24.6 Cystic adenoma FNA

should be performed. This protocol ensures that an inadvertent metastatic neck lymph node is not misdiagnosed during the evaluation of a suspected parathyroid adenoma. It is best to contact the clinical laboratory in each hospital to determine the preferred specimen processing for the red top tube; the details above are included here for the reader's awareness of relevant issues. The syringe washout PTH levels are typically elevated in the several thousand pg/ml range. The lowest PTH that was observed in one study is 40 pg ml [21]. Parathyroid cytology is of limited value in the diagnosis and can often mimic and be misinterpreted by pathologists as a thyroid "follicular neoplasm," especially if the parathyroid tissue source of origin is not communicated to the lab. Thyroid follicular cells and colloid, furthermore, are often encountered on the specimen, due to the inadvertent sampling of thyroid tissue during FNA of superior adenomas [24].

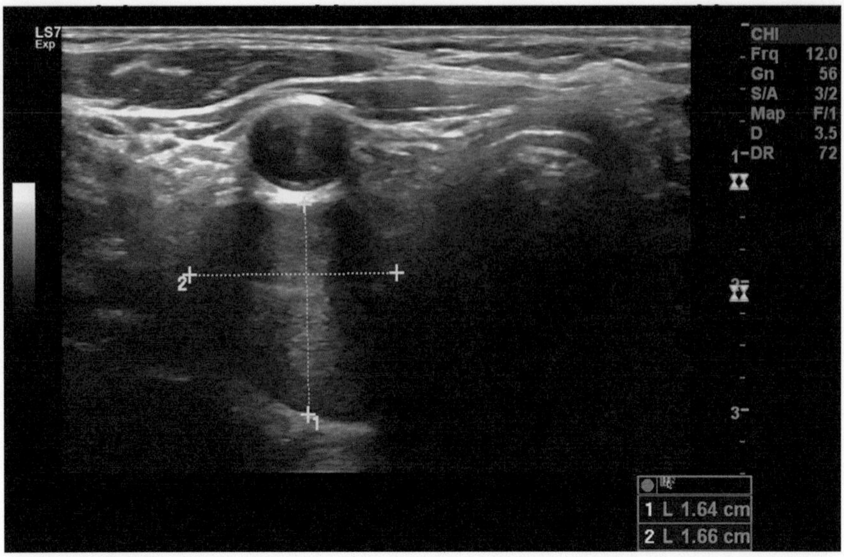

Fig. 24.7 Upper PA atypical location

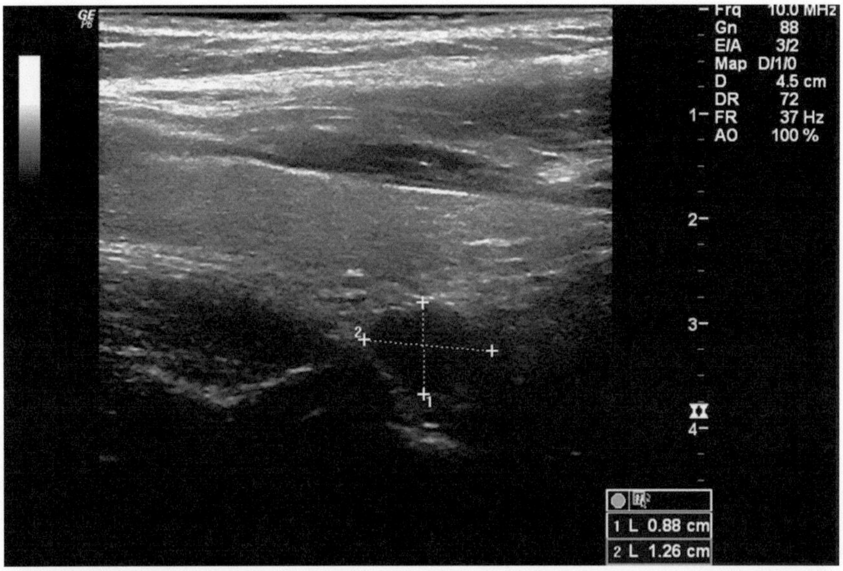

Fig. 24.8 Caudal displacement of superior adenoma

24.10 Indications and Procedure of ETOH Ablation

Surgery is the mainstay for the definitive treatment of PHPT. In an occasional patient, who is deemed to have high surgical risk, percutaneous ethanol ablation may be an alternative option. The indications and contraindications to alcohol ablation are listed in Table 24.1. The procedure is performed in the following manner. The skin and subcutaneous tissue is anesthetized using 2 cm^3 of lidocaine under guidance. Lidocaine infiltration is performed under vision, using US transducer along the facial planes anterior to the parathyroid lesion. Once lidocaine infiltration is complete, the lesion is entered with a 27 or 25 g

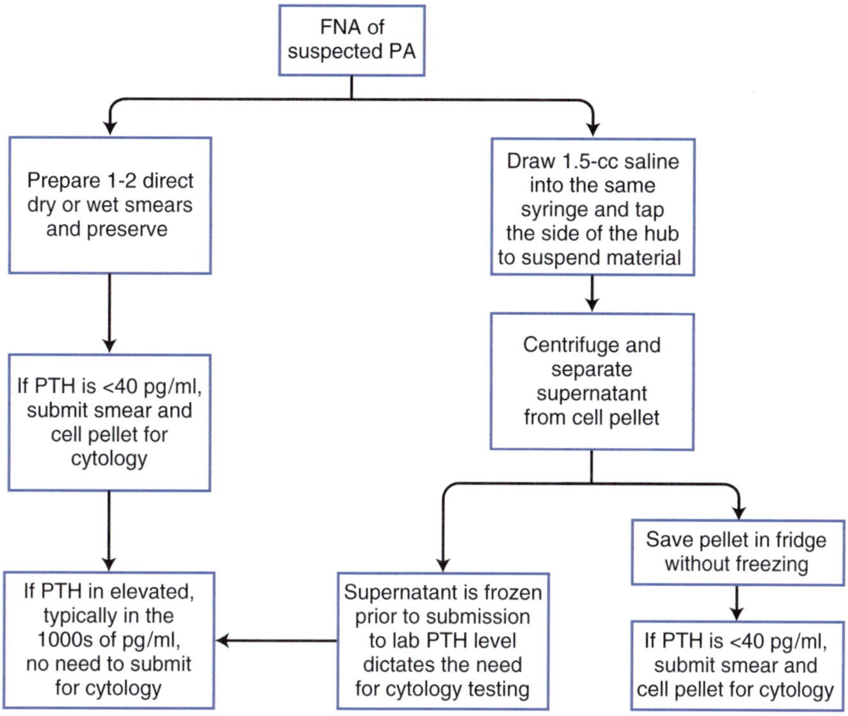

Fig. 24.9 Specimen processing flow chart

Table 24.1 Indications and contraindications of parathyroid FNA

Indications	Contraindications
Failed surgery	Anticoagulation (relative)
Multiple lesions	Morbid obesity (relative)
Intrathyroidal location	Deeply located lesion (relative)
Atypical location or appearance	Partial or complete obscuration by vital structures
Ethanol ablation	Suspected parathyroid carcinoma (absolute)

needle that is loaded with 0.5–1 cm^3 of alcohol. The alcohol is injected into the target lesion in question (Video 24.2). Great care should be taken to avoid injection outside the parathyroid lesion. This can result in tissue necrosis. Similarly, puncturing of the posterior or medial aspect of the capsule should be avoided altogether. The risk for injury to recurrent laryngeal nerve is greater in such situations. Patients sometimes complain of a twinge or dull ache for 5–10 min. The disappearance of blood flow by Doppler predicts success of injection. If blood flow into the gland is unaffected by the injection 5–10 min following the first injection, a second injection may be administered. Ethanol ablation can be effective in multiple endocrine neoplasia patients who have recurrent primary hyperparathyroidism [25].

24.11 Special Considerations: Multigland Disease, Atypical Adenomas, and Parathyroid Carcinomas

The use of ultrasound localization in multiple endocrine neoplasia and renal failure patients has utility, but it is unlikely to reveal the location of all abnormal glands. Whether the USA detects only one or multiple glands, the underlying clinical biology is four-gland hyperplasia and these patients require bilateral neck exploration [19]. Hence, the utility of ultrasound is to identify where a parathyroid gland has not been seen and to correlate with other imaging studies, so that surgery can proceed efficiently and focus on ensuring glands are not missed in these locations. Furthermore, the identification of concomitant thyroid disease remains important in these subgroups of patients.

Parathyroid carcinomas and atypical adenomas present in a rapidly progressive fashion [26]. The long lag time of gradual development of hypercalcemia is typically absent. The CDC-73 gene codes for a tumor suppressor protein called parafibromin. A common syndrome related to CDC-73 mutation is the Hyperparathyroidism—Jaw Tumor Syndrome (JPT-JT) syndrome. These patients are often in their late adolescence or young adulthood and manifest other findings such as ossifying fibromas of the maxilla or mandible, renal, and uterine tumors. The vast majority of individuals with HPT-JT present with benign single parathyroid adenomas (85 %), which require careful biochemical monitoring for recurrence in other glands. In suspected parathyroid carcinoma patients, the surgery should aim to remove the parathyroid tumor en-bloc along with the adjacent thyroid lobe and intraoperative clear margins with respect to other adjacent anatomy (thus, the procedure is a parathyroidectomy with ipsilateral thyroid lobectomy and often ipsilateral central neck lymph node removal). Genetic testing is recommended in subjects diagnosed with atypical adenoma or parathyroid carcinomas. Germline CDC-73 related disorders are inherited in an autosomal dominant fashion. About 20 % of individuals with sporadic parathyroid carcinomas harbor CDC-73 mutation. About 15 % of subjects with CDC-73 germline mutations present with parathyroid carcinomas [23]. Parathyroid carcinomas often manifest calcifications, cystic changes, or irregular margins.

24.12 Parathyroid Incidentalomas and Confounders

Parathyroid like lesions encountered incidentally during neck or thyroid imaging are not uncommon in clinical practice. These tumors have the imaging phenotype and likeness of a parathyroid adenoma but actually represent other tissues such as lymph nodes or thymus. Serum chemistry testing can reveal calcium or PTH elevation to determine previously undiagnosed PHPT subjects. The confirmatory test is FNA PTH measurement from the lesion following a biopsy [27].

24.13 Summary

Parathyroid ultrasonography is a valuable tool for the assessment of diseased parathyroid glands in patients with primary hyperparathyroidism. It serves as a valuable tool to assess the thyroid gland prior to parathyroid surgery. Also, it enables the conduct of percutaneous ethanol ablation.

References

1. Owen R. On the anatomy of the Indian Rhinoceros (Rh. Unicornis L.). Trans Zool Soc Lond. 1862;4:31–58.
2. Johansson H. The Uppsala anatomist Ivar Sandström and the parathyroid gland. Upsala J Med Sci. 2015;112:72–7.
3. Rogers-Stevane J, Kauffman GL. A historical perspective on surgery of the thyroid and parathyroid glands. Otolaryngol Clin N Am. 2008;41(6):1059–67.
4. Spence HM. The life and death of Captain Charles Martell and kidney stone disease. J Urol. 1984;132(6):1204–7.
5. Udelsman R, Donovan PI. Open minimally invasive parathyroid surgery. World J Surg. 2004;28(12):1224–6.
6. Yao K, Singer FR, Roth SI, Sassoon A, Ye C, Giuliano AE. Weight of normal parathyroid glands in patients with parathyroid adenomas. J Clin Endocrinol Metab. 2004;89:320–3213.
7. Akerstrom T, Makmaeus J, Bergstrom R. Surgical anatomy of human parathyroid glands. Surgery. 1984;95:14–21.
8. Gilmore JR. The gross anatomy of parathyroid glands. J Pathol. 1938;46:133.
9. Alveryd A. Parathyroid glands in thyroid surgery. Acta Chir Scand. 1968;389:1.
10. Wang CA, Mahaffey JE, Axelrod L, et al. Hyperfunctioning supernumerary parathyroid glands. Surg Gynecol Obstet. 1979;148:711.
11. Heath III H, Hodgson SF, Kennedy M. Primary hyperparathyroidism: incidence, morbidity and potential economic impact in a community. N Engl J Med. 1980;302:189–93.
12. Yeh MW, Ituarte PHG, Zhou HC, et al. Incidence and prevalence of primary hyperparathyroidism in a racially mixed population. J Clin Endocrinol Metab. 2013;98(3):1122–9.
13. Abdulla AG, Ituarte P, Harari A, Wu JX, Yeh MW. Trends in the frequency and quality of parathy-

roid surgery: analysis of 17,082 cases over 10 years. Ann Surg. 2015;261(4):746–50.
14. Eastell R, Brandi ML, Costa AG, D'Amour P, Shoback DM, Thakker RV. Diagnosis of asymptomatic primary hyperparathyroidism: Proceedings of the Fourth International Workshop. J Clin Endocrinol Metab. 2014;99:3570–9.
15. Kamaya A, Quon A, Jeffrey RB. Sonography of the abnormal parathyroid gland. Ultrasound Q. 2006;22(4):253–62.
16. Lane MJ, Desser TS, Weigel RJ, Jeffrey Jr RB. Use of color and power Doppler sonography to identify feeding arteries associated with parathyroid adenomas. AJR Am J Roentgenol. 1998;171(3):819–23.
17. Wolf RJ, Cronan JJ, Monchik JM. Color Doppler sonography: an adjunctive technique in assessment of parathyroid adenomas. J Ultrasound Med. 1994;13(4):303–8.
18. Lappas D, Noussios G, Anagnostis P, Adamidou F, Chatzigeorgiou A, Skandalakis P. Location, number and morphology of parathyroid glands: results from a large anatomical series. Anat Sci Int. 2012;87:160–4.
19. Schneider R, Waldmann J, Ramaswamy A, Fernández ED, Bartsch DK, Schlosser K. Frequency of ectopic and supernumerary intra-thymic parathyroid glands in patients with renal hyperparathyroidism: analysis of 461 patients undergoing initial parathyroidectomy with bilateral cervical thymectomy. World J Surg. 2011;35(6):1260–5.
20. Doppman JL, Krudy AG, Marx SJ, Saxe A, Schneider P, Norton JA, Spiegel AM, Downs RW, Schaaf M, Brennan ME, Schneider AB, Aurbach GD. Aspiration of enlarged parathyroid glands for parathyroid hormone assay. Radiology. 1983;148(1):31–5.
21. Abraham D, Sharma PK, Bentz J, Gault PM, Neumayer L, McClain DA. The utility of ultrasound guided FNA of parathyroid adenomas for preoperative localization prior to minimally invasive parathyroidectomy. Endocr Pract. 2007;13(4):333–7.
22. Norman J, Politz D, Browarski E. Diagnostic aspiration of parathyroid adenomas causes severe fibrosis complicating surgery and final histologic diagnosis. Thyroid. 2007;17(12):1251–5.
23. Abraham D, Duick AS, Baskin HJ. Appropriate administration of fine-needle aspiration (FNA) biopsy on selective parathyroid adenomas is safe. Thyroid. 2008;18(5):581–2.
24. Agarwal AM, Bentz JS, Hungerford R, Abraham D. Parathyroid fine-needle aspiration cytology in the evaluation of parathyroid adenoma: cytologic findings from 53 patients. Diagn Cytopathol. 2009;37:407–10.
25. Naykky SO, Thompson GB, Lee RA, Reading CC, Young Jr WF. Safety and efficacy of percutaneous parathyroid ethanol ablation in patients with recurrent primary hyperparathyroidism and multiple endocrine neoplasia type 1. J Clin Endocrinol Metab. 2015;100(1):E87–90.
26. Sharretts JM, Kebebew E, Simonds WF. Parathyroid cancer. Semin Oncol. 2010;37(6):580–90.
27. Pesenti M, Frasoldati A, Azzarito C, Valcavi R. Parathyroid incidentaloma discovered during thyroid ultrasound imaging. J Endocrinol Invest. 1999;22(10):796–9.

Ultrasound as a Localization Technique in Hyperparathyroidism

25

Colleen M. Kiernan and Carmen C. Solórzano

25.1 Introduction

Bilateral neck exploration for the treatment of sporadic primary hyperparathyroidism (HPT) has a success rate ranging from 94 to 98 % when performed by experienced parathyroid surgeons [1–3]. Minimally invasive focused parathyroidectomy, with its potential advantages of smaller incisions, lesser dissection, and eligibility for outpatient surgery, has become the preferred surgical approach to HPT [4]. To allow a focused dissection while maintaining the same success rate as the gold standard bilateral exploration (BE), focused parathyroidectomy requires accurate preoperative imaging and intraoperative adjuncts. Furthermore, surgeons who perform BE routinely will also use imaging studies to identify the dominant gland, speed the efficiency of the operation, and avoid extensive dissection.

While imaging studies guide the surgeon to the precise location of the abnormal parathyroid gland, intraoperative parathyroid hormone monitoring (IPM) assures the surgeon that all the hyperfunctioning tissue has been removed before leaving the operating room thereby avoiding higher failure rates [5]. Localization studies should not be used to diagnose hyperparathyroidism or to indicate operative intervention. Rather, once the patient has a secure biochemical diagnosis, the surgeon depends on accurate localization to allow a focused imaged guided approach or to speed up the completion of a bilateral approach. Most experienced parathyroid surgeons are proponents of localization studies with the most commonly used method being a combination of ultrasonography (US) and Technitium-99m sestamibi scintigraphy (MIBI). Four-dimensional computed tomography (4DCT) is, however, gaining popularity as a primary localization study [6]. This review will focus on the use of US as a localization technique in HPT and will discuss its practical utility particularly when performed by the parathyroid surgeon.

Electronic supplementary material: The online version of this chapter (doi:10.1007/978-3-319-44100-9_25) contains supplementary material, which is available to authorized users Videos can also be accessed at http://link.springer.com/chapter/10.1007/978-3-319-44100-9_25.

C.M. Kiernan, M.D., M.P.H.
Department of General Surgery, Vanderbilt University, 1161 21st Ave S, CCC-4312 MCN, Nashville, TN 37232, USA
e-mail: colleen.m.kiernan@vanderbilt.edu

C.C. Solórzano, M.D., F.A.C.S. (✉)
Division of Surgical Oncology and Endocrine Surgery, Department of Surgery, Vanderbilt University Medical Center, 597 PRB, 2220 Pierce Ave, Nashville, TN 37232, USA
e-mail: Carmen.solorzano@vanderbilt.edu

M. Milas et al. (eds.), *Advanced Thyroid and Parathyroid Ultrasound*,
DOI 10.1007/978-3-319-44100-9_25

25.2 Education of Surgeons in Parathyroid Ultrasound

In the mid 1990s, US began to be adopted in general surgical practice. Residents in general surgery today are increasingly exposed to ultrasound for central line placement, FAST examinations in trauma (Focused Assessment with Sonography in Trauma), assessment of hernias, liver, gallbladder and appendix, and less commonly exposed to breast, thyroid, parathyroid, and cervical/axillary lymph node examination. Formal training in ultrasound for surgeons is provided by the American College of Surgeons and consists of a postgraduate course with didactic lectures, hands-on skill sessions with formal US examination of patient volunteers, practice fine needle aspiration biopsy (FNA) on phantoms, and faculty observation and written examination [7]. Commercially available US units are now readily available; they are portable and easy to use in clinician's offices, emergency and operating rooms [8].

25.3 Ultrasound in Patients with Primary Hyperparathyroidism: Why Not?

To obtain the best results, US for parathyroid localization should be performed with high-resolution probes and by a dedicated parathyroid ultrasonographer. This method of parathyroid gland localization is convenient, does not involve radiation exposure, is noninvasive, provides the surgeon with excellent detailed topographic information, identifies concomitant thyroid pathology, and it is the least costly parathyroid localization. In the author's opinion, US should be performed in all patients undergoing parathyroidectomy due to the following:

1. High incidence of concomitant thyroid disease in patients with primary hyperparathyroidism (HPT)
2. US can accurately localize the abnormal parathyroid and assess its relationship to the thyroid and surrounding structures, thus helping the surgeon with operative planning
3. Parathyroid US is cost effective.

25.3.1 Concomitant Thyroid Disease

Thyroid disease occurs in up to two thirds of patients with HPT [9]. Compared to intraoperative evaluation, preoperative assessment of thyroid nodules leads to a higher sensitivity for discovery and a lower rate of non-indicated thyroid procedures than intraoperative evaluation alone [10]. Newly encountered thyroid pathology should be identified and addressed preoperatively modifying the surgical procedure accordingly [11, 12]. US is also useful to avoid possible pitfalls during parathyroidectomy, such as in a patient with prior ablative radioiodine (RAI) treatment for Graves' and MIBI uptake in the right neck (Figs. 25.1, 25.2, and 25.3) or a patient who has an intra-thyroidal parathyroid (Figs. 25.4 and 25.5).

25.3.2 US to Localize the Parathyroid and Help with Operative Planning

When US is performed by an experienced sonographer it can accurately identify the parathyroid abnormality in 76–89 % of cases and help the surgeon direct the exploration [13–19]. A parathyroid that is behind the mid or upper portion of the thyroid lobe on ultrasound is usually a superior gland and it will likely be in a posterior location at exploration. An enlarged parathyroid that is near the lower pole of the thyroid or near the clavicle is most likely an inferior gland and the surgeon should look in a more anterior location near the lower thyroid pole, the thyro-thymic ligament, or the thymus (see the next section for interpretation of US images). A "negative" US can inform the surgeon on "what is not there." For instance, with a "negative" US, the surgeon can surmise that the adenoma may be in a posteriorly located para-esophageal/tracheoesophageal position, which is not easily imaged by US, and direct the exploration to such area first. In this patient the MIBI could show a "low cervical adenoma" confirming that this is a superior gland that has moved to the low neck by growth (Fig. 25.6). Furthermore, the sonographer should not accept a "negative" US unless the upper neck, the carotid sheath, and the area just under the

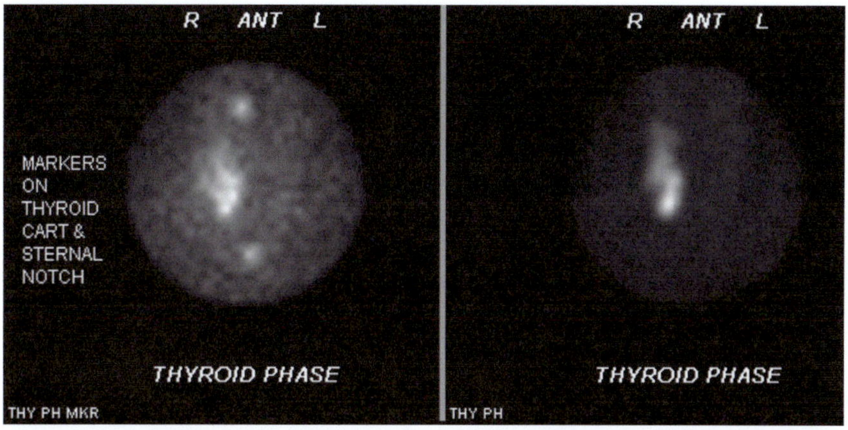

Fig. 25.1 Early planar Sestamibi scan in a patient with Graves' disease treated with RAI. Notice absence of uptake in the left thyroid lobe and positive uptake in the right thyroid and lower cervical parathyroid

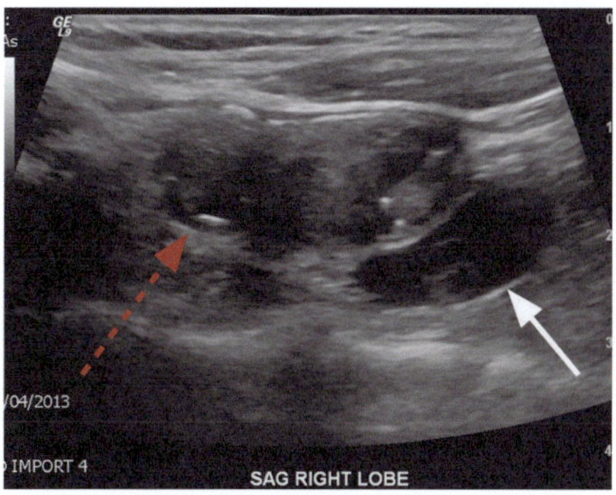

Fig. 25.2 Ultrasound sagittal view of the right lobe confirms the presence of multiple thyroid nodules (*red arrow*) and a right inferior parathyroid (*white arrow*) in a patient with Graves' who had prior RAI ablation

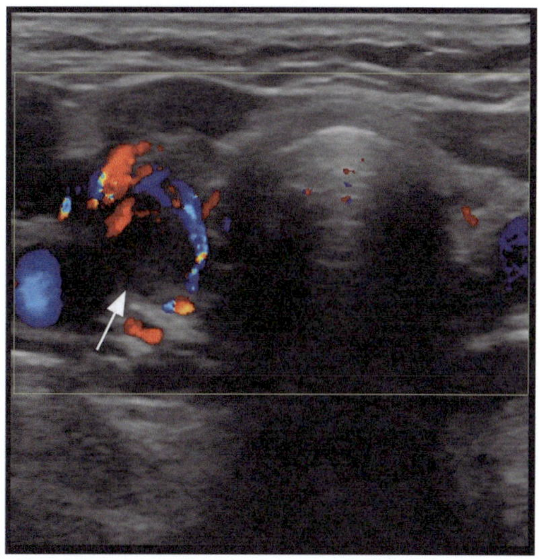

Fig. 25.3 Ultrasound in transverse view showing an arc of vascularity around the right inferior parathyroid in a patient with Graves' treated with RAI ablation

clavicle and sternal notch have been carefully imaged (see below).

In patients with prior thyroid operations or after ablative RAI (Figs. 25.1, 25.2, and 25.3) US is critical to evaluate whether thyroid tissue is still present in the neck and to correlate with MIBI scan (if one was performed). The radiologist reading the MIBI scan and without clinical history may assume incorrectly that what is imaged in the para-tracheal space is thyroid when in fact it is parathyroid tissue in the setting of ablated, surgically removed, or agenesis of the thyroid lobe (Fig. 25.7, Video 25.1).

A contemporary meta-analysis evaluated the accuracy of common preoperative localization techniques in patients with primary hyperparathyroidism against the gold standard of intraoperative visualization and histology. The pooled sensitivity and positive predictive value of US was 76.1 % (57–89 %) and 93.2 % (85–100 %), respectively [20]. Ruda et al. reviewed the literature from 1995 to 2003 and reported US sensitivity of 79 % in localizing abnormal parathyroid glands [21]. It is important to know that the results of US are operator dependent and can be negatively influenced by the presence of thyroid nodular disease, increased body mass index, presence of multiglandular/ectopic parathyroid

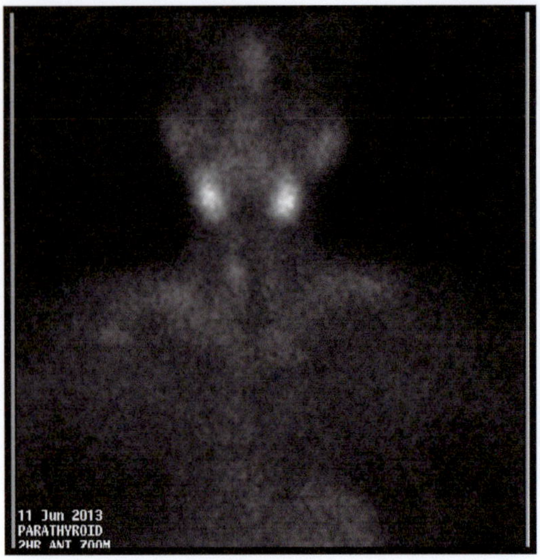

Fig. 25.4 Planar Sestamibi scan showing a right-sided likely superior parathyroid

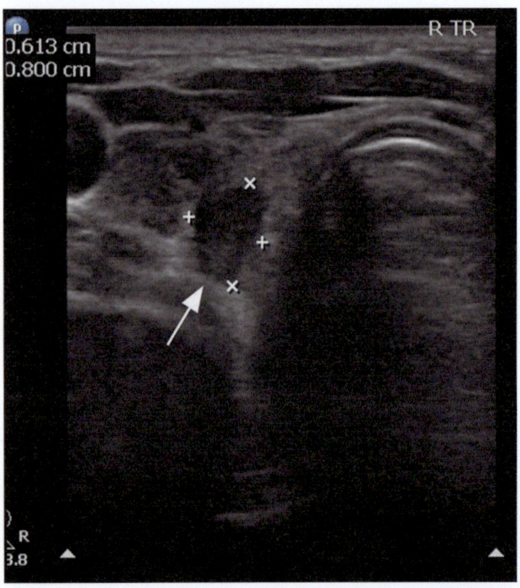

Fig. 25.5 Transverse view ultrasound indicating that the parathyroid gland, which was identified on Sestamibi scan, is intra-thyroidal (*arrow*)

disease, and small parathyroid size [22]. Posterior thyroid nodules and cysts can be mistaken for a parathyroid adenoma and visa-versa. US is less sensitive when parathyroids are located behind the trachea, esophagus, in the superior mediastinum and in patients with thyroiditis who may have extensive reactive adenopathy.

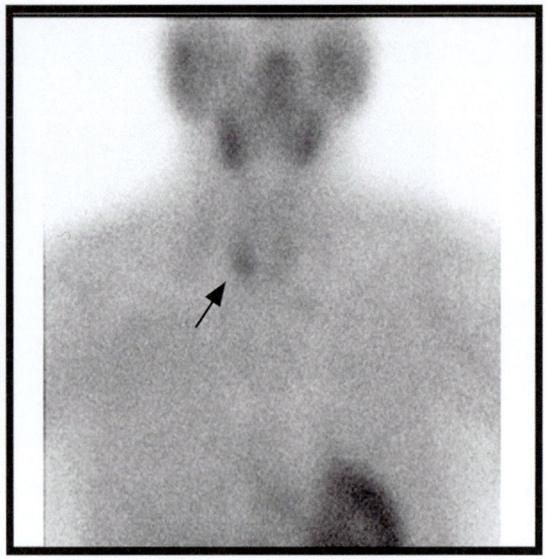

Fig. 25.6 Planar delayed view of Sestamibi scan showing a lower cervical parathyroid adenoma (*arrow*). Because the ultrasound was "negative" (not shown) the surgeon should suspect this to be a superior gland deep in the tracheoesophageal groove

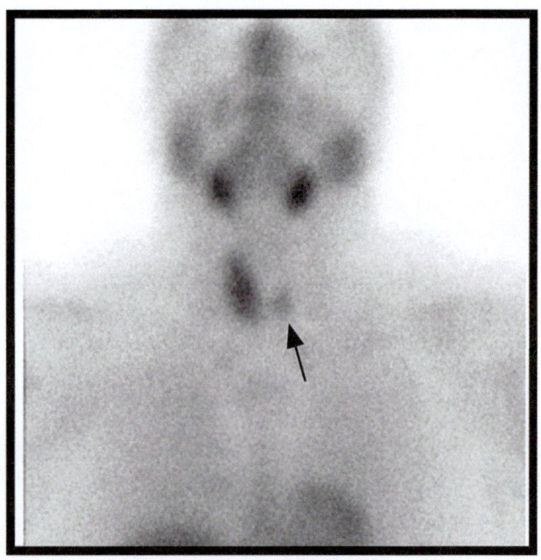

Fig. 25.7 Planar early phase Sestamibi showing an "atrophic" left lobe (*arrow*)

25.3.3 Cost-Effectiveness of Ultrasound

Wang et al. reported on a cost-utility analysis to optimize preoperative imaging for HPT [23]. A decision tree was constructed to determine the incremental cost-utility ratio of five localization strategies: (1) US; (2) MIBI with single photon emission tomography (SPECT); (3) 4DCT; (4) MIBI-SPECT and US; and (5) MIBI-SPECT and US ± 4DCT (4DCT added when MIBI and US were discordant). The authors concluded that US is the least expensive imaging modality. Yet, the most cost-effective strategy involved the use of US combined with MIBI-SPECT and if needed 4DCT. This strategy costs less and accrued more "utility" (a measure of quality of life) mostly because BE was avoided, hence decreasing the overall cost of parathyroidectomy. Interestingly, utilizing MIBI-SPECT as the sole localization study was the least cost-effective strategy.

In another economic analysis of preoperative localization strategies for HPT, Lubitz and colleagues constructed a decision-analytic model to evaluate eight different localization strategies [24]. The authors concluded that US followed by 4DCT when the US results were indeterminate, was the least costly strategy. Differences in cost were largely based on improved sensitivity for detecting single-gland disease and, therefore, on the proportion of patients able to undergo minimally invasive focused procedures with shorter operating time and same-day discharge.

Both studies mentioned above concluded that the cost of BE without localization was always higher, even when the sensitivity of localization studies was lowest (i.e., localization studies were least useful). Most cost-effectiveness studies assume that the majority of patients undergoing BE will require longer operating times and overnight stays in the hospital, therefore driving the costs of parathyroidectomy higher. Currently, a growing number of high-volume parathyroid surgeons who perform BE via small incisions will discharge their patients the same day, possibly neutralizing the cost of such approach when compared to minimally invasive procedures [25, 26].

The authors use surgeon-performed US (SUS) in all patients with HPT who are scheduled for parathyroidectomy. When a clear parathyroid adenoma is localized by SUS, patients are explored using US as the only localization study [14, 27]. However, the authors always use IPM to avoid missing multiple gland disease. Recently, Untch et al. confirmed previous findings that SUS has the same sensitivity as MIBI scans and can be used as the only localization study resulting in excellent operative success when parathyroidectomy is guided by IPM [17].

25.4 Parathyroid Embryology and Anatomy as It Relates to Parathyroid Ultrasound Interpretation

Ideally, the sonographer and the operating surgeon should have a thorough understanding of parathyroid embryology and anatomy. Most patients will have four parathyroid glands (two superior and two inferior), although <4 glands and supernumerary glands can be encountered in up to 3–13 % of cases, respectively [28, 29]. Understanding the parathyroid glands eutopic and ectopic locations is of utmost importance in the interpretation of imaging studies as it relates to the surgical procedure. The surgeon should always review all the radiologic images when planning the operative approach never relying on the radiology report alone. The superior glands are derived from the fourth branchial pouch along with the lateral lobes of the thyroid. The inferior glands arise from the third pouch along with the thymus (further discussion below). Superior and inferior glands are typically symmetric to each other (80 % and 70 % of the time respectively).

25.4.1 Typical Ultrasound Appearance and Location of Parathyroid Adenomas

The typical US appearance and location of an inferior parathyroid adenoma is depicted in Figs. 25.8 and 25.9 and Video 25.2. On grayscale imaging, parathyroid adenomas are predominantly solid lesions with well-defined margins. Internal echo texture is nearly always homogenous and hypoechoic when compared to the thyroid (Table 25.1). A parathyroid is usually separated from the thyroid by a well-defined echogenic tissue plane [30]. Enlarged parathyroids are almost always >1 cm, oval but can also be kidney shaped, bilobed, or multi-lobulated.

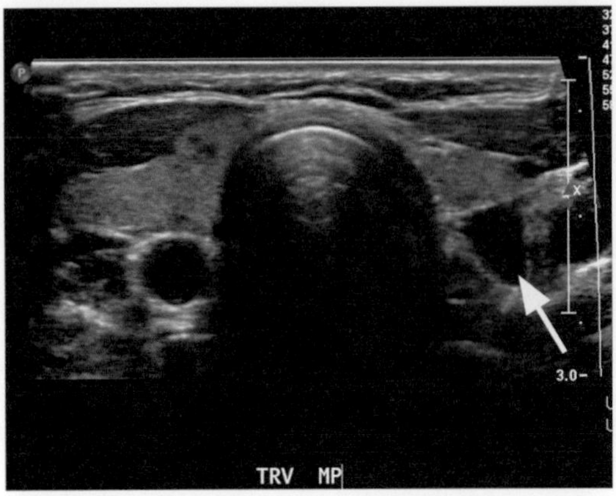

Fig. 25.8 Transverse ultrasound view of a typical wedge-shaped inferior parathyroid adenoma (*arrow*)

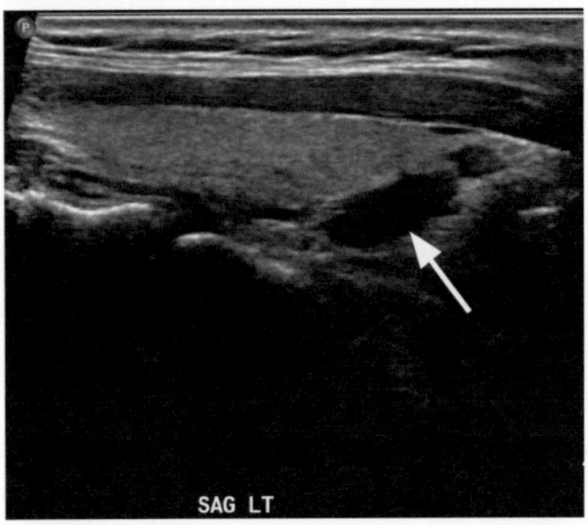

Fig. 25.9 Longitudinal ultrasound view of a typical inferior parathyroid adenoma (*arrow*)

Table 25.1 Typical and atypical ultrasound characteristics of abnormal parathyroids

Typical	Atypical
Solid	Cystic areas
Homogenous	Heterogenous
Smooth well defined borders	Infiltrative or irregular borders
Oblong, tear drop, or oval shaped	Lobulated
Not calcified	Calcified
Polar artery on Doppler	Highly vascular on Doppler
Single	Multiple
Located along the margins of the thyroid gland	Ectopic locations: retro-esophagus, high in the neck above the thyroid, in the thymic tongue, deep in the mediastinum, in the thyroid

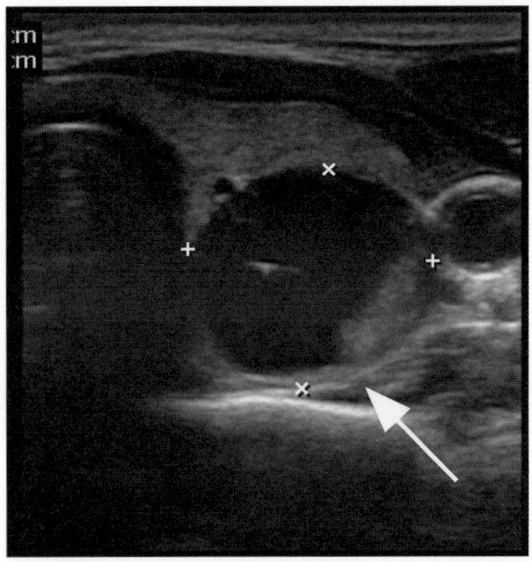

Fig. 25.10 Transverse ultrasound view of a cystic and heterogenous left parathyroid adenoma

On color Doppler sonography, parathyroid adenomas are very vascular. Color Doppler usually shows a peripheral vascular arc arising from the inferior thyroid artery and encircling the gland 90–270° (Fig. 25.3). This feature may help distinguish a parathyroid from a lymph node. The polar artery usually arborizes around the parathyroid vs. a lymph node will have a more hilar vascular flow (Video 25.3). Atypical parathyroids may be cystic (Figs. 25.10 and 25.11), heterogenous, echogenic, have a dual concentric sign and/or calcified (Fig. 25.12) [31–33].

The three most common locations for the inferior parathyroid can be easily imaged by US (see below). Sonographers should always scan posterior to the clavicle by angling the US probe under it and asking the patient to swallow. This maneuver is helpful in localization of thymic or thoracic inlet parathyroid glands. Such glands can be common in patients with secondary hyperparathyroidism due to renal failure (Fig. 25.13a, b; Video 25.3). When US fails to reveal an abnormal parathyroid in its eutopic location, the lateral high neck, particularly the area medial to the carotid artery (Level II lymph node basin/carotid bulb area) should be carefully scanned looking for a rare ectopic and/or undescended gland.

The location of the superior parathyroid is less variable, yet its posterior position can be challenging to visualize with US, particularly in obese patients, male patients, those with goiters, or in the presence of thyroiditis (Fig. 25.14).

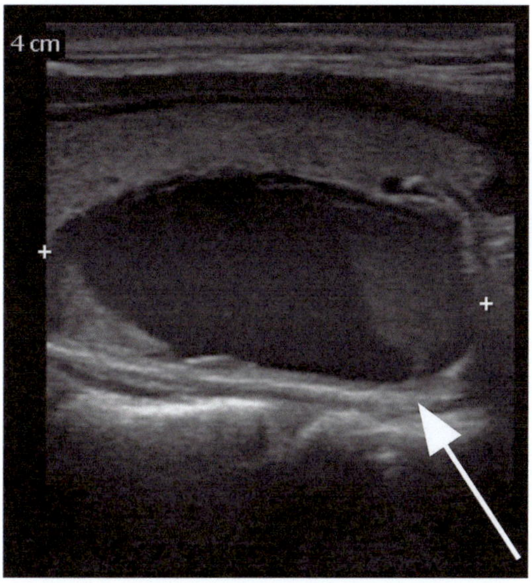

Fig. 25.11 Longitudinal ultrasound view of a cystic and heterogenous left parathyroid adenoma

25.4.2 Superior Parathyroid Anatomic and Imaging Location

The superior parathyroids are usually located in a posterior plane when compared to the inferior glands. The possible location of the superior para-

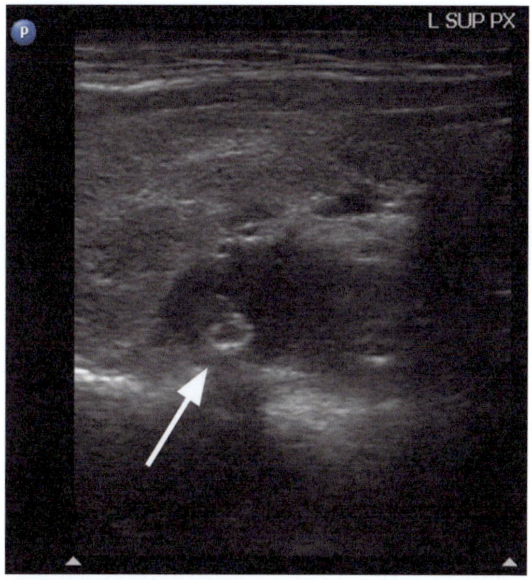

Fig. 25.12 Longitudinal ultrasound view of a calcified left superior parathyroid in a renal failure patient (*arrow* on calcium)

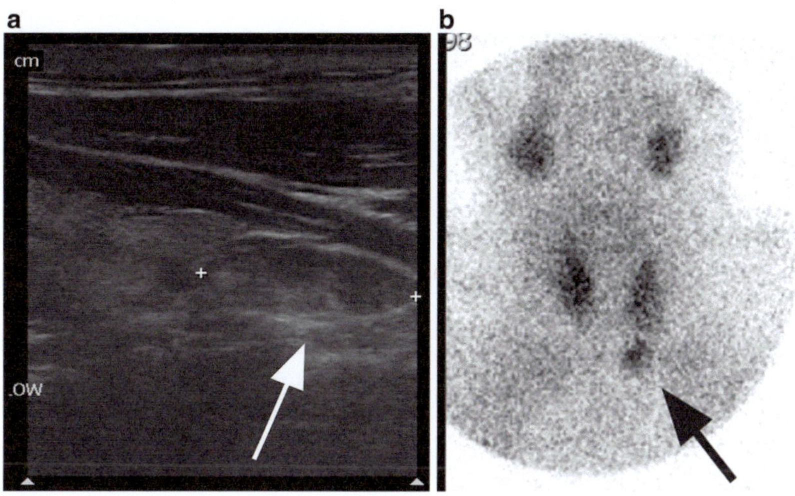

Fig. 25.13 (**a**) Longitudinal ultrasound view of a heterogenous thyro-thymic parathyroid in a patient with renal failure. Note that the overlying strap muscles are seen to diverge toward the right side of the panel (caudad on the patient)—this is a clue that the longitudinal image captured is from a location close the clavicles. (**b**) Dual phase planar sestamibi on the same patient confirming the thyro-thymic left-sided parathyroid

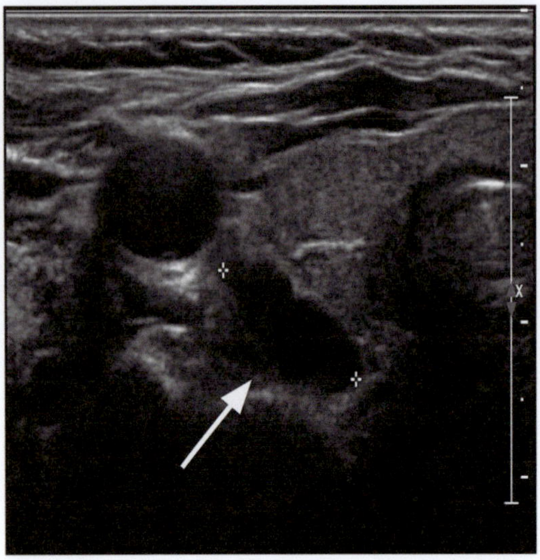

Fig. 25.14 Transverse ultrasound view of a typical hypoechoic oblong superior right-sided parathyroid (*arrow*)

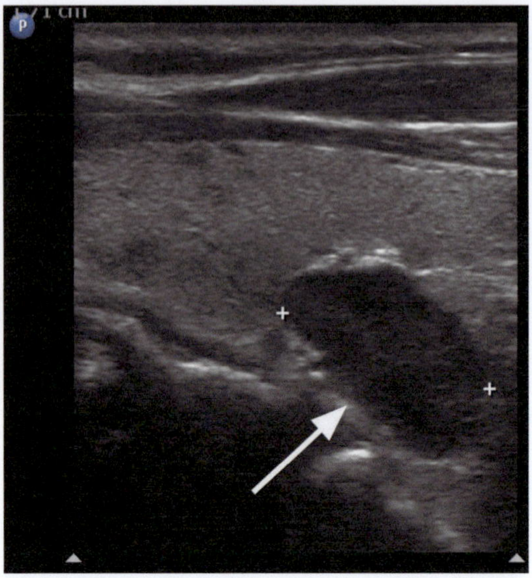

Fig. 25.16 Longitudinal ultrasound view of a superior right-sided parathyroid adenoma (*arrow*)

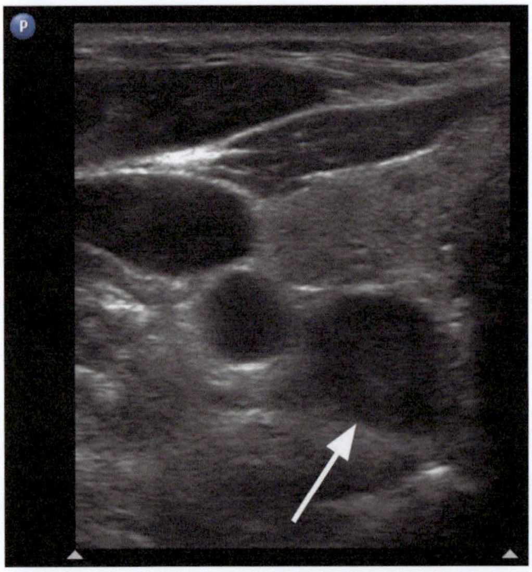

Fig. 25.15 Transverse ultrasound view of a superior right-sided parathyroid adenoma (*arrow*)

thyroid is posterior to the mid portion of the superior thyroid lobe near the cricothyroid junction (>90 %) posterior to the mid thyroid lobe (4 %) (Figs. 25.15 and 25.16), superior to the thyroid lobe (3 %) (Fig. 25.17a–c), in the retropharyngeal/retroesophageal location (1 %), or intra-thyroidal (0.2 %) [28, 29, 34]. A superior gland that has "fallen down" due to growth and gravity into the tracheoesophageal groove or para-esophageal area can be imaged in a relatively low cervical location [35] (Fig. 25.18). The inexperienced radiologist or surgeon may interpret this as an inferior gland when in fact it is a superior gland that has grown enough to migrate low in the neck [36]. In effect, one of the most common locations of a missed parathyroid during a prior failed parathyroidectomy is a superior gland in the posterior and low paraesophageal area [37]. The posterior location of the superior gland can, therefore, be confirmed on ultrasound (Fig. 25.18, Video 25.4), 4DCT, SPECT/CT MIBI images, or the oblique images of a planar dual phase MIBI scan. Similarly, a retropharyngeal/retroesophageal superior gland may not be apparent on US while 4DCT and MIBI with SPECT or MIBI SPECT/CT are more suitable to image such posterior/deep locations. An intrathyroidal parathyroid gland can be localized with MIBI scans; however, ultrasound is ideal in assisting the surgeon to determine if the abnormality is indeed parathyroid tissue (Fig. 25.5).

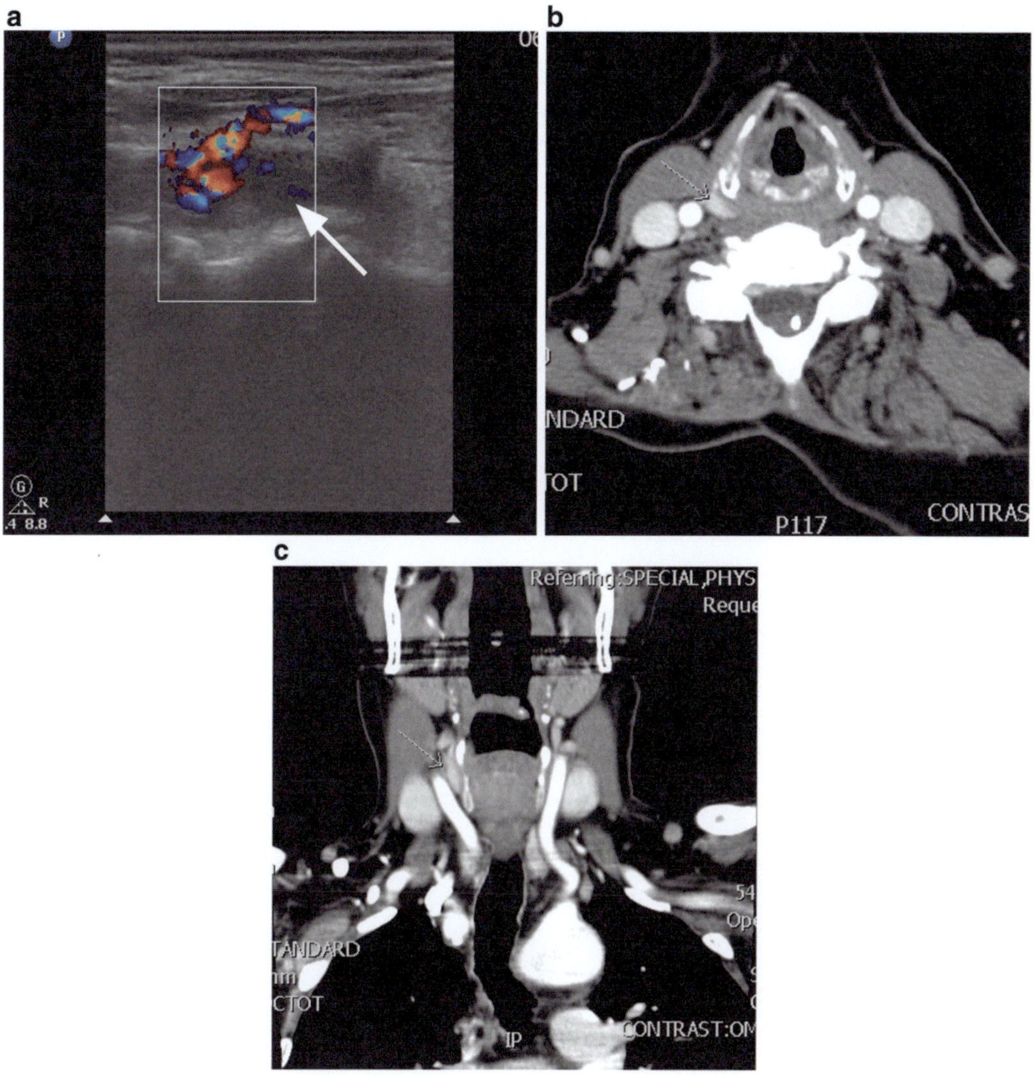

Fig. 25.17 (**a**) Longitudinal ultrasound view showing a superior parathyroid (*arrow*) above the upper right thyroid lobe with a single feeding vessel. (**b**) Transverse CT scan in arterial phase of the same parathyroid (*arrow*). (**c**) Coronal CT scan in arterial phase of the same right superior parathyroid (*arrow*)

25.4.3 Inferior Parathyroid Anatomic and Imaging Location

The possible locations of the inferior parathyroid are caudad, posterior, or lateral to the lower thyroid pole (69 %) (Figs. 25.8 and 25.9), in the thyro-thymic ligament or thymic tongue (26 %) (Fig. 25.13a, b), superior to the superior parathyroid gland as an undescended inferior parathyroid (<1 %), in the mediastinal thymus or in the mediastinum outside the thymus (2 %) [28, 29, 34]. On ultrasound an inferior gland is usually located in a lower and generally more anterior cervical location when compared to a superior gland [38]. Many times, it appears to protrude out of the lower pole of the thyroid (Figs. 25.13 and 25.19) or sometimes it is "tucked" under the lobe (Fig. 25.20). An extremely rare deep mediastinal

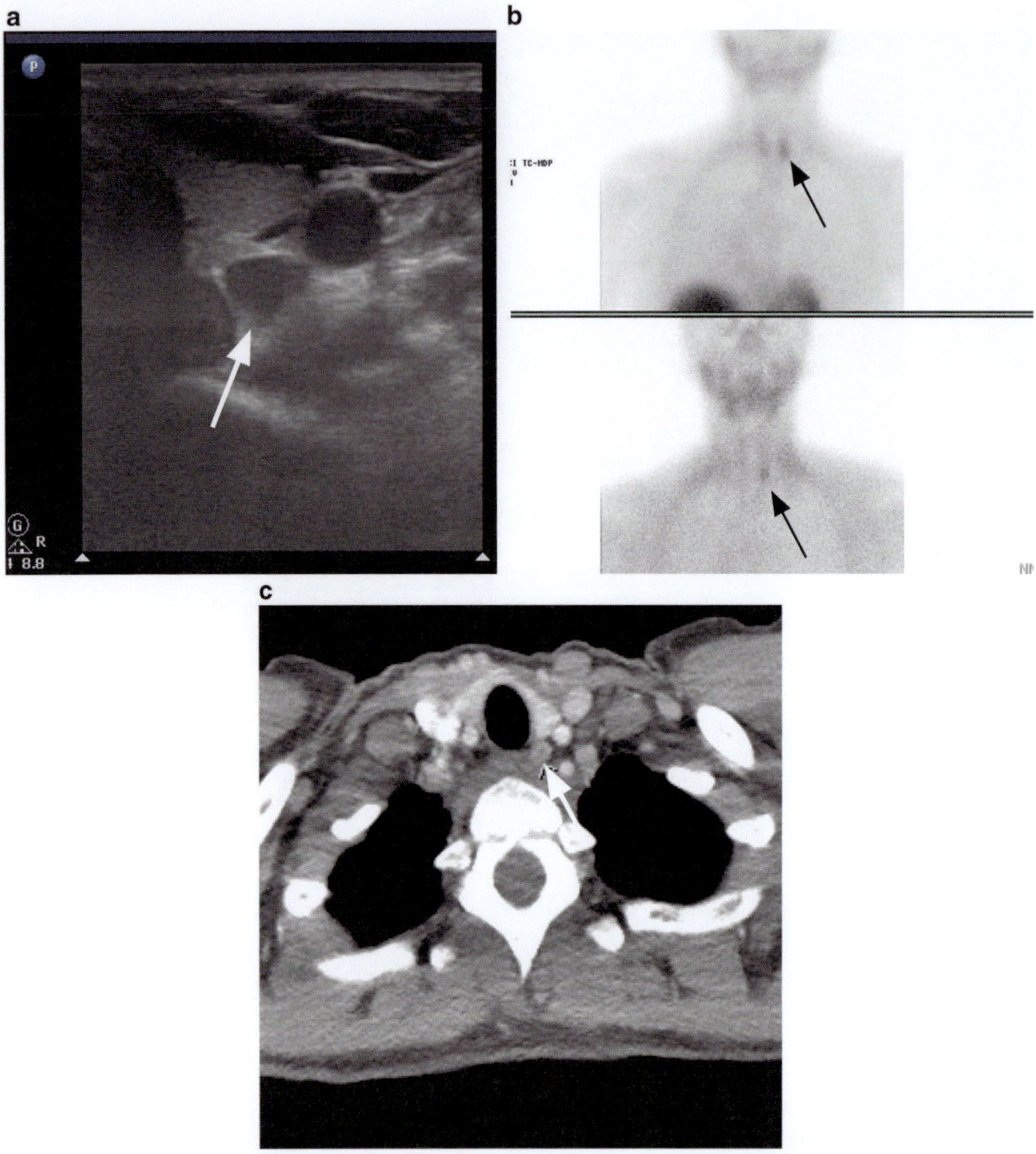

Fig. 25.18 (**a**) Transverse ultrasound view of a left superior parathyroid. Notice its posterior location near the esophagus (*arrow*). (**b**) Planar dual phase Sestamibi scan showing the lower cervical location of the same superior parathyroid (*arrow*). (**c**) Transverse view of a CT scan showing the posterior location by the esophagus of the same superior left sided parathyroid (*arrow*)

parathyroid would be impossible to image with US but 4DCT and and/or SPECT/CT MIBI are usually successful. An inferior parathyroid that failed to descend will remain with a variable amount of thymic tissue high in the neck and the sonographer should always image the area near the hyoid bone, carotid bifurcation, and the submandibular gland to find such glands [39, 40].

25.5 A Suggested Algorithm for the Use of Ultrasound as a Localization Technique in Hyperparathyroidism

Drawing from our own experience and from reviewing the literature, US is the least expensive localization study in patients with HPT. When

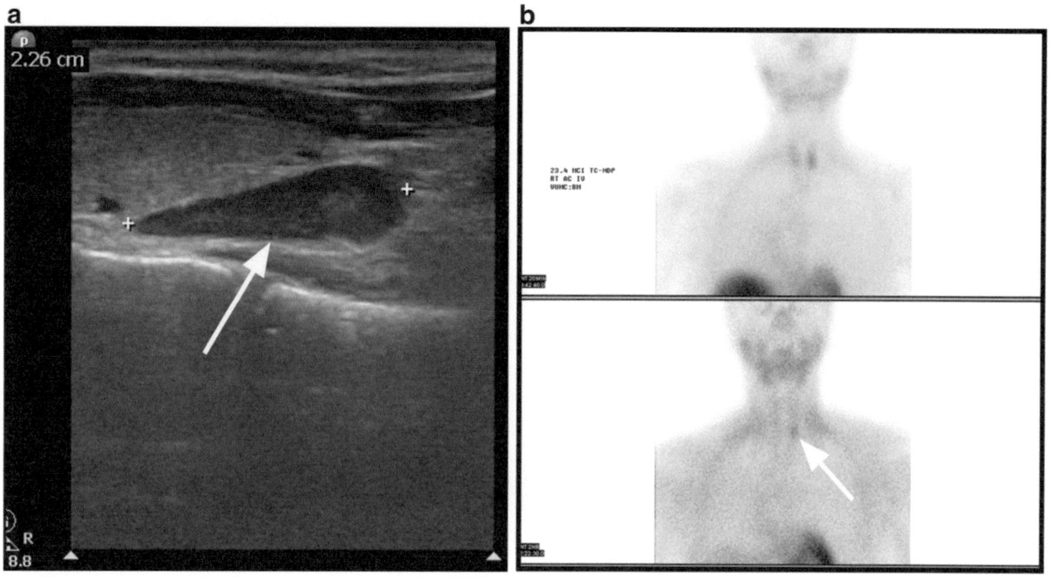

Fig. 25.19 (**a**) Longitudinal ultrasound view of a superior parathyroid that has descended low in the neck by growth (figure). (**b**) Planar dual phase Sestamibi showing the lower cervical position of the superior parathyroid. Do not confuse this with an inferior parathyroid

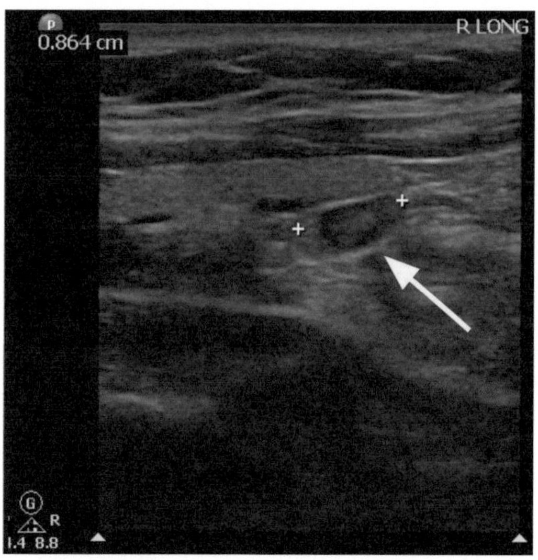

Fig. 25.20 Longitudinal ultrasound view of an inferior parathyroid "tucked" under the lower thyroid lobe. This parathyroid position can be missed during a surgical procedure because the parathyroid hides in a partially intrathyroid position (*arrow*)

the surgeon can rely on accurate and clear US results to localize the parathyroid gland, he or she can proceed with parathyroidectomy solely guided by the US results and intraoperative PTH. When the parathyroid gland is not clearly identified or the images are equivocal, an additional study such as MIBI or 4DCT can be obtained. The choice, of which additional localization study to obtain, will depend on local expertise, surgeon's comfort level with such study, and experience. The authors' algorithm for parathyroid localization is shown in Fig. 25.21.

25.6 Ultrasound in the Reoperative Setting

Persistent or recurrent hyperparathyroidism is not infrequent after parathyroid operations. The most common cause of parathyroidectomy failure is missed multiglandular disease or the inability to find the abnormal single parathyroid gland [37, 41–44]. After confirmation of the diagnosis and consideration of the risks and benefits of reoperative intervention, the surgeon must have accurate localization before embarking in this more technically challenging procedure that can be fraught with higher complication and lower cure rates. The success rates of reoperative parathyroidectomy procedures are highest in patients

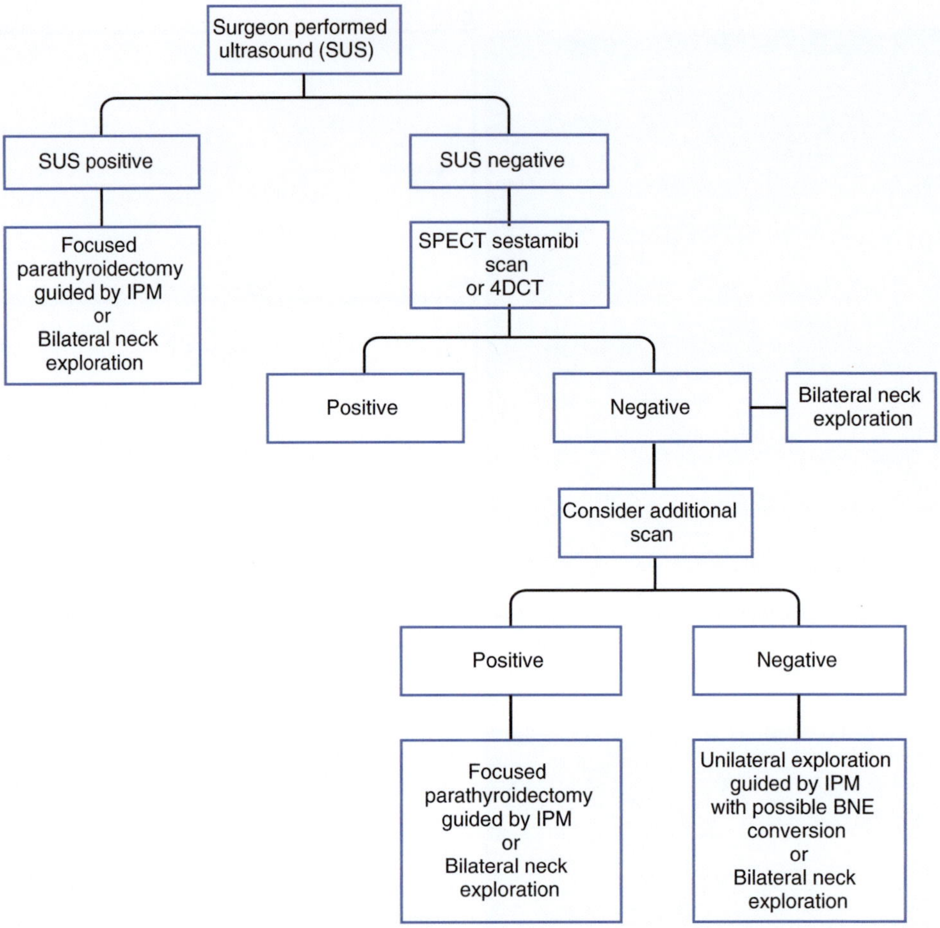

Fig. 25.21 Authors' imaging algorithm prior to parathyroidectomy in patients with primary hyperparathyroidism

with positive imaging (up to 98 %) [45]. When two or more positive and correlating studies can be obtained, the success of reoperative parathyroidectomy is higher [41]. Recently, 4DCT has been shown to be very accurate in the setting of reoperative parathyroidectomy [46].

In reoperative cases, US is an excellent first localization modality. The reasons for US in the reoperative setting are the same as for first-time cases. Commonly, the missed parathyroid is in an eutopic or ectopic cervical location. Such locations include: normal cervical locations, intrathyroidal, retroesophageal, anterior trachea, undescended high neck, or carotid sheath. In reoperative cases, US has a sensitivity ranging from 55 to 75 % [41, 47]. Frequently, an US was never obtained prior to the first operation. The "old" localization studies (usually a MIBI) should be reviewed by the surgeon and correlated with any new images. As mentioned above, one of the most common missed "eutopic" parathyroid locations is a superior parathyroid in a posterior position behind the inferior thyroid artery and RLN. In our practice, we begin with US of the neck and soft tissues, if there is an obvious parathyroid abnormality on US and we can correlate it to the outside MIBI images obtained prior to the failed exploration, we do not repeat the MIBI, but a 4DCT is always obtained. Two positive localization studies are preferred but they are not always possible.

Ultrasound combined with cytologic and biochemical confirmation by FNA of the suspected parathyroid can improve the accuracy and sensitivity of US alone from 65 to 85 % and 75–90 %, respectively [41]. This procedure can be successfully performed by clinicians in office settings and has been shown to be valuable for directing parathyroid exploration in challenging cases [48]. The authors refrain from using this technique in first-time cases because of the possible inflammatory reaction associated with FNA [49]. Patients who have undergone previous parathyroid or thyroid surgery and those with ectopic parathyroid glands may benefit from this technique. Ultrasound can also be used to screen for vocal cord paralysis in reoperative patients (see the chapter on transcutaneous vocal cord US) [50].

25.7 Clinical Scenarios and Lessons Learned

25.7.1 Case 1: Ultrasound to Avoid Radiation Exposure

A 31 year old G3P2 female at 11 weeks gestation was admitted to the hospital for refractory nausea and vomiting and hypercalcemia. Calcium was 14.6 mg/dL, and PTH was 103 pg/mL and 25-OH vitamin D was 25 ng/mL. Amylase and lipase levels were elevated, demonstrating concomitant pancreatitis. Endocrine surgery was consulted and parathyroidectomy was planned. Ultrasound was obtained showing a right-sided parathyroid adenoma (Fig. 25.14). No other localization studies were obtained. She underwent urgent parathyroidectomy with removal of the imaged gland and adequate PTH drop. Her calcium and PTH levels remain normal 1 year later.

25.7.2 Case 2: Is It a Thyroid Nodule or a Parathyroid?

A 52 year old female presents with severe hypercalcemia (16 mg/dL, PTH 1829 pg/mL), dehydration, and renal insufficiency. The outside evaluating physician obtains an MIBI scan that is read as negative. A noncontrasted CT scan was read as a “thyroid cyst.” The patient was transferred to our hospital and US revealed a large cystic parathyroid posterior to the thyroid with a solid component and this was correlated with the MIBI images that showed the solid portion was uptaking sestambi. The left lobe of the thyroid and large cystic parathyroid were resected en block. Final pathology was consistent with a benign 7 g solid/cystic parathyroid adenoma (Fig. 25.22a–c).

25.7.3 Case 3: Parathyroid Cancer Confused with a Goiter: Avoid FNA When Not Absolutely Necessary

A 60 year old female presented to the emergency department complaining of weakness, fatigue, constipation, abdominal pain, 30 lb weight loss, and increased thirst. She had a soft mobile 8 cm right neck mass with tracheal deviation. Her creatinine was 2.3 mg/dL, calcium 18.3 mg/dL, and PTH of 1762 pg/mL. Ultrasound read by radiology showed a heterogenous solid 5.2 cm vascular right “thyroid” mass (Fig. 25.23a) and a 1.6 cm solid hypoechoic mass posterior to the left thyroid lobe suspicious for a parathyroid adenoma. Sestamibi SPECT/CT showed heterogenous uptake on the right side of the neck and correlated with a mass crossing the midline and extending into the upper mediastinum (Fig. 25.23b). Fine needle aspirate was ordered by the medicine team and revealed bland epithelial cells. On neck exploration there was an enlarged right-sided parathyroid densely attached to surrounding tissues including the recurrent laryngeal nerve, thyroid lobe, and the cervical esophagus. The recurrent laryngeal nerve was preserved and the mass was removed en bloc with the thyroid lobe and a small portion of the anterior esophageal wall. Pathology revealed a 6.3 cm parathyroid carcinoma with capsular and lymphovascular invasion as well as focal extension to the thyroid tissue (Fig. 25.23c). Her postoperative calcium remains normal but her PTH has risen from 27 to 227 pg/mL.

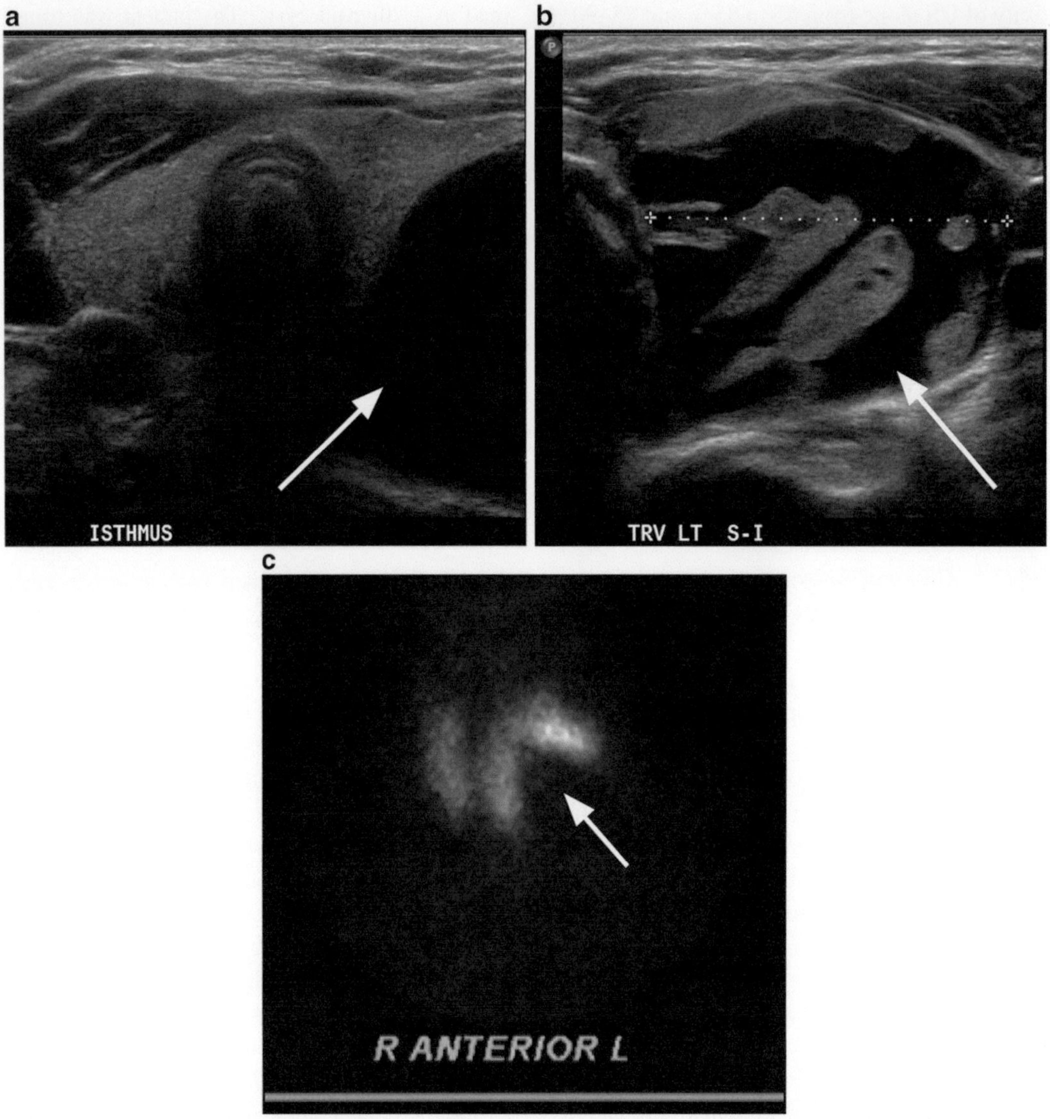

Fig. 25.22 (**a**) Transverse ultrasound view of the entire thyroid at the level of the isthmus showing a large cystic mass behind the left thyroid lobe (*arrow* points to mass). (**b**) Large left cystic and solid parathyroid (*arrow*). (**c**) Planar sestamibi images of the same parathyroid. Notice that only the top of the parathyroid "lights" up with sestamibi and there is a large "cold" area correlating with the cystic component of the parathyroid. This sestamibi was read as "negative"

25.7.4 Lessons Learned

1. Parathyroids can look like thyroid nodules
2. Parathyroids can be located posterior to the thyroid and esophagus
3. FNA should be avoided particularly when parathyroid cancer is suspected. Unlike thyroid FNA, parathyroid FNA causes more troublesome scarring that can interfere with surgery. A scarred parathyroid may need to be handled and grasped (actions that are otherwise avoided in routine parathyroidectomy), thus making it more prone to fragmentation, which in turn can lead to parathyromatosis. With the additional background of parathyroid cancer, parathyromatosis can become even more problematic.

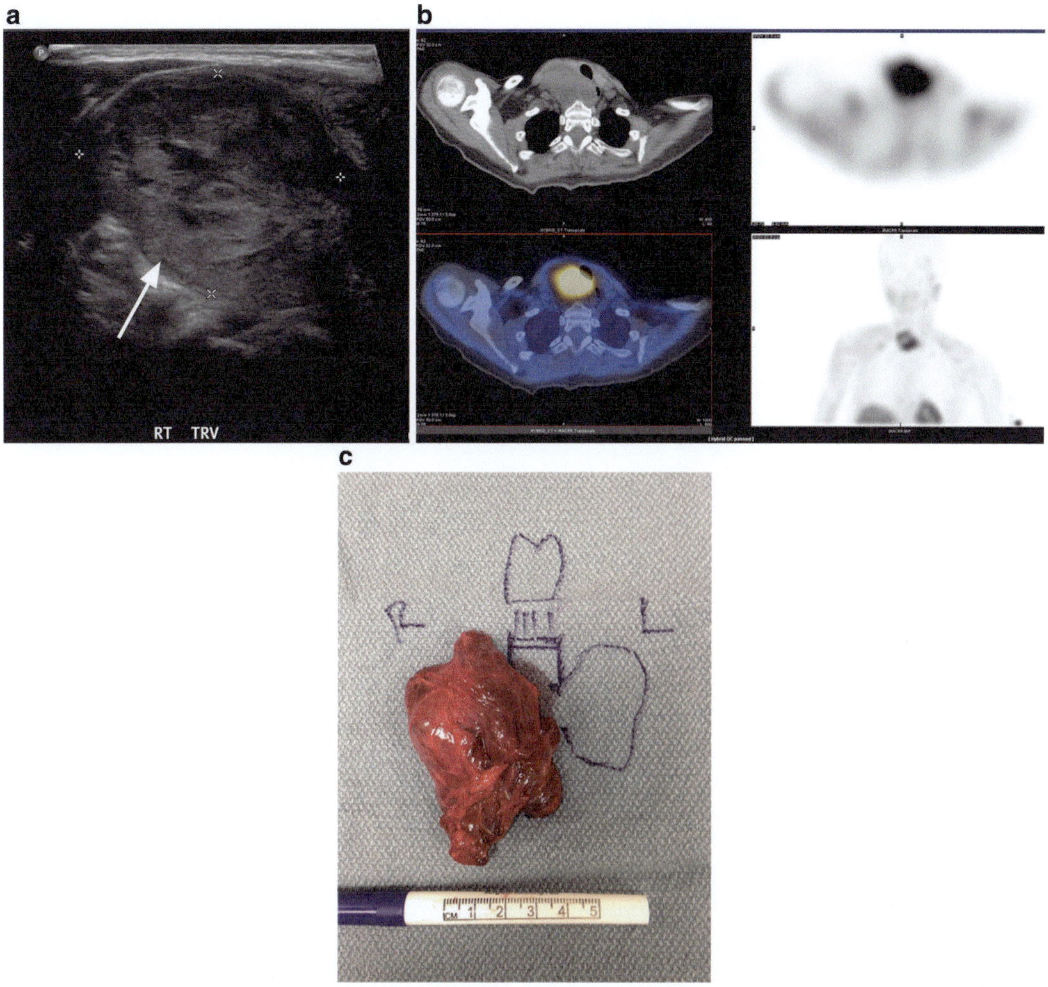

Fig. 25.23 (**a**) Transverse ultrasound view demonstrating a large heterogenous mass in the right paratracheal space. This was a parathyroid cancer. The ultrasonographer read it as a thyroid mass (*arrow*). (**b**) SPECT/CT Sestamibi showing marked uptake of the right paratracheal mass with extension to the esophagus and crossing midline. (**c**) Gross intraoperative picture of the en block specimen (right thyroid lobe and large parathyroid cancer). This parathyroid carcinoma was involving the wall of the cervical esophagus

4. The surgeon should be involved early in the evaluation of the patient, the images, and the plan.

25.7.5 Case 4: Thinking Outside the Box: Case of a Missing Parathyroid

A 50 year old female with a previous total thyroidectomy in 2008 presented with primary hyperparathyroidism. She denied any symptoms. Dexa scan was consistent with osteoporosis. Her calcium was 11 mg/dL, PTH 118 pg/mL, and Vitamin D 25-0H 27 ng/mL. On exam, she had a well-healed 5 cm neck incision and no evidence of masses or lymphadenopathy. Prior operative report could not be obtained but pathology revealed micro papillary thyroid carcinoma and one benign parathyroid. Ultrasound of the neck showed no thyroid or parathyroid tissue and mobile vocal cords. Sestamibi was negative. A 4DCT showed an ectopic parathyroid in the right retropharyngeal space (Fig. 25.24a). On exploration of the right neck, she was noted to

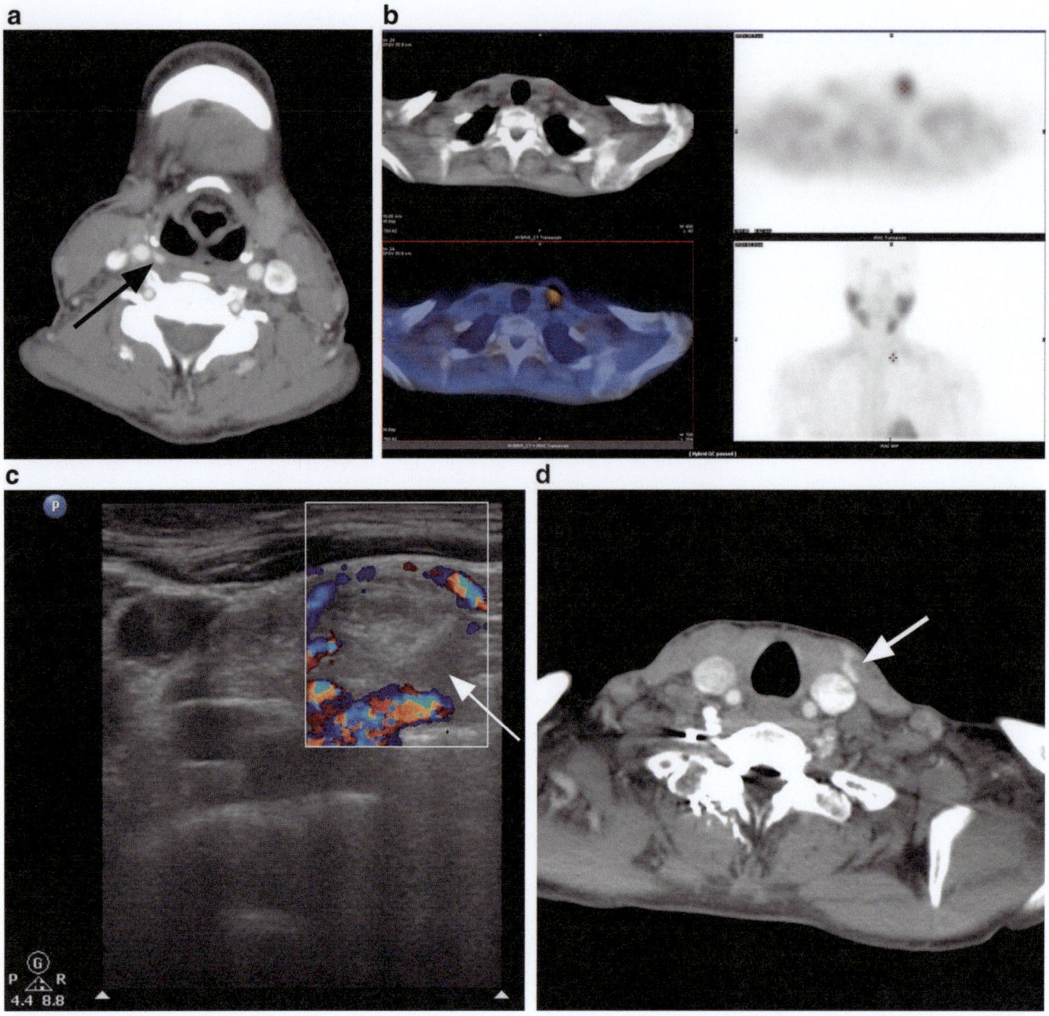

Fig. 25.24 (**a**) 4DCT showing a possible parathyroid in the retropharyngeal position (*arrow*). This patient had a prior total thyroidectomy and presented with hyperparathyroidism (*arrow*). (**b**) SPECT/CT Sestamibi showing uptake in the left sternocleidomastoid muscle. (**c**) Transverse ultrasound view of parathyroid tissue with arc of vascularity in the left sternocleidomastoid muscle (*arrow*). (**d**) 4DCT showing parathyroid tissue in the left sternocleidomastoid muscle (*arrow*)

have extensive adhesions. The mass in the retropharyngeal space was removed; PTH did not drop, and frozen section was consistent with thyroid tissue. Further extensive exploration of the right paratracheal area revealed a normal parathyroid, which was spared, and the operation was concluded. A SPECT/CT MIBI was performed 1 month postoperatively and showed no abnormal uptake. She was followed clinically, and 6 months postoperatively fell and broke her tibia. Her calcium rose to 12.5 mg/dL and PTH remained elevated at 127 pg/mL. MIBI 1 year later showed a focus of uptake within the lateral left neck (Fig. 25.24b). Ultrasound showed vascular tissue in the sternocleidomastoid muscle (Fig. 25.24c). Upon review, this lesion was present on the previous 4DCT and was easily correlated with US (Fig. 25.24c, d). This lesion most likely represented parathyroid tissue implanted (autotransplanted) during the 2008 surgery, typically as a maneuver to preserve normal parathyroid gland that had been devascularized during thyroidectomy. She underwent removal of the implanted parathyroid tissue and her calcium and PTH are now normal.

25.7.6 Lesson Learned

With any prior thyroidectomy or parathyroidectomy look at the sternocleidomastoid muscle for possible implanted parathyroid tissue. This is usually at the level of the prior incision.

25.8 Parathyroid Ultrasound Pearls

- Use compression to increase visibility
- Look for polar artery and arc of vascularity
- Always look in ectopic places even when you think you found the parathyroid on US
- Beware of the inferior parathyroid “Tucked” and hidden under the lower thyroid lobe
- Do not get distracted by a large parathyroid, always look for others
- When the patient had a prior parathyroid and or thyroid operation always look at the SCM for possible parathyroid implants

References

1. Bergenfelz A, Jansson S, Martensson H, Reihner E, Wallin G, Kristoffersson A, et al. Scandinavian quality register for thyroid and parathyroid surgery: audit of surgery for primary hyperparathyroidism. Langenbecks Arch Surg. 2007;392(4):445–51.
2. Irvin 3rd GL, Carneiro DM, Solorzano CC. Progress in the operative management of sporadic primary hyperparathyroidism over 34 years. Ann Surg. 2004;239(5):704–8. discussion 8-11.
3. Siperstein A, Berber E, Barbosa GF, Tsinberg M, Greene AB, Mitchell J, et al. Predicting the success of limited exploration for primary hyperparathyroidism using ultrasound, sestamibi, and intraoperative parathyroid hormone: analysis of 1158 cases. Ann Surg. 2008;248(3):420–8.
4. Wang TS, Pasieka JL, Carty SE. Techniques of parathyroid exploration at North American endocrine surgery fellowship programs: what the next generation is being taught. Am J Surg. 2014;207(4):527–32.
5. Irvin 3rd GL, Solorzano CC, Carneiro DM. Quick intraoperative parathyroid hormone assay: surgical adjunct to allow limited parathyroidectomy, improve success rate, and predict outcome. World J Surg. 2004;28(12):1287–92.
6. Starker LF, Mahajan A, Bjorklund P, Sze G, Udelsman R, Carling T. 4D parathyroid CT as the initial localization study for patients with de novo primary hyperparathyroidism. Ann Surg Oncol. 2011;18(6):1723–8.
7. Staren ED, Knudson MM, Rozycki GS, Harness JK, Wherry DC, Shackford SR. An evaluation of the American College of Surgeons' ultrasound education program. Am J Surg. 2006;191(4):489–96.
8. Sofferman R. The history of clinical ultrasound. In: Sofferman RA, Ahuja AT, editors. Ultrasound of the thyroid and parathyroid glands. New York, NY: Springer; 2012. p. 3–8.
9. Arciero CA, Shiue ZS, Gates JD, Peoples GE, Dackiw AP, Tufano RP, et al. Preoperative thyroid ultrasound is indicated in patients undergoing parathyroidectomy for primary hyperparathyroidism. J Cancer. 2012;3:1–6.
10. Milas M, Mensah A, Alghoul M, Berber E, Stephen A, Siperstein A, et al. The impact of office neck ultrasonography on reducing unnecessary thyroid surgery in patients undergoing parathyroidectomy. Thyroid. 2005;15(9):1055–9.
11. Adler JT, Chen H, Schaefer S, Sippel RS. Does routine use of ultrasound result in additional thyroid procedures in patients with primary hyperparathyroidism? J Am Coll Surg. 2010;211(4):536–9.
12. Morita SY, Somervell H, Umbricht CB, Dackiw AP, Zeiger MA. Evaluation for concomitant thyroid nodules and primary hyperparathyroidism in patients undergoing parathyroidectomy or thyroidectomy. Surgery. 2008;144(6):862–6. discussion 6-8.
13. Jabiev AA, Lew JI, Solorzano CC. Surgeon-performed ultrasound: a single institution experience in parathyroid localization. Surgery. 2009;146(4):569–75. discussion 75-7.
14. Solorzano CC, Carneiro-Pla DM, Irvin 3rd GL. Surgeon-performed ultrasonography as the initial and only localizing study in sporadic primary hyperparathyroidism. J Am Coll Surg. 2006;202(1):18–24.
15. Solorzano CC, Lee TM, Ramirez MC, Carneiro DM, Irvin GL. Surgeon-performed ultrasound improves localization of abnormal parathyroid glands. Am Surg. 2005;71(7):557–62. discussion 62-3.
16. Tublin ME, Pryma DA, Yim JH, Ogilvie JB, Mountz JM, Bencherif B, et al. Localization of parathyroid adenomas by sonography and technetium tc 99m sestamibi single-photon emission computed tomography before minimally invasive parathyroidectomy: are both studies really needed? J Ultrasound Med. 2009;28(2):183–90.
17. Untch BR, Adam MA, Scheri RP, Bennett KM, Dixit D, Webb C, et al. Surgeon-performed ultrasound is superior to 99Tc-sestamibi scanning to localize parathyroid adenomas in patients with primary hyperparathyroidism: results in 516 patients over 10 years. J Am Coll Surg. 2011;212(4):522–9. discussion 9-31.
18. Van Husen R, Kim LT. Accuracy of surgeon-performed ultrasound in parathyroid localization. World J Surg. 2004;28(11):1122–6.
19. Deutmeyer C, Weingarten M, Doyle M, Carneiro-Pla D. Case series of targeted parathyroidectomy with surgeon-performed ultrasonography as the only preoperative imaging study. Surgery. 2011;150(6):1153–60.
20. Cheung K, Wang TS, Farrokhyar F, Roman SA, Sosa JA. A meta-analysis of preoperative localization techniques for patients with primary hyperparathyroidism. Ann Surg Oncol. 2012;19(2):577–83.

21. Ruda JM, Hollenbeak CS, Stack Jr BC. A systematic review of the diagnosis and treatment of primary hyperparathyroidism from 1995 to 2003. Otolaryngol Head Neck Surg. 2005;132(3):359–72.
22. Berber E, Parikh RT, Ballem N, Garner CN, Milas M, Siperstein AE. Factors contributing to negative parathyroid localization: an analysis of 1000 patients. Surgery. 2008;144(1):74–9.
23. Wang TS, Cheung K, Farrokhyar F, Roman SA, Sosa JA. Would scan, but which scan? A cost-utility analysis to optimize preoperative imaging for primary hyperparathyroidism. Surgery. 2011;150(6):1286–94.
24. Lubitz CC, Stephen AE, Hodin RA, Pandharipande P. Preoperative localization strategies for primary hyperparathyroidism: an economic analysis. Ann Surg Oncol. 2012;19(13):4202–9.
25. Norman J, Lopez J, Politz D. Abandoning unilateral parathyroidectomy: why we reversed our position after 15,000 parathyroid operations. J Am Coll Surg. 2012;214(3):260–9.
26. Kiernan CM, Isom C, Kavalukas S, Schlegel C, Peters MF, Solorzano CC. Outpatient parathyroidectomy: bilateral neck exploration compared to focused approach. World Congress of Surgery -- International Association of Endocrine Surgeons; 8/25/2015; Bangkok, Thailand, p. 132. Available from http://www.isw2015.com/files/wcs2015_abstracts.pdf2015.
27. Solorzano CC, Carneiro-Pla D. Minimizing cost and maximizing success in the preoperative localization strategy for primary hyperparathyroidism. Surg Clin North Am. 2014;94(3):587–605.
28. Akerstrom G, Malmaeus J, Bergstrom R. Surgical anatomy of human parathyroid glands. Surgery. 1984;95(1):14–21.
29. Wang C. The anatomic basis of parathyroid surgery. Ann Surg. 1976;183(3):271–5.
30. Kamaya A, Quon A, Jeffrey RB. Sonography of the abnormal parathyroid gland. Ultrasound Q. 2006;22(4):253–62.
31. Acar T, Ozbek SS, Ertan Y, Kavukcu G, Tuncyurek M, Icoz RG, et al. Variable sonographic spectrum of parathyroid adenoma with a novel ultrasound finding: dual concentric echo sign. Med Ultrason. 2015;17(2):139–46.
32. Johnson NA, Yip L, Tublin ME. Cystic parathyroid adenoma: sonographic features and correlation with 99mTc-sestamibi SPECT findings. AJR Am J Roentgenol. 2010;195(6):1385–90.
33. Meola M, Petrucci I, Cupisti A. Ultrasound in clinical setting of secondary hyperparathyroidism. J Nephrol. 2013;26(5):848–55.
34. Johnson NA, Tublin ME, Ogilvie JB. Parathyroid imaging: technique and role in the preoperative evaluation of primary hyperparathyroidism. AJR Am J Roentgenol. 2007;188(6):1706–15.
35. Rodgers SE, Hunter GJ, Hamberg LM, Schellingerhout D, Doherty DB, Ayers GD, et al. Improved preoperative planning for directed parathyroidectomy with 4-dimensional computed tomography. Surgery. 2006;140(6):932–40. discussion 40-1.
36. Melton GB, Somervell H, Friedman KP, Zeiger MA, Cahid CA. Interpretation of 99mTc sestamibi parathyroid SPECT scan is improved when read by the surgeon and nuclear medicine physician together. Nucl Med Commun. 2005;26(7):633–8.
37. Udelsman R, Donovan PI. Remedial parathyroid surgery: changing trends in 130 consecutive cases. Ann Surg. 2006;244(3):471–9.
38. Moreno MA, Callender GG, Woodburn K, Edeiken-Monroe BS, Grubbs EG, Evans DB, et al. Common locations of parathyroid adenomas. Ann Surg Oncol. 2011;18(4):1047–51.
39. Billingsley KG, Fraker DL, Doppman JL, Norton JA, Shawker TH, Skarulis MC, et al. Localization and operative management of undescended parathyroid adenomas in patients with persistent primary hyperparathyroidism. Surgery. 1994;116(6):982–9. discussion 9-90.
40. Fraker DL, Doppman JL, Shawker TH, Marx SJ, Spiegel AM, Norton JA. Undescended parathyroid adenoma: an important etiology for failed operations for primary hyperparathyroidism. World J Surg. 1990;14(3):342–8.
41. Thompson GB, Grant CS, Perrier ND, Harman R, Hodgson SF, Ilstrup D, et al. Reoperative parathyroid surgery in the era of sestamibi scanning and intraoperative parathyroid hormone monitoring. Arch Surg. 1999;134(7):699–704. discussion -5.
42. Lee S, Ryu H, Morris LF, Grubbs EG, Lee JE, Harun N, et al. Operative failure in minimally invasive parathyroidectomy utilizing an intraoperative parathyroid hormone assay. Ann Surg Oncol. 2014;21(6):1878–83.
43. Lew JI, Rivera M, Irvin 3rd GL, Solorzano CC. Operative failure in the era of focused parathyroidectomy: a contemporary series of 845 patients. Arch Surg. 2010;145(7):628–33.
44. Rodriquez JM, Tezelman S, Siperstein AE, Duh QY, Higgins C, Morita E, et al. Localization procedures in patients with persistent or recurrent hyperparathyroidism. Arch Surg. 1994;129(8):870–5.
45. Shin JJ, Milas M, Mitchell J, Berber E, Ross L, Siperstein A. Impact of localization studies and clinical scenario in patients with hyperparathyroidism being evaluated for reoperative neck surgery. Arch Surg. 2011;146(12):1397–403.
46. Mortenson MM, Evans DB, Lee JE, Hunter GJ, Shellingerhout D, Vu T, et al. Parathyroid exploration in the reoperative neck: improved preoperative localization with 4D-computed tomography. J Am Coll Surg. 2008;206(5):888–95. discussion 95-6.

47. Parikh PP, Farra JC, Allan BJ, Lew JI. Long-term effectiveness of localization studies and intraoperative parathormone monitoring in patients undergoing reoperative parathyroidectomy for persistent or recurrent hyperparathyroidism. Am J Surg. 2015;210(1):117–22.
48. Stephen AE, Milas M, Garner CN, Wagner KE, Siperstein AE. Use of surgeon-performed office ultrasound and parathyroid fine needle aspiration for complex parathyroid localization. Surgery. 2005;138(6):1143–50. discussion 50-1.
49. Norman J, Politz D, Browarsky I. Diagnostic aspiration of parathyroid adenomas causes severe fibrosis complicating surgery and final histologic diagnosis. Thyroid. 2007;17(12):1251–5.
50. Carneiro-Pla D, Solorzano CC, Wilhelm SM. Impact of vocal cord ultrasonography on endocrine surgery practices. Surgery. 2016;159(1):58–64.

26 Ultrasound Case Vignettes: Multigland Parathyroid Disease

Vijayaratna Chockalingham, Mira Milas, and Cord Sturgeon

26.1 Introduction

Ultrasound, 99Tc-Setsamibi scans, and 4DCT scans are complementary radiology modalities for the evaluation of parathyroid disease [1–3]. When the initial modality selected to evaluate a patient with parathyroid disease fails to localize abnormal parathyroids, one or more of the other radiology exams are often recommended [2, 3]. Each imaging technique has unique advantages and limitations [4]. Many studies have demonstrated that cervical ultrasound by a dedicated parathyroid sonographer improves the accuracy of parathyroid localization [5–11]. Although cervical ultrasound detects possible MGD in only 2–7 % of cases [7, 12, 13], MGD is found in 96 % of cases where it is suggested on ultrasound [14]. When the cervical ultrasound is nonlocalizing, MGD is found in approximately 50 % of cases [14].

Several studies suggest that ultrasound should be the initial (or perhaps only) localization study obtained in primary hyperparathyroidism [7, 13]. Ultrasound is versatile, provides anatomic orientation similar to the views seen from surgical exposure, and can examine the entire neck and some portions of thymus; yet, even large parathyroids may be hard to detect in areas close to the trachea, esophagus, and high parapharyngeal zones where ultrasound waves propagate poorly [15]. A few studies have demonstrated that ultrasound is the least costly imaging modality and that combining it with another complementary form of imaging, such as sestamibi or 4DCT, is a cost-effective strategy [2, 16, 17]. 99Tc-Sestamibi and 4DCT both image the mediastinum and ectopic areas that are inaccessible by ultrasound [2, 18, 19]. 99Tc-Sestamibi is well recognized to detect only some but rarely all glands in MGD [4, 7, 20]. 4DCT scanning poses concerns for radiation exposure and intravenous iodine contrast in select patients.

Electronic supplementary material: The online version of this chapter (doi:10.1007/978-3-319-44100-9_26) contains supplementary material, which is available to authorized users. Videos can also be accessed at http://link.springer.com/chapter/10.1007/978-3-319-44100-9_26.

V. Chockalingham, M.D.
Department of Endocrinology, Banner - University Medical Center Phoenix, University of Arizona College of Medicine – Phoenix, 1300 N 12th Street Suite 612, Phoenix, AZ 85006, USA
e-mail: Vijayaratna.chockalingam@bannerhealth.com

M. Milas, M.D., F.A.C.S.
Department of Surgery and the Endocrinology & Metabolism Institute, University of Arizona College of Medicine - Phoenix, Banner - University Medical Center Phoenix, 1441 North 12th Street 2nd floor, Phoenix, AZ 85006, USA
e-mail: Mira.Milas@bannerhealth.com

C. Sturgeon, M.D., M.S., F.A.C.S. (✉)
Department of Surgery, Northwestern University, 676 N. St. Clair Street, Suite 650, Chicago, IL 60611, USA
e-mail: csturgeo@nm.org

M. Milas et al. (eds.), *Advanced Thyroid and Parathyroid Ultrasound*,
DOI 10.1007/978-3-319-44100-9_26

Table 26.1 Biochemical profile for routine diagnostic evaluation of parathyroid disease. The units and reference ranges apply to the case vignettes

Laboratory value	Unit	Normal reference range
Calcium, serum	mg/dl	8.3–10.4
Calcium, ionized	mg/dl	4.57–5.21
Parathyroid hormone, intact (PTH)	pg/ml	12–88
Phosphorus	mg/dl	2.5–4.5
Creatinine	mg/dl	0.6–1.5
Albumin	g/dl	3.4–5.0
24 h calcium, urine	mg/day	50–300
24 h creatinine, urine	g/day	0.8–2.0
25-hydroxy vitamin D (VitD25)	ng/ml	30–100
1,25-dihydroxy vitamin D (VitD1,25)	pg/ml	18–72
Magnesium, serum	mg/dl	1.7–2.4

The following patient scenarios illustrate the value of a thoughtful and comprehensive evaluation of patients when MDG is known or suspected in advance of surgery. While some clinicians may suggest that no imaging is necessary in such cases, because bilateral, four-gland exploration will be necessary, these cases illustrate that imaging nevertheless provides information that can change the conduct of surgery. Table 26.1 lists the names, abbreviations, normal laboratory range values, and units of biochemical parameters cited in the clinical descriptions. For clarity and simplicity of presentation only numbers without the units are used in the case descriptions, omitting mention of values if normal or not directly relevant to the case.

26.2 Case Vignette 1: Hypercalcemic Crisis

A 64 year old man was hospitalized from his primary physician's office after routine laboratory tests were obtained in follow-up of a recent admission for stroke. These were his presenting lab values: serum calcium 14.5, ionized calcium 8.5, PTH 94, 25 hydrroxy vitamin D level 17.6, phosphorus 2.2, creatinine 1.6, 24 h urinary calcium 296, and creatinine 1.0. Serum protein electrophoresis and PTH-related peptide were both normal. He was aware of potential parathyroid disease since 2011 and remembers undergoing a 99Tc-Sestamibi. He denied typical symptoms and side effects of parathyroid disease—kidney stones, polyuria/nocturia, neurocognitive changes, extreme fatigue, and arthralgias. Several months prior he had sustained an ankle fracture from a motorcycle accident. The patient denied childhood radiation exposure to the head and neck area or a family history of parathyroid disease. His exam was unremarkable for parathyroid disease-related abnormalities.

A report of the Sestamibi scan performed in 2011 indicated that there were four abnormal foci of uptake with the largest focus in the right lower neck. The same findings were re-demonstrated on the Sestamibi scan obtained during the current hospitalization (Fig. 26.1a, b). A bedside clinician-performed ultrasound detected four abnormal parathyroid glands, appreciating that the largest focus was actually a large superior parathyroid that descended into the tracheoesophageal groove, thus appearing to have a "lower" location (Fig. 26.1c, d; Videos 26.1, 26.2, 26.3, 26.4, 26.5, 26.6, and 26.7).

Four-gland exploration was planned once the patient was medically stable and transitioned off of anticoagulation for the stroke. The imaging findings were helpful in determining the sequence in which the parathyroid glands were exposed and which one could be fashioned into a viable remnant. All were histologically hypercellular parathyroid glands with the following sizes: right upper 4025 mg; right lower 120 mg; left upper 118 mg. The left lower parathyroid was biopsied (not weighed), since it was least abnormal in appearance and most suitable to leave in situ as a viable remnant. Normal parathyroid size is 15–50 mg, with mean weights approximately 30 mg. Intraoperative PTH declined by >50 % following excision of the large right upper parathyroid gland and would not have predicted MGD had imaging shown a single focus of disease.

This patient's imaging findings are interesting because rarely do all four abnormal parathyroid glands appear clearly, and even rarer is the chance

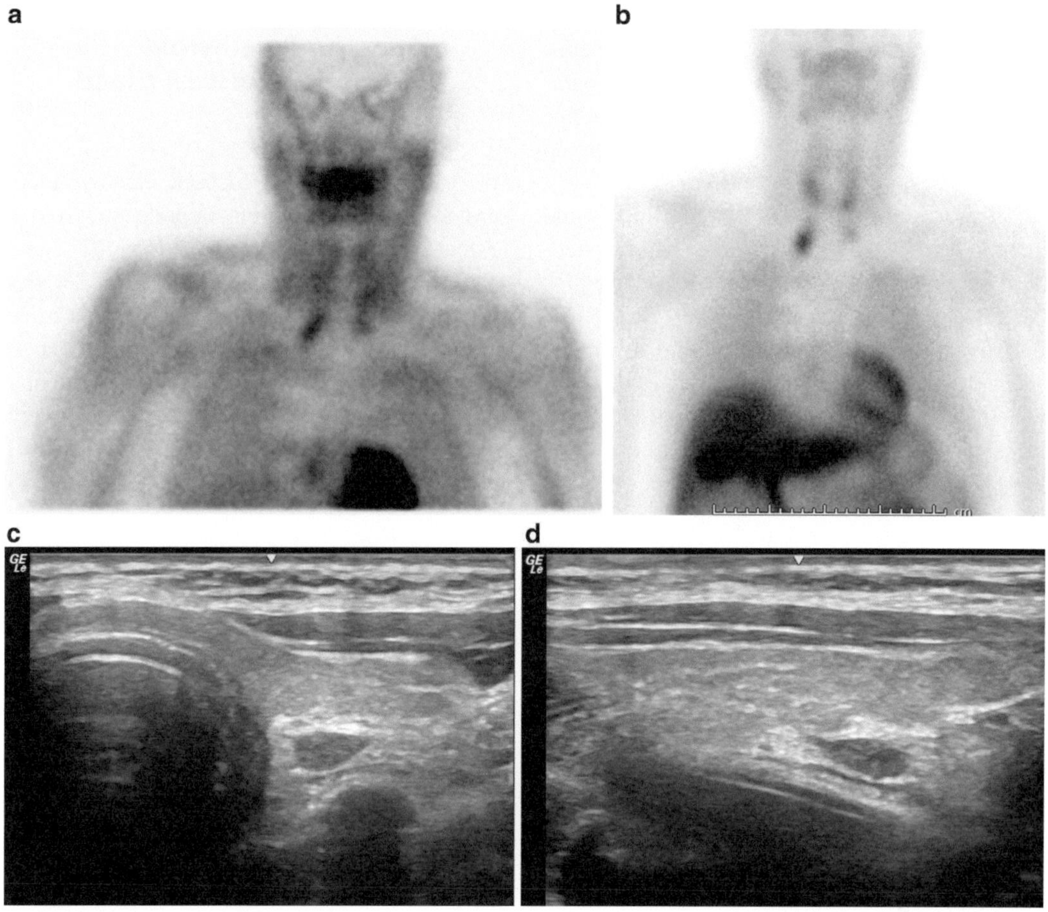

Fig. 26.1 (**a**) Sestamibi scan demonstrating four gland MGD, after initial injection of radiotracer. (**b**) Sestamibi scan clearly demonstrating four gland MGD, after delayed acquisition of images allowing radiotracer to wash out of thyroid gland. (**c**) Ultrasound image left upper parathyroid gland, transverse view. (**d**) Ultrasound image left upper parathyroid gland, longitudinal view

that two imaging studies agree on the same locations for MGD [12]. This case also illustrates how MGD in primary hyperparathyroidism can manifest with asymmetrical sizes and shapes of parathyroid glands.

26.3 Case Vignette 2: Tertiary Hyperparathyroidism and Thyroid Cancer

One month following kidney transplantation, a 55 year old woman was found to have serum calcium levels of 11–12 during a routine nephrology follow-up visit. She had been on dialysis for 10 years and this was her second kidney transplant. PTH level prior to transplant was approximately 2000 and had declined to 650 at presentation with hypercalcemia. Ultrasound detected markedly enlarged upper parathyroid glands that mimicked thyroid nodules because of their partial intrathyroidal positioning (Videos 26.8, 26.9, and 26.10). Furthermore, discreet thyroid nodules were also detected and classified into a high risk for malignancy category by sonographic features of interrupted peripheral calcifications and irregular margins (Videos 26.11 and 26.12). The patient underwent total thyroidectomy with central neck lymph node dissection and concomitant subtotal parathyroidectomy, leaving a small in-situ parathyroid fragment. Histology confirmed multifocal bilateral papillary thyroid cancer and four hyperplastic parathyroid glands. She has no evidence of recurrence for both conditions at nearly 1 year of follow-up after surgery.

This case illustrates the fact that ultrasound identifies previously unrecognized thyroid nodules and thyroid cancer. Coexistent pathology is identified in approximately 30–50 % of cases [21, 22]. In one study ultrasound identified previously silent thyroid nodules in one-third of patients with hyperparathyroidism, and the rate of thyroid cancer in patients with hyperparathyroidism was 7 % [12].

26.4 Case Vignette 3: Double Superior Parathyroid Adenomas Versus 4-Gland Hyperplasia

Two years following a focused parathyroidectomy to remove a 5 cm right upper parathyroid, a 71 year old man was found to be hypercalcemic. At the initial operation, intraoperative PTH was not available. His biochemical serum and urine parameters were diagnostic of primary hyperparathyroidism at the original time of presentation and were confirmed at this recent presentation. Sestamibi scan (Fig. 26.2a) detected only a single strong focus of radiotracer uptake in

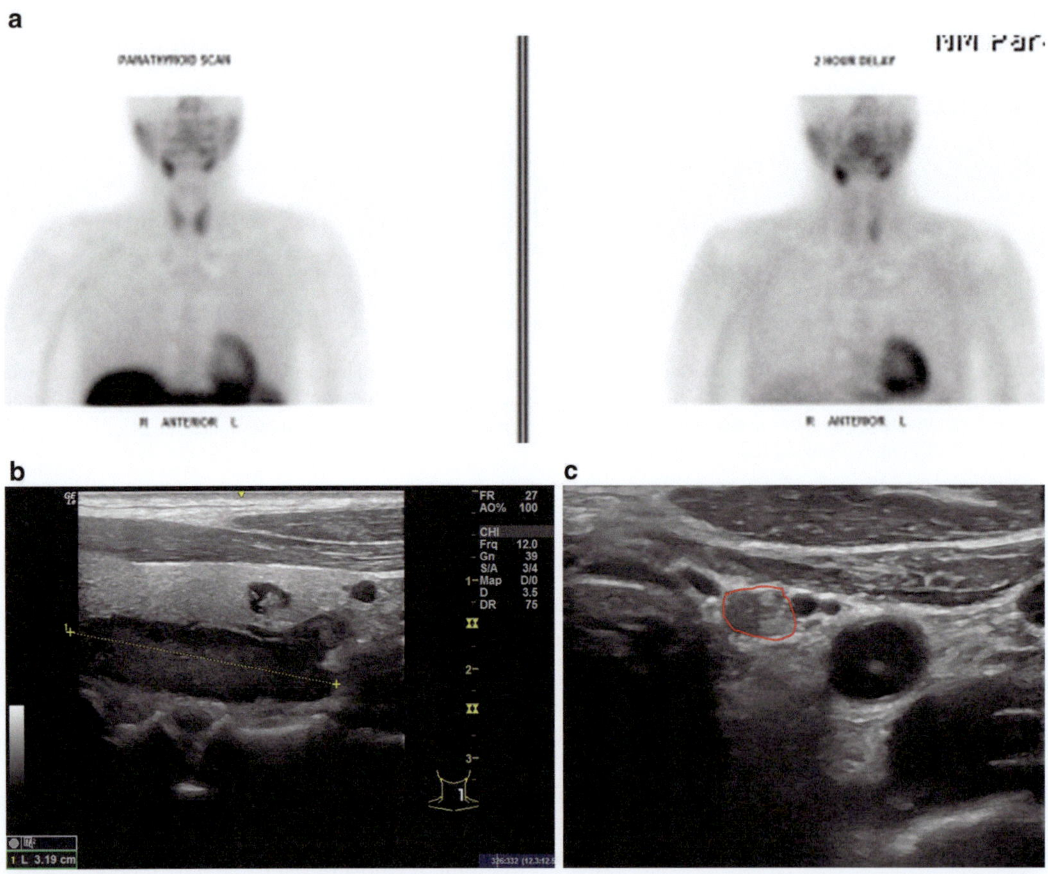

Fig. 26.2 (**a**) Sestamibi scan showing only large single focus of radiotracer in left neck. (**b**) Ultrasound image left upper parathyroid, longitudinal view, showing extent of enlargement nearly as long as the thyroid lobe itself. (**c**) Ultrasound image left lower parathyroid (*circled* in *red*). Keeping this image in mind, viewing of Video 26.15 cine clip may be helpful

the left neck prior to reoperative surgery. This corresponded to a large (3–4 cm) left upper parathyroid gland on ultrasound (Fig. 26.2b, Videos 26.13, 26.14, and 26.15). A subtle echogenicity was also appreciated at the tip of the left lower pole (Fig. 26.2c, Video 26.15) and alerted the surgeon to explore this area as well. Intraoperatively, both the left upper and lower parathyroid glands were abnormally enlarged. Exploration of the right lower parathyroid revealed a third abnormal parathyroid gland. A portion of this parathyroid was fashioned into a remnant while the remaining parathyroid tissue was excised. Histology confirmed hypercellular parathyroid glands with the following sizes: left upper 2673 mg, left lower 80 mg with cystic degeneration; right lower fragment confirmed as hypercellular. Intraoperative PTH level declined from 262 to 30 following excision of only the large left upper gland, hence failing to predict the additional abnormal glands. In follow-up, calcium and PTH levels are 9.1 and 10, respectively.

This case illustrates the more typical clinical situation where Sestamibi scan detects only one gland in MGD. Ultrasound and a low threshold to suspect MGD were essential to this patient avoiding a third surgery for persistent hyperparathyroidism. Because of the sestamibi results the surgeon might have considered that the patient actually had two large superior parathyroid adenomas, which are the most commonly encountered double adenoma combination [23]; however, the subtle findings on ultrasound helped clarify the presence of 4-gland disease.

26.5 Case Vignette 4: Primary Hyperparathyroidism in Pregnancy

A 37 year old woman presented during her second pregnancy with fluctuating calcium values. She had been told 5 years previously during her first pregnancy that she has primary hyperparathyroidism. Lack of medical insurance had prevented her from seeking additional treatment previously and there were no adverse effects from maternal hypercalcemia on the first baby. The patient had multiple kidney stones over the last several years, fatigue and osteopenia. Her biochemical profile was unusual and the following laboratory values are grouped in brackets by two separate dates tested: [calcium 10.7, ionized calcium 6.0, PTH 43, 25 hydroxy vitamin D 22.7, 1,25 dihydroxy vitamin D 102, 24 h urinary calcium 631] and [calcium 11.6, ionized calcium 6.31, PTH 26, 25 hydroxy vitamin D 13.4, 1,25 dihydroxy vitamin D 133, creatinine 0.58, albumin 4.4].

She was referred for evaluation at 17 weeks estimated gestational age (EGA). Multidisciplinary coordination of maternal-fetal specialists and adult endocrinologists was engaged. The patient also was formally tested for hereditary syndromes associated with hyperparathyroidism and found to have none (excluding among others, multiple endocrine neoplasia type 1). Her family history was unknown as she was adopted as a child. Twenty years ago, she had radioiodine ablation for Graves' disease. Parathyroid surgery was performed at 26 weeks EGA.

Ultrasound in the outpatient setting performed separately by both surgeon and endocrinologist failed to detect enlarged parathyroid glands. Because radiotracers are contraindicated in pregnancy, Sestamibi scanning was not performed. Thus, the patient had 4DCT scan that showed a fairly large right upper parathyroid and possibly also an enlarged right lower parathyroid (Fig. 26.3a, b). While the right lower parathyroid abnormality was not particularly large, it had the correct imaging characteristics of abnormal parathyroid tissue on 4DCT scanning: hypoechoic on pre-contrast CT scan, hyperechoic on arterial phase CT scan, and slow contrast washout on venous CT scan phase. With this new knowledge, ultrasound performed at the time of surgery revealed a possible right upper parathyroid (Fig. 26.3c, Video 26.16). However, this density, almost isoechoic to the thyroid gland, was rather subtle and the atrophic nature of the thyroid gland

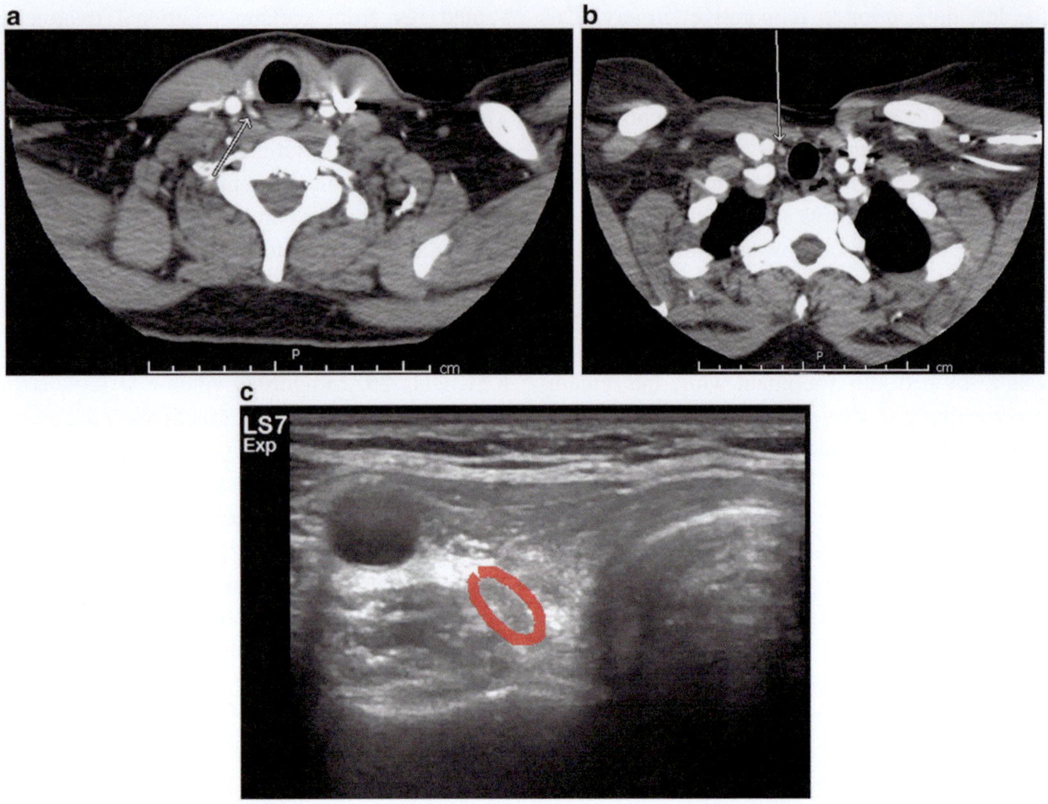

Fig. 26.3 (**a**) 4DCT scan with *arrow* marking right upper parathyroid. (**b**) 4DCT scan with *arrow* marking right lower parathyroid. (**c**) Ultrasound image with suspected right upper parathyroid *circled*

also likely obscured ultrasound imaging. The intraoperative ultrasound was performed after the patient was under anesthesia with the neck hyperextended and more pressure with the transducer probe than is possible in an office setting.

The morning of surgery, preoperative levels were calcium 9.6, ionized calcium 5.21, and PTH 45. Intraoperatively, baseline PTH was 111 but failed to decline by >50 % after excision of the largest right lower parathyroid gland: the 10-min post-excision PTH value was 77. Four-gland exploration revealed all abnormal glands with the following size measurements during surgery:

Right upper parathyroid 15×12×7 mm and 320 mg, right lower 10×6×4 mm and 97 mg, left upper 8×6×4 mm and 112 mg, left lower approximately 8×4×3 mm. As indicated above, a normal parathyroid gland is approximately 6×4×2 mm in size and weighs approximately 30 mg.

Histologically, all glands were described as hypercellular except for the left lower remnant biopsy that was only focally hypercellular and supported the decision of selecting it as the remnant. Subtotal parathyroidectomy with an in-situ remnant of left lower parathyroid was the surgical management. At the completion of surgery, intraoperative PTH was 13. Postoperative levels were calcium 8.0 and PTH 11. Fetal monitoring throughout the procedure and in the postoperative period revealed healthy parameters for the baby. The patient describes feeling "back to her normal self for the first time in ages."

The imaging results for this patient illustrate the limitations of ultrasound and the complementary value of additional imaging in suspected MGD. In this case, the findings of the 4DCT scan were critical because they lateralized the most abnormal parathyroids to the right side of the neck, and indicated that there might be two abnormal glands, thereby maximizing efficiency during surgery and reducing the time under anesthesia for a pregnant patient and her baby. While the intraoperative PTH levels correctly predicted MDG, the surgeon was actually able to rely on the clues from 4DCT and perform a bilateral exposure of all glands without waiting for the post-excision PTH to be resulted from the lab.

26.6 Case Vignette 5: Multiple Endocrine Neoplasia Type 1 (MEN-1)

Ultrasound images presented here reveal mild parathyroid enlargement of only the right-sided parathyroid glands in a 26 year old woman with known MEN1 and minimal elevation of calcium and PTH levels (10.8 and 90 respectively). She postponed undergoing surgery until finishing college studies. Therefore, only her ultrasound is available for case illustration (Fig. 26.4, Videos 26.17, 26.18, 26.19, and 26.20). In MEN-1 there is a nearly 100 % penetrance of primary hyperparathyroidism, which always manifests as asymmetric 4 gland hyperplasia. In addition, they may also have a higher risk of supernumerary glands, usually located in the thymus. For these reasons, the standard surgical approach for patients who are known to have MEN-1 is a bilateral exploration, subtotal parathyroidectomy, and bilateral cervical thymectomy. In most cases, sestamibi scanning will not indicate four or more abnormal parathyroid glands, and in many cases only one abnormal parathyroid will be demonstrated. Sestamibi scanning, therefore, has the potential of misguiding the surgeon. Ultrasound will continue to yield useful information regarding size, depth, and location of some, but not necessarily all, of the abnormal glands, and will identify coexistent thyroid pathology.

26.7 Conclusions

Ultrasound is the essential imaging modality for evaluating the soft tissue in the central and lateral cervical compartments. Due to the high resolution of ultrasound, a skilled sonographer can frequently distinguish the parathyroid glands from the lymph nodes, thymus, thyroid, and other soft tissues of the central compartment. The true parathyroid anatomy may be obscured in cases of high BMI, coexistent thyroid pathology, and parathyroid ectopia. Ultrasound also has poorer performance with MGD and deep gland locations [15]. Migrated superior glands, especially those in the retroesophageal or retrotracheal positions,

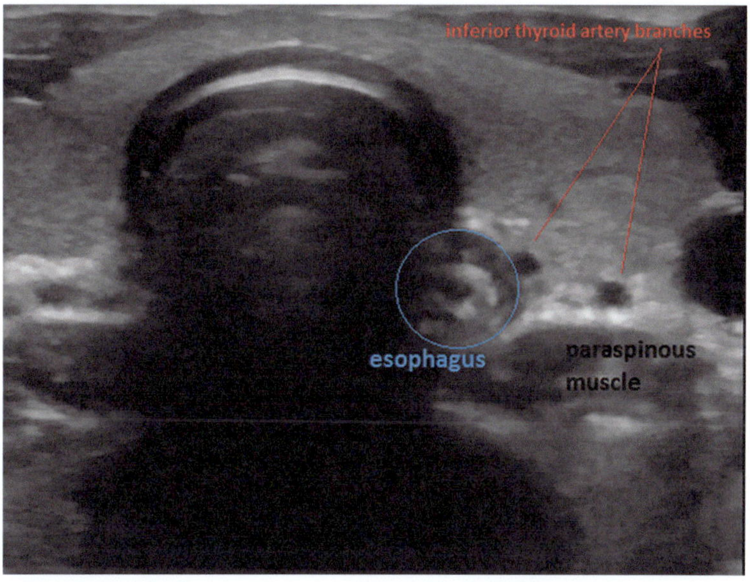

Fig. 26.4 Ultrasound image of normal thyroid anatomy in transverse view centered around trachea. Consider the normal anatomical structures that are labeled. In the subsequent cine clips, these structures are visible and can sometimes be misinterpreted as parathyroid abnormalities

may not be visible due to depth and impeded sound transmission through the esophagus or trachea. Inferior parathyroid glands located in the thymus, or in kyphotic patients, may be obscured by overlying bone.

Parathyroid imaging is done for the purpose of planning a parathyroid operation. Sestamibi scanning is a functional study designed to locate areas of hyperfunctioning parathyroid tissue, but is often limited by poor resolution and a relatively high rate of false positive and false negative results. Sestamibi may also misguide the surgeon, such as in cases where there is a high probability of multigland disease. In contrast, ultrasound and 4DCT yield anatomic data about the soft tissue structures within the neck, but cannot confirm the function of those tissues. Regardless, sonographic data are essential to the surgeon. Several studies suggest that ultrasound should be the initial, or perhaps only, localization study obtained in primary hyperparathyroidism [7, 13]. Whenever the history of the patient or the preoperative imaging studies indicate that there is a high risk of multigland disease a bilateral exploration should be performed.

References

1. Sepahdari AR, Bahl M, Harari A, Kim HJ, Yeh MW, Hoang JK. Predictors of multigland disease in primary hyperparathyroidism: a scoring system with 4D-CT imaging and biochemical markers. AJNR Am J Neuroradiol. 2015;36:987–92.
2. Lubitz CC, Hunter GJ, Hamberg LM, et al. Accuracy of 4-dimensional computed tomography in poorly localized patients with primary hyperparathyroidism. Surgery. 2010;148:1129–37. discussion 37-8.
3. Cham S, Sepahdari AR, Hall KE, Yeh MW, Harari A. Dynamic parathyroid computed tomography (4DCT) facilitates reoperative parathyroidectomy and enables cure of missed hyperplasia. Ann Surg Oncol. 2015;22:3537–42.
4. Alkhalili E, Tasci Y, Aksoy E, et al. The utility of neck ultrasound and sestamibi scans in patients with secondary and tertiary hyperparathyroidism. World J Surg. 2015;39:701–5.
5. Van Husen R, Kim LT. Accuracy of surgeon-performed ultrasound in parathyroid localization. World J Surg. 2004;28:1122–6.
6. Deutmeyer C, Weingarten M, Doyle M, Carneiro-Pla D. Case series of targeted parathyroidectomy with surgeon-performed ultrasonography as the only preoperative imaging study. Surgery. 2011;150:1153–60.
7. Untch BR, Adam MA, Scheri RP, et al. Surgeon-performed ultrasound is superior to 99Tc-sestamibi scanning to localize parathyroid adenomas in patients with primary hyperparathyroidism: results in 516 patients over 10 years. J Am Coll Surg. 2011;212:522–9. discussion 9-31.
8. Jabiev AA, Ikeda MH, Reis IM, Solorzano CC, Lew JI. Surgeon-performed ultrasound can predict differentiated thyroid cancer in patients with solitary thyroid nodules. Ann Surg Oncol. 2009;16:3140–5.
9. Lew JI, Solorzano CC, Irvin 3rd GL. Long-term results of parathyroidectomy for hypercalcemic crisis. Arch Surg. 2006;141:696–9. discussion 700.
10. Solorzano CC, Lee TM, Ramirez MC, Carneiro DM, Irvin GL. Surgeon-performed ultrasound improves localization of abnormal parathyroid glands. Am Surg. 2005;71:557–62. discussion 62-3.
11. Tublin ME, Pryma DA, Yim JH, et al. Localization of parathyroid adenomas by sonography and technetium tc 99m sestamibi single-photon emission computed tomography before minimally invasive parathyroidectomy: are both studies really needed? J Ultrasound Med. 2009;28:183–90.
12. Aliyev S, Agcaoglu O, Aksoy E, et al. An analysis of whether surgeon-performed neck ultrasound can be used as the main localizing study in primary hyperparathyroidism. Surgery. 2014;156:1127–31.
13. Solorzano CC, Carneiro-Pla DM, Irvin 3rd GL. Surgeon-performed ultrasonography as the initial and only localizing study in sporadic primary hyperparathyroidism. J Am Coll Surg. 2006;202:18–24.
14. Siperstein A, Berber E, Mackey R, Alghoul M, Wagner K, Milas M. Prospective evaluation of sestamibi scan, ultrasonography, and rapid PTH to predict the success of limited exploration for sporadic primary hyperparathyroidism. Surgery. 2004;136:872–80.
15. Ruda JM, Hollenbeak CS, Stack Jr BC. A systematic review of the diagnosis and treatment of primary hyperparathyroidism from 1995 to 2003. Otolaryngol Head Neck Surg. 2005;132:359–72.
16. Solorzano CC, Carneiro-Pla D. Minimizing cost and maximizing success in the preoperative localization strategy for primary hyperparathyroidism. Surg Clin North Am. 2014;94:587–605.
17. Wang TS, Cheung K, Farrokhyar F, Roman SA, Sosa JA. Would scan, but which scan? A cost-utility analysis to optimize preoperative imaging for primary hyperparathyroidism. Surgery. 2011;150:1286–94.
18. Bahl M, Sepahdari AR, Sosa JA, Hoang JK. Parathyroid adenomas and hyperplasia on four-dimensional ct scans: three patterns of enhancement relative to the thyroid gland justify a three-phase protocol. Radiology. 2015;277:454–62.

19. Ellika S, Patel S, Aho T, Marin H. Preoperative localization of parathyroid adenomas using 4-dimensional computed tomography: a pictorial essay. Can Assoc Radiol J. 2013;64:258–68.
20. Galvin L, Oldan JD, Bahl M, Eastwood JD, Sosa JA, Hoang JK. Parathyroid 4D CT and scintigraphy: what factors contribute to missed parathyroid lesions? Otolaryngol Head Neck Surg. 2016;154:847–53.
21. Morita SY, Somervell H, Umbricht CB, Dackiw AP, Zeiger MA. Evaluation for concomitant thyroid nodules and primary hyperparathyroidism in patients undergoing parathyroidectomy or thyroidectomy. Surgery. 2008;144:862–6. discussion 6-8.
22. Adler JT, Chen H, Schaefer S, Sippel RS. Does routine use of ultrasound result in additional thyroid procedures in patients with primary hyperparathyroidism? J Am Coll Surg. 2010;211:536–9.
23. Milas M, Wagner K, Easley KA, Siperstein A, Weber CJ. Double adenomas revisited: nonuniform distribution favors enlarged superior parathyroids (fourth pouch disease). Surgery. 2003;134:995–1003. discussion -4.

27 Parathyroid Ultrasound Imaging: Pearls, Pitfalls, and Tips

Manjiri K. Dighe and David Steward

27.1 Typical Appearance on US

The normal parathyroid gland is not seen due to its small size and deep location, when seen, they appear as small hypoechoic nodule. Parathyroid adenomas are typically solid lesions with well-defined margins. They are hypoechoic relative to the thyroid gland and appear as well-circumscribed ovoid nodules (Fig. 27.1a, Video 27.1). They can appear bilobed or lobulated when large and can develop cystic changes. A well-defined echogenic tissue plane can be seen separating the thyroid gland from the parathyroid adenoma (Videos 27.2 and 27.3). Color and power Doppler shows the parathyroid adenomas to be highly vascular lesions supplied by a prominent extra-thyroidal feeding artery (Fig. 27.1b). The feeding artery encircles 90–270° around the gland and will enter the adenoma at one pole along its long axis [1] and arborize around the periphery before smaller branches penetrate deeper [1, 2] (Fig. 27.2). Increased vascularity can be seen in the overlying thyroid gland, which can hint at the presence of an underlying adenoma [2]. This is seen in 85 % of adenomas when compared with the normal contralateral side [3].

Electronic supplementary material: The online version of this chapter (doi:10.1007/978-3-319-44100-9_27) contains supplementary material, which is available to authorized users. Videos can also be accessed at http://link.springer.com/chapter/10.1007/978-3-319-44100-9_27.

M.K. Dighe, M.D. (✉)
Department of Radiology, University of Washington, Seattle, WA, USA
e-mail: dighe@u.washington.edu

D. Steward, M.D. (✉)
University of Cincinnati, Cincinnati, OH, USA
e-mail: stewardd@ucmail.uc.edu

27.2 Elusive Adenoma

While usually scanning for parathyroid adenomas is straightforward, identification of adenomas may be challenging in some cases. Some of the atypical appearances and abnormal locations are described below along with the imaging pitfalls and scanning technique to be used.

27.3 Atypical Findings

Although most adenomas are less than 2 cm in size, large adenomas greater than 5 cm can occur [4]. Most adenomas are oval in shape; however, some can have an asymmetric shape as well (Fig. 27.3) especially when large. Occasionally, parathyroid adenomas may be echogenic or heterogeneous in echotexture rather than displaying the usual homogenous hypoechoic appearance. This is especially possible when the adenomas are larger than 2 cm (Fig. 27.4, Video 27.4) [5]. Cystic adenomas are seen to occur in 2 % of cases and may be difficult to differentiate from rare

M. Milas et al. (eds.), *Advanced Thyroid and Parathyroid Ultrasound*,
DOI 10.1007/978-3-319-44100-9_27

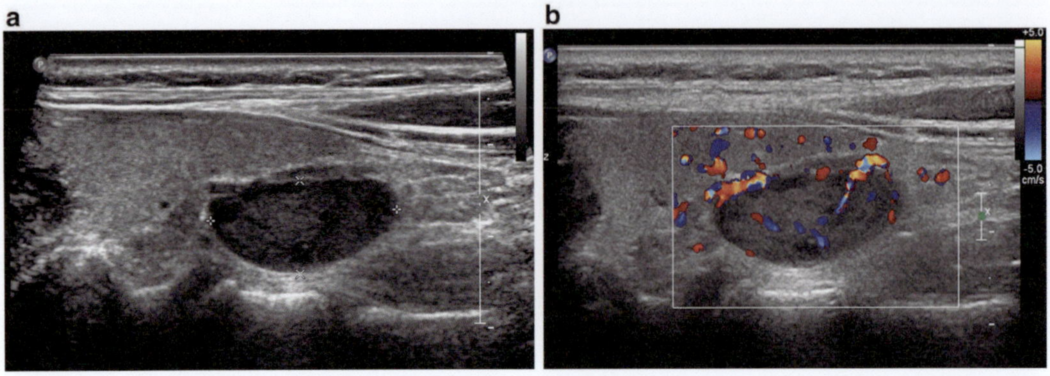

Fig. 27.1 Typical appearance of a parathyroid adenoma seen as a (**a**) solid oval lesion with well-defined margins and hypoechoic relative to the thyroid gland (*calipers* in image). Color Doppler shows the typical arborization of blood supply in the parathyroid adenoma (**b**)

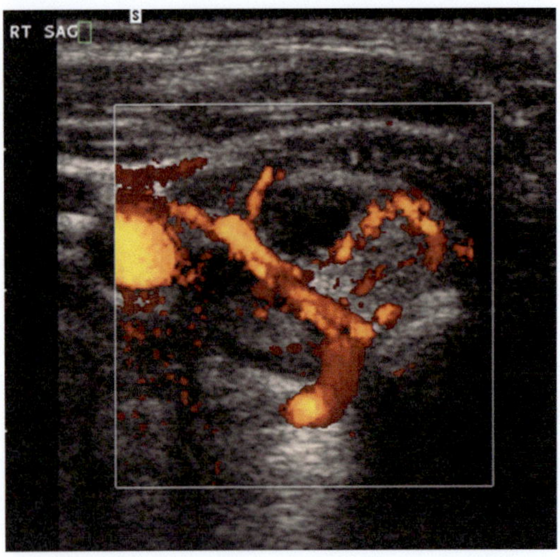

Fig. 27.2 Enlarged extra-thyroidal artery (*arrow*) seen arising from the inferior thyroidal artery and supplying the parathyroid adenoma (*)

true parathyroid cyst (Fig. 27.5, Video 27.5) [4]. In patients with parathyroid hyperplasia, all four glands are enlarged to varying degrees with the glands being usually smaller in size than in patients with parathyroid adenomas (Fig. 27.6). Hence, they are not as readily visible [6]. Hyperplasia is more commonly seen in patients with familial syndromes such as Multiple Endocrine Neoplasia (MEN) 1 and MEN 2A [5].

Multiple adenomas are seen to occur in 5 % of patients (Fig. 27.7, Video 27.6). In these cases, the surgical management will change from unilateral minimally invasive operation to bilateral neck dissection; identification of these patients is crucial. Hence, it is imperative that all the four quadrants and potential ectopic locations are evaluated, even if one abnormal parathyroid gland has already been identified [7–9].

Intrathyroidal adenomas are impossible to differentiate from thyroid nodules, however should be suspected in patients with non-localized parathyroid adenomas and presence of primary hyperparathyroidism. Intrathyroidal adenomas are seen in only 6 % of cases [10]. On imaging, a homogenously hypoechoic nodule is seen within the thyroid capsule (Fig. 27.8). A large feeding artery may be seen; however, in the review by Yabuta et al., feeding artery was not commonly seen and only an echogenic line between the parathyroid adenoma and the surrounding thyroid tissue on the ventral surface of the parathyroid gland was seen [11].

27.4 Abnormal Location

The parathyroid glands develop from the third and fourth pharyngeal pouches and usually two glands develop on each side, one superior and one inferior. This can range from 2 to 6 glands with some authors reporting up to 12 glands [12, 13]. Since the thymus and the inferior parathyroid glands arise from the third pharyngeal pouch and since the thymus descends into the mediasti-

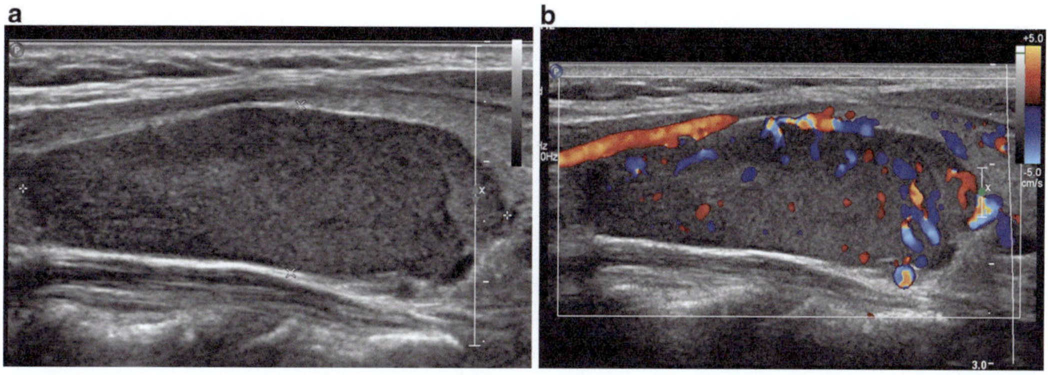

Fig. 27.3 Large parathyroid adenoma measuring 4.5 cm seen posterior to the thyroid with a homogenous hypoechoic appearance on Bmode image (**a**) and peripheral vascularity on Color Doppler (**b**)

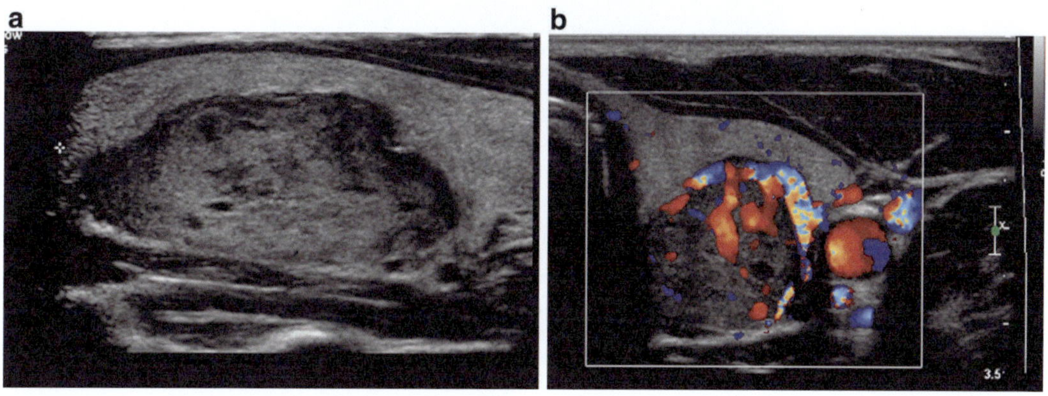

Fig. 27.4 Large parathyroid adenoma with a heterogenous appearance and lobulated margins. Note the cystic areas (*arrow*) in the adenoma (**a**) and prominent vascularity on color Doppler (**b**)

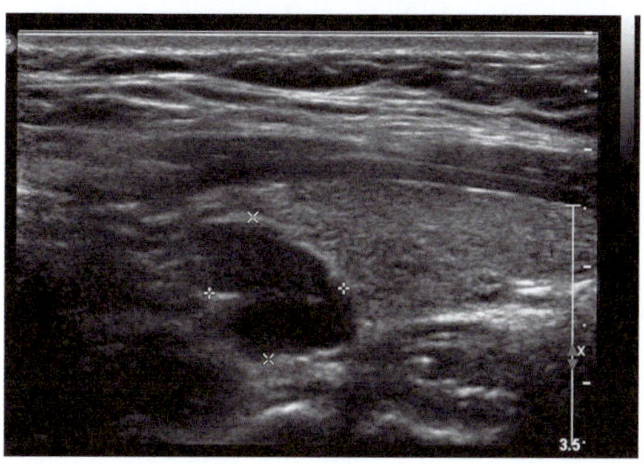

Fig. 27.5 Superior parathyroid adenoma with a partially cystic appearance (*calipers* in image)

num, ectopic inferior parathyroid glands may be located anywhere along this pathway (Fig. 27.9, Videos 27.7 and 27.8). The superior parathyroid glands arise from the fourth pharyngeal pouch along with part of the thyroid gland [14].

27.5 Parathyroid Carcinoma

Parathyroid carcinomas are rare seen in less than 1 % of patients with an abnormal parathyroid gland. Differentiation from a parathyroid adenoma is difficult. Imaging may show a parathyroid gland more than 2 cm in size with a thicker capsule and marked vascularity (Fig. 27.10). Local tissue invasion may be seen in advanced cases and metastasis may occur in lungs, liver, and bone. Local recurrence after surgery is seen in approximately one third patients [5, 9].

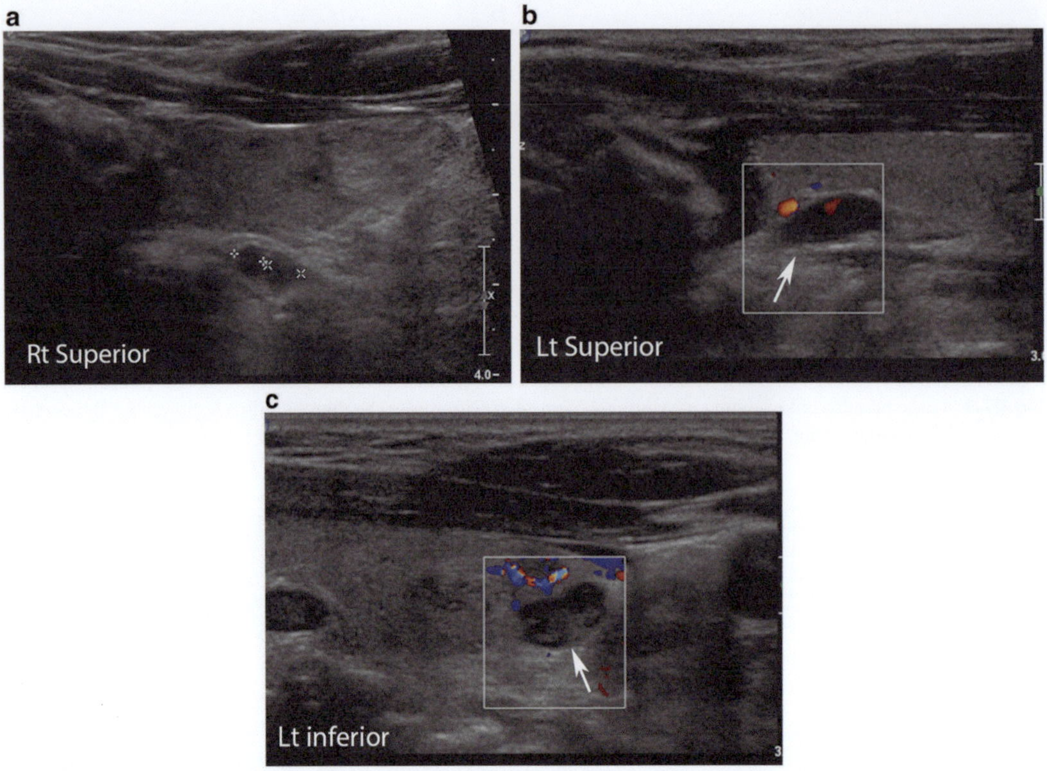

Fig. 27.6 Parathyroid hyperplasia in primary hyperparathyroidism. 54 year old female with a persistently elevated parathyroid hormone level. Ultrasound showed small right superior (*calipers* in **a**), left superior (*arrow* in **b**) and left inferior (*arrow* in **c**) hypoechoic nodules posterior to the thyroid gland suggesting multiple adenomas or parathyroid hyperplasia

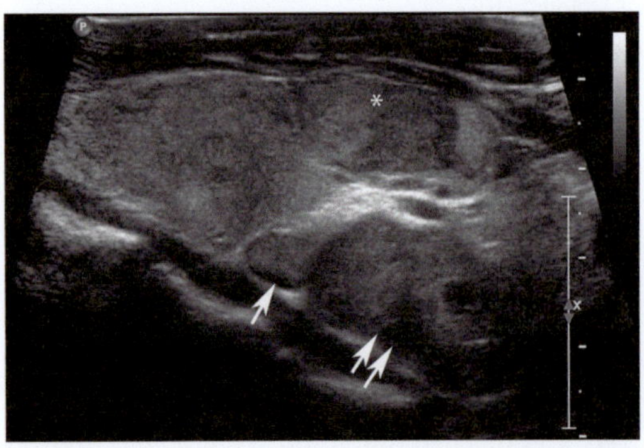

Fig. 27.7 Multiple parathyroid adenomas. Two large hypoechoic nodules seen posterior to the right thyroid gland in a patient with elevated parathyroid hormone levels (*arrow* and *double arrows*) suggesting multiple adenomas

27.6 Imaging Pitfalls

Enlarged lymph nodes can mimic parathyroid adenomas. The presence of an echogenic hilum and central hilar vascular supply allows accurate differentiation from parathyroid adenoma [15].

Small parathyroid adenomas may be difficult to detect. In a study by Stucken et al., modified 4-D computed tomography/ultrasound had lower sensitivity in detecting glands less than 150 mg in weight [16]. Meticulous scanning technique may be necessary for localization of these small parathyroid adenomas.

Presence of thyroid nodules may decrease the sonographic and scintigraphic accuracy in detecting parathyroid adenomas. A large multinodular goiter may displace adjacent structures, (Video 27.9) cause refractile shadows or sound attenuation, and hence decrease the visibility of structures posterior to the thyroid [4]. In a study with 142 patients, preoperative ultrasound yielded accuracy of 79 % with an 11.3 % false-negative rate. Thyroid nodularity was significantly more common (81.8 %) in patients with a false-positive or false-negative finding on ultrasound than in the total

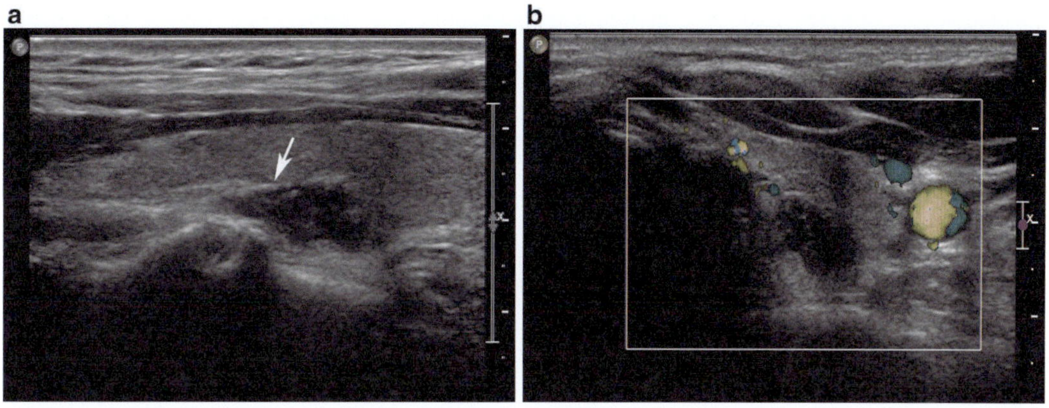

Fig. 27.8 Intrathyroidal parathyroid adenoma. Hypoechoic nodule seen along the posterior aspect of the left thyroid lobe on B-mode image (**a**). Color Doppler image did not show any polar vessel blood supply (**b**). Presence of echogenic line in between the adenoma and the thyroid (*arrow*) suggested a parathyroid adenoma. This was confirmed by fine needle aspiration

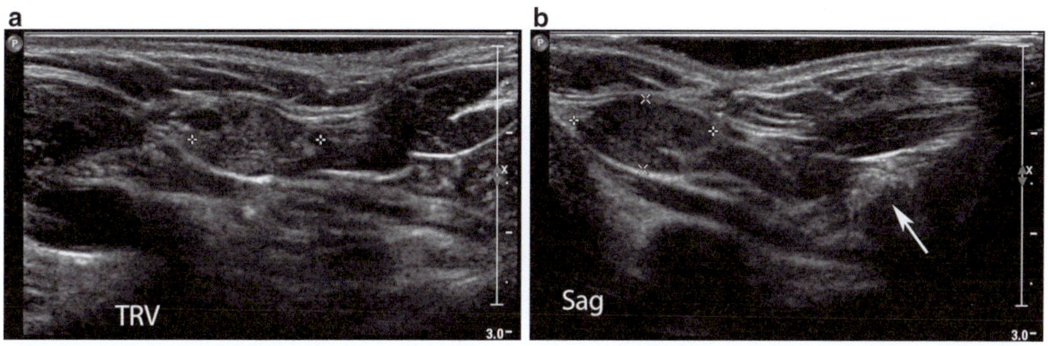

Fig. 27.9 Ectopic parathyroid adenoma. 44 year old male with persistently elevated parathyroid hormone and serum calcium levels. Ultrasound of the thyroid region did not reveal a parathyroid adenoma, hence the inferior part of the neck was scanned to assess for ectopic adenomas. A heterogenous partially cystic lesion was seen in the supraclavicular region. This was confirmed to be an ectopic parathyroid adenoma on seistamibi scan. *Arrow*—clavicle

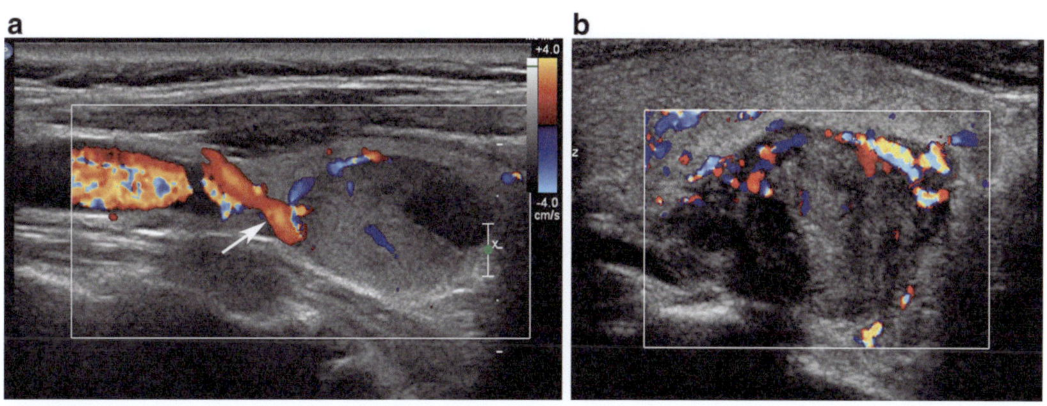

Fig. 27.10 Parathyroid carcinoma. 53 year old female with a PTH level of 275 and serum calcium level of 12.4. Ultrasound showed a large lobulated lesion in the right neck posterior to the thyroid (**a**) with vascularity seen on color Doppler (**b**) image

population (61.3 %) [17]. Exophytic thyroid nodules can mimic parathyroid adenomas, presence of thyroid capsule, or extra-thyroidal fat separating thyroid from adjacent structures and presence of enlarged polar feeding artery can be seen associated with parathyroid adenoma. Most thyroid nodules will be heterogenous in echotexture and not have a polar vascular pedicle [5]. If necessary, percutaneous biopsy may be helpful in differentiating the two entities. Patients with underlying inflammation of the thyroid gland such as Hashimoto's thyroiditis are more likely to have mildly enlarged adjacent lymph nodes, which can be mistaken for parathyroid adenomas [15].

In some patients, the esophagus and longus colli can be mistaken for a parathyroid adenoma. Turning the head from one side to the next and swallowing will show movement of the esophagus and longus colli muscle independent of the adjacent structures and help in differentiating them from an abnormal parathyroid gland [18].

27.7 Optimizing Scanning Technique

Parathyroid sonography should be performed with high frequency linear array transducers 10 MHz or higher with patient in supine position with the neck extended and a pillow placed beneath the shoulders to slightly extend the neck. Scanning is performed in transverse and longitudinal planes focusing to identify the structures anterior of the longus colli muscles, the esophagus and trachea and then scrutinize the retrothyroidal region medial to the carotid artery where many parathyroid adenomas are located. Knowledge of the parathyroid embryology is essential to evaluate the appropriate locations in case of ectopic adenomas. Most adenomas are eutopic with superior glands located posteriorly at the level of the midthyroid and the inferior glands located just posterior and below the lower pole. Evaluation should be performed from the level of the superior pole of the thyroid continuing inferiorly to the sternal notch. Just above the clavicle, the probe should be angled inferiorly to visualize the neck to the level of the subclavian vein.

In addition to real-time gray scale imaging, color and power Doppler imaging and graded compression gray scale imaging should also be performed. Color and power Doppler imaging should be used to evaluate for presence of prominent extra-thyroidal feeding artery usually the inferior thyroid artery with polar distribution to the parathyroid adenoma (Fig 27.11a). This is in contrast to an enlarged lymph node in which the feeding vessels enter the node at its hilum (Fig. 27.11b). In addition, flow to the thyroid lobes should be evaluated since the side with the parathyroid adenoma may have increased vascularity. This is helpful in cases

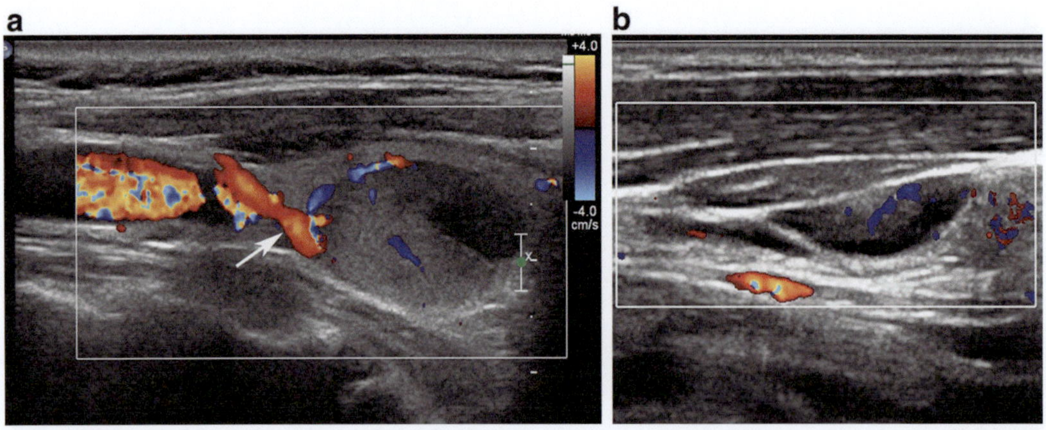

Fig. 27.11 Polar blood supply in parathyroid adenoma. Note the enlarged blood vessel (*arrow*) entering the adenoma at the superior aspect (**a**) compared to a lymph node with hilar blood supply (**b**)

with an elusive parathyroid adenoma. In the presence of asymmetric thyroid lobe vascularity, anatomic side with the greatest vascularity should be scanned with color Doppler to identify an enlarged extra-thyroidal artery feeding the parathyroid adenoma [1].

Increasing amounts of pressure are gradually applied, sufficient to deform the strap muscles and subcutaneous tissue contour. Deep regions such as the tracheoesophageal groove and carotid sheath should be scanned in this manner so that deeply positioned adenomas may become visible. This technique is especially useful in patients with thick necks, those with adenomas less than 1 cm, ectopic glands in the lower neck and adenomas in the tracheoesophageal groove or along the longus colli [3].

27.8 Conclusion

In conclusion, sensitivity of ultrasound for detection of parathyroid adenomas can be increased with a meticulous scanning technique. Both the typical locations and potential sites of ectopic parathyroid adenomas in the neck should be carefully scrutinized in gray-scale and color Doppler modes using the scanning technique described above.

References

1. Lane MJ, Desser TS, Weigel RJ, Jeffrey RB. Use of color and power Doppler sonography to identify feeding arteries associated with parathyroid adenomas. AJR Am J Roentgenol. 1998;171:819–23.
2. Wolf RJ, Cronan JJ, Monchik JM. Color Doppler sonography: an adjunctive technique in assessment of parathyroid adenomas. J Ultrasound Med. 1994;13: 303–8.
3. Reeder SB, Desser TS, Weigel RJ, Jeffrey RB. Sonography in primary hyperparathyroidism: review with emphasis on scanning technique. J Ultrasound Med. 2002;21:539–52. quiz 553-534.
4. Huppert B, Reading C. The parathyroid glands. In: Rumack C, Wilson S, Charboneau JW, Levine D, editors. Diagnostic ultrasound. 4th ed. St. Louis, MO: Mosby; 2011. p. 750–72.
5. Shawker T, Avila N, Premkumar A, Bradford M, Doppman J. Ultrasound evaluation of primary hyperparathyroidism. Ultrasound Q. 2000;16:73–87.
6. Khati N, Adamson T, Johnson KS, Hill MC. Ultrasound of the thyroid and parathyroid glands. Ultrasound Q. 2003;19:162–76.
7. Chen H, Pruhs Z, Starling JR, Mack E. Intraoperative parathyroid hormone testing improves cure rates in patients undergoing minimally invasive parathyroidectomy. Surgery. 2005;138:583–7. discussion 587-590.
8. Braunwald E, Fauci A, Kasper D, Hauser S, Longo D, Jameson JL. Disorders of the endocrine system. In: Harrison's principles of internal medicine. 15th ed. New York, NY: McGraw-Hill Professional Publishing; 2001. p. 2192–244.
9. DeLellis R. Tumors of parathyroid glands. In: Atlas of tumor pathology: American Registry of Pathology. Washington, DC: Armed Forces Institute of Pathology; 1993.
10. Low RA, Katz AD. Parathyroidectomy via bilateral cervical exploration: a retrospective review of 866 cases. Head Neck. 1998;20:583–7.
11. Yabuta T, Tsushima Y, Masuoka H, Tomoda C, Fukushima M, Kihara M, Inoue H, et al. Ultrasonographic features of intrathyroidal parathyroid adenoma causing primary hyperparathyroidism. Endocr J. 2011;58:989–94.
12. Loevener L. Anatomy and pathology of thyroid and parathyroid glands. In: Peter S, Hugh C, editors. Head and neck imaging. 5th ed. St. Louis, MO: Mosby; 2011.
13. O'Rahilly R, Müller F. The endocrine system. In: Human embryology & teratology. 3rd ed. New York, NY: Wiley-Liss; 2001. p. 345.
14. Grevellec A, Tucker AS. The pharyngeal pouches and clefts: development, evolution, structure and derivatives. Semin Cell Dev Biol. 2010;21:325–32.
15. Solivetti FM, Nasrollah N, Paganelli C, De Majo A. Lymphadenopathy as specific ultrasonography index of subacute thyroiditis. Preliminary data. Radiol Med. 1998;96:596–8.
16. Stucken EZ, Kutler DI, Moquete R, Kazam E, Kuhel WI. Localization of small parathyroid adenomas using modified 4-dimensional computed tomography/ultrasound. Otolaryngol Head Neck Surg. 2012;146:33–9.
17. Ghaheri BA, Koslin DB, Wood AH, Cohen JI. Preoperative ultrasound is worthwhile for reoperative parathyroid surgery. Laryngoscope. 2004;114:2168–71.
18. Meilstrup JW. Ultrasound examination of the parathyroid glands. Otolaryngol Clin North Am. 2004;37:763–78. ix.

Part VII

Interventional Ultrasound

The Procedure of Ultrasound-Guided Percutaneous Biopsy of Thyroid and Cervical Lymph Nodes: Technical Steps, Pitfalls, and Pearls

28

Robert A. Levine and John Interlandi

28.1 Introduction

Fine needle aspiration (FNA) of thyroid nodules (TN) was first reported in 1930 by Martin and Ellis [1] who described aspirating a thyroid mass with a 22-gauge needle. Nondiagnostic specimens due to bloody aspirates and concerns about spread of cancer along the needle track prevented prompt adoption of this technique. In 1977, Walfish [2] recommended combining FNA with ultrasound guidance (USGFNA) to decrease the number of inadequate samples. Subsequent studies confirmed his hypothesis that ultrasound guidance on the initial FNA could reduce the nondiagnostic rate by 50 % [3, 4]. USGFNA has evolved into the diagnostic procedure of choice for thyroid nodules [5]. USGFNA has been adapted to include evaluation of cervical lymph nodes, parathyroid glands, and other neck masses.

The goal of USGFNA on solid nodules is to provide specimens that are adequate for diagnosis. An adequate number of thyroid cells that are unobscured by excessive blood, and do not have crush or clot artifact must be obtained. The procedure should minimize patient discomfort and be performed safely without excessive bleeding, pain, bruising, infection, or damage to vital structures.

Inherent to thyroid cytology is the difficulty in distinguishing well-differentiated follicular carcinoma or follicular variant of papillary carcinoma from benign follicular adenoma. This results in approximately 15 % of samples being categorized as indeterminate. Recommended approaches to an indeterminate biopsy include repeating the biopsy in 2–3 months, integration of other B-mode and Doppler features, elastography, and the use of molecular markers [5]. Obtaining sufficient cellular groups from cystic, highly vascular, or calcified nodules adds difficulty and will be addressed in this chapter. Poor sampling, improper slide-making, or incomplete on-site analysis can result in inaccurate diagnosis or excessively high rate of indeterminate or nondiagnostic samples [6].

A full diagnostic ultrasound should be performed prior to FNA of palpable thyroid nodules [5]. Studies have shown that many palpable abnormalities are not true nodules [7]. Conversely, nonpalpable nodules of clinical significance are often

Electronic supplementary material: The online version of this chapter (doi:10.1007/978-3-319-44100-9_28) contains supplementary material, which is available to authorized users. Videos can also be accessed at http://link.springer.com/chapter/10.1007/978-3-319-44100-9_28.

R.A. Levine, M.D., F.A.C.E., E.C.N.U. (✉)
Thyroid Center of New Hampshire, St. Joseph Hospital Endocrinology, Geisel School of Medicine at Dartmouth College, Nashua, NH, USA
e-mail: thyroidmd2@gmail.com

J. Interlandi, M.D., F.A.C.E., E.C.N.U. (✉)
Department of Endocrinology, Advanced Health Partners, 5651 First Blvd, #415, Hermitage, TN 37076, USA
e-mail: foslman1950@gmail.com

M. Milas et al. (eds.), *Advanced Thyroid and Parathyroid Ultrasound*,
DOI 10.1007/978-3-319-44100-9_28

detected upon US evaluation of an index nodule. US performed prior to biopsy creates an accurate record of the size and characteristics of the nodules, assists in selection of the most suspicious nodule(s) in a multinodular thyroid, and is used for selection of needle size and length. Finally, the ultrasound assessment for cervical lymphadenopathy is essential prior to biopsy of a thyroid nodule, as the presence of suspicious lymph nodes necessitates biopsy of both the lymph node and the nodule.

This chapter will address FNA only. Core needle biopsy is rarely needed for thyroid diagnosis. There are reports of hemorrhage and tumor needle tracking with large core needle biopsy. Core biopsy requires extensive local anesthesia, proper training, and is associated with increased patient discomfort. Some studies have shown the value of core needle biopsy following inadequate fine needle aspiration biopsy, but it does not consistently improve the diagnostic quality of indeterminate biopsies on follicular neoplasms [8–10]. Core biopsy should be performed only by clinicians trained in the technique, in a setting with ability to deal with potential complications.

28.2 Preparation of the Patient

To prepare a patient for USFNA, the operator should:

(a) Give a detailed explanation of the procedure, including the small needle used, the brief dwell time, what the oscillations feel like, the expected discomfort (including possible referred pain to the ipsilateral ear), and discussion of not swallowing during the brief needle dwell time.
(b) Allow discussion. Patient anxiety regarding the procedure can usually be alleviated with proper reassurance.
(c) Allow the patient to assist in positioning. Discuss whether he/she can tolerate being supine with the neck hyperextended. Explain that pillows are available for back/neck comfort.
(d) Discuss the option of local anesthesia (see below), including an explanation of what the anesthetic feels like.
(e) Obtain any history of cardiac or pulmonary disease, bleeding disorders, anticoagulant use, vasovagal syncope, or other conditions that may affect the procedure.
(f) Discuss the potential diagnoses to be obtained (insufficient, benign, indeterminate, suspicious, or malignant) and how the results will be communicated to the patient.
(g) Have the patient sign an informed consent document. Consider additional consent for molecular markers if this may be performed after reviewing the FNA cytology results.

The decision whether to use local anesthesia is individualized. Most patients state after the biopsy that their anticipation of pain was greater than the actual discomfort of the FNA. In a study of FNA with 25-gauge needles and no local anesthetic in 218 patients, the amount of pain increased with younger age, female sex, patient anxiety, and the number of nodules biopsied [11, 12]. Since the injection of lidocaine is painful itself, most patients will tolerate FNA of a single nodule without anesthetic. However in select patients, including those with marked anxiety, local anesthesia can be offered (Table 28.1 "Steps for Local Anesthesia").

28.3 The Biopsy-Planning Ultrasound and the "Time Out"

Immediately prior to the FNA, the patient's vital signs should be reviewed and recorded. Image each nodule considering the order in which the nodules will be biopsied, the optimal patient positioning and angle(s) of approach for each nodule, and the location of anesthetic to be placed, if desired. The anatomy, vascularity, capsule thickness, and calcifications in each nodule should be reviewed.

Prior to the biopsy, using light pressure on the transducer, the vessels between the skin and each target nodule should be interrogated with Doppler, and a route avoiding them planned. Although a 27-gauge needle will rarely cause a bleeding complication, traversing a vessel may introduce blood into the specimen, and should be avoided. Similarly, a Doppler image of the target nodule will provide information regarding the vascularity of the nodule, influencing the choice

Table 28.1 Steps for local anesthesia

1. Put 1.5 cm^3 of 1 % Xylocaine into a 3 cm^3 syringe and change the needle to a fresh 27-gauge needle.
2. Squirt a few drops out of the end to make sure the needle lumen is open.
3. Using ultrasound guidance, locate the path to the target and make sure it is clear of large veins or any arteries. Leave the transducer in this location.
4. With the bevel up, spread the skin taut and insert the needle all the way through the skin with a quick motion and inject a small amount of Xylocaine (0.1–0.25 cm^3) under the dermis into the subcutaneous fat. The injection should not meet resistance. If it does, the needle tip is still in the dermis and do not inject until you push through to the sq fat. You will not be able to see the needle tip during step 4—it is all by feel since the bevel is to the side of the US beam.
5. Advance the needle slowly until the bevel appears on the ultrasound screen, then push it through the strap muscles and directly onto the capsule of the thyroid.
6. Slowly inject 0.75–1 cm^3 of Xylocaine as the needle is withdrawn under direct visualization. The operator should be able to see the tissues spreading apart and the muscles becoming hyperechoic as the Xylocaine is injected.
7. Once the bevel disappears off the side of the ultrasound image, stop injecting and this will avoid injecting Xylocaine into the dermis, which is painful. Wait several minutes for the Xylocaine to diffuse.
8. Make a mental note of the angle the needle path traveled and use it to adjust your angle to the target for the actual FNA.
9. The most pain-sensitive areas for thyroid FNA are the dermis and the fascia of the strap muscles. Sufficient anesthetic needs to be applied directly to the fascia, and just underneath the dermis, to achieve the desired effect.

of entry site, biopsy technique (suction versus non-suction), needle size, and dwell time.

A brief "time-out" is held prior to the procedure to reconfirm the patient identity, planned procedure, location of the nodule(s), allergies, and answer any remaining questions. The informed consent document should be reviewed for completeness.

28.4 Performing the FNA: Technical Aspects

Proper room setup and availability of all necessary equipment is essential. A probe cover, several 10 cm^3 syringes, biopsy needles, alcohol, povidone-iodine, gauze pads, sterile ultrasound gel or Surgilube, and a hemostat or needle driver should be present on the biopsy tray. The hemostat or needle driver is used to hold needles for slide making, and to transfer used biopsy needles to the needle disposal device. 22 and 25-gauge spinal needles should be available for deep targets or if a stylet is necessary, as discussed later. Extension tubing and stopcocks should be available.

Whether local anesthesia is chosen or not, 27-gauge needles are optimal for FNA and will minimize pain. A 27-gauge needle results in far less discomfort than larger needles, and will allow sampling of complete small follicles, sheets of cells from walls of macrofollicles, and may even provide tissue fragments (Fig. 28.1). Larger gauge or spinal needles are for special situations or for draining cyst fluid (see below). Echogenic needles and needle guides mounted on the probe are available but typically not needed. Before using any needles, the operator should confirm that the lumen of each is functional by pushing air through the needles.

FNA is an antiseptic, not a sterile procedure. As with venipuncture, full sterile preparation is unnecessary. The skin should be cleaned with either alcohol, or with povidone-iodine followed by alcohol. Sterile draping of the patient is not necessary. Gloves are worn to protect the operator and to prevent contamination of the puncture site. A small amount of ultrasound coupling gel is placed on the uncovered probe, its cover applied, then cleaned with alcohol.

If local anesthesia is to be used, it can be applied at this time. The skin entry site should be anesthetized and a track to the nodule infiltrated with very slow injection. Allow adequate time for the anesthetic to take effect prior to the procedure (Table 28.1 "Steps for Local Anesthesia")

To minimize discomfort, avoid going through the sternocleidomastoid muscle (SCM) whenever possible. This is usually achievable with diagonal orientations of the biopsy needle or transducer, or with techniques including medial to lateral needle direction, but will be impossible in a small number of nodules and cervical lymph nodes or in very muscular individuals. When the head is

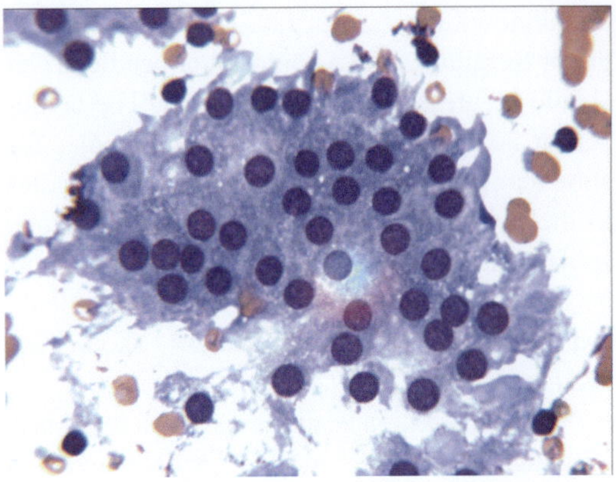

Fig. 28.1 *Fragment of follicle*. This segment of a benign macro-follicle was obtained through a 27-gauge needle

Table 28.2 Suction versus suction-less biopsy

Suction	Suction-less
1. Larger volume of sample	1. Smaller volume of sample
2. More blood	2. Less blood
3. Begin sampling once in target	3. Simpler
4. Avascular nodules	4. Vascular nodules
5. Lymph nodes	5. Superficial nodules
6. Parathyroids	6. Most nodules
7. Complex cysts	
8. Drain cysts	

rotated significantly away from the side of the FNA, the ipsilateral SCM will be pulled over the target site, and this position should be avoided. If avoiding the SCM is not possible, its superficial fascia, belly, and deep fascia may be anesthetized. A spinal needle may rarely be necessary for the USGFNA in muscular or obese individuals if the SCM must be traversed.

As shown in Videos 28.1, 28.2, 28.3, and 28.4, holding the skin taut at the time of needle entry, puncturing quickly, then slowly advancing to the target with US imaging will minimize patient discomfort and maximize visualization. The suction, rotation, or fine oscillations of the needle after the needle tip has entered the target will typically not cause discomfort, but the patient may describe pressure or referred pain to the ipsilateral ear at this time.

In solid thyroid nodules, FNA can be done using a suction technique (ST), or a non-suction technique (NST). The capillary action required for the NST depends on the distance the needle is moved forward as well as surface tension within the lumen, both of which allow material to travel up the needle. In solid nodules over 2 cm, the larger oscillations using NST are usually enough to drive the cell fragments up the needle quickly. In smaller solid thyroid nodules the oscillations must be shorter, so suction may be necessary. ST results in a larger volume, but more blood is introduced to the sample, potentially causing clot artifact and obscuration, whereas NST will result in a smaller volume that contains less blood and is often of better quality. With ST, sampling begins ***after*** the needle tip is within the target, whereas NST will result in acquisition of some cells from the intervening tissues.

The advantages and disadvantages of ST versus NST are summarized in Table 28.2. The initial biopsy can be performed without suction, or with very light (1–2 cm^3) suction. If the first aspiration yields insufficient material, suction can be applied or increased during subsequent passes. If excessive blood or material is aspirated, the suction can be decreased or eliminated on subsequent passes. Suctionless techniques using a bare needle or a needle attached to a syringe without the plunger are shown in Videos 28.1, 28.2, 28.3, and 28.4. There are several devices and methods for applying suction during USGFNA. These are illustrated in Videos 28.5, 28.6, 28.7, 28.8, 28.9, and 28.10.

In a palpation-based biopsy study using two passes with each technique in 260 thyroid nodules there was no difference in adequacy or accuracy when comparing aspiration (ST) with capillary action (NST). In an ultrasound-guided biopsy study, 88 nodules underwent fine needle aspiration with ST, and 92 underwent fine needle NST, with no difference between the results in terms of adequacy and quality of specimen. The authors concluded that the NST technique may offer more technical ease [13, 14].

Rotating the needle, without suction or oscillations, may reduce blood contamination in large or vascular nodules because it minimizes the number of vessels that are traversed. A combination of spinning and small oscillations can also be used (Videos 28.1, 28.2, 28.3, and 28.4). Avoid long oscillation strokes in nodules with high grade vascularity.

While some authors recommend covering the hub or syringe after the biopsy and prior to withdrawing the needle, this does not appear to be necessary to achieve adequate samples. However, covering the needle hub or syringe barrel is typically used when performing biopsy of complex cysts, so that capillary pressure does not draw cyst fluid into the needle prior to entering the solid target. Suction can then be applied once the needle tip is well within the solid component. Suction is always used in the drainage of cysts, and movement of the needle tip within the cyst may help if there is solid tissue plugging the bevel.

Adequacy of technique can be confirmed with rapid on-site cytologic analysis.

28.5 Imaging for FNA

Proper room setup and availability of equipment is essential to maximize the contribution of US to FNA procedures. Ideally, the monitor for the US should be across the patient from the operator, allowing the operator to visualize the patient's neck and the monitor simultaneously. A second monitor connected to the ultrasound machine can be placed on the contralateral side attached to the wall with a C-arm, or on a movable table to allow visualizing the procedure from either side of the patient (Figs. 28.2 and 28.3).

Visualization of the needle can be performed using either a parallel or perpendicular technique. In the parallel technique, the needle is inserted along the axis of the ultrasound beam (Fig. 28.4a, b, Videos 28.11 and 28.12) and is visualized throughout its course through the tissue and into the target. In the perpendicular technique, the needle is inserted perpendicular to the axis of the beam, and is visualized only at the point that it intersects the beam (Fig. 28.5, Video 28.13). Advantages of the parallel approach include visualization of the needle tip at all times during the biopsy, decreasing the probability of the needle tip leaving the target or traversing blood vessels. Multiple spots within the nodule can be sampled, and the needle can be redirected while being inserted. The perpendicular approach does not require accurate alignment of the needle and ultrasound beam, and may be simpler to perform, especially for superficial nodules.

Operators should become skilled in all techniques, as the nodule size and location often will dictate which technique is preferred. There are several techniques to improve needle visualization when using the parallel approach. It is essential that the needle and the long axis of the transducer perfectly line up. Positioning yourself so that you can see the relationship between the

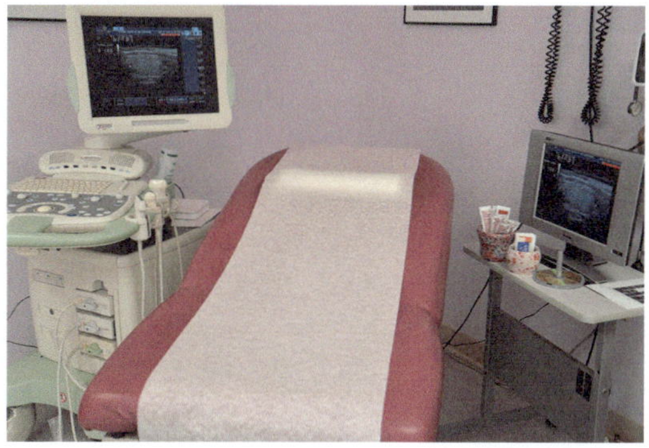

Fig. 28.2 *Room setup*. The use of an additional monitor allows the operator to line up the patient's neck and the monitor, and observe both simultaneously

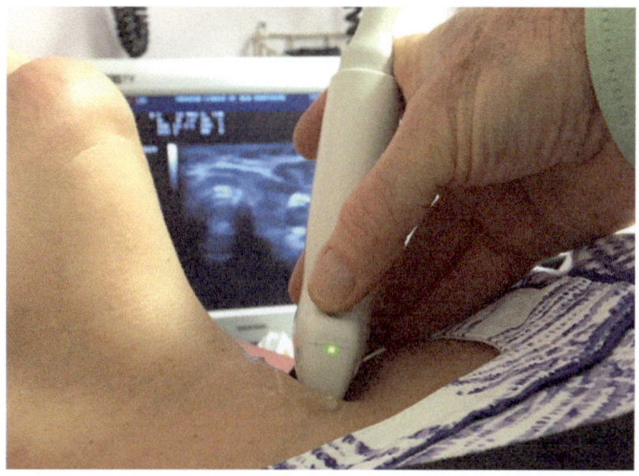

Fig. 28.3 *Line-up transducer*. Achieving perfect alignment of the needle and the long axis of the transducer is much easier when looking down the axis of the transducer

a b

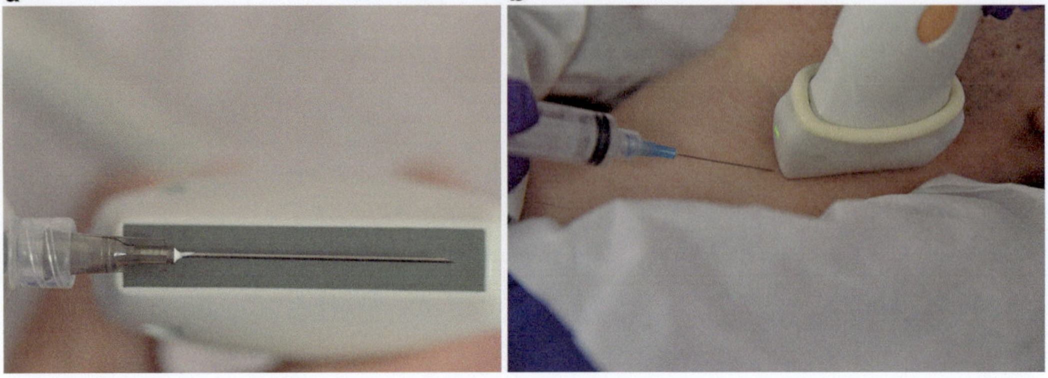

Fig. 28.4 (**a**, **b**). *Parallel approach*. In the parallel technique, the needle is inserted along the axis of the ultrasound beam and is visualized throughout its course through the tissue and into the target

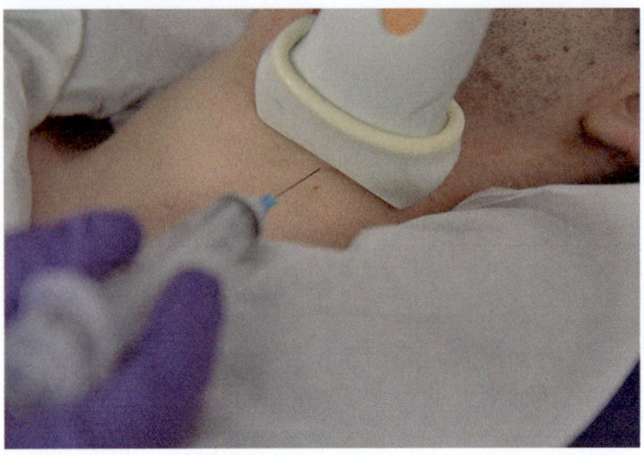

Fig. 28.5 *Perpendicular approach*. In the perpendicular technique, the needle is inserted perpendicular to the axis of the beam, and is visualized only at the point that it intersects the beam

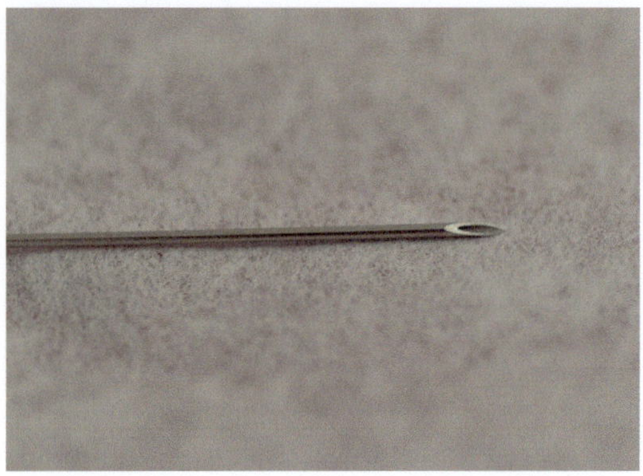

Fig. 28.6 *Bevel up*. The strongest refection off of the needle will be from the flat bevel. The bevel, shown in this image, should be "up," pointing toward the transducer

needle and transducer head is essential. Having the transducer placed so that you can look down the needle and the transducer head (Fig. 28.3) will improve the ability to line the two items up. The bevel of the needle should be pointed toward the ultrasound transducer in all techniques (Fig. 28.6). Fine adjustments of the transducer, both rotation and lateral movement, will bring the needle into view if the axis is off by a small amount. The most important part of developing skill in properly lining up the needle is practice. It is highly recommended that the operator begin with work on phantoms until sufficient skill in lining up the needle is obtained, prior to performing biopsy in a clinical setting.

Beam steering can be applied during the parallel approach to improve needle visualization. Beam steering will decrease the angle of incidence between the ultrasound beam and the needle, making the needle more conspicuous. This may be useful in deep nodules (Fig. 28.7a, b).

Most biopsies are performed using a linear probe as this is the transducer typically used for diagnostic imaging. However, a micro-convex probe may also be used for biopsy and is preferred by some experts. Figure 28.8 and Video 28.14 demonstrate the technique using a micro-convex (curvilinear) probe. The probe is placed directly over the target and the target is centered within the ultrasound screen. The probe is then

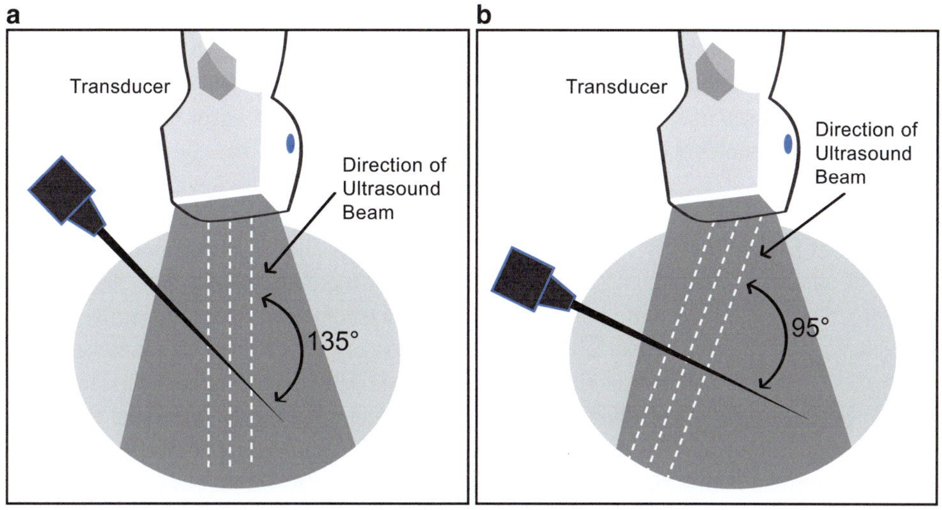

Fig. 28.7 (**a**, **b**). *Beam Steering*. Beam steering will decrease the angle of incidence between the ultrasound beam and the needle, making the needle more conspicuous. This may be useful in deep nodules

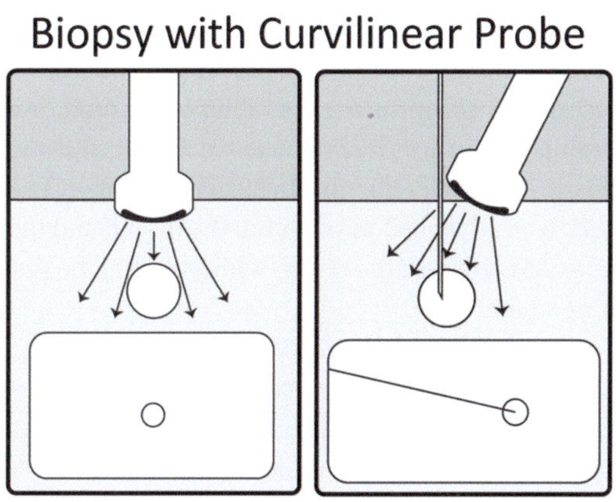

Fig. 28.8 *Curvilinear transducer biopsy*. The probe is placed directly over the target and the target is centered within the ultrasound screen. The probe is then slid laterally and rotated medially, continuing to point toward the target. The needle is then introduced directly perpendicular to the skin, aiming straight down from the prior initial center of the ultrasound probe. See also Video 28.15

slid laterally and rotated medially, continuing to point toward the target. The needle is then introduced directly perpendicular to the skin, aiming straight down from the prior initial center of the ultrasound probe. If performed adequately, the needle will enter the target as the skin entry site is directly above the target.

For most solid nodule biopsies, the briefest dwell time possible is preferred. The longer the needle remains within the target, the more hemorrhage will occur, and the specimen will become diluted by blood and develop clot artifact. In general, 2–5 s of dwell time within the nodule utilizing gentle oscillation and rotation will be adequate. When material is seen within the hub, the biopsy needle should be removed immediately. The assistant can watch the hub of the needle while the operator is visualizing the ultrasound, and notify the operator immediately upon noting any material in the needle hub.

In nodules larger than 2 cm, the needle tip should be placed in the peripheral aspect of the nodule rather than the center since the central area has the least cellular growth, and the most potential for cystic degeneration. Subsequent aspirations should be directed to different quadrants of the nodule while continuing to avoid the center and the most peripheral 2–3 mm of the nodule, as it contains fibrous material and blood vessels.

The number of passes performed is operator dependent, and should be based on the adequacy rate achieved. If rapid on-site evaluation of cytology is available, often two passes by an experienced operator may be sufficient with adequacy confirmed. Additional passes should be performed if an adequate number of cells are not present (typically defined as more than six groups containing more than ten thyroid follicular cells).

Further passes should be performed until adequacy is ascertained. When on-site adequacy is not utilized, typically three or four passes are performed. Additional passes may be necessary for special studies such as molecular markers.

28.6 Special Situations

Hypervascular Nodules. When significant vascularity is observed on the pre-biopsy ultrasound power Doppler analysis, the non-suction technique should be used to decrease blood contamination. A much briefer dwell time is also important, often utilizing only one or two oscillations or rotations after gentle positioning of the needle within the nodule. Subsequent passes should be performed at different areas within the nodule to decrease blood within the subsequent specimens.

Nodules with peripheral calcification. Nodules may demonstrate peripheral eggshell calcification. In general, continuous uninterrupted eggshell calcification is a relatively reassuring finding, whereas interrupted eggshell calcification implies growth of previously calcified nodule and indicates a higher degree of suspicion. When interrupted eggshell calcification is present, the needle should be inserted through areas of interruption. For uninterrupted calcification a 22-gauge needle can be used, and local anesthesia may be needed. The patient should be informed that they may feel very intense pressure during the biopsy. The needle is positioned at the edge of the nodule and pressure is applied until a pop is felt as the needle enters through the calcification. Suction aspiration is then performed with oscillation of the needle tip. If multiple passes are made, the subsequent passes should enter through the original puncture site if possible, but the needle should be re-angled to sample different areas within the nodule.

Occasionally heavily calcified nodules will not permit entry of a 22-gauge needle. In this situation, a 22 or 25-gauge needle is used to "drill" a hole in the side of the nodule using a combination of rotation and pressure until the nodule is punctured. Subsequently, the drilling needle is removed and a 27-gauge needle can be used to complete the FNA.

Predominantly cystic nodules. The target area should be the most suspicious solid component, especially one that has vascular supply evident. Suction is typically used with complex nodules, to avoid capillary pressure filling the needle with cyst fluid. The needle should be mounted on a syringe with no suction applied until the tip traverses through the fluid into the solid portion, with suction applied only after the needle tip is well within the solid component. It is preferable to biopsy the solid component prior to draining the cyst, since the image of the solid component is often distorted after cyst drainage. However, if cyst fluid fills the hub in the first pass, it may be necessary to drain the cyst and then biopsy the residual solid component.

Deep biopsies. The technique of utilizing a spinal needle for deep biopsy is illustrated in Video 28.15. This video demonstrates using a spinal needle with a parallel approach. Beam steering is recommended as the needle direction may be close to the axial axis of the ultrasound beam and not well visualized (Fig. 28.6). The needle is advanced until within the target, and the assistant removes the stylet, with sampling beginning at that time.

For nodules that are deep and medial (e.g., close to the trachea), the operator can stand opposite from the side of the nodule and use a parallel approach with neck rotation. Rotation of the neck about 45° toward the operator will bring the nodule closer to the surface without bringing the ipsilateral SCM muscle too close, and will often create a much shorter distance to travel to the target nodule (Fig. 28.9).

High Lateral Nodules. Thyroid nodules that are very high in the superior pole may be difficult to reach using a straight transverse position of the transducer due to protrusion of the cornu of the larynx, especially in thin patients. FNA may be best performed using a parallel needle approach, with both the transducer and needle held in an oblique orientation, and the patient's head rotated 45° away from the biopsy side (Fig. 28.10). Entering the needle inferior and slightly lateral to the thyroid cartilage will permit access to this area of the thyroid.

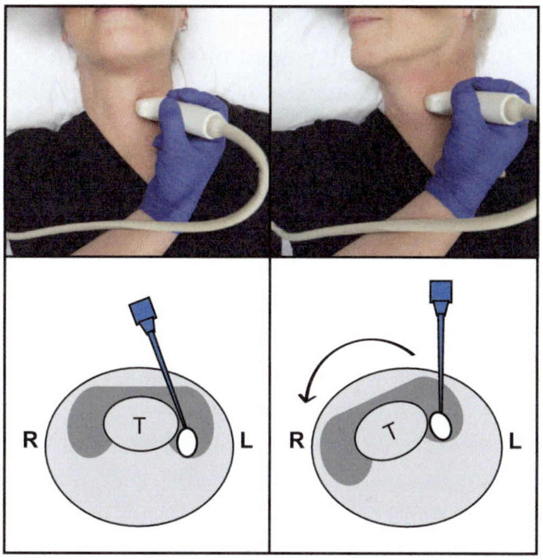

Fig. 28.9 *Deep medial position nodule.* For nodules that are deep and medial (e.g., close to the trachea), the operator can stand opposite from the side of the nodule and use a parallel approach with partial neck rotation. Rotation of the neck about 45° toward the operator will bring the nodule closer to the surface without bringing the ipsilateral SCM muscle too close, and will often create a much shorter distance to travel to the target nodule

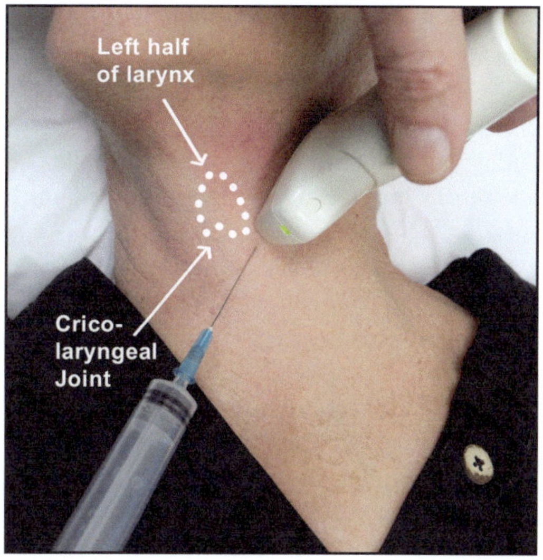

Fig. 28.10 *High lateral nodule.* Thyroid nodules that are very high in the superior pole may be difficult to reach due to the cornu of the larynx and may be best performed with a parallel-style needle approach, with the transducer held in an oblique orientation, with the patient's head rotated 45° away from the biopsy side

Insufficient biopsy results. If the operator has a high rate of insufficient biopsy samples there are several remedial techniques. Using rapid on-site assessment to determine adequacy may improve results. It should be determined whether the insufficient biopsies are due to not obtaining enough thyroid follicular epithelial cells or whether the sample is obscured by excessive blood. This information will help determine if an adjustment in needle size is indicated: using a smaller needle if excessive blood is present, or changing from non-suction technique to suction technique if inadequate cells are being obtained. If samples are excessively hemorrhagic rotation rather than oscillation can be used. Excessive blood will also be present if veins are repeatedly punctured during the procedure. Repeating the biopsy using a different approach to the target may improve the sample.

Taking a course to learn proper slide making technique may be useful. If inadequate cells are being obtained with slide preparation, considering changing to liquid-based cytology. If there are overt suspicious findings on ultrasound, proceeding directly to surgery may be preferable. It is essential that the operator discuss all insufficient biopsies with the pathologist to determine why the sample was inadequate. If multiple attempts at biopsy are insufficient consider a referral to an expert for repeat fine needle aspiration biopsy or core needle biopsy.

28.7 Complications: Prevention and Treatment

Bleeding complications are rare following USGFNA. Patients receiving anticoagulation or antiplatelet therapy including aspirin, heparin, clopidogrel, or Coumadin may have superficial ecchymosis if subcutaneous vessels are punctured [15]. This can be minimized by careful planning of the entry route during the pre-biopsy ultrasound.

In patients treated with a platelet inhibitor or Coumadin, it may be useful to pretreat the biopsy site for 10 min with a cold compress to reduce the blood blow. A cold compress can also decrease the discomfort associated with injection of Lidocaine.

To avoid injury to the thyroid, the patient should be advised to swallow immediately prior to each needle puncture and then to not swallow during the dwell time. If the patient swallows during the procedure the needle should be allowed to travel with the thyroid to minimize shear.

If a subcutaneous hematoma appears after a puncture, the procedure should be temporarily stopped and pressure applied until the bleeding stops.

In patients treated with anticoagulants it is advisable to observe the patient for 10 min following biopsy for hematoma formation and to repeat a quick limited ultrasound before discharge. Subcutaneous ecchymosis does not require an US for confirmation. However, if a deep hematoma is seen in the strap muscles or thyroid gland, a cold compress should be applied with a repeat ultrasound approximately 30 min later to be sure that there is no expansion of the hematoma. Also, the ultrasonographer should be aware that muscles into which lidocaine is introduced will appear temporarily wider and more hyperechoic from the lidocaine.

After-care instructions will include the use of a cold compress and acetaminophen if any local pain or bruising occurs. Thyroid biopsy should be easy and relatively painless for the patient. If this is not the case in most biopsies, additional education in biopsy technique is strongly recommended.

28.8 Slide Preparation

The goal of quality slide preparation is to obtain a monolayer dispersion of cells and to avoid distortion or crush artifact of the cells. The technique used for slide preparation and staining is at the discretion of the cytopathologist and the operator should perform whatever technique the expert cytopathologist prefers. Some studies suggest that slide preparation is preferable to liquid-based preparation. The technique of smearing the sample on a slide is demonstrated in Videos 28.16, 28.17, and 28.18. In the typical smear technique, the second microscope slide is introduced in a perpendicular dimension and contact is made between the edge of the slide and the below the target on the index slide. The top slide is then lightly and gradually lowered until it lightly makes contact with the sample, at which time it is lightly dragged down, avoiding crush artifact. An alternative method of slide preparation is referred to as "bookends" (Videos 28.19 and 28.20). In this technique, the second slide is lightly placed in a parallel orientation to the first and capillary action spreads the sample out over the slides. They are then separated as in opening a book. This technique provides two slides with "mirror image" samples. The first slide may be used for rapid on-site assessment, and the second slide can be used for definitive staining.

During slide preparation, all material should be extracted from the needle, hub, and syringe. Initially, the sample should be expressed from the needle by a forcefully pressing on the plunger. If material remains within the needle hub, a technique of snapping the hub onto the slide to extract the material should be utilized (Video 28.21).

In liquid-based preparation the entire sample is introduced into a preservative rather than preparing slides directly. This is then centrifuged and slides are prepared by the pathologist. While studies have suggested that slide preparation is superior [16], several prestigious medical centers use liquid-based preparation with excellent results. As stated, the ultimate decision on how to present the material obtained from biopsy should be at the discretion of the expert cytopathologist.

28.9 Cervical Lymph Node FNA

FNA of cervical lymph nodes with analysis of cytology and thyroglobulin of the needle hub washing is the recommended approach for the evaluation of abnormal lymph nodes in a preoperative or postoperative thyroid cancer patient [5, 17]. Thyroglobulin analysis is not impacted by the presence of serum anti-thyroglobulin antibodies.

At the time of initial thyroid nodule evaluation, any suspicious lymph nodes should undergo biopsy. In patients with biopsy proven or suspected thyroid cancer a comprehensive cervical ultrasound should be performed for lymph node assessment, and any suspicious lateral nodes should undergo biopsy. In patients with a history of thyroid cancer, lymph nodes larger than 1 cm in smallest axis with suspicious ultrasonographic features should undergo biopsy if a positive result will affect management [5].

Similar considerations to biopsy of nodules apply when considering local anesthesia for lymph nodes. Deep lymph node biopsies may benefit from local anesthesia, especially when performing biopsy on lymph nodes deep to the SCM muscle or in level VI. Muscles and fascia that are to be traversed may be anesthetized.

Prior to the biopsy US should be used to plan the shortest, most avascular route to the target node. Nodes in levels II–V may require positioning the patient on their side with extra pillows for support.

A parallel imaging method should be used so the operator can be sure that the needle tip is in the area of interest of the lymph node. This may require oblique or sagittal orientation of the transducer depending on the location in the neck and the orientation of the lymph node. Occasionally, there may be focal involvement of the lymph node by tumor, and it is essential that the needle tip be in the involved area. Areas of calcification, cystic necrosis, or disordered vascularity should be targeted (Fig. 28.11).

Suction should be applied in all lymph node FNA procedures since it will maximize sample obtained. Blood contamination is less of a concern, as thyroglobulin analysis will complement cytology. Rapid on-site assessment may be useful to ascertain if it is an adequate sample. Typically, one or two passes are made during a lymph node biopsy. Accurate ultrasonographic determination that the needle tip is well placed in the lymph node is essential.

Following preparation of a single slide, rinse the needle and hub with 1 cm^3 of saline and send the sample for thyroglobulin analysis. If hematologic or lymphocytic neoplasms are suspected additional specimens should be sent for flow cytometry.

Bleeding after FNA of cervical nodes may occur when muscles are involved and can be minimized by adhering to the previous recommendations. Patients on Coumadin or platelet inhibitors should have a cold compress applied for 15 min before and 15 min after the procedure. Any patient with an obvious hematoma should have a cold compress applied after the procedure.

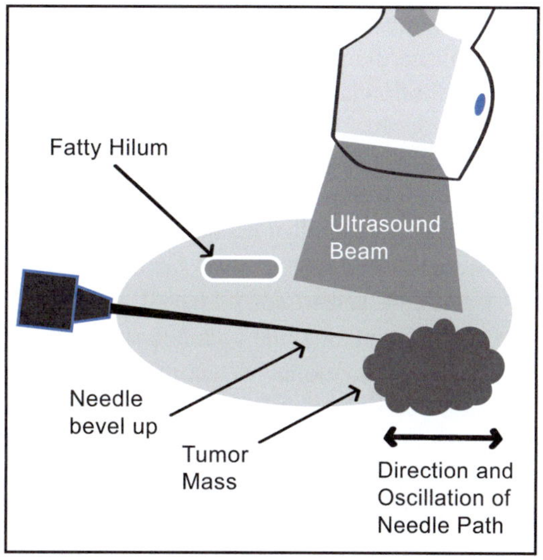

Fig. 28.11 *Node biopsy*. A parallel imaging method should be used so the operator can be sure that the needle tip is in the area of interest of the lymph node. Occasionally, there may be focal involvement of the lymph node by tumor, and it is essential that the needle tip be in the involved area. Areas of calcification, cystic necrosis, or disordered vascularity should be targeted

28.10 Top 10 Pearls Regarding Biopsy

1. *Enter quickly—Advance slowly*. Hold tension on the skin and puncture it quickly. A slow skin puncture will cause discomfort. Advance slowly through deeper structures.
2. *Have biopsy trays pre-prepared*. To save time have trays set up with povidone-iodine, alcohol, probe cover, sterile coupling gel, gauze pads, needles, syringes, slides, and bandages.
3. *Reassurance as effective anesthesia*. When using a 27-gauge needle local anesthesia is not absolutely needed for most patients if the patient is adequately reassured prior to the

procedure. Reassure the patient that with a small needle and brief dwell time, the local anesthesia may cause more discomfort than the biopsy.

4. *The needle itself as a diagnostic instrument.* The needle can provide information regarding the "hardness" of the nodule. If the target nodule permits entry, then seems to "grab" the needle and to not release it easily with needle oscillation, the nodule is more suspicious for carcinoma. When this occurs, the needle must be oscillated more slowly than usual through the nodule in order for the oscillations to yield cells. If the oscillations are too quick, the nodule will move with the needle.
5. *Use your assistant.* When performing a biopsy with suction, the first flash of sample into the needle hub may be missed if the operator is watching the monitor for needle localization. Instruct your assistant to observe the needle hub and immediately indicate (verbally or with nonverbal signal) when sample is in the hub. Withdraw the needle immediately to avoid additional blood contamination.
6. *Brief dwell time.* Keeping the time that the needle is in the target under 6 s will minimize blood contamination and decrease the likelihood of the patient swallowing during the procedure. Often the dwell time can be as brief as 2 or 3 s.
7. *IV tubing and stopcocks.* When draining large cysts the volume of fluid removed may exceed the capacity of the syringe. Placement of a three way stopcock at the distal end of IV tubing will allow switching the syringe without fluid leaking during syringe exchange.
8. *Mobile Nodules*—Nodules in the Isthmus and Pyramidal Lobes of the Thyroid are very mobile because they are not held in place by strap muscles or surrounding thyroid tissue. An extra drop of ultrasound gel put under the edge of the transducer just lateral to the nodule on the side of the needle entry (parallel approach) will allow better ultrasound visualization and prevent "dropoff" of the image. The operator can stretch the skin tightly over the nodule to help immobilize it.
9. *Avoid excessive head rotation*—Having the patient turn their head more than 45° from the side of the biopsy may result in the sternocleidomastoid muscle shifting over the nodule. Keeping the patient's head as close as possible to a neutral position can help avoid going through the muscle, and decrease discomfort from the biopsy.
10. *Warn the lab.* When submitting samples for thyroglobulin, PTH, or calcitonin, let the lab know that the sample is a syringe washing in 1 cm^3 of saline, to avoid having a sample discarded as "quantity not sufficient."

References

1. Martin HE, Ellis EB. Biopsy by needle puncture and Aspiration. Ann Surg. 1930;92:169–81.
2. Walfish PG, Hazani E, Strawbridge HTG, Miskin M, Rosen IB. Combined ultrasound and needle aspiration cytology in the assessment and management of hypofunctioning thyroid nodule. Ann Intern Med. 1977;87(3):270–4.
3. Gharib H. Fine-needle aspiration biopsy of thyroid nodules: advantages, limitations, and effect. Mayo Clin Proc. 1994;69:44–9.
4. Danese D, Sciacchitano S, Farsetti A, Andreoli M, Pontecorvi A. Diagnostic accuracy of conventional versus sonography guided fine-needle aspiration biopsy in the management of non-palpable and palpable thyroid nodules. Thyroid. 1998;8:511–5.
5. Haugen BR, Alexander EK, Bible KC, Doherty G, Mandel S, Nikiforov YE, Pacini F, Randolph G, Sawka A, Schlumberger M, Schuff KG, Sherman SI, Sosa JA, Steward D, Tuttle RM, Wartofsky L. 2015 American Thyroid Association Management Guidelines for adult patients with thyroid nodules and differentiated thyroid cancer: the American Thyroid Association Guidelines Task Force on thyroid nodules and differentiated thyroid cancer. Thyroid. 2016;26:1.
6. Abele JS, Levine RA. Diagnostic criteria and risk-adapted approach to indeterminate thyroid cytodiagnosis. Cancer Cytopathol. 2010;118(6):415–22.
7. Marqusee E, Benson C, Frates MC, Doubilet PM, Larsen PR, Cibas ES, Mandel SJ. Usefulness of ultrasonography in the management of nodular thyroid disease. Ann Intern Med. 2000;133(9):696–700.
8. Samir AE, Vij A, Seale MK, Desai G, Halpern E, Faquin WC, Parangi S, Hahn PF, Daniels GH. Ultrasound-guided percutaneous thyroid nodule core biopsy: clinical utility in patients with prior nondiagnostic fine-needle aspirate. Thyroid. 2012;22(5): 461–7.

9. Park KT, Ahn SH, Mo JH, Park YJ, Park DJ, Choi SI, Park SY. Role of core needle biopsy and ultrasonographic finding in management of indeterminate thyroid nodules. Head Neck. 2011;33(2):160–5.
10. Hahn SY, Shin JH, Han BK, Ko EY, Ko ES. Ultrasonography-guided core needle biopsy for the thyroid nodule: does the procedure hold any benefit for the diagnosis when fine-needle aspiration cytology analysis shows inconclusive results? Br J Radiol. 2013;86:1025.
11. Lo WC, Cheng PW, Wang CT, Yeh ST, Liao LJ. Pain levels associated with ultrasound-guided fine-needle aspiration biopsy for neck masses. Head Neck. 2014;36(2):252–6.
12. Leboulleux S, Borget I, Labro S, Bidault S, Vielh P, Hartl D, Dauchy S, Chougnet CN, Girard E, Azoulay S, Mirghani H, Berdelou A, Lumbroso J, Deandreis D, Baudin E, Schlumberger M, Laurent S. Frequency and intensity of pain related to thyroid nodule fine-needle aspiration cytology. Thyroid. 2013;23(9):1113–8.
13. de Carvalho GA, Paz-Filho G, Cavalcanti TC, Graf H. Adequacy and diagnostic accuracy of aspiration vs. capillary fine needle thyroid biopsies. Endocr Pathol. 2009;20:204–8.
14. Tublin ME, Martin JA, Rollin LJ, Pealer K, Kurs-Lasky M, Ohori NP. Ultrasound-guided fine-needle aspiration versus fine-needle capillary sampling biopsy of thyroid nodules. does technique matter? J Ultrasound Med. 2007;26(12):1697–701.
15. Abu-Yousef MM, Larson JH, Kuehn DM, Wu AS, Laroia AT. Safety of ultrasound-guided fine needle aspiration biopsy of neck lesions in patients taking antithrombotic/anticoagulant medications. Ultrasound Q. 2011;27(3):157–9.
16. Nagarajan N, Schneider EB, Ali SZ, Zeiger MA, Olson MT. How do liquid-based preparations of thyroid fine-needle aspiration compare with conventional smears? An analysis of 5475 specimens. Thyroid. 2015;25(3):308–13.
17. Baskin HJ. Detection of recurrent papillary thyroid carcinoma by thyroglobulin assessment in the needle washout after fine-needle aspiration of suspicious lymph nodes. Thyroid. 2004;14(11):959–63.

The Preparation of Biopsy Specimens for Routine and Molecular Cytology: Technical Steps, Pearls, and Pitfalls

29

Nicole A. Massoll

29.1 Introduction

The importance of optimal specimen preparation cannot be over emphasized. Poor specimen preparation hinders the optimal cytopathologic evaluation. Cytopathology specimens have numerous methods of collection, preparation, fixation, and staining.

29.2 Collection

One method for thyroid fine-needle aspiration (FNA) collection is as a rinse for liquid based fixation samples. The rinse collection method may be used for a liquid based cytology preparation such as ThinPrep®. This liquid based cytology preparation allows for the FNA samples to be rinsed directly into a liquid fixative. Each pass from the same nodule is rinsed into the same vial. It is important to repeat the aspirating, rinsing, and expressing of the needle in the liquid fixative to elute all of the sample from the needle hub.

Liquid based collection can be used to prepare a cell block. In this collection method, the aspirated specimens are expressed into a formalin fixative cup. Although not necessary for thyroid FNA, this method allows the sample to be processed as a paraffin-embedded block, which may be helpful when immunohistochemical stains are needed to exclude metastatic disease.

For techniques using slides, prepared as classic smears or bookends, the FNA specimen is procured in the same fashion. However the specimen is placed directly on the glass slides instead of into a liquid. This method allows for multiple slides to be prepared for different types of fixation and stains. Since the slides can be made at the bedside and stained rapidly, it allows for immediate assessment of adequacy or ROSE (Rapid on Site Evaluation).

29.3 Preparation

To prepare the liquid based slide, the vial containing the sample is sent to the lab and placed on an instrument to process the sample. The vial is centrifuged to form a concentrated pellet. The pellet is then resuspended and an aliquot placed into the PreservCyt solution vial. This solution is left to stand for 15 min and then processed on the ThinPrep ® machine using the non-gyn sequence. From this vial, generally a single slide is made that is a representative cellular collection from all the FNA passes rinsed into the container. This resulting slide is a monolayer of the aspirated

N.A. Massoll, M.D., F.A.S.C.P. (✉)
Division of Cytopathology, University of Arkansas for Medical Sciences, 4301 W Markham St, Slot 604, Little Rock, AR 72205, USA
e-mail: namassoll@uams.edu

M. Milas et al. (eds.), *Advanced Thyroid and Parathyroid Ultrasound*,
DOI 10.1007/978-3-319-44100-9_29

cells. The fact that this method typically produces only one slide may be considered as a drawback. Since only one slide is produced, only one staining method can be utilized, so the ability to evaluate the specimen with two stains, both a Papanicolaou and Romanowsky, is lost [1]. In this setting, the single slide is stained with a Papanicolaou stain (Fig. 29.1). This method has been gaining in popularity; however, its utilization has been controversial particularly in thyroid where extracellular matrix (colloid or amyloid) and architectural features are important. From the collection perspective, it is very simple to rinse the entire specimen into the vial and lack of smearing eliminates possible crush artifact. From the diagnostic perspective, the mechanical distribution results in an even monolayer of specimen to be evaluated in a smaller area of the slide. The downside is that background elements, such as blood and colloid, are decreased, resulting in a higher concentration of the cellular elements; this makes the diagnosis of hyperplasia versus neoplasia more challenging. Another concern with liquid based preparations is the lack of optimal cytologic features needed for the diagnosis of papillary thyroid carcinoma. This lack of crisp nuclear diagnostic features led to a false negative diagnosis in 7% of liquid based cases compared to smear methods [2].

Some liquid specimens can be used for a cytospin preparation. This method concentrates the liquid sample and a portion is placed in a cyto-funnel on a cyto-centrifuge machine. This method produces a monolayer of cells within a well-defined area of the slide. Depending on the amount of the sample, multiple slides can be made for different types of stains, though the Papanicolaou stain is the most common. This method is most commonly used when the cellularity of a sample is scant (Fig. 29.2).

Cell blocks are made from the formalin-fixed collection sample. The cell block can be prepared via several different methods, based on the techniques available to the specific lab. The sediment, clot, or tissue fragments are processed and embedded in paraffin. The paraffin block is cut on a microtome that makes thin tissue sections subsequently placed on glass slides. The end product is

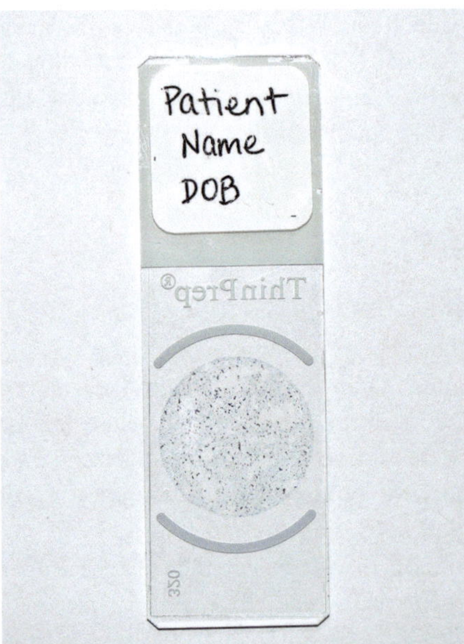

Fig. 29.1 Liquid-based slide prepared on Thinprep machine and stained with Papanicolaou stain. The single slide provides a representative monolayer of the aspirated material

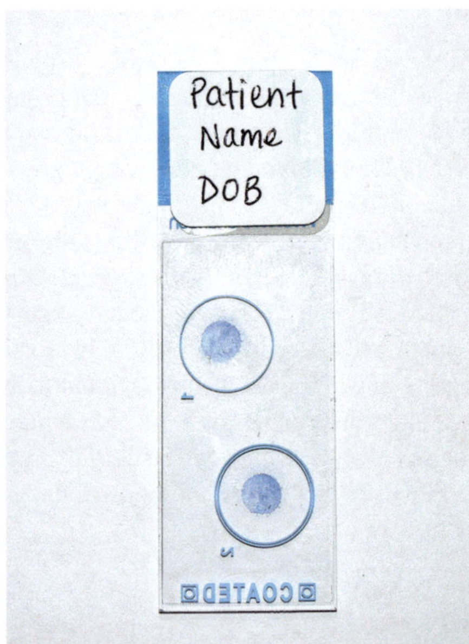

Fig. 29.2 A Cytospin preparation stained with Papanicolaou stain after liquid fixative collection method. This method is often performed when the sample collected is small

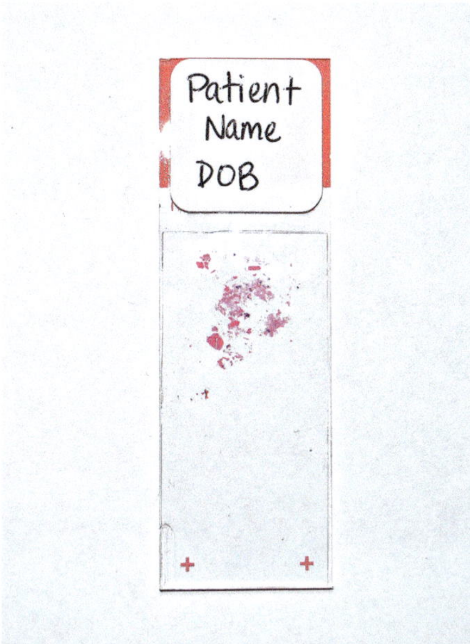

Fig. 29.3 A representative slide of hematoxylin and eosin stained cell block specimen. These samples are collected in a liquid fixative and paraffin embedded for cutting sections to place on slides

the traditionally hematoxylin and eosin (H&E) stained slides. The author's laboratory does not routinely use cell blocks. In our experience this method does not add additional information unless metastatic carcinoma needs to be confirmed with immunohistochemical stains (Fig 29.3).

There are numerous methods for direct slide preparation. To prepare smears the aspirate is expelled onto the slide with the needle tip bevel down touching the glass to minimize spraying of the sample and possible air-dry artifact for any alcohol-fixed slides.

29.3.1 Classic Smear Technique

1. Label frosted end with two patient identifiers (name, date of birth, medical record, etc.) using a #2 pencil
2. Place a small drop of the aspirate a few millimeters from the frosted end
3. Place another slide at the edge of the drop at a 45° angle and allow the sample drop to spread along the edge of the second slide
4. Decrease the angle, then gently and quickly, push the specimen evenly away from the frosted end down the slide, trying to keep the smear at least 1 mm from the edges of the glass
5. Immediately alcohol or spray fix one slide for Papanicolaou stain to be performed in the lab. The other slide can be air-dried and stained with a modified Romanowsky for ROSE or in the lab (Fig. 29.4a, b).

Depending on the amount of material aspirated, multiple slides can be made. Optimally, one air-dried and one alcohol-fixed slide should be made from each pass. This allows for ROSE to be performed if desired and allows for evaluation of the specimen using both stains.

29.3.2 Bookend Smear Technique

1. Label two slides at the frosted end with two patient identifiers (name, date of birth, medical record, etc.) using a #2 pencil.
2. Place a small drop of the aspirate in the middle of one slide.
3. Place the labeled, frosted side of the second slide face down onto the slide with the sample drop.
4. Allow the sample to spread by capillary action, do not apply pressure.
5. When the sample stops spreading, open the slides like a book, or pop them open. DO NOT SLIDE THEM ACROSS EACH OTHER.
6. This will produce two mirror image slides. Immediately alcohol or spray fix one slide for Papanicolaou stain to be performed in the lab. The other slide can be air-dried and stained with a modified Romanowsky for ROSE or in the lab (Fig. 29.5a, b).

This method ensures that each FNA pass results in one slide for an air-dried and one slide for an alcohol fixation method. ROSE can be performed if desired on the air-dried slide. Bookend smears render slides as mirror images of each other allowing mates for the Papanicolaou and Romanowsky stained slides from each pass. This unique feature provides the ability to evaluate atypical cells seen on the Romanowsky slide again on the Papanicolaou

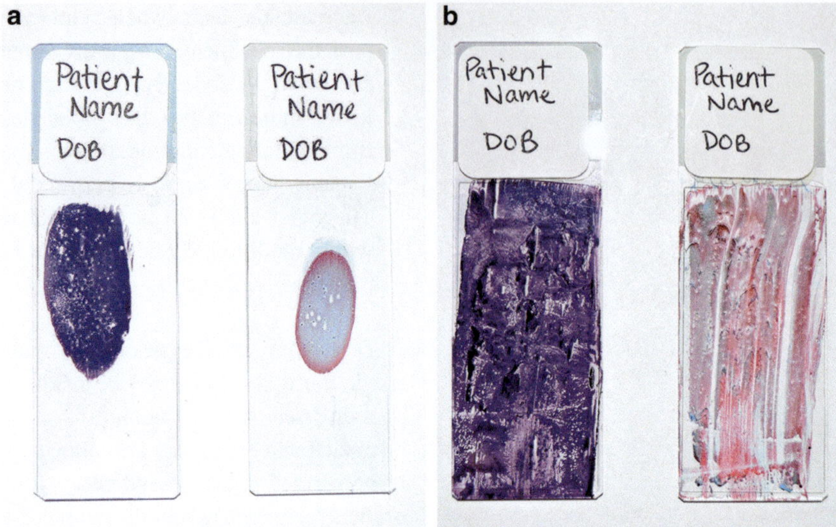

Fig. 29.4 (**a**) Properly prepared direct slide preparation with classic smears. The left slide is a Romanowsky stain stained smear and the right is a Papanicolaou stained smear that has the proper amount of specimen and keeps the smear edges at least 1 mm from the edges of the glass slide. (**b**) Improperly prepared direct slide preparation with classic smears. The left slide is a Romanowsky stain stained smear and the right is a Papanicolaou stained smear. Both slides have too much specimen causing the sample to cover the entire slide. The smearing pressure was uneven causing irregularities in the smear as well

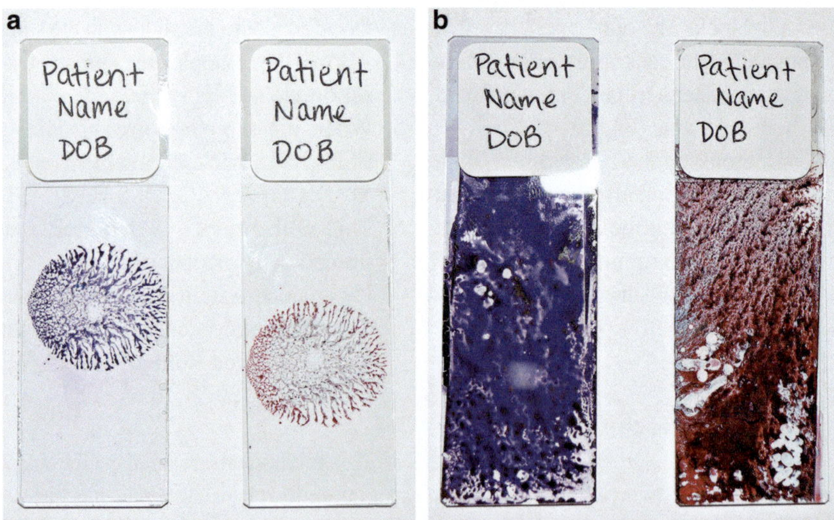

Fig. 29.5 (**a**) Properly prepared direct slide preparation with bookends method. The left slide is a Romanowsky stain stained smear and the right is a Papanicolaou stained smear that has the proper amount of specimen and creates mirror image slides from one pass. (**b**) Improperly prepared direct slide preparation with bookends. The left slide is a Romanowsky stain stained smear and the right is a Papanicolaou stained smear. Both slides have too much specimen causing the sample to cover the entire slide. The cover slip does not sit well on the specimen due to the increased thickness of the sample. The thickness issue could have been fixed by applying an additional slide to remove the excess sample, thus providing additional better prepared slides

Table 29.1 Comparison of different specimen preparation and fixation techniques

Differences in thyroid FNA preparations		
Prep and fixation		
Liquid based	Classic smears	Bookends
Liquid vial collection	Slide collection	Slide collection
Wet fixation only	Wet and/or dry fixation	Wet and/or dry fixation
Papanicolaou stain only	Pap and/or Romanowsky stain	Pap and/or Romanowsky stain
Single slide to evaluate	multiple individual slides	Multiple slides (mirror images for Pap and Romanowsky)
Consistent slide quality	Quality dependent on practice	Quality less dependent on practice
Even monolayer	Uneven with larger area to screen	Uneven with moderate area to screen
ROSE[a] not eligible	ROSE eligible	ROSE eligible
Diagnostic features		
Decreased colloid	Colloid visible on Romanowsky	Colloid visible on Romanowsky
Decreased background blood	Some blood lysis on wet fixed slide	Some blood lysis on wet fixed slide
Large fragments are broken	Large papillae retained	Large papillae retained
Intranuclear inclusions reduced	Intranuclear inclusions retained	Intranuclear inclusions retained
Loss of psammoma bodies	Psammoma bodies visible	Psammoma bodies visible

[a]*ROSE* rapid onsite evaluation

slide. The area of atypia on the Romanowsky slide should be matched to the area on the mirror image Papanicolaou slide to try to clarify the atypia. While this method causes some increase in three dimensional features it has minimal overall effect on the cytologic features used for thyroid FNA diagnoses.

For either of the smear methods, more sample does not yield more diagnostic material or better slides. For the non-pathologist, this may seem counterintuitive but only a small quantity of appropriately obtained sample is required to make adequate slides for evaluation. Either preparation method may result in too thick a sample if too much is placed on the slide. It is harder to correct a poorly made classic smear than a bookend smear. If the bookend smear is too thick, an additional labeled slide can be touched to the original slide to remove excess sample and all slides can be stained as desired (See Table 29.1).

29.4 Fixation

Cytopathologists' preferences for fixation methods differ depending on the type of stain they prefer to use for specimen interpretation. The author prefers to use both alcohol wet fixed slides and air-dried slides because some cytologic features are more readily appreciated from one stain over the other. Certain specimen preparation methods allow for a single aspiration to be split into two or more slides allowing at least one slide to be fixed wet and one to be fixed dry.

Once smears or bookends have been made, it is imperative that the slides to be wet fixed are processed rapidly. There are several methods for wet fixation of the specimen. Spray fixative for the slides that will undergo Papanicolaou staining is quick and easy to perform; however, it requires additional prep time in the lab. The spray fixative must be soaked off in 95 % ethyl alcohol prior to the staining of the slides. If this is not done, poor staining quality is noticed. Spray fixative does not lyse any of the blood in the slide, which can be detrimental if the specimen is bloody. The slide should be held 12 in. from the spray, and the spray should be applied without delay, well coating the specimen. Any delay will cause air-dry artifact when performing the Papanicolaou stain. Well coated follicular cells will be well preserved and well visualized if the smear in not too bloody and thick.

Fixation in 95 % ethyl alcohol is quick and easy. Since the slide is placed directly into the 95 % alcohol container, the process is faster and the specimen has a more even appearance on the slide vs the droplet appearance of the spray fixative. The slides do not have to be sent in the alcohol as long as they have been soaked for at least 15 min [3]. Since some FNA specimens are bloody, the fact that alcohol lyses some of the background blood can be beneficial. Cell sizes are similar to that seen in tissue specimens; however, smaller than the enlarged cells of air-dried slides.

A less commonly used wet fixative is saccomannos. It is composed of 2 % carbowax or polyethylene glycol in ethyl alcohol. Cell block samples and slides can be fixed with this method.

Whichever of the wet fixative methods used, it is imperative that it happens rapidly. When cells dry, they swell and appear larger and the nuclear detail is lost. The edges of well-fixed smears can even become air-dried causing these cells to be unsuitable for interpretation.

The last technique in slide fixation is the air-dry method. While wet fixed slides provide better nuclear detail, air-dried slides provide better visualization of cytoplasm and extracellular components such as colloid or amyloid. Air-dried slides also allow for ROSE to be performed in the clinic or at the bedside. Once the smear or book-end slides are made, the sample can be left to dry or can be fanned dry. It is critical that the slide is completely dry before staining.

Table 29.2 Differences in Papanicolaou and Romanowsky stains for thyroid aspiration

Papanicolaou stain	Romanowsky stain
Wet fix preparation	Air-dried preparation
Air-dry artifact possible	No fixation artifacts
Cell size shrinkage	Cell size enlargement
Some cellularity loss possible in fixation	No cell loss in fixation
Crisp nuclear grooves and inclusions	Poor nuclear grooves and inclusions
Poor intracytoplasmic features	Cytoplasmic features (granules) preserved
Squamoid cytoplasmic features prominent	Squamoid cytoplasmic features noticeable
Extracellular material (colloid) not well visualized	Extracellular material easily visualized

29.5 Staining

Wet fixed specimens are most often stained with a Papanicolaou stain. The Papanicolaou stain is a polychromatic stain with multiple dyes that stain various parts of the cell differently [4]. The hematoxylin component stains the nucleus a dark blue and the three acidic components of the dye stain the cytoplasm giving it a paler cyanophilic type appearance. The Papanicolaou stain is a vital component of thyroid FNA diagnosis because it effectively highlights the nuclear alterations of papillary thyroid cancer, such as grooves and inclusions. It also aids in the diagnosis for Hurthle cell and C-cell lesions because nuclear changes can be more easily appreciated.

The air-dried slides are stained with one of the many Romanowsky stains. The two components of the dye include methylene blue and eosin Y [4]. The combination of these two dyes causes the nucleus and nucleolus to stain shades of deep purple and the cytoplasm to stain pale purple-blue. The metachromatic nature of this stain allows for a spectrum of reddish-purple color that is beneficial in evaluating some secretory granules and extracellular components, such as colloid and amyloid, which do not stain as well with the Papanicolaou stain. This stain is simple and rapid making it the stain of choice for ROSE. See Table 29.2.

29.6 Ancillary Studies

On rare occasion, additional testing is needed to characterize the nodule. This can require different types of specimen collection techniques depending on the ancillary tests. Immunohistochemical studies can be performed depending on the cellularity of the specimen. From the cell block, additional sections can be cut from the block. Liquid based and cytospin slides can sometimes have an additional prepared slide. If using previously stained slides, the slide must be destained prior to the immunohistochemistry being performed.

When the differential diagnosis includes lymphoid lesions, flow cytometry can be of benefit. This specimen should be a rinse of the multiple passes made into the nodule or dedicated passes rinsed into a dedicated flow cytometry media such as RPMI (Roswell Park Memorial Institute medium). This can be used for thyroid nodules as well as lymph nodes. If being shipped overnight to a lab, flow cytometry specimens should be sent cold.

If the thyroid FNA diagnosis is one of the indeterminate categories, thyroid molecular tests may be of use according to American Thyroid Association Guidelines [5]. These tests have different collection and/or shipping requirements depending on the test used and the reader is referred to the manufacturer's instructions.

At times non-thyroid specimens are biopsied. To evaluate a parathyroid lesion, FNA slides should be prepared in the usual fashion and the remainder of the sample can be rinsed into a sterile red top chemistry tube containing 1 cc of normal saline for measurement of PTH level. This is referred to as a PTH washout. This same procedure is used to evaluate neck lymph nodes suspected of metastatic papillary thyroid carcinoma involvement. After preparation of the slides for cytologic evaluation, the remainder of the specimen is rinsed into 1 cc of normal saline for a thyroglobulin analysis.

References

1. Kini SR. Thyroid cytopathology: an atlas and text. Philadelphia, PA: Lippincott Williams & Wilkins; 2008. p. 487.
2. Andrew H, et al. Performance differences between conventional smears and liquid-based preparations of thyroid fine-needle aspiration samples analysis of 47076 responses in the College of American Pathologists Interlaboratory Comparison Program in Non-Gynecologic Cytology. Arch Pathol Lab Med. 2013;137:26–31.
3. McKee GT. Cytopathology. London: Mosby-Wolfe; 1997. p. 80.
4. Boon ME, Drijver JS. Routine cytologic staining techniques and theoretical background practice. London: MacMillan Education; 1986.
5. Haugen BR. 2015 American Thyroid Association Management Guidelines for adult patients with thyroid nodules and differentiated thyroid cancer: the American Thyroid Association Guidelines task force on thyroid nodules and differentiated thyroid cancer. Thyroid. 2016;26:1.

Cytomorphology of Fine Needle Aspiration of Thyroid

30

Zubair W. Baloch

30.1 Introduction and General Considerations

Fine-needle aspiration (FNA) biopsy is considered an essential tool in providing a rational approach to the clinical management of thyroid nodules. The results of FNA can determine whether a thyroid nodule should be followed clinically or undergo surgical excision [1, 2].

Thyroid FNA specimens can be prepared by making air-dried and alcohol-fixed smears for staining with Romanowsky (Diff-Quik®, Wright-Geimsa stains) and Papanicolaou stains, respectively. The smears can be processed alone or with a liquid based monolayer preparation or cell-block [3]. The Romanowsky staining method is the method of choice for immediate evaluation of FNA specimens. This stain highlights the background watery colloid and cell architecture (papillary, monolayer sheets, and macro- and micro-follicles), and distinguish between cell types (follicular and oncocytic cells, lymphocytes, macrophages, crystals and calcifications). Liquid based monolayer preparations can be used either alone or as an adjunct to smears [3].

The ***leading cause of a non-diagnostic thyroid FNA specimen*** is failure to procure a sufficient number of cells required to render a definite diagnosis. Several studies have proposed different ***numbers of cells or cell groups as criteria for specimen adequacy***. The presence of six well-preserved follicular or epithelial cell groups on two slides with at least 10–20 cells in each group is considered to be the best criterion [4, 5].

Thyroid FNA specimens are usually classified by employing a tiered system (3–6 diagnostic categories) [1, 6]. In 2007, the National Cancer Institute sponsored the “Thyroid Fine Needle Aspiration State of the Science Conference” to develop consensus criteria for cytology classification, “The Bethesda System for Reporting Thyroid Cytology” (TBSRTC). A key contribution of this system was to define three specific categories for indeterminate interpretation, each correlating with a more narrow range of malignancy risk, resulting in a six-tiered cytology classification.

To date the TBSRTC is commonly used in the USA and has served to generate a body of cytopathology and clinical literature. Furthermore, the recent paradigms for ancillary testing of thyroid FNA specimens have been proposed based on diagnostic categories of TBSRTC. Nonetheless, besides its wide applicability and usage, controversies have risen over the use of diagnostic

Z.W. Baloch, M.D., Ph.D. (✉)
Department of Pathology and Laboratory Medicine, Perelman School of Medicine, University of Pennsylvania Medical Center, 3400 Spruce Street, 6 Founders Pavilion, Philadelphia, PA 19104, USA
e-mail: baloch@mail.med.upenn.edu

M. Milas et al. (eds.), *Advanced Thyroid and Parathyroid Ultrasound*,
DOI 10.1007/978-3-319-44100-9_30

Table 30.1 The Bethesda System for Reporting Thyroid Cytopathology (TBSRTC): diagnostic categories and implied risk of malignancy

Diagnostic category	ROM(%)[a] [6]	ROM(%)[b] [7, 8]
Nondiagnostic or unsatisfactory	1–4	11–26
Benign	0–3	4–9
Atypia of undetermined significance or follicular lesion of undetermined significance	~5–15	19–38
Follicular neoplasm or suspicious for a follicular neoplasm	15–30	26–40
Suspicious for malignancy	60–75	50–79
Malignant	97–99	98–99

ROM risk of malignancy
[a]2007—calculated based on available literature
[b]Calculated based on current literature

designations of AUS/FLUS and FN/SFN, recommended follow-up, i.e., repeat FNA vs. surgery and implied risk of malignancy. It has been shown that the risk of malignancy of cases diagnosed as AUS/FLUS is approximately the same or even higher in some studies to cases diagnosed as FN/SFN (Table 30.1) [7–9].

The brief description of the diagnostic categories in the Bethesda Classification is as follows:

1. **Nondiagnostic or Unsatisfactory**:
   (a) This diagnostic category applies to specimen which are nondiagnostic due to limited cellularity, no follicular cells and adequate specimen which are uninterpretable due to poor fixation and preservation, i.e., obliteration of cellular details.
   (b) In some cases of solid nodules it may be prudent to process and examine the entire specimen.
2. **Benign**:
   (a) The diagnostic terms in this category include but are not limited to nodular goiter, hyperplastic/adenomatoid nodule in goiter, chronic lymphocytic thyroiditis, and sub-acute thyroiditis.
   (b) A thyroid nodule with a benign diagnosis should be followed periodically by US examination; a repeat FNA may be considered if the nodule increases in size (as per thyroid nodule management guidelines).
3. **Atypia of undetermined significance/ Follicular lesion of undetermined significance (AUS/FLUS)**:
   (a) This is a heterogeneous diagnostic category (a true Gray Zone). The reported malignancy risk for cases diagnosed as such in large case series published after Bethesda Classifications ranges from 6 to 38 % [7, 9–12].
   (b) It is recommended that the number of cases diagnosed as such should be kept to minimum; 7 % of the total diagnoses.
   (c) Some authors have shown that subclassifying this diagnosis, i.e., reason for AUS/ FLUS further stratifies the risk of malignancy [12, 13].
   (d) Molecular studies with high negative and positive predictive value are recommended in cases diagnosed as AUS/FLUS.
4. **Follicular/Follicular neoplasm with oncocytic features (AKA Hurthle cell) neoplasm or Suspicious for Follicular or Follicular neoplasm with oncocytic features (AKA Hurthle cell) neoplasm**:
   (a) These diagnostic terms encompasses both benign and malignant tumors, i.e., follicular adenoma and carcinoma and oncocytic follicular adenoma and carcinoma. The cytologic diagnosis of "neoplasm" reflects the limitations of thyroid cytology, since the diagnosis of follicular carcinoma is

only based on the demonstration of capsular and/or vascular invasion. Several authors have shown that, at most, only 20–30 % of cases diagnosed as "follicular neoplasm" are diagnosed as malignant on histological examination and the rest are either follicular adenomas or cellular adenomatoid nodules, i.e., benign [11].

   (b) Several studies have shown that half or more of the malignant cases diagnosed as follicular neoplasm or suspicious for follicular neoplasm (FON/SFON) are found to be either invasive follicular variant of papillary thyroid carcinoma (FVPC) and noninvasive FVPC (also known as noninvasive follicular tumor with papillary like nuclear features—NIFTP) on surgical excision [11, 14, 15].

5. **Suspicious for malignancy**:
   (a) This term includes suspicious for: papillary carcinoma, medullary carcinoma, other malignancies, lymphoma (flow cytometry can be recommended with repeat FNA), metastatic carcinoma/secondary tumor, and carcinoma (includes poorly differentiated and anaplastic carcinoma).
6. **Malignant**:
   (a) The thyroid FNA cases diagnosed as such carry a 97–100 % risk of malignancy. The malignant tumors of the thyroid diagnosed on FNA include: papillary carcinoma and variants, medullary carcinoma, poorly differentiated carcinoma, anaplastic carcinoma, metastatic carcinoma (with immunohistochemistry), and lymphoma (combined with flow cytometry).

30.2 Cytomorphology of Thyroid Lesions

30.2.1 Benign Lesions

30.2.1.1 Nodular Goiter

The term goiter encompasses both nodular and diffuse enlargement of the thyroid, and clinically can be divided into toxic and nontoxic variants based on the clinical symptoms and thyroid function tests (hypothyroid, euthyroid, or hyperthyroid) and isotope uptake on scintigraphy [16, 17].

The cytology specimen from a benign nodule shows (depending upon the preparation method) abundant watery colloid, small, round to oval shaped follicular cells with scant cytoplasm (may contain small blue lysosome granules) and dark nuclei arranged in monolayer sheets, groups with follicle formation or as single cells [18] (Fig. 30.1). Macrophages are usually present and their number depends upon the presence or absence of degenerative changes or a cystic component [18, 19]. The aspirates from a hyperplastic/adenomatoid nodule tend to be more cellular and contain an admixture of follicular cells and oncocytic cells arranged in monolayer sheets in a background of watery colloid and macrophages [18–20].

Solitary papillary hyperplastic nodules frequently occur in children and teenagers and can be hyper-functioning on radionuclide scan. By histologic examination these lesions are encapsulated and often demonstrate cystic change, papillary architecture and the lesional cells lack nuclear cytology of papillary thyroid carcinoma [21, 22]. The FNA specimens of solitary papillary hyperplastic nodules tend to be cellular and show papillary clusters, nuclear atypia and pleomorphism, nuclear grooves, multinucleated giant cells, and cells with vacuolated cytoplasm. In view of these features, some of these cases could be misclassified as "suspicious of" or consistent with papillary carcinoma [23].

30.2.2 Diffuse Toxic Goiter (Graves' disease)

Patients with Graves' disease (GD) usually do not undergo FNA; however, cytology material may be obtained from a hypo-functioning or enlarging nodule arising in a background of GD. These specimens are usually cellular, show features similar to hyperplastic goiter, and may contain lymphocytes and oncocytic cells [24–27].

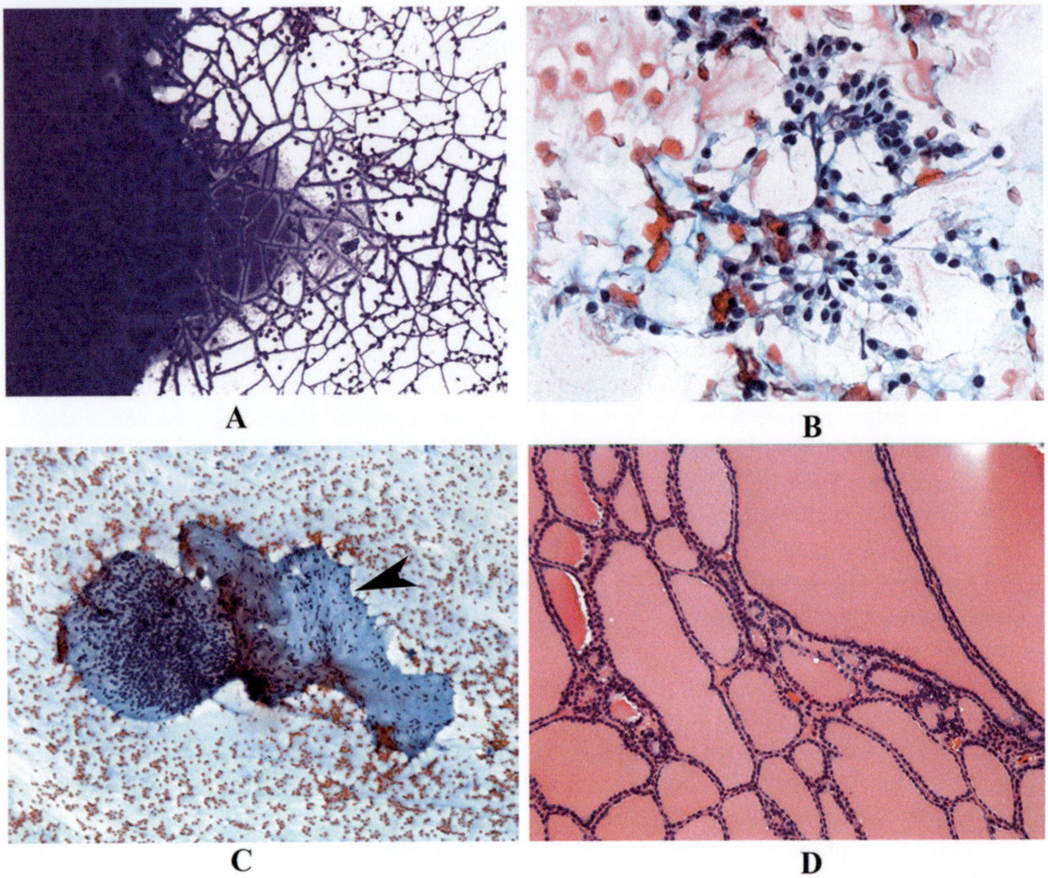

Fig. 30.1 A case of nodular goiter demonstrating back watery colloid—onsite air-dried smear ("chicken wire appearance") (**a**—Diff Quik® stain). The alcohol-fixed smear from the same case demonstrates follicular cells with small round nuclei arranged in flat sheets (**b**—Papanicolaou stain) and cohesive clusters with associated stroma (*arrowhead*) (**c**—Papanicolaou stain). The histology of nodular goiter demonstrates macrofollicles filled with watery colloid (**d**)

30.2.3 Autoimmune Thyroiditis/Chronic Lymphocytic Thyroiditis

FNA is usually performed in patients with chronic lymphocytic thyroiditis who present with distinct nodules. The specimens usually show scant colloid, oncocytes (Hürthle), follicular cells, lymphocytes, and a few plasma cells. The lymphocytes are usually seen in the background, interspersed among cell groups and in some cases one may see an intact lymphoid follicle (Fig. 30.2) [28]. The oncocytic follicular (Hürthle) cells may display nuclear atypia and similarly follicular cells may show some chromatin clearing and intranuclear grooves; however, one should refrain from interpreting these changes as malignant [29, 30]. Papillary thyroid carcinoma (PTC) arising in the background of thyroiditis often seen as a separate population of tumor cells, devoid of a lymphocytic infiltrate and with diagnostic nuclear features [22].

An extensive lymphocytic infiltrate which may appear monotonous can be mistaken for malignant lymphoma arising in lymphocytic thyroiditis. If lymphoma is suspected, an aliquot of specimen can be submitted for flow cytometry to confirm the morphologic suspicion [31, 32].

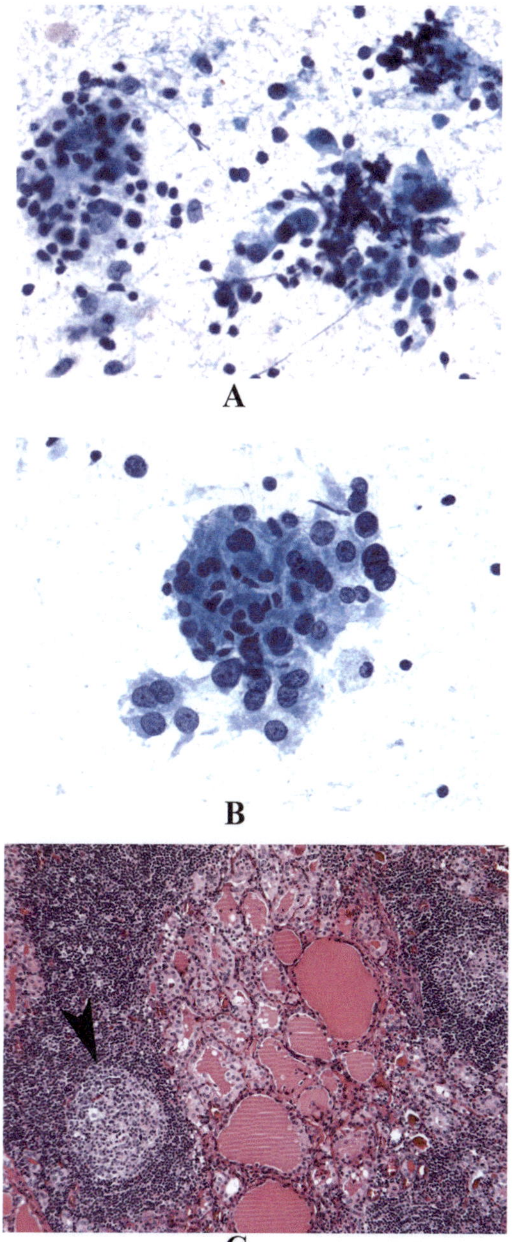

Fig. 30.2 A case of chronic lymphocytic thyroiditis on low power showing cells and lymphocytes in background and among oncocytic follicular cells (**a**—alcohol-fixed smear, Papanicolaou stain). On high power the cells are oncocytic follicular cells showing dense cytoplasm and round nuclei (**b**—alcohol-fixed smear, Papanicolaou stain). The histology of chronic lymphocytic thyroiditis is evident by oncocytic follicular nodules surrounded by lymphocytes and some areas show "lymphoid germinal center formation" (*arrowhead*) (**c**—hematoxylin and eosin stain)

30.2.4 Follicular Neoplasm/Suspicious for Follicular Neoplasm

Thyroid (FNA) cannot distinguish between benign and malignant follicular patterned lesions, i.e., follicular adenoma and carcinoma [33], because the diagnosis of follicular carcinoma is based on the demonstration of capsular and/or vascular invasion [34–36]. Several authors have shown that, at most, 20–30 % of cases diagnosed as "follicular neoplasm" are diagnosed as malignant on histological examination and the rest are either follicular adenomas or cellular adenomatoid nodules, i.e., benign [37, 38]. Interestingly half of the malignant cases are diagnosed as follicular variant of papillary thyroid carcinoma. However, this rate of malignancy will dramatically change in the future due to reclassification of noninvasive follicular variant of PTC as noninvasive follicular tumor with papillary like nuclei—NIFTP [39].

The FNA specimen of a follicular neoplasm is usually hyper-cellular and shows a monotonous population of follicular cells. The watery colloid seen in the aspirates of nodular goiter is usually lacking. The colloid in the aspirates of follicular neoplasm appears as round dense eosinophilic deposits on Romanowsky stain with or without surrounding cells [33, 40]. The lesional cells can be seen as three dimensional groups or microfollicles with prominent nuclear overlapping and crowding [36, 40] (Fig. 30.3).

30.2.5 Oncocytic Follicular (AKA Hürthle Cell) Neoplasm/Suspicious for Oncocytic Follicular (AKA Hürthle Cell) Neoplasm

The Oncocytic cells (oxyphil, Askanazy cells, Hürthle cells) are usually larger than follicular cells and have distinct cell borders, voluminous granular eosinophilic cytoplasm, and an eccentrically or centrally placed round nuclei with a

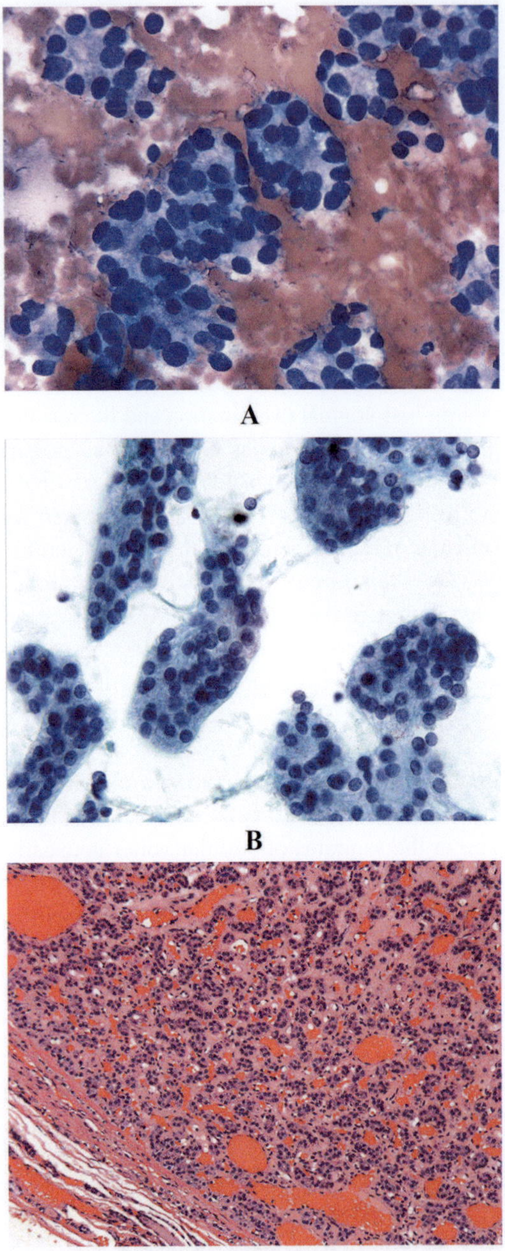

Fig. 30.3 A case diagnosed as follicular neoplasm/suspicious for follicular neoplasm demonstrating a monotonous population of follicular cells arranged in follicular patterned groups—onsite air-dried smear (**a**—Diff Quik® stain). The alcohol-fixed smear stained with Papanicolaou stain shows round nuclei lacking nuclear features of papillary carcinoma (**b**). On surgical excision this case showed an encapsulated follicular patterned nodule without any evidence of invasive characteristics; diagnosed as follicular adenoma (**c**—hematoxylin and eosin stain)

prominent nucleolus. A majority of oncocytic follicular/Hürthle cell neoplasms of the thyroid are solitary mass lesions that show complete or partial encapsulation. Oncocytic follicular neoplasms are defined as being composed of at least 75 % oncocytic cells. These can be divided into adenoma and carcinoma based on the same pathologic criteria as applied in the diagnosis of follicular carcinoma, i.e., the identification of capsular and/or vascular invasion [41, 42].

FNA specimens obtained from an oncocytic follicular neoplasm usually demonstrate a monotonous population of oncocytic cells arranged in cohesive groups/tissue fragments and as single cells [43, 44]. Neoplastic oncocytic follicular cells, i.e., obtained from either adenoma or carcinoma are usually large and round to oval or polygonal in shape with well-defined cell borders [34, 45]. Random nuclear atypia is commonly observed in oncocytic follicular lesions; this can be seen in the form of nuclear enlargement, multi-nucleation, cellular pleomorphism and prominent "cherry red" nucleoli. Intranuclear grooves are common in non-papillary oncocytic follicular lesions, however, the nuclei maintain a round shape with prominent nucleoli and other major diagnostic features of papillary carcinoma are not seen [46–48]

The FNA specimens of oncocytic neoplasms usually contain thick colloid that appears as circular deposits representing the lumen of thyroid follicles. It should be noted that similar atypical nuclear features can also be seen in aspirates of nonneoplastic oncocytic lesion seen in longstanding goiter, toxic nodular goiter, and chronic lymphocytic thyroiditis.

The differential diagnosis of oncocytic follicular neoplasm includes other tumors of the thyroid gland with oncocytic cytoplasm. These include: variants of papillary thyroid carcinoma such as ***oncocytic variant***, ***Warthin-like variant and tall cell variant of papillary carcinoma***; ***oncocytic variant of medullary thyroid carcinoma and granular cell tumor of the thyroid***. An occasional ***intra-thyroidal oncocytic parathyroid adenoma*** can also mimic an oncocytic follicular neoplasm.

30.2.6 Malignant Neoplasms

30.2.6.1 Papillary Thyroid Carcinoma and Its Variants

Papillary thyroid carcinoma (PTC) is the most common form of thyroid malignancy in non-endemic goiter regions. The ***classic variant of papillary carcinoma*** predominantly consists of true papillae, i.e., finger like projection with cores containing vessel(s) and connective tissue surrounded by tumor cells. The papillae are of different sizes and can display a complex branching pattern. It is not uncommon to encounter a few follicles intermixed with papillae in this variant of PTC. Minor cystic changes are common. By light microscopy, the tumor cells are larger and are cuboidal to short columnar and contain amphophilic to slightly eosinophilic cytoplasm. Nuclei are relatively large and oval in shape and show nuclear indentations/grooves and round intranuclear cytoplasmic pseudoinclusions. Nucleoli are usually small and situated close to the nuclear membranes (eccentric), and much of the interior of the nucleus to be "empty," "clear," or "ground glass" in appearance. Follicles may be colloid-filled or empty and occur as small or large follicles, i.e., micro- or macro-follicles [49].

The cytology diagnosis of PTC is based on major and minor cytologic criteria. The major diagnostic feature is the characteristic nuclear morphology regardless of cytoplasmic features and architecture. The FNA specimen of PTC is usually cellular and shows tumor cells arranged in papillary groups, three-dimensional clusters or as single cells in a background of watery or thick "ropy" colloid (i.e., chewing gum colloid), nuclear or calcific debris, macrophages and stromal fragments. The cell groups may show a typical concentric arrangement of lesional cells described as "cellular swirls" [5, 50].

The individual tumor cells are enlarged, elongated, i.e., oval in shape with eosinophilic cytoplasm (cytoplasmic eosinophilia is common in Romanowsky stained preparations but is usually indistinct in alcohol-fixed Papanicolaou stained preparations; this also holds true for monolayer preparations). The nuclei show elongation, membrane thickening, chromatin clearing, grooves, and inclusions. The nucleoli are usually small and eccentric. Intranuclear grooves and inclusions can be seen in other benign and malignant conditions of the thyroid (Fig. 30.4). These include Hashimoto's thyroiditis, nodular goiter, hyalinizing trabecular neoplasm, oncocytic follicular tumors, and medullary carcinoma [22, 51].

Psammoma bodies occur in about 20 % of cases of papillary thyroid carcinoma. These are lamellated round to oval calcified structures that represent the "ghosts" of dead papillae. Multinucleated histiocytes are common in FNA specimens of papillary thyroid carcinoma [52, 53]. The cytologic features of papillary thyroid carcinoma may not be readily evident in monolayer preparations [54].

The **follicular variant of papillary thyroid carcinoma (FVPTC)** is the second most common variant of PTC. Its diagnosis may be made when more than 70 % of the tumor consists of neoplastic follicles lined by cells demonstrating diagnostic nuclear morphology of PTC. Three distinct types of follicular variant exist represented by: the infiltrative type, the diffuse follicular variant, and the encapsulated follicular variant. The encapsulated FVPTC is characterized by the presence of a capsule around the lesion and is associated with an excellent prognosis. In some cases the diagnosis of this particular variant of papillary carcinoma can be difficult due to the presence of multifocal rather than a diffuse distribution of nuclear features of papillary thyroid carcinoma. Because of this peculiar morphologic presentation, these tumors can be misdiagnosed as adenomatoid nodule or follicular adenoma. Due to their excellent prognosis, the noninvasive forms of FVPTC are now recommended to be designated as noninvasive follicular tumor with papillary like nuclei—NIFTP, i.e., neoplasms but not carcinomas [39].

The cytologic interpretation of **FVPTC** can be challenging due to a paucity of diagnostic nuclear features [55]. The cytologic samples from FVPTC usually show enlarged follicular cells arranged in monolayer sheets and follicular

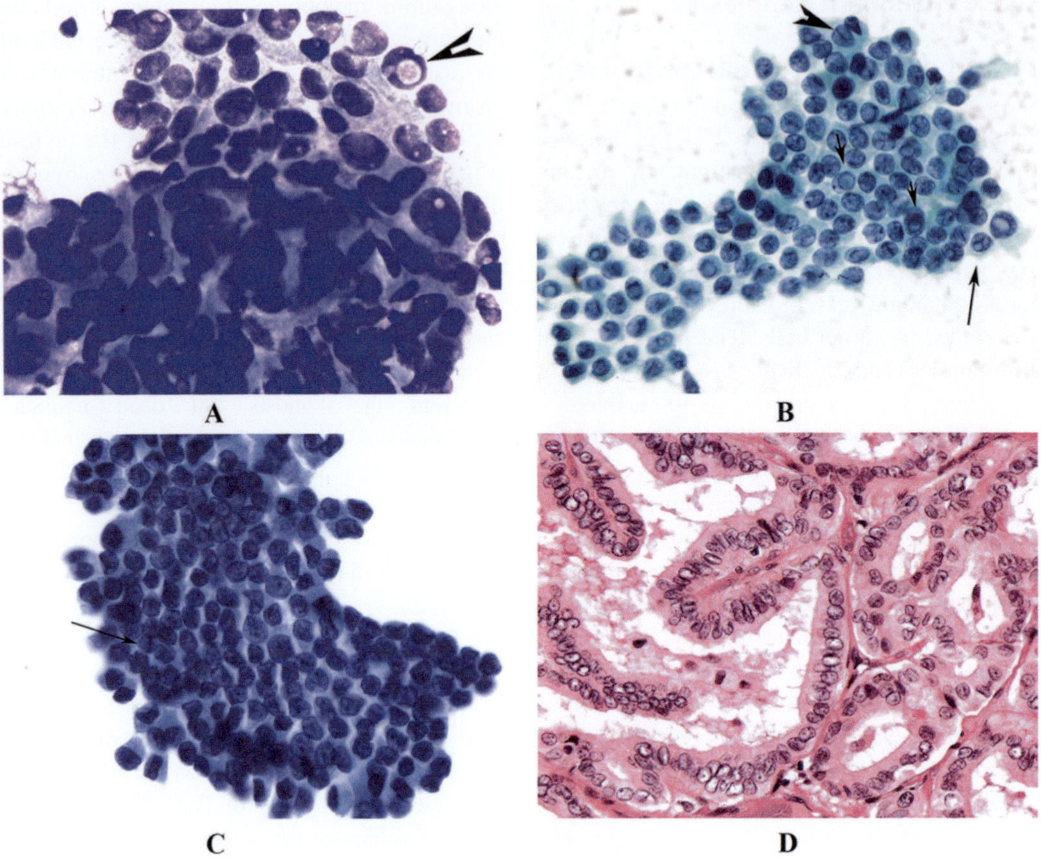

Fig. 30.4 A case of classic variant of papillary thyroid carcinoma showing lesional cells with arranged in papillary configuration demonstrating a single intranuclear inclusion—onsite air-dried smear (*arrowhead*) (**a**—Diff Quik® stain). The tumor cells demonstrate enlarged oval nuclei intranuclear grooves (*arrowhead*), eccentric nucleoli and intranuclear inclusions (*arrows*) (**b**—Papanicolaou stain). The ThinPrep® slide shows tumor cells arranged similar to a "Jigsaw Puzzle" with intranuclear grooves (*arrow*) (**c**). The histology demonstrates well formed papillae with vascular core lined by cells with nuclear features of papillary carcinoma (**d**—hematoxylin and eosin stain)

groups in a background of thin and thick colloid. The individual tumor cells show nuclear elongation, chromatin clearing and thick nuclear membranes. The intranuclear grooves in FVPTC are delicate and do not traverse the entire length of nucleus; however, nuclear grooves and inclusions are very scarce. Thus, a majority of cytologic samples of FVPTC are diagnosed as either follicular neoplasm or suspicious for papillary carcinoma [56, 57].

Cystic papillary thyroid carcinomas are often encapsulated and the cystic component usually ranges from 50 % to occupying most of the lesion. The papillary fronds lining the cyst wall may be visible on gross examination. FNA specimens of this tumor contain large numbers of hemosiderin-laden histiocytes and considerable cellular debris. Sheets of intact follicular cells may be seen, which resemble those from cellular adenomatoid nodules; however, these will demonstrate nuclear cytology suspicious or diagnostic of PTC. Squamous metaplasia has been reported in cases of cystic PTCs. Dense globules of pink-staining colloid may be present [58–60].

Tall cell variant of papillary thyroid carcinoma is an aggressive form of PTC and can lead to multiple local recurrences, distant metastases and even death. This tumor shows oncocytic cells which are at least three times as tall as their width [61]. The cytologic samples from this tumor contain elongated cells with sharp cytoplasmic borders, granular eosinophilic cytoplasm, and variably sized nuclei with nuclear features of papillary carcinoma [62, 63]. The diagnostic nuclear features of PTC are readily found in aspirates of this variant. The intranuclear inclusions can be multiple within the same nucleus giving rise to a "soap-bubble-like" appearance [63].

30.2.7 Diffuse Sclerosis Variant of PTC

The diffuse sclerosis variant of papillary thyroid carcinoma (DSV-PTC) is rare, representing only approximately 3 % of all papillary carcinomas. The tumor, which most often affects children and young adults, may present as a bilateral goiter. In histologic section, the tumor cells permeate the gland outlining the intra-glandular lymphatics. Tumor papillae have associated areas of squamous metaplasia. Numerous psammoma bodies are found; lymphocytic infiltrates are also found around the tumor foci. This particular feature gives rise to a "snow storm" appearance on ultrasound examination. Cytological preparations shows tumor cells with nuclear features of papillary carcinoma arranged in nests and numerous psammoma bodies. Some cases may also demonstrate a brisk lymphocytic infiltrate around the tumor cell groups and in the background. Squamous metaplasia is commonly seen in aspirates of DSV-PTC [64–66].

The cytologic features of less common variants of PTC such as **Warthin-like variant**, **columnar cell variant**, **clear cell variant,** and others have been described in the [64, 67, 68].

30.2.8 Medullary Thyroid Carcinoma

Medullary thyroid carcinoma (MTC) arises from the C-cells of the thyroid and constitutes about 10 % of all malignant thyroid neoplasms. This thyroid tumor is peculiar among thyroid neoplasms due to its clinical presentation, familial incidence, association with lesions of other endocrine organs, and variable morphology [16]. In the absence of genetic predisposition, no epidemiologic factors have been identified for medullary cancer. Germ line mutations lead to C-cell hyperplasia, which has been implicated as the precursor/in situ lesions of the medullary carcinoma in the genetically determined subset of cases [69].

Medullary carcinoma usually presents as a firm painless thyroid nodule. Approximately 50 % of patients show lymph node metastases and up to 15 % can show distant metastases at presentation (commonly bone and liver).

Typically, in histologic sections MTC consists of sheets and solid nests of round cells with granular eosinophilic cytoplasm and a prominent eccentric nucleus with evenly dispersed chromatin. The tumor nests can contain randomly distributed pleomorphic nuclei or even multinucleated tumor cells. In some cases the tumor cells can show prominent nuclear grooves and even inclusions. The tumor cells may exhibit marked nuclear pleomorphism, prominent central nucleoli and eosinophilic granular cytoplasm; such cases can be mistaken for oncocytic follicular neoplasms. MTC also exhibit a spindle cell morphology and mimic either primary or metastatic mesenchymal tumors of the thyroid or anaplastic carcinoma or tumors of thymic origin. Several other histologic patterns of this tumor have been described, which include: small cell, oncocytic and squamous cell, giant cell, pseudo-papillary, carcinoid-like, insular, and mixed medullary and papillary. Amyloid can be seen in up to 80 % of medullary cancers; therefore Congo red staining and polarized light microscopy are used to diagnose these tumors. The gold standard for the diagnosis of MTC is the immunostain for calcitonin which stains both the tumor cells and the amyloid. However, calcitonin negative MTC have been reported in the familial setting. Another marker which can be used to highlight MTC is CEA. Increased levels of serum CEA; along with calcitonin values are often used for follow-up in patients at risk for recurrent or metastatic disease.

Lymph node metastases involving regional and mediastinal nodes can be seen in up to 50 %

of MTC cases. These tumors also show a propensity towards extra-thyroidal extension and involvement of the contralateral lobe. The common sites for distant metastasis include lung, bone, liver, and adrenals [70, 71].

FNA specimens of MTC display a spectrum of morphologic patterns similar to surgical pathology specimens. The majority of MTC FNA specimens are cellular consisting of round to oval cells arranged mainly as single cells or loosely cohesive groups. The tumor cells show ample granular cytoplasm with eccentric nuclei imparting a "plasma cell like/plasmacytoid" appearance to the cells. The nuclear chromatin is similar to that seen in neuroendocrine tumors; intranuclear inclusions and multinucleated cells may be seen. Marked nuclear pleomorphism is uncommon; however, when present the cases are indistinguishable from aspirates of anaplastic thyroid carcinoma. The neoplastic cells can assume a "spindle shape" and appear mesenchymal in origin. Amyloid may be observed as acellular material and can be distinguished from the thick colloid of papillary carcinoma by performing a Congo-red stain. The diagnosis of MTC can be confirmed by performing immunostains for calcitonin and thyroglobulin [72].

The cytomorphologic diagnosis of MTC can be challenging due to morphologic variability. The differential diagnosis of MTC includes: hyalinizing trabecular neoplasm, oncocytic follicular neoplasm (AKA Hürthle cell neoplasm), papillary thyroid carcinoma, follicular neoplasm with solid and trabecular growth pattern, poorly differentiated carcinoma/insular carcinoma, anaplastic carcinoma, plasmacytoma, and metastatic tumors to the thyroid especially melanoma.

30.2.9 Poorly Differentiated Carcinoma

The poorly differentiated thyroid carcinoma (PDTC) is a follicular cell derived neoplasm that shows limited evidence of structural follicular cell architecture and occupies both morphologically and behaviorally an intermediate position between differentiated and undifferentiated (anaplastic) carcinoma [61]. Insular growth pattern with areas of coagulative necrosis, nuclear pleomorphism, and greater than 3 mitoses per 10 high power field (HPF) is considered by many experts as diagnostic features of PDTC. Lymphovascular invasion, metastases to regional lymph nodes, lung, and bones are commonly associated with PDTC [73–75].

Aspirates of these tumors are cellular and demonstrate a monotonous population of cells arranged in large solid groups with cell crowding and overlapping, mitoses, and apoptotic bodies. On high power examination nuclear pleomorphism is readily evident. Endothelial wrapping of the tissue fragment can be seen in some cases. Since this growth pattern can also be encountered in MTC and secondary tumors of the thyroid such as metastatic neuroendocrine carcinoma; it is prudent to confirm the diagnosis of PDTC by performing immunostains for TTF-1, thyroglobulin, and calcitonin [76, 77].

30.2.10 Anaplastic Carcinoma

Anaplastic carcinoma of the thyroid is one of the most aggressive and fatal human tumors. It usually presents in older individuals and is more common in regions of endemic goiter. The aspirates from anaplastic carcinoma usually do not pose any diagnostic difficulties; they can be readily classified as malignant due to extreme cellular pleomorphism and obvious malignant features [17].

30.3 Rare Tumors of Thyroid Gland

Hyalinizing trabecular neoplasm (HTN) is a rare tumor of the thyroid. Aspirates of HTN which show cohesive lesional cells with easily identifiable well-formed intranuclear inclusions and grooves embedded or closely associated with an acellular matrix [78].

Primary thyroid lymphoma is a rare but well-recognized thyroid neoplasm [79–81]. It virtually always arises in a gland that is immunologically abnormal and most lymphomas occur in the background of chronic lymphocytic thyroiditis [82, 83]. The thyroid gland is recognized as a MALT organ and many of the primary lymphomas are MALTOMAS [80]. The diagnosis can be made by FNA of the mass and if lymphoma is suspected, a specimen can be sent for special studies including flow cytometry and molecular analysis in order to characterize the subtype of lymphoma [84].

The incidence of **Secondary Tumors of Thyroid** ranges from 1.25 to 25 %. Breast, lung, and kidney (mostly renal cell carcinoma) represent the most common primary sites that can give rise to metastases to thyroid [85–89]. In some cases secondary tumors can present as solitary nodules and may be mistaken for a primary thyroid tumor. Similarly on histology and FNA some metastatic tumors can also be difficult to differentiate from primary thyroid neoplasms; however, immunohistochemistry and a detailed history are always helpful for differentiation between primary and secondary tumors of thyroid [88, 90].

30.4 Conclusions

This chapter discusses and illustrates the cytopathology of common and uncommon thyroid lesions, stressing key cytomorphologic and histopathologic features and differential diagnosis.

Although the past several years have witnessed the development of ancillary testing to refine diagnostic cytology in the thyroid, it is still the role of the cytopathologist to identify those "indeterminant" nodules which should be tested. Thus, the cytopathologist contributes both an essential diagnostic and an important cost-saving role which hopefully will continue in the future.

References

1. Baloch ZW, Cibas ES, Clark DP, Layfield LJ, Ljung BM, Pitman MB, Abati A. The National Cancer Institute Thyroid fine needle aspiration state of the science conference: a summation. Cytojournal. 2008;5:6.
2. Cooper DS, Doherty GM, Haugen BR, Kloos RT, Lee SL, Mandel SJ, Mazzaferri EL, McIver B, Sherman SI, Tuttle RM. Management guidelines for patients with thyroid nodules and differentiated thyroid cancer. Thyroid. 2006;16:109–42.
3. Baloch ZW, Tam D, Langer J, Mandel S, LiVolsi VA, Gupta PK. Ultrasound-guided fine-needle aspiration biopsy of the thyroid: role of on-site assessment and multiple cytologic preparations. Diagn Cytopathol. 2000;23:425–9.
4. Zhu W, Michael CW. How important is on-site adequacy assessment for thyroid FNA? An evaluation of 883 cases. Diagn Cytopathol. 2007;35:183–6.
5. Kini SR. Thyroid cytopathology: an atlas and text. 1st ed. Philadelphia, PA: Lippincott Williams & Wilkins; 2008.
6. Cibas ES, Ali SZ. The Bethesda system for reporting thyroid cytopathology. Thyroid. 2009;19:1159–65.
7. Sheffield BS, Masoudi H, Walker B, Wiseman SM. Preoperative diagnosis of thyroid nodules using the Bethesda System for Reporting Thyroid Cytopathology: a comprehensive review and meta-analysis. Exp Rev Endocrinol Metab. 2014;9: 97–110.
8. Bongiovanni M, Spitale A, Faquin WC, Mazzucchelli L, Baloch ZW. The Bethesda System for reporting thyroid cytopathology: a meta-analysis. Acta Cytol. 2012;56:333–9.
9. Wong LQ, Baloch ZW. Analysis of the Bethesda system for reporting thyroid cytopathology and similar precursor thyroid cytopathology reporting schemes. Adv Anat Pathol. 2012;19:313–9.
10. Bongiovanni M, Krane JF, Cibas ES, Faquin WC. The atypical thyroid fine-needle aspiration: past, present, and future. Cancer Cytopathol. 2012;120:73–86.
11. Faquin WC, Baloch ZW. Fine-needle aspiration of follicular patterned lesions of the thyroid: diagnosis, management, and follow-up according to National Cancer Institute (NCI) recommendations. Diagn Cytopathol. 2010;38:731–9.
12. Krane JF, Vanderlaan PA, Faquin WC, Renshaw AA. The atypia of undetermined significance/follicular lesion of undetermined significance: malignant ratio: a proposed performance measure for reporting in The Bethesda System for thyroid cytopathology. Cancer Cytopathol. 2012;120:111–6.
13. VanderLaan PA, Marqusee E, Krane JF. Usefulness of diagnostic qualifiers for thyroid fine-needle aspirations with atypia of undetermined significance. Am J Clin Pathol. 2011;136:572–7.
14. Strickland KC, Howitt BE, Marqusee E, Alexander EK, Cibas ES, Krane JF, Barletta JA. The impact of noninvasive follicular variant of papillary thyroid carcinoma on rates of malignancy for fine-needle aspiration diagnostic categories. Thyroid. 2015;25:987–92.
15. Maletta F, Massa F, Torregrossa L, Duregon E, Casadei GP, Basolo F, Tallini G, Volante M, Nikiforov

YE, Papotti M. Cytological features of "non-invasive follicular thyroid neoplasm with papillary-like nuclear features" and their correlation with tumor histology. Hum Pathol. 2016;54:134.
16. Murray D. The thyroid gland. Malden, MA: Blackwell Science; 1998.
17. Baloch Z, LiVolsi VA. Pathology of the thyroid gland. Philadelphia, PA: Churchill Livingston; 2002.
18. Layfield LJ, Wax T, Jones C. Cytologic distinction of goiterous nodules from morphologically normal thyroid: analyses of cytomorphologic features. Cancer. 2003;99:217–22.
19. Baloch ZW, Sack MJ, Yu GH, Livolsi VA, Gupta PK. Fine-needle aspiration of thyroid: an institutional experience. Thyroid. 1998;8:565–9.
20. Oertel YC, Oertel JE. Thyroid cytology and histology. Baillieres Best Pract Res Clin Endocrinol Metab. 2000;14:541–57.
21. Vickery Jr AL. Thyroid papillary carcinoma. Pathological and philosophical controversies. Am J Surg Pathol. 1983;7:797–807.
22. Baloch ZW, LiVolsi VA. Cytologic and architectural mimics of papillary thyroid carcinoma. Diagnostic challenges in fine-needle aspiration and surgical pathology specimens. Am J Clin Pathol. 2006; 125(Suppl):S135–44.
23. Khurana KK, Baloch ZW, LiVolsi VA. Aspiration cytology of pediatric solitary papillary hyperplastic thyroid nodule. Arch Pathol Lab Med. 2001; 125:1575–8.
24. Centeno BA, Szyfelbein WM, Daniels GH, Vickery Jr AL. Fine needle aspiration biopsy of the thyroid gland in patients with prior Graves' disease treated with radioactive iodine. Morphologic findings and potential pitfalls. Acta Cytol. 1996;40:1189–97.
25. Anderson SR, Mandel S, LiVolsi VA, Gupta PK, Baloch ZW. Can cytomorphology differentiate between benign nodules and tumors arising in Graves' disease? Diagn Cytopathol. 2004;31:64–7.
26. Kim WB, Han SM, Kim TY, Nam-Goong IS, Gong G, Lee HK, Hong SJ, Shong YK. Ultrasonographic screening for detection of thyroid cancer in patients with Graves' disease. Clin Endocrinol (Oxf). 2004;60:719–25.
27. Cantalamessa L, Baldini M, Orsatti A, Meroni L, Amodei V, Castagnone D. Thyroid nodules in Graves disease and the risk of thyroid carcinoma. Arch Intern Med. 1999;159:1705–8.
28. Fadda G, LiVolsi VA. Histology and aspiration cytology of benign thyroid diseases. Rays. 1999;24:182–96.
29. Kumar N, Ray C, Jain S. Aspiration cytology of Hashimoto's thyroiditis in an endemic area. Cytopathology. 2002;13:31–9.
30. Kumarasinghe MP, De Silva S. Pitfalls in cytological diagnosis of autoimmune thyroiditis. Pathology. 1999;31:1–8.
31. Aozasa K, Tajima K, Tominaga N, Katagiri S, Yonezawa T, Matsuzuka F, Kuma K, Sawada M. Immunologic and immunohistochemical studies on chronic lymphocytic thyroiditis with or without thyroid lymphoma. Oncology. 1991;48:65–71.
32. Babu N, Dey P. Fine needle aspiration cytology of non-Hodgkin's lymphoma of thyroid. Cytopathology. 2002;13:188.
33. Baloch ZW, Fleisher S, LiVolsi VA, Gupta PK. Diagnosis of "follicular neoplasm": a gray zone in thyroid fine-needle aspiration cytology. Diagn Cytopathol. 2002;26:41–4.
34. Pu RT, Yang J, Wasserman PG, Bhuiya T, Griffith KA, Michael CW. Does Hurthle cell lesion/neoplasm predict malignancy more than follicular lesion/neoplasm on thyroid fine-needle aspiration? Diagn Cytopathol. 2006;34:330–4.
35. Deveci MS, Deveci G, LiVolsi VA, Baloch ZW. Fine-needle aspiration of follicular lesions of the thyroid. Diagnosis and follow-Up. Cytojournal. 2006;3:9.
36. Clary KM, Condel JL, Liu Y, Johnson DR, Grzybicki DM, Raab SS. Interobserver variability in the fine needle aspiration biopsy diagnosis of follicular lesions of the thyroid gland. Acta Cytol. 2005;49:378–82.
37. Tuttle RM, Lemar H, Burch HB. Clinical features associated with an increased risk of thyroid malignancy in patients with follicular neoplasia by fine-needle aspiration. Thyroid. 1998;8:377–83.
38. Yang J, Schnadig V, Logrono R, Wasserman PG. Fine-needle aspiration of thyroid nodules: a study of 4703 patients with histologic and clinical correlations. Cancer. 2007;111:306–15.
39. Nikiforov YE, Seethala RR, Tallini G, Baloch ZW, Basolo F, Thompson LD, Barletta JA, Wenig BM, Al Ghuzlan A, Kakudo K, Giordano TJ, Alves VA, Khanafshar E, Asa SL, El-Naggar AK, Gooding WE, Hodak SP, Lloyd RV, Maytal G, Mete O, Nikiforova MN, Nose V, Papotti M, Poller DN, Sadow PM, Tischler AS, Tuttle RM, Wall KB, LiVolsi VA, Randolph GW, Ghossein RA. Nomenclature revision for encapsulated follicular variant of papillary thyroid carcinoma: a paradigm shift to reduce overtreatment of indolent tumors. JAMA Oncol. 2016;2:1023.
40. Carpi A, Ferrari E, Sagripanti A, Nicolini A, Iervasi G, De Gaudio C, Romani R, Di Coscio G. Aspiration needle biopsy refines preoperative diagnosis of thyroid nodules defined at fine needle aspiration as microfollicular nodule. Biomed Pharmacother. 1996;50:325–8.
41. Asa SL. My approach to oncocytic tumours of the thyroid. J Clin Pathol. 2004;57:225–32.
42. Montone KT, Baloch ZW, LiVolsi VA. The thyroid Hurthle (oncocytic) cell and its associated pathologic conditions: a surgical pathology and cytopathology review. Arch Pathol Lab Med. 2008;132:1241–50.
43. Giorgadze T, Rossi ED, Fadda G, Gupta PK, Livolsi VA, Baloch Z. Does the fine-needle aspiration diagnosis of "Hurthle-cell neoplasm/follicular neoplasm with oncocytic features" denote increased risk of malignancy? Diagn Cytopathol. 2004;31:307–12.

44. Yang GC, Schreiner AM, Sun W. Can abundant colloid exclude oncocytic (Hurthle cell) carcinoma in thyroid fine needle aspiration? Cytohistological correlation of 127 oncocytic (Hurthle cell) lesions. Cytopathology. 2013;24:185.
45. Nasuti JF, Benedict C, Hurford M, Bibbo M. Differential diagnosis of oncocytic lesions of the breast and thyroid utilizing a semiquantitative approach. Acta Cytol. 1999;43:544–51.
46. Nguyen GK, Husain M, Akin MR. Cytodiagnosis of benign and malignant Hurthle cell lesions of the thyroid by fine-needle aspiration biopsy. Diagn Cytopathol. 1999;20:261–5.
47. Cochand-Priollet B, Prat JJ, Polivka M, Thienpont L, Dahan H, Wassef M, Guillausseau PJ. Thyroid fine needle aspiration: the morphological features on ThinPrep slide preparations. Eighty cases with histological control. Cytopathology. 2003;14:343–9.
48. Ford L, Rasgon BM, Hilsinger Jr RL, Cruz RM, Axelsson K, Rumore GJ, Schmidtknecht TM, Puligandla B, Sawicki J, Pshea W. Comparison of ThinPrep versus conventional smear cytopreparatory techniques for fine-needle aspiration specimens of head and neck masses. Otolaryngol Head Neck Surg. 2002;126:554–61.
49. Carcangiu ML, Zampi G, Rosai J. Papillary thyroid carcinoma: a study of its many morphologic expressions and clinical correlates. Pathol Annu. 1985;20 (Pt 1):1–44.
50. Szporn AH, Yuan S, Wu M, Burstein DE. Cellular swirls in fine needle aspirates of papillary thyroid carcinoma: a new diagnostic criterion. Mod Pathol. 2006;19:1470–3.
51. Albores-Saavedra J, Wu J. The many faces and mimics of papillary thyroid carcinoma. Endocr Pathol. 2006;17:1–18.
52. Riazmontazer N, Bedayat G. Psammoma bodies in fine needle aspirates from thyroids containing nontoxic hyperplastic nodular goiters. Acta Cytol. 1991;35:563–6.
53. Das DK, Mallik MK, Haji BE, Ahmed MS, Al-Shama'a M, Al-Ayadhy B, George SS, Sathar SA, Junaid TA. Psammoma body and its precursors in papillary thyroid carcinoma: a study by fine-needle aspiration cytology. Diagn Cytopathol. 2004;31: 380–6.
54. Saleh H, Bassily N, Hammoud MJ. Utility of a liquid-based, monolayer preparation in the evaluation of thyroid lesions by fine needle aspiration biopsy: comparison with the conventional smear method. Acta Cytol. 2009;53:130–6.
55. Baloch ZW, Shafique K, Flannagan M, Livolsi VA. Encapsulated classic and follicular variants of papillary thyroid carcinoma: comparative clinicopathologic study. Endocr Pract. 2010;16:952–9.
56. Gallagher J, Oertel YC, Oertel JE. Follicular variant of papillary carcinoma of the thyroid: fine-needle aspirates with histologic correlation. Diagn Cytopathol. 1997;16:207–13.
57. Zacks JF, de las Morenas A, Beazley RM, O'Brien MJ. Fine-needle aspiration cytology diagnosis of colloid nodule versus follicular variant of papillary carcinoma of the thyroid. Diagn Cytopathol. 1998;18:87–90.
58. Ruiz-Velasco R, Waisman J, Van Herle AJ. Cystic papillary carcinoma of the thyroid gland. Diagnosis by needle aspiration with transmission electron microscopy. Acta Cytol. 1978;22:38–42.
59. Castro-Gomez L, Cordova-Ramirez S, Duarte-Torres R, Alonso de Ruiz P, Hurtado-Lopez LM. Cytologic criteria of cystic papillary carcinoma of the thyroid. Acta Cytol. 2003;47:590–4.
60. Yang GC, Stern CM, Messina AV. Cystic papillary thyroid carcinoma in fine needle aspiration may represent a subset of the encapsulated variant in WHO classification. Diagn Cytopathol. 2010;38:721–6.
61. DeLellis RA, Lloyd RD, Heitz PU, Eng C, editors. WHO: pathology and genetics. Tumours of endocrine organs. Lyon: IARC Press; 2004. Kleihues P, Sobin LE, eds. WHO Classification of Tumours.
62. Bocklage T, DiTomasso J, Ramzy I, Ostrowski M. Tall cell variant of papillary thyroid carcinoma: cytologic features and differential diagnostic considerations. Diagn Cytopathol. 1997;17:25–9.
63. Solomon A, Gupta PK, LiVolsi VA, Baloch ZW. Distinguishing tall cell variant of papillary thyroid carcinoma from usual variant of papillary thyroid carcinoma in cytologic specimens. Diagn Cytopathol. 2002;27:143–8.
64. Gupta S, Sodhani P, Jain S, Kumar N. Morphologic spectrum of papillary carcinoma of the thyroid: role of cytology in identifying the variants. Acta Cytol. 2004;48:795–800.
65. Kumarasinghe MP. Cytomorphologic features of diffuse sclerosing variant of papillary carcinoma of the thyroid. A report of two cases in children. Acta Cytol. 1998;42:983–6.
66. Triggiani V, Ciampolillo A, Maiorano E. Papillary thyroid carcinoma, diffuse sclerosing variant, with abundant psammoma bodies. Acta Cytol. 2003;47:1141–3.
67. Hui PK, Chan JK, Cheung PS, Gwi E. Columnar cell carcinoma of the thyroid. Fine needle aspiration findings in a case. Acta Cytol. 1990;34:355–8.
68. Ylagan LR, Dehner LP, Huettner PC, Lu D. Columnar cell variant of papillary thyroid carcinoma. Report of a case with cytologic findings. Acta Cytol. 2004;48:73–7.
69. Wu LS, Roman SA, Sosa JA. Medullary thyroid cancer: an update of new guidelines and recent developments. Curr Opin Oncol. 2011;23:22–7.
70. Albores-Saavedra J, LiVolsi VA, Williams ED. Medullary carcinoma. Semin Diagn Pathol. 1985;2:137–46.
71. Asa SL. C-cell lesions of the thyroid. Pathol Case Rev. 1997;2:210–7.
72. Collins BT, Cramer HM, Tabatowski K, Hearn S, Raminhos A, Lampe H. Fine needle aspiration of medullary carcinoma of the thyroid. Cytomorphology,

immunocytochemistry and electron microscopy. Acta Cytol. 1995;39:920–30.
73. Asioli S, Erickson LA, Righi A, Jin L, Volante M, Jenkins S, Papotti M, Bussolati G, Lloyd RV. Poorly differentiated carcinoma of the thyroid: validation of the Turin proposal and analysis of IMP3 expression. Mod Pathol. 2010;23:1269–78.
74. Tallini G. Poorly differentiated thyroid carcinoma. Are we there yet? Endocr Pathol. 2011;22:190–4.
75. Sadow PM, Faquin WC. Poorly differentiated thyroid carcinoma: an incubating entity. Front Endocrinol. 2012;3:77.
76. Bongiovanni M, Bloom L, Krane JF, Baloch ZW, Powers CN, Hintermann S, Pache JC, Faquin WC. Cytomorphologic features of poorly differentiated thyroid carcinoma: a multi-institutional analysis of 40 cases. Cancer Cytopathol. 2009;117:185–94.
77. Ohori NP, Schoedel KE. Cytopathology of high-grade papillary thyroid carcinomas: tall-cell variant, diffuse sclerosing variant, and poorly differentiated papillary carcinoma. Diagn Cytopathol. 1999;20:19–23.
78. Bishop JA, Ali SZ. Hyalinizing trabecular adenoma of the thyroid gland. Diagn Cytopathol. 2011;39:306–10.
79. Hamburger JI, Miller JM, Kini SR. Lymphoma of the thyroid. Ann Intern Med. 1983;99:685–93.
80. Kossev P, Livolsi V. Lymphoid lesions of the thyroid: review in light of the revised European-American lymphoma classification and upcoming World Health Organization classification. Thyroid. 1999;9:1273–80.
81. Straus DJ. Primary thyroid lymphoma, a rare disease with a good treatment outcome. J Surg Oncol. 2010;101:543–4.
82. Sarinah B, Hisham AN. Primary lymphoma of the thyroid: diagnostic and therapeutic considerations. Asian J Surg. 2010;33:20–4.
83. Graff-Baker A, Sosa JA, Roman SA. Primary thyroid lymphoma: a review of recent developments in diagnosis and histology-driven treatment. Curr Opin Oncol. 2010;22:17–22.
84. Morgen EK, Geddie W, Boerner S, Bailey D, Santos Gda C. The role of fine-needle aspiration in the diagnosis of thyroid lymphoma: a retrospective study of nine cases and review of published series. J Clin Pathol. 2010;63:129–33.
85. Hughes JH, Jensen CS, Donnelly AD, Cohen MB, Silverman JF, Geisinger KR, Raab SS. The role of fine-needle aspiration cytology in the evaluation of metastatic clear cell tumors. Cancer. 1999;87:380–9.
86. Papi G, Fadda G, Corsello SM, Corrado S, Rossi ED, Radighieri E, Miraglia A, Carani C, Pontecorvi A. Metastases to the thyroid gland: prevalence, clinicopathological aspects and prognosis: a 10-year experience. Clin Endocrinol (Oxf). 2007;66:565–71.
87. Owens CL, Basaria S, Nicol TL. Metastatic breast carcinoma involving the thyroid gland diagnosed by fine-needle aspiration: a case report. Diagn Cytopathol. 2005;33:110–5.
88. Bula G, Waler J, Niemiec A, Koziolek H, Bichalski W, Gawrychowski J. Diagnosis of metastatic tumours to the thyroid gland by fine needle aspiration biopsy. Endokrynol Pol. 2010;61:427–9.
89. Cozzolino I, Malapelle U, Carlomagno C, Palombini L, Troncone G. Metastasis of colon cancer to the thyroid gland: a case diagnosed on fine-needle aspirate by a combined cytological, immunocytochemical, and molecular approach. Diagn Cytopathol. 2010;38:932–5.
90. Lam KY, Lo CY. Metastatic tumors of the thyroid gland: a study of 79 cases in Chinese patients. Arch Pathol Lab Med. 1998;122:37–41.
91. Cibas ES, Ali SZ. The Bethesda system for reporting thyroid cytopathology. Thyroid. 2009;19:1159–65.

31 Transcutaneous Laryngeal Ultrasonography: Clinical Variables

Brian H. Lang

31.1 Background

Thyroidectomy is one of the most commonly performed surgical procedures worldwide and because vocal cord paresis or palsy (VCP) is an important outcome measure of the procedure itself, surgeons should have the knowledge of a patient's vocal cord (VC) function before and after the procedure [1, 2]. However, the gold standard examination for VC function, namely the flexible nasopharyngeal laryngoscopy (FLS) or better still video-laryngo-stroboscopy, is only available in some general or endocrine surgical practices and therefore, if a patient requires a formal VC examination, further consultation to an otolaryngologist is necessary. This not only increases cost but also causes inconvenience and disrupts patient flow [3]. In addition, many patients find FLS to be uncomfortable and unpleasant leading to poor patient compliance and cooperation [4].

Transcutaneous laryngeal ultrasound (TLUSG), on the other hand, is a less-invasive and more convenient method of assessing the VCs. With increasing number of surgical practices now equipped with an ultrasound (USG) machine, TLUSG has become more applicable for surgeons and could potentially reduce many additional consultations and FLS [3, 5]. Furthermore, learning the skills of TLUSG is not difficult and it is clear that even individuals who do not routinely perform USG could quickly overcome the learning curve and become competent [6]. A recent study involving three high-volume independent endocrine surgeons reported that by adopting TLUSG in their clinical practice, 107 additional consultations and FLS were prevented over 1 year period and there was a net saving of USD $7918 to $21,507 [5]. Although TLUSG is never meant to be a replacement or an alternative to FLS because it does not allow a full visualization of the larynx, it is highly accurate in determining the VC function before and after thyroidectomy [7, 8]. In fact, instead of thinking of it as a replacement, a more pragmatic approach would be to use TLUSG as a screening tool for FLS. One study has shown that if TLUSG is used as a screening tool for FLS, the total number of routine FLS could potentially be reduced by up to 86 % without having to miss a clinically significant VCP [7].

Electronic supplementary material: The online version of this chapter (doi:10.1007/978-3-319-44100-9_31) contains supplementary material, which is available to authorized users. Videos can also be accessed at http://link.springer.com/chapter/10.1007/978-3-319-44100-9_31.

B.H. Lang, M.S., F.R.A.C.S., F.C.S.H.K., F.H.K.A.M. (✉)
Division of Endocrine Surgery, Department of Surgery, Queen Mary Hospital, The University of Hong Kong, Room 1401, Block K, 102 Pokfulam Road, Hong Kong, SAR, China
e-mail: blang@hku.hk

M. Milas et al. (eds.), *Advanced Thyroid and Parathyroid Ultrasound*,
DOI 10.1007/978-3-319-44100-9_31

It is worth pointing out that TLUSG is not a particularly novel technique. In fact, the earliest reports could be traced back in the 1980s [9, 10]. However, since most of the earlier reports were published in the radiology literature, surgeons were simply either unaware of this technique or did not recognize its clinical importance to thyroid surgery. One of the earlier reports by surgeons was published by an Australian group in 2001 [11]. In that study, TLUSG only correctly identified the side of the lesion in four of six VCPs and therefore, the overall sensitivity was only 67 %. As a result, the authors concluded that TLUSG was not a reliable alternative to FLS in the assessment of VC function after thyroid or parathyroid surgery [11]. However, perhaps with advances in the quality of USG as well as improving skills over time, recent studies reported better success with some even reporting a sensitivity of up to 100 % [7, 8, 12–14]. In a large prospective assessor-blind evaluation of TLUSG, one group reported a VC visualization rate of 94.5 % with an overall sensitivity of detecting a VCP of 93.3 % [7]. Therefore, the chance of missing an actual VCP when one could clearly see movement in both VCs on TLUSG is very low [7].

31.2 How Does TLUSG Work?

TLUSG essentially relies on the propagation of USG waves from the anterior neck skin to VCs via the ventral part of the thyroid cartilage and then back again. Although the laryngeal box has air in and around it, the movement of the VCs and the arytenoids are still visible and imageable on TLUSG. This is believed to be due to the fact that the thyroid cartilage can act as an acoustic window for USG waves to propagate. On actual imaging, the true VCs usually appear hypoechoic while the false VCs appear hyperechoic. This is because the former are made of muscles while the latter comprise fibro-fatty tissues. In addition to these two landmarks, the other landmark is the arytenoids. Because the arytenoids are made of hyaline cartilage and elastic cartilage, they normally would appear almost echoless with a hyperechoic rim at the posterior end of the VCs. Figure 31.1 shows the true and false VCs.

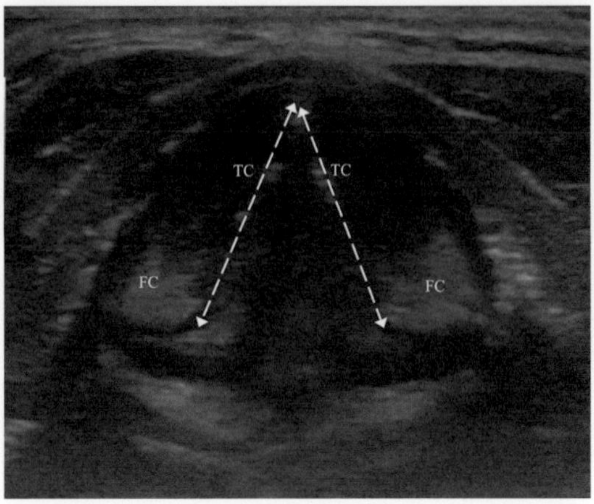

Fig. 31.1 This is an image depicting the true (TC) and false (FC) vocal cords on transcutaneous laryngeal ultrasound using the ventral approach

31.3 Steps and Tips in Carrying Out a TLUSG of the VCs

Similar to performing an USG for the thyroid or parathyroid gland, it is recommended that the patient should be placed in a supine position with the neck slightly extended and arms resting on the side. After applying ample amount of gel over the thyroid cartilage area, a linear transducer is placed transversely in the middle of the thyroid cartilage. It is important that the transducer is placed gently on the cartilage rather than pressing too forcefully onto the cartilage. The reason for using ample amount of gel is maximize the physical contact while avoiding air between the linear probe and the concavity of the cartilage. This is particularly crucial in male patients because the thyroid cartilage is usually more angulated in the middle than female patients and so there is less direct contact between the probe and cartilage. In terms of selecting the most appropriate USG probe for TLUSG, we believe the lower the frequency (i.e., 5–10 MHz) the better because the lower frequency helps with the tissue penetration and as mentioned earlier, the quality of the images depends on how well the USG waves could propagate through the thyroid cartilage. After placing the probe transversely on the body of the cartilage, the region is scanned cranio-caudally along the sagittal plane until either the true or false VCs are clearly visualized.

In the transverse plane, the false VCs are located immediately above the true VCs while the arytenoids are usually in the same transverse plane as the false VCs. To enhance visualization, it is recommended to turn up the gain or gray-scale during examination until the false VCs become hyperechoic. Based on the experience of previous authors, probably among the three moving landmarks on TLUSG (namely, false VCs, true VCs and arytenoids), the most easily visible landmark (at least initially) is the false VCs [15]. This is supported by a study that showed the rate of visualization of false VCs is almost three times higher than that of true VCs (92.7 % vs. 36.7 %, $p<0.05$) and is also slightly higher than that of the arytenoids (89.8 %) [16]. Once one or more landmarks are visualized on TLUSG, there are two types of VC movement that one should observe to determine if the function of the VCs has been compromised. First is passive (where a patient is breathing normally) and the other is active (where a patient is instructed to either phonate or perform a Valsalva maneuver). To date, there is no consensus on which type of VC movement or active maneuver provides the most reliable assessment. However, given that passive movement is technically the easiest to do, most clinicians prefer passive movement alone to determine if a patient has a unilateral VCP or not. For a patient without VCP, during passive movement, one could observe spontaneous, subtle symmetrical movement of both VCs with each cord moving in a rhythmic matter along with respiration while for a patient with an unilateral VCP, this passive movement either becomes asymmetrical or completely absent on the affected side. However, it should be noted that there is a small percentage of patients who do not have spontaneous passive movement in their VCs and so, it is not unreasonable to combine the finding of passive movement with at least one other active maneuver to confirm the motility in both VCs. In terms of active maneuvers, the recommended technique is the Valsalva maneuver because it is the technically easiest to learn [5, 17]. During Valsalva maneuver, if the patient has normal VCs, one could see both VCs adducting symmetrically to the midline (see Video 31.1). On the other hand, when a patient suffers from a unilateral VCP, one would see either reduced (Video 31.2) or completely absent movement (Video 31.3) on the affected side (i.e., asymmetrical movement). Other maneuvers such as active phonation at times may induce movement in other laryngeal muscles and therefore not prefer. The other trick one could also try to induce voluntary movement of VCs is to ask the patient to swallow his or her own saliva for a few times.

31.4 Factors Leading to Non-visualization of VCs

Since visualization of the VCs really depends on whether the USG waves could travel from the skin to the VCs and the landmarks via the thyroid cartilage, the presence of ossification in the thyroid cartilage is the major reason for unclear VC visualization. There is little controversy that patients with ossified thyroid cartilage are not good candidates for TLUSG. Ossification itself blocks the propagation of USG waves onto the VCs and therefore, on imaging, one could see that there is a large acoustic shallow over the VCs and arytenoids making evaluation of VCs impossible (Fig. 31.2). Nevertheless, there are patient factors that could help to predict the presence of ossification. First is age. It has been well demonstrated that the extent of ossification gradually increases with age. This is compatible with our and others' experience that it is much easier to image VCs in young patients [12–15]. In fact, a previous study found that almost 100 % of patients aged <30 years old had clear VC visualization while this rate dropped to <90 % in patients aged >70 years old [15]. A recent anatomical study of 200 healthy individuals of all ages have shown that this ossification process begins at the age of 18–20 years in the posterior part of the thyroid cartilage regardless of sex and over time, the ossification process slowly moves in an anteromedial direction until the entire cartilage has been completely replaced by bone (i.e., ossified) [18]. In this study, the authors found that the thyroid cartilage is not consistently denser (as measured by Hounsfield units) on CT scan until

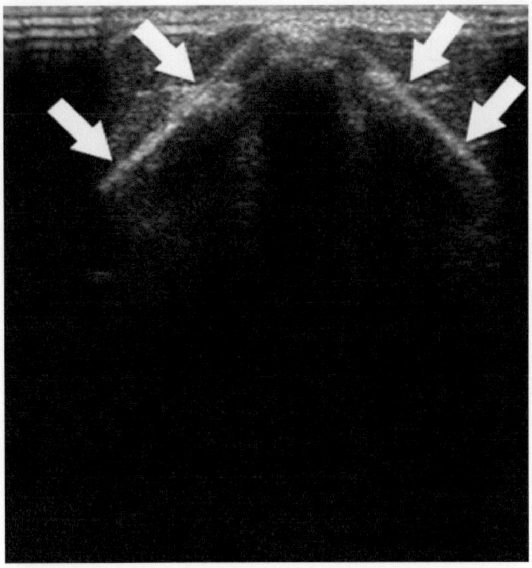

Fig. 31.2 This is an image depicting the presence of ossification at both lamina of the thyroid cartilage. Please also note the large post-acoustic shallow posterior to the cartilage

after the age 40 [18]. Consistent with this, some studies have reported that the entire cartilage only becomes replaced by bone by age of 65 [19]. Fortunately, this process appears to be less complete in females and therefore, some females may still have a small non-ossified ventral window in their thyroid cartilage making TLUSG possible [20]. Partly because of this difference in ossification between the two sexes, male patients generally have significantly lower rate of VC visualization than female patients. By adjusting for other significant clinical variables, one study found male patients to be 13 times more likely to have non-visualized VCs than females [15]. The other reason for this gender difference might be due to the thickness of the thyroid cartilage as males tend to have thicker and larger thyroid cartilage than females leading to poorer propagation of USG waves.

In addition to age and sex, patient height and the placement of neck incision in relation to the cricoid cartilage have also been found to be independent factors for non-visualization of VCs in postoperative TLUSG. For patient height, it was shown that even after adjusting for sex and age, those who were taller were significantly less likely to have non-visualized VCs on TLUSG than those who were shorter in height. Using a median cutoff of 158 cm, the non-visualization rate for patients taller than 158 cm was significantly higher than those shorter than 158 cm (9.0 % vs. 1.0 %, $p<0.001$). Similarly, using a median distance of 60 mm from skin incision to the cricoid cartilage, those with distance less than 60 mm were significantly more likely to have non-visualized VCs than those with distance ≥60 mm (6.9 % vs. 3.9 %, $p=0.050$) [15]. The reason why the distance between wound and cricoid cartilage is an independent factor for non-visualization is probably related to the presence of subplatysmal swelling or edema after thyroidectomy. Therefore, it may still be possible to visualize the VCs in patients with short distance between wound and cricoid cartilage provided that a longer waiting period is allowed for the resolution of swelling and edema.

31.5 Ventral vs. Lateral Approach

To date, two general approaches for TLUSG had been described in the literature and they were the ventral and lateral approaches. For the ventral approach, the USG probe is placed transversely in front of the middle of the thyroid cartilage. The advantages with this approach are the symmetrical view and the better appreciation of the three landmarks in the larynx as this is the same view as in FLS. The symmetrical view is important in TLUSG particularly when one relies on seeing symmetrical passive movement as a criterion to rule out unilateral VCP. However, the ventral approach may not always be possible because male patients sometimes have very prominent and angular cartilage making a full contact between the probe and cartilage almost impossible. More recently, another group of investigators suggested the lateral approach could be one way to overcome this drawback for male patients [8]. Using the lateral approach, the authors were able to achieve 100 % visualization rate and a sensitivity and specificity of 100 % and 98.7 %, respectively, in male patients. Unlike the ventral approach, the lateral approach

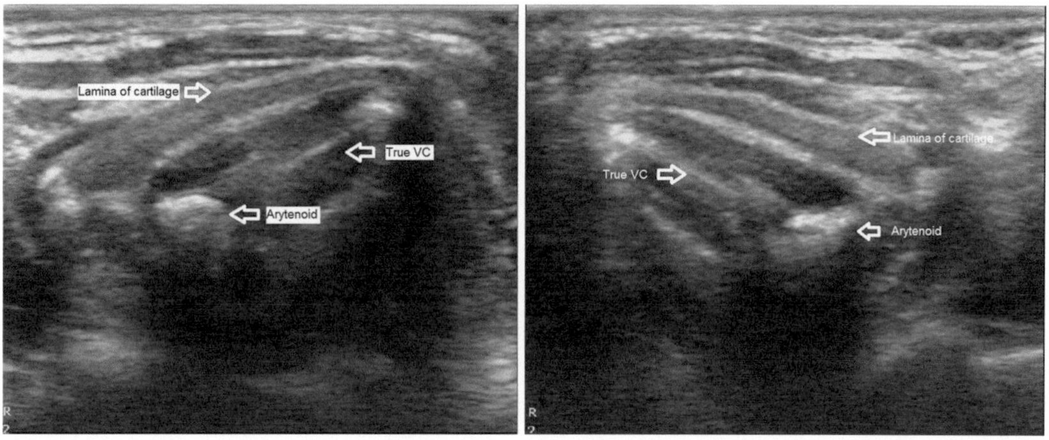

Fig. 31.3 These are two images showing the right and left true vocal cords and arytenoids via the lateral approach

involves placing the USG probe on the lateral surface of the thyroid lamina (Fig. 31.3). The authors believed the lateral approach could significantly improve the efficacy of TLUSG in male patients and postulated that placing the probe on the lateral surface of the larynx improves not only the physical contact but also shorten the distance between the probe and the laryngeal landmarks [8]. However, it is worth pointing out that in their comparison, the actual visualization rate of both the true VCs and arytenoids in the lateral approach tended to be lower than those in the ventral approach. Furthermore, based on anatomical studies, the ossification process actually starts posteriorly and moves slowly in the anteromedial direction and so the chance of encountering ossification using the lateral approach might actually be higher than the ventral approach. Nevertheless, more studies are needed to confirm their findings.

31.6 Conclusions

TLUSG is a noninvasive and convenient method of evaluating the motility of VCs before and after thyroidectomy. In our opinion, provided appropriate training has been given, the skills of TLUSG could be quickly learned even by individuals who do not routinely perform USG in their clinical practice. Ossification of thyroid cartilage remains the main reason for clear VC visualization. Given the association between age, sex, and presence of ossification, TLUSG is most applicable in young, female patients. Ventral approach remains the preferred approach over the lateral approach in the assessment of VC function.

Acknowledgments I would like to take this opportunity to thank Dr. KP Wong and Dr. JW Woo for providing some of the wonderful images and videos used in this chapter.

Competing Interests The author declares that he has no competing interests.

Author Contributions BHH Lang was involved in the review of literature, acquisition of data, and drafting and completing the chapter. BHH Lang was also involved in the review of literature and drafting the chapter. BHH Lang conceived the study, participated in the coordination and the acquisition of data and helped to draft the chapter. He read and approved the chapter.

References

1. Lang BH, Wong CK, Tsang RK, Wong KP, Wong BY. Evaluating the cost-effectiveness of laryngeal examination after elective total thyroidectomy. Ann Surg Oncol. 2014;21(11):3548–56.
2. Lang BH, Chu KK, Tsang RK, Wong KP, Wong BY. Evaluating the incidence, clinical significance

and predictors for vocal cord palsy and incidental laryngopharyngeal conditions before elective thyroidectomy: is there a case for routine laryngoscopic examination? World J Surg. 2014;38(2):385–91.
3. Parangi S. Translaryngeal vocal cord ultrasound: ready for prime time. Surgery. 2016;159:67. doi:10.1016/j.surg.2015.10.014. pii: S0039-6060(15)00841-7.
4. Paul BC, Rafii B, Achlatis S, Amin MR, Branski RC. Morbidity and patient perception of flexible laryngoscopy. Ann Otol Rhinol Laryngol. 2012; 121(11):708–13.
5. Carneiro-Pla D, Solorzano CC, Wilhelm SM. Impact of vocal cord ultrasonography on endocrine surgery practices. Surgery. 2016;159:58. doi:10.1016/j.surg.2015.06.067. pii: S0039-6060(15)00743-6.
6. Wong KP, Lang BH, Lam S, Au KP, Chan DT, Kotewall NC. Determining the learning curve of transcutaneous laryngeal ultrasound in vocal cord assessment by CUSUM analysis of eight surgical residents: when to abandon laryngoscopy. World J Surg. 2016;40:659.
7. Wong KP, Lang BH, Ng SH, Cheung CY, Chan CT, Lo CY. A prospective, assessor-blind evaluation of surgeon-performed transcutaneous laryngeal ultrasonography in vocal cord examination before and after thyroidectomy. Surgery. 2013;154(6):1158–64. discussion 1164-5.
8. Woo JW, Suh H, Song RY, Lee JH, Yu HW, Kim SJ, Chai YJ, Choi JY, Lee KE. A novel lateral-approach laryngeal ultrasonography for vocal cord evaluation. Surgery. 2016;159:52. doi:10.1016/j.surg.2015.07.043. pii: S0039-6060(15)00705-9.
9. Raghavendra BN, Horii SC, Reede DL, Rumancik WM, Persky M, Bergeron T. Sonographic anatomy of the larynx, with particular reference to the vocal cords. J Ultrasound Med. 1987;6(5):225–30.
10. Garel C, Legrand I, Elmaleh M, Contencin P, Hassan M. Laryngeal ultrasonography in infants and children: anatomical correlation with fetal preparations. Pediatr Radiol. 1990;20(4):241–4.
11. Sidhu S, Stanton R, Shahidi S, Chu J, Chew S, Campbell P. Initial experience of vocal cord evaluation using grey-scale, real-time. B-mode ultrasound. ANZ J Surg. 2001;71(12):737–9.
12. Cheng SP, Lee JJ, Liu TP, Lee KS, Liu CL. Preoperative ultrasonography assessment of vocal cord movement during thyroid and parathyroid surgery. World J Surg. 2012;36(10):2509–15.
13. Wang CP, Chen TC, Yang TL, Chen CN, Lin CF, Lou PJ, Hu YL, Shieh MJ, Hsieh FJ, Hsiao TY, Ko JY. Transcutaneous ultrasound for evaluation of vocal fold movement in patients with thyroid disease. Eur J Radiol. 2012;81(3):e288–91.
14. Dedecjus M, Adamczewski Z, Brzeziński J, Lewiński A. Real-time, high-resolution ultrasonography of the vocal folds--a prospective pilot study in patients before and after thyroidectomy. Langenbecks Arch Surg. 2010;395(7):859–64.
15. Wong KP, Woo JW, Youn YK, Chow FC, Lee KE, Lang BH. The importance of sonographic landmarks by transcutaneous laryngeal ultrasonography in post-thyroidectomy vocal cord assessment. Surgery. 2014;156(6):1590–6. discussion 1596.
16. Wong KP, Lang BH, Chang YK, Wong KC, Chow FC. Assessing the validity of transcutaneous laryngeal ultrasonography (TLUSG) after thyroidectomy: what factors matter? Ann Surg Oncol. 2015;22(6):1774–80.
17. Carneiro-Pla D, Miller BS, Wilhelm SM, Milas M, Gauger PG, Cohen MS, Hughes DT, Solorzano CC. Feasibility of surgeon-performed transcutaneous vocal cord ultrasonography in identifying vocal cord mobility: a multi-institutional experience. Surgery. 2014;156(6):1597–602. doi:10.1016/j.surg.2014.08.071. discussion 1602-4.
18. Wenaas AE, Tran B, Ongkasuwan J. The progression of thyroid cartilage calcification as it relates to the utilization of laryngeal ultrasound. Laryngoscope. 2016;126:913. doi:10.1002/lary.25582.
19. Gray H. The larynx. In: Anatomy of the human body. Philadelphia, PA: Lea & Febiger; 1918. http://www.bartleby.com/107/236.html. Accessed April 22, 2014.
20. Kirsch T, Claassen H. Matrix vesicles mediate mineralization of human thyroid cartilage. Calcif Tissue Int. 2000;66(4):292–7.

Transcutaneous Laryngeal Ultrasonography: Technical Performance and Interpretation

32

Denise Carneiro-Pla

32.1 Introduction

Recurrent laryngeal nerve injury during cervical procedures leading to true vocal cord (TVC) paralysis is fortunately infrequent; however, identification of TVC immobility before cervical reexploration is critical to determine the risk of bilateral vocal cord paralysis and tracheostomy. Because a paralyzed vocal cord (VC) can be clinically not evident when it is medialized, it is recommended that all patients with previous neck operations or suspicious to have VC dysfunction have vocal cord mobility evaluation before neck reexploration. Yet, some surgeons are not as selective recommending VC visualization to all patients before and after any neck exploration. With that in mind, a simple and noninvasive method of VC mobility evaluation would be valuable in the workup of patients undergoing thyroid and parathyroidectomy.

Electronic supplementary material: The online version of this chapter (doi:10.1007/978-3-319-44100-9_32) contains supplementary material, which is available to authorized users. Videos can also be accessed at http://link.springer.com/chapter/10.1007/978-3-319-44100-9_32.

D. Carneiro-Pla, M.D., F.A.C.S. (✉)
Division of Oncologic & Endocrine Surgery, Department of Surgery, Medical University of South Carolina, 114 Doughty Street, Suite 240, Charleston, SC 29425, USA
e-mail: carneiro@musc.edu

Vocal cord ultrasonography (VCUS) has been shown useful and accurate in demonstrating vocal mobility in most patients with a sensitivity ranging from 62 to 100 % [1–12]. This convenient technique can be an asset for surgeons and endocrinologists who perform US routinely during evaluation of thyroid and parathyroid disease as part of their physical examination. When it was used prospectively, VCUS changed the preoperative evaluation significantly by safely avoiding FL in 76 % of patients who otherwise would have required an FL preoperatively [8].

32.2 Larynx Anatomy

The structures visualized on VCUS are the thyroid cartilage anterior to the vocal cords, TVCs as hyperechoic lines connecting the thyroid cartilage to the arytenoid cartilages, false vocal cords (FVC) which are hyperechoic muscular structures lateral to the TVC bilaterally and the arytenoids cartilages as shown on Fig. 32.1, Videos 32.1 and 32.2.

It is important to clarify the orientation of the VC visualization on US versus FL which can be confusing because the right VC is displayed on the right of the screen on both studies, although the arytenoids are on the opposite sides of the screen. On VCUS, the arytenoids are on the inferior portion of the screen, and on FL it is on the

M. Milas et al. (eds.), *Advanced Thyroid and Parathyroid Ultrasound*,
DOI 10.1007/978-3-319-44100-9_32

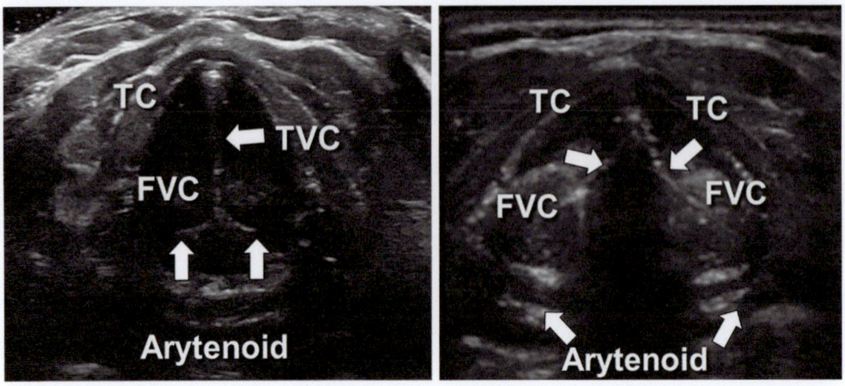

Fig. 32.1 Laryngeal anatomy on ultrasonography

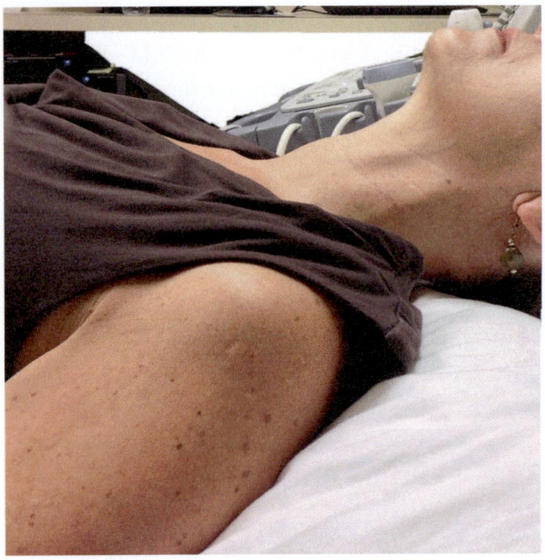

Fig. 32.2 Patient's position for vocal cord ultrasonography

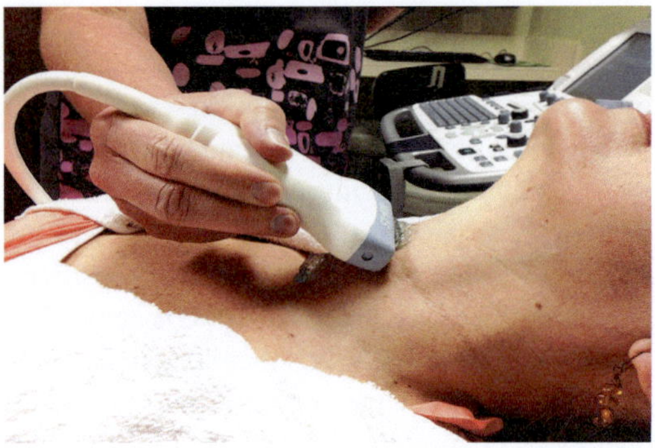

Fig. 32.3 Probe position on the patient's neck for VCUS

superior portion of the screen. This orientation of VC visualization between both studies is further explained on Video 32.3.

32.3 Technique and Material

The patient's position for VCUS is similar to the cervical hyperextension used for scanning of the thyroid gland (Fig. 32.2). The probe is placed just inferior to the thyroid cartilage angling superiorly (Fig. 32.3). Ample gel should be used to obtain ideal probe contact with the trachea and thyroid cartilage.

Ultrasound probe for small parts scanning with capability to decrease its frequency from 15 to 12 MHz to 8–9 MHz is necessary to improve the visualization of TVC. Higher frequencies will decrease the ability to visualize the arytenoids and the hyperechoic TVC, especially posteriorly. Furthermore, the gain should be increased to enhance the visualization of the structures posterior to the thyroid cartilage.

TVCs can be visualized during passive breathing and phonation; however, localization and rapid evaluation of bilateral VC movement can be accomplished by asking the patient to perform a Valsalva maneuver. During Valsalva, the TVC will adduct on the midline allowing the ultrasonographer to easily localize the VC by slightly moving the probe superiorly and inferiorly. When the TVCs are found closed on the midline, the patient is asked to take a normal breath and TVC,

FVC and arytenoids will abduct, therefore confirming bilateral vocal cord mobility as seen on Videos 32.4 and 32.5.

Usually when a TVC is paralyzed, ipsilateral FVC and arytenoid cartilage are also immobile as seen on Video 32.6 where the right TVC is paralyzed. A valuable hint of vocal cord dysfunction is the asymmetry of the arytenoids as seen on this clip. Video 32.7 shows left immobile TVC demonstrating similar findings. On both videos, arytenoid cartilage asymmetry and immobility of TVC, FVC, and arytenoid are easily visualized.

Frequently, not all structures can be visualized at the same time which might be one of the reasons for the variation TVC visualization rates among ultrasonographers. It is more challenging to demonstrate the TVC than the FVC and arytenoids. While the arytenoids are anatomically accurate predictors of TVC function, Wong et al. have shown that FVC movement on US also predicted the TVC mobility [13]. Further studies are needed to validate this finding since FVC can be hyperfunctioning when there is a TVC paralysis. In the author's opinion, arytenoid cartilages asymmetry is an accurate marker of abnormal vocal fold movement and it should raise the suspicion for VC mobility dysfunction; however, immobility of TVC and/or arytenoids should be used as diagnostic of VC paralysis.

32.4 Pearls and Pitfalls of Vocal Cord Ultrasound

VCUS has significant limitations which are mainly associated with inability of vocal folds visualization in patients with thyroid cartilage calcification (TCC) (Fig. 32.4). Because most men have thyroid cartilage ossification, VCUS has a very low visualization rate in men.

Although some studies have shown decreased visualization of VC on US in older and in obese patients, these finding were not reproduced in other studies.

For VCUS some basic US skills are necessary; however, the learning curve with proper training is steep.

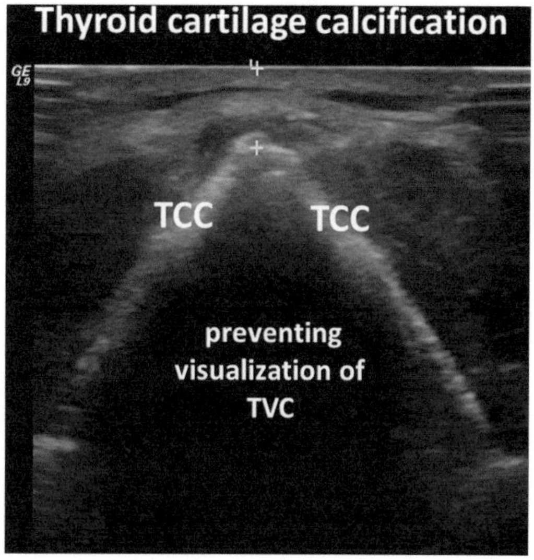

Fig. 32.4 Demonstrate thyroid cartilage calcification

Technical tips include the decrease of frequency to lower ranges such as 8–9 MHz and increase in the gain. These two scanning technical factors could be the reason for discrepancies in vocal visualization rates available in the literature.

VCUS is not as accurate in identifying paresis and mild changes in vocal cord mobility. As the ultrasonographer becomes more experienced, subtle abnormalities of mobility can be seen, however, not as accurately as vocal cord paralysis. For identification of vocal fold paresis, arytenoid asymmetry is the easiest landmark to point out VC dysfunction.

32.5 Conclusion

Flexible laryngoscopy remains the gold standard study to evaluate vocal cord mobility; however, vocal cord ultrasonography is accurate in predicting VC paralysis in most patients, especially in females. True vocal cord ultrasonography can be a great asset to surgeons and endocrinologists performing cervical US routinely. This technique can potentially prevent FL in most patient who require FL before neck reexploration and to confirm TVC mobility postoperatively. VCUS is a great screening test which can guide the clinician to obtain an FL only selectively on patients with higher risk for vocal cord paralysis, poor VC visualization on US, or significant VC dysfunction.

References

1. Wong KP, Woo JW, Li JY, Lee KE, Youn YK, Lang BH. Using Transcutaneous Laryngeal Ultrasonography (TLUSG) to assess post-thyroidectomy patients' vocal cords: which maneuver best optimizes visualization and assessment accuracy? World J Surg. 2016;40:652.
2. Wong KP, Lang BH, Lam S, Au KP, Chan DT, Kotewall NC. Determining the learning curve of transcutaneous laryngeal ultrasound in vocal cord assessment by CUSUM analysis of eight surgical residents: when to abandon laryngoscopy. World J Surg. 2016;40:659.
3. Wong KP, Lang BH, Chang YK, Wong KC, Chow FC. Assessing the validity of transcutaneous laryngeal ultrasonography (TLUSG) after thyroidectomy: what factors matter? Ann Surg Oncol. 2015;22(6):1774–80.
4. Vats A, Worley GA, de Bruyn R, Porter H, Albert DM, Bailey CM. Laryngeal ultrasound to assess vocal fold paralysis in children. J Laryngol Otol. 2004;118(6):429–31.
5. Amis RJ, Gupta D, Dowdall JR, Srirajakalindini A, Folbe A. Ultrasound assessment of vocal fold paresis: a correlation case series with flexible fiberoptic laryngoscopy and adding the third dimension (3-D) to vocal fold mobility assessment. Middle East J Anaesthesiol. 2012;21(4):493–8.
6. Wang CP, Chen TC, Yang TL, Chen CN, Lin CF, Lou PJ, et al. Transcutaneous ultrasound for evaluation of vocal fold movement in patients with thyroid disease. Eur J Radiol. 2012;81(3):e288–91.
7. Carneiro-Pla D, Miller BS, Wilhelm SM, Milas M, Gauger PG, Cohen MS, et al. Feasibility of surgeon-performed transcutaneous vocal cord ultrasonography in identifying vocal cord mobility: a multi-institutional experience. Surgery. 2014;156(6):1597–602. discussion 602-4.
8. Carneiro-Pla D, Solorzano CC, Wilhelm SM. Impact of vocal cord ultrasonography on endocrine surgery practices. Surgery. 2016;159:58.
9. Cheng SP, Lee JJ, Liu TP, Lee KS, Liu CL. Preoperative ultrasonography assessment of vocal cord movement during thyroid and parathyroid surgery. World J Surg. 2012;36(10):2509–15.
10. Dedecjus M, Adamczewski Z, Brzezinski J, Lewinski A. Real-time, high-resolution ultrasonography of the vocal folds--a prospective pilot study in patients before and after thyroidectomy. Langenbecks Arch Surg. 2010;395(7):859–64.
11. Lai PK, Wang YA, Welsh AW. Reproducibility of regional placental vascularity/perfusion measurement using 3D power Doppler. Ultrasound Obstet Gynecol. 2010;36(2):202–9.
12. Sidhu S, Stanton R, Shahidi S, Chu J, Chew S, Campbell P. Initial experience of vocal cord evaluation using grey-scale, real-time. B-mode ultrasound. ANZ J Surg. 2001;71(12):737–9.
13. Wong KP, Woo JW, Youn YK, Chow FC, Lee KE, Lang BH. The importance of sonographic landmarks by transcutaneous laryngeal ultrasonography in post-thyroidectomy vocal cord assessment. Surgery. 2014;156(6):1590–6. discussion 6.

The Role of Ultrasound in Determining Eligibility for Remote Access/Robotic Surgery and Cosmetic Incision Placement

33

William S. Duke and David J. Terris

33.1 Introduction

Advances in surgical techniques and technology have revolutionized endocrine surgery over the last several decades. These improvements have decreased operative morbidity and ushered in an era of individualized thyroid and parathyroid surgery, in which the procedure is customized to each specific patient and their disease. At the same time, the rise of minimally invasive surgery and corresponding evolution of patient expectations have mandated that surgeons give increasing attention to the cosmetic outcome of these procedures. Ultrasound plays a key role in the evaluation of structural endocrine disease in the neck, and helps the surgeon determine if the patient is a candidate for a cosmetically favorable small-incision minimally invasive procedure or for a remote access operation.

W.S. Duke, M.D., F.A.C.S.
D.J. Terris, M.D., F.A.C.S., F.A.C.E. (✉)
Department of Otolaryngology—Head and Neck Surgery, Augusta University, 1120 Fifteenth Street, BP-4109, Augusta, GA 30912-4060, USA
e-mail: William.Duke@multicare.org; dterris@augusta.edu

33.2 Ultrasound for Incision Planning

33.2.1 Thyroid

Incisions for thyroid surgery have traditionally been placed either a specified distance from a fixed reference point (such as 2 cm or 2 fingerbreadths above the sternal notch or below the cricoid cartilage) or in a more variable but still rigidly defined location, such as at the midpoint between the cricoid cartilage and sternal notch [1–5]. The incisions are generally placed in the center of the neck, although laterally based incisions have also been described for unilateral or reoperative thyroid surgery [3]. Incisions may be placed higher on the neck if difficulty accessing the superior pole is anticipated [6, 7]. Although an incision too low in the neck increases the risk of hypertrophy or keloid formation [8], incisions high in the neck are more difficult to conceal with clothing or the shadowing from the natural hollow between the sternocleidomastoid muscles. It is now recognized that the optimal location for a thyroidectomy incision is centered on the midline in a naturally occurring skin crease that is selected with the patient in a neutral upright position (Fig. 33.1) [9]. This location offers the best balance between access to the thyroid gland and minimizing the cosmetic impact of the scar.

M. Milas et al. (eds.), *Advanced Thyroid and Parathyroid Ultrasound*,
DOI 10.1007/978-3-319-44100-9_33

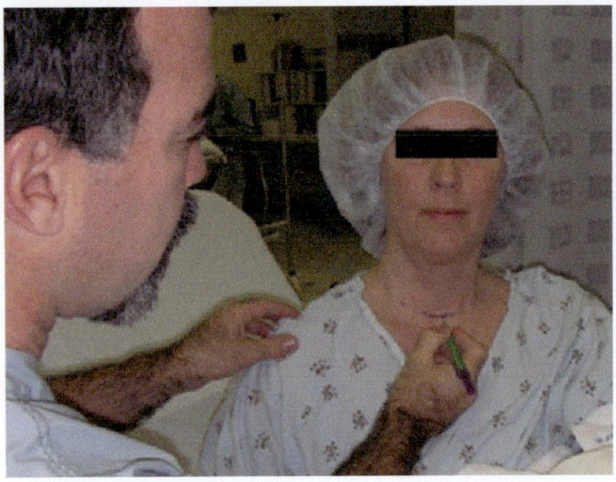

Fig. 33.1 Marking the incision in a naturally occurring skin crease while the patient is in an upright position ensures optimal positioning of the scar. Reproduced with permission from: Terris DJ. Novel surgical maneuvers in modern thyroid surgery. *Operative Techniques in Otolaryngology*. 2009;20:23–28

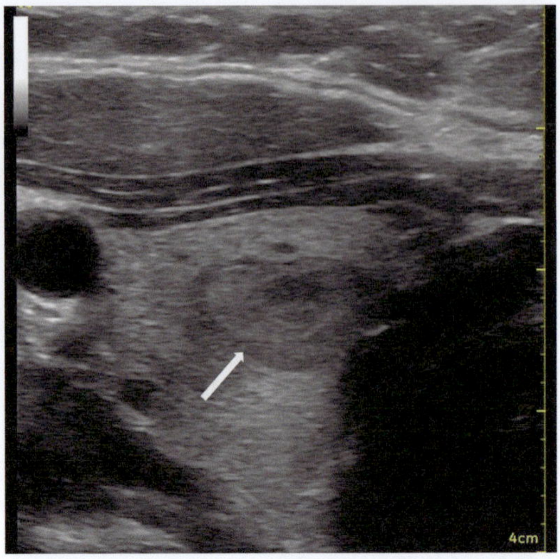

Fig. 33.2 Thyroid nodule (*white arrow*) that is suitable for minimally invasive video-assisted thyroidectomy approach

Since the ideal location of the scar is primarily determined by the patient's skin creases, the ultrasonographic findings do not generally alter the recommended position of the thyroidectomy incision. Although a slightly higher incision may be contemplated to improve the exposure of the superior aspect of the gland, it is often more cosmetically favorable to extend the incision within an ideal skin crease than to increase the visibility of the scar by creating a shorter incision higher in the neck in an unfavorable skin crease.

Ultrasound is more helpful in determining the type of surgical approach utilized and the length of the incision [10], particularly when directly performed by the surgeon [11]. Patients with small nodules ($\leq$30 mm) and normal size glands (volume $\leq$ 20 mL) with no substernal or extrathyroidal extension on ultrasound may be candidates for a minimally invasive video-assisted thyroidectomy approach (Fig. 33.2) [12]. This procedure is routinely performed through a 20 mm incision, and is associated with less postoperative pain, a faster recovery, and improved cosmetic outcomes when compared to conventional thyroid surgery [13, 14]. Depending on their body habitus and associated conditions such as thyroiditis (Fig. 33.3) or prior central neck surgery, patients with larger nodules or glands, or with extrathyroidal or substernal extension on ultrasound may need larger incisions.

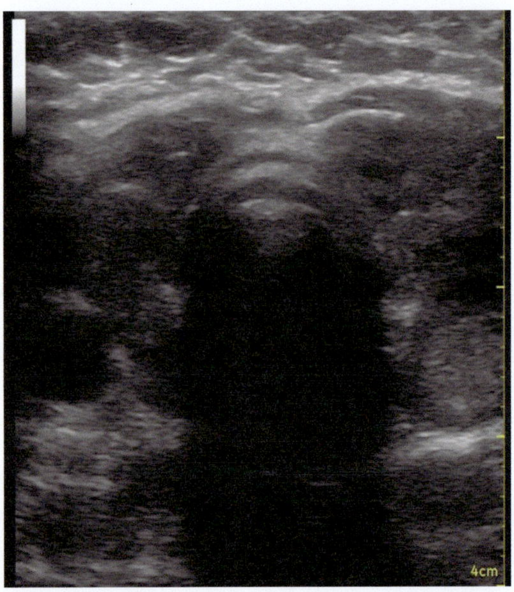

Fig. 33.3 Ultrasound appearance of Hashimoto's thyroiditis. This condition makes minimally invasive video-assisted and remote access thyroidectomy approaches challenging

Ultrasound is also particularly useful in evaluating for metastatic lymphadenopathy in the central and lateral neck in patients with known or suspected thyroid cancer. Suspicious lymph nodes can be biopsied using ultrasound guidance, and if metastatic disease is confirmed the incision can be adjusted as necessary to permit dissection of these nodal compartments at the time of the initial thyroid surgery.

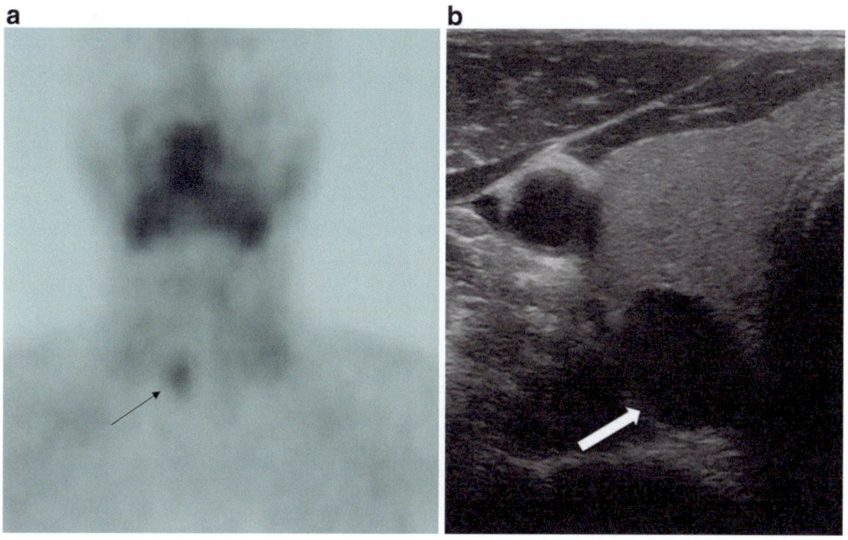

Fig. 33.4 Concordant sestamibi (**a**) and ultrasound (**b**) imaging showing a right inferior parathyroid adenoma (*arrow*), appropriate for minimally invasive parathyroid surgery

33.2.2 Parathyroid

Parathyroid surgery has historically necessitated a long cervical incision and bilateral neck exploration to evaluate all four parathyroid glands, even though the majority of cases of primary hyperparathyroidism are caused by a solitary adenoma. Advances in intraoperative parathyroid hormone (PTH) assessment and preoperative imaging techniques have rendered many patients with primary hyperparathyroidism eligible for minimally invasive, single gland surgery.

This image-directed approach relies largely on complementary information provided by technetium-99m (^{99m}Tc)-sestamibi (sestamibi) scanning and ultrasound (Fig. 33.4). If both the sestamibi and ultrasound co-localize an abnormal parathyroid gland in the same central neck quadrant, the operation may be performed through an inconspicuous 20 mm (or less) midline incision [15, 16]. As in thyroid surgery, this small incision is hidden in a preexisting neck crease to optimize the long-term cosmetic outcome of the procedure. Both sides of the neck are accessible through these small central incisions, so failure to localize the adenoma with preoperative ultrasound is not a contraindication to small incision surgery.

Alternatively, some authors prefer a laterally based incision for parathyroid surgery depending on the imaging results [17]. While this incision placement may offer a more direct approach for superior adenomas and avoid some of the central scar tissue when pursuing reoperative procedures, it sacrifices the cosmetic symmetry of a centrally placed incision, and requires a second incision if contralateral disease is suggested by intraoperative PTH assessment.

33.3 Ultrasound for Remote Access Approaches

Remote access thyroid surgery removes the incision from the visible portion of the anterior neck, concealing the scar in a distant, hidden location. These approaches generally access the thyroid compartment using axillary, chest, or postauricular incisions. While these procedures were initially performed using endoscopic assistance, the application of robotic surgical technology has increased their global popularity. The two most commonly performed robotic-assisted remote access thyroid operations are the robotic axillary thyroidectomy (RAT) and the robotic facelift thyroidectomy (RFT) (Fig. 33.5) [18, 19].

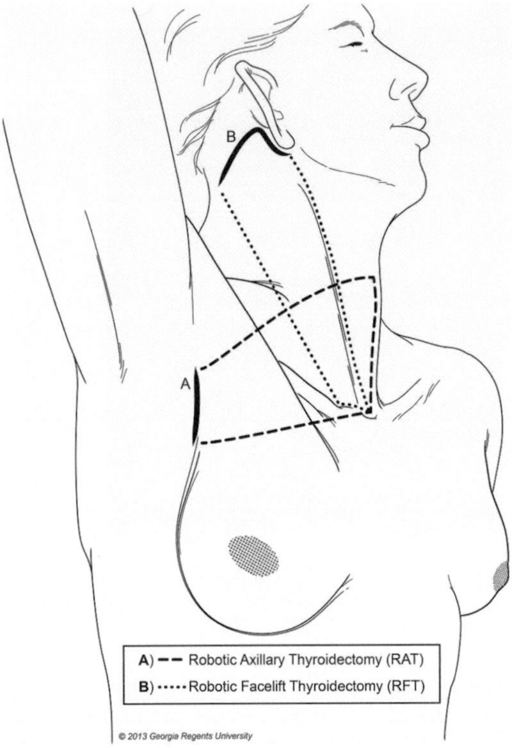

Fig. 33.5 Comparison of the incision location and approach for the robotic facelift thyroidectomy (RFT) and the robotic axillary thyroidectomy (RAT). Reproduced with permission from Duke WS, Terris DJ. Alternative approaches to the thyroid gland. *Endocrinol Metab Clin N Am*. 2014;43:459–474

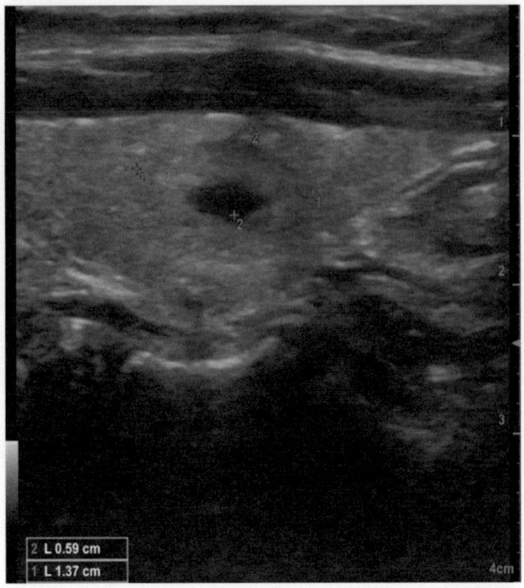

Fig. 33.6 The ideal nodules for remote access surgery are positioned within the midportion of the thyroid gland, as demonstrated in this longitudinal view

Ultrasound is critical in determining a patient's candidacy for remote access thyroid surgery. While there are no uniform selection criteria for RAT [20, 21], the procedure was initially reserved for patients with benign nodules ≤5 cm or malignant lesions ≤2 cm [18, 22]. RFT requirements are more firmly defined, recommending that nodules be <4 cm and presumed benign for consideration [23]. For both approaches, ultrasound findings of extrathyroidal, substernal, or retropharyngeal extension exclude patients from consideration [18, 23]. A history of or ultrasound findings consistent with Hashimoto's thyroiditis are also contraindications to remote access thyroid surgery [23], and RFT is not indicated in the setting of metastatic disease [23]. Total thyroidectomy through a single incision has been reported using RAT [24]. With RFT, bilateral thyroidectomy may be accomplished [25]; however, we prefer a staged bilateral procedure if the ultrasound shows bilateral disease.

The location of the nodule on ultrasound also influences the decision to perform remote access robotic-assisted thyroid surgery. An ideal nodule is located in the midportion of the lobe (Fig. 33.6). This allows the superior pole to be easily grasped to manipulate the gland, permits safe transection of the isthmus, and makes it easier to work around the inferior aspect of the lobe. Lesions located in the dorsal aspect of the gland may be challenging to dissect, particularly with the RAT approach [26]. These posterior nodules, especially in the setting of malignancy, may be associated with proximity to the recurrent laryngeal nerve, which may be adherent to or even focally invaded by the tumor.

33.4 Conclusion

Ultrasound provides critical anatomic information in patients undergoing thyroid and parathyroid surgery. The size and extent of the structural disease, findings suggestive of metastatic nodal disease, and the likelihood of Hashimoto's thyroiditis all influence the decision to offer patients small-incision, minimally invasive procedures or remote access surgery. Ultrasound is most beneficial for surgical planning when performed directly by the operating surgeon.

References

1. Khatri V, Asensio J. Thyroidectomy. In: Khatri V, Asensio J, et al., editors. Khatri: operative surgery manual. 1st ed. Philadelphia, PA: Saunders; 2003. p. 3–9.
2. Sturgeon C, Corvera C, Clark O. The missing thyroid. J Am Coll Surg. 2005;201(6):841–6.
3. Pinchot S, Chen H, Sippel R. Incisions and exposure of the neck for thyroidectomy and parathyroidectomy. Oper Tech Gen Surg. 2008;10(2):63–76.
4. Lai S, Mandel S, Weber R. Management of thyroid neoplasms. In: Flint PW, Haughey BH, Lund VJ, Niparko JK, Richardson MA, Robbins KT, Thomas JR, et al., editors. Flint: cummings otolaryngology: head & neck surgery. 5th ed. Philadelphia, PA: Mosby; 2010. p. 1750–72.
5. Smith P, Salomone L, Hanks J. Thyroid. In: Townsend CM, Beauchamp RD, Evers M, Mattox KL, et al., editors. Townsend: Sabiston textbook of surgery. 19th ed. Philadelphia, PA: Elsevier Saunders; 2012. p. 886–923.
6. Gil Z, Fliss DM. Hemi and total thyroidectomy. In: Gil Z, Fliss DN, et al., editors. Atlas of head and neck surgery. New Delhi: Jaypee Brothers Medical Publishers; 2013. p. 332–44.
7. Sinha P, Inabnet WB. Cancer of the thyroid. In: Matteotti R, Ashley SW, et al., editors. Minimally invasive surgical oncology: state-of-the-art cancer management. Heidelberg: Springer Science & Business Media; 2011. p. 331–54.
8. Kim JH, Sung JY, Kim YH, et al. Risk factors for hypertrophic surgical scar development after thyroidectomy. Wound Repair Regen. 2012;20(3):304–10.
9. Duke WS, Bush CM, Singer MC, et al. Incision planning in thyroid compartment surgery: getting it perfect. Endocr Pract. 2015;21(2):107–14.
10. Daly AP, Romanelli-Gobbi M, Miller JL, et al. Using ultrasonic preoperative thyroid volume to determine incision length for minimally invasive thyroid surgery. Ear Nose Throat J. 2015;94(8):346–52.
11. Coltrera MD. Clinician-performed thyroid ultrasound. Otolaryngol Clin North Am. 2014;47(4):491–507.
12. Miccoli P, Berti P, Raffaelli M, et al. Minimally invasive video-assisted thyroidectomy. Am J Surg. 2001;181(6):567–70.
13. Miccoli P, Berti P, Raffaelli M. Comparison between minimally invasive video-assisted thyroidectomy and conventional thyroidectomy: a prospective randomized study. Surgery. 2001;130:1039–43.
14. Miccoli P, Berti P, Materazzi G, Minuto M, Barellini L. Minimally invasive video-assisted thyroidectomy: five years of experience. J Am Coll Surg. 2004;199:243–8.
15. Barczyński M, Cichoń S, Konturek A, Cichoń W. Minimally invasive video-assisted parathyroidectomy versus open minimally invasive parathyroidectomy for a solitary parathyroid adenoma: a prospective, randomized, blinded trial. World J Surg. 2006;30(5):721–31.
16. Miccoli P, Berti P, Materazzi G, et al. Endoscopic bilateral neck exploration versus quick intraoperative parathormone assay (qPTHa) during endoscopic parathyroidectomy: a prospective randomized trial. Surg Endosc. 2008;22(2):398–400.
17. Shindo ML, Rosenthal JM. Minimal access parathyroidectomy using the focused lateral approach: technique, indication, and results. Arch Otolaryngol Head Neck Surg. 2007;133(12):1227–34.
18. Kang SW, Lee SC, Lee SH, et al. Robotic thyroid surgery using a gasless, transaxillary approach and the da Vinci S system: the operative outcomes of 338 consecutive patients. Surgery. 2009;146: 1048–55.
19. Terris DJ, Singer MC, Seybt MW. Robot facelift thyroidectomy: II. Clinical feasibility and safety. Laryngoscope. 2011;121:1636–41.
20. Kuppersmith R, Holsinger F. Robotic thyroid surgery: an initial experience with North American patients. Laryngoscope. 2011;121:521–6.
21. Lin H, Folbe A, Carron M, et al. Single-incision transaxillary robotic thyroidectomy: challenges and limitations in a North American population. Otolaryngol Head Neck Surg. 2012;147(6):1041–6.
22. Kang SW, Jeong JJ, Yun JS, et al. Robot-assisted endoscopic surgery for thyroid cancer: experience with the first 100 patients. Surg Endosc. 2009;23:2399–406.
23. Terris D, Singer MC, Seybt MW. Robotic facelift thyroidectomy: patient selection and technical considerations. Surg Laparosc Percutan Tech. 2011;21(4):237–42.
24. Ryu HR, Kang SW, Lee SH. Feasibility and safety of a new robotic thyroidectomy through a gasless, transaxillary single-incision approach. J Am Coll Surg. 2010;211(3):e13–9.
25. Byeon HK, Holsinger FC, Tufano RT. Robotic total thyroidectomy with modified radical neck dissection via unilateral retroauricular approach. Ann Surg Oncol. 2014;21:3872–5.
26. Kang SW, Jeong JJ, Nam KH, et al. Robot-assisted endoscopic thyroidectomy for thyroid malignancies using a gasless transaxillary approach. J Am Coll Surg. 2009;209:e1–7.

Intraoperative Use of Ultrasound in Thyroid, Parathyroid, and Cervical Lymph Node Surgery

34

Vikram D. Krishnamurthy, Eren Berber, and Joyce J. Shin

34.1 Introduction

In the operating room surgeons have greatest access to their armamentarium, including ultrasonography. Intraoperative ultrasound (IOUS) has proven to be useful for localization, planning extent of surgery, and analyzing completeness of intervention in procedures including hepatectomy, ablation of metastatic neuroendocrine tumors to the liver, pancreatic resections, and laparoscopic adrenalectomy [1–4]. Surgeons can use this technology in a similar fashion during thyroid, parathyroid, and cervical lymph node operations. Using ultrasound requires a baseline proficiency to optimize its full potential during an operation. The ultrasound should be performed after the patient has been administered anesthetics and the neck is gently hyperextended (Fig. 34.1). This exposes the neck contents and allows for gentle pressure with the probe, potentially providing more information than the ultrasound in the office setting. This chapter provides examples and suggestions for how ultrasound can be implemented in both an extracorporeal and intracorporeal capacity during operations for the thyroid, the parathyroid glands, and lymph nodes.

V.D. Krishnamurthy, M.D. (✉) • E. Berber, M.D.
J.J. Shin, M.D., F.A.C.S.
Department of Endocrine Surgery, The Cleveland Clinic, 9500 Euclid Ave, F20, Cleveland, OH 44195, USA
e-mail: krishnv3@ccf.org; berbere@ccf.org; shinj2@ccf.org

34.2 Thyroid

Surgeons often review cervical ultrasonography results, whether performed by the surgeon themselves or by another provider, prior to an operation. However, useful information can be obtained when the surgeon repeats the ultrasound in the operating room for several reasons. The surgeon can re-familiarize herself or himself with the unique anatomy of the patient's gland including size, location of the poles and isthmus, and involvement of adjacent structures such as the trachea, esophagus, or strap muscles. In addition, the surgeon can assess the gland's firmness and vascularity, which is helpful when operating on patients with Graves' disease or Hashimoto's thyroiditis. Moreover, ultrasound has high sensitivity for identifying vascular anomalies associated with a nonrecurrent laryngeal nerve, such as an aberrant right subclavian artery [5]. Re-familiarization with the anatomy is useful for shaping intraoperative expectations and tailoring the operative approach.

Furthermore, the surgeon may detect new findings when repeating the ultrasound in the operating room. With the patient's neck

M. Milas et al. (eds.), *Advanced Thyroid and Parathyroid Ultrasound*,
DOI 10.1007/978-3-319-44100-9_34

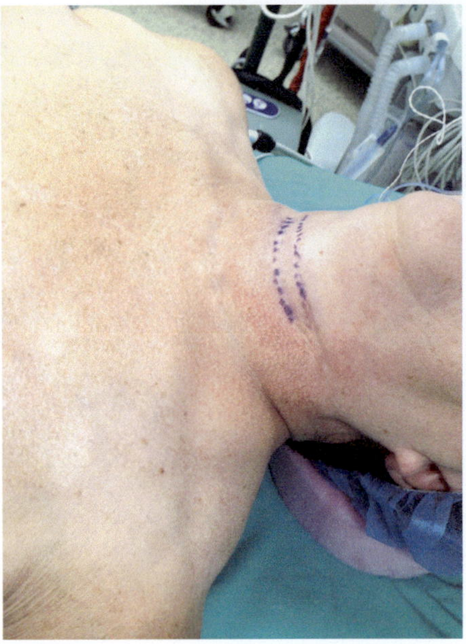

Fig. 34.1 Positioning: The neck hyperextended after potential sites for the incision were mapped in the preoperative holding area

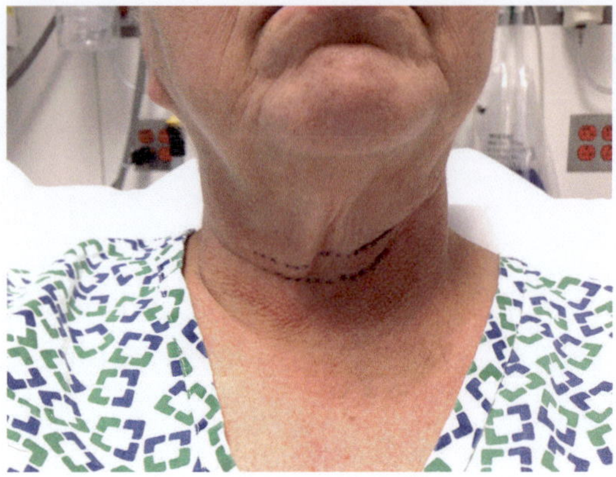

Fig. 34.2 Incisional mapping: The patient's natural skin creases are marked in the preoperative holding area

hyperextended, the central neck is better visualized, enhancing the detection of enlarged lymph nodes. Additionally, if there has been a significant time interval between the preoperative ultrasound to the operation or if there is particularly aggressive malignant behavior, the ultrasound may demonstrate advancement of disease. Lastly, the ultrasound findings can influence where and how large to make the incision. Ideally, the incision is centered over the gland and/or isthmus, is appropriately sized to access all poles, and is placed in a natural skin crease. The surgeon can mark all natural skin creases in the preoperative holding area with the patient sitting upright and awake (Fig. 34.2), and once the patient is under anesthesia and the neck is extended, the ultrasound is used to identify which crease will be most favorable given the patient's unique gland anatomy (Fig. 34.3).

34.3 Parathyroid

Surgeon-performed ultrasound is a highly sensitive preoperative localization study for patients with primary hyperparathyroidism [6]. Occasionally, repeating the ultrasound in the operating room after the patient has been optimally positioned can identify parathyroid adenomas that were not visible in the office (Fig. 34.4). The necessary amount of pressure with the transducer can be obtained because the patient has received anesthetics. Applying pressure with the transducer on the neck can distinguish the relationship of parathyroid adenomas to the thyroid, elucidating the likely embryologic origin of the gland and producing real-time information to target the dissection. Similar to IOUS of the thyroid, repeating the exam can re-familiarize the surgeon with the patient's unique anatomy to identifying the relationship of enlarged parathyroid adenomas to the thyroid gland, tubercle of Zuckerkandl, vasculature, thymus, and sternothyroid muscle. In the event that no abnormal parathyroid gland is found during exploration, IOUS can be performed to scrutinize the remainder of the neck, especially regions historically known to harbor ectopic glands. For example, IOUS can reidentify thyroid nodules and their laterality, prompting the consideration of an intrathyroidal parathyroid adenoma if the intraoperative findings warrant this possibility (Fig. 34.5).

Perhaps the most valuable use of IOUS for parathyroid operations is in setting of a previous neck operation, referred to as reoperative parathyroidectomy. Reoperative parathyroidectomy is a challenging clinical scenario, and many surgeons require more than one preoperative localizing study to plan parathyroidectomy.

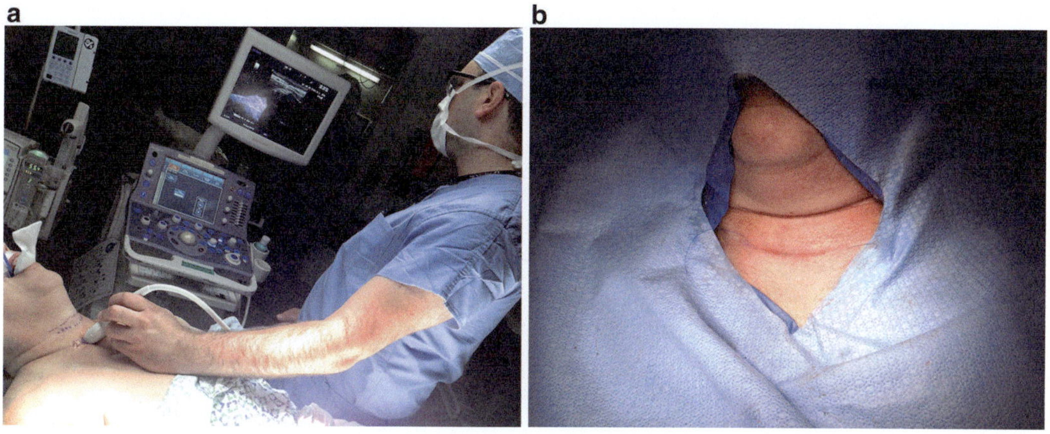

Fig. 34.3 Individualized incision-making: (**a**) The choice of incision location is influenced by intraoperative ultrasound, which reveals each patient's unique anatomy. The incision that grants adequate access and also enhances the cosmetic result is used. (**b**) The appearance of the incision after closure

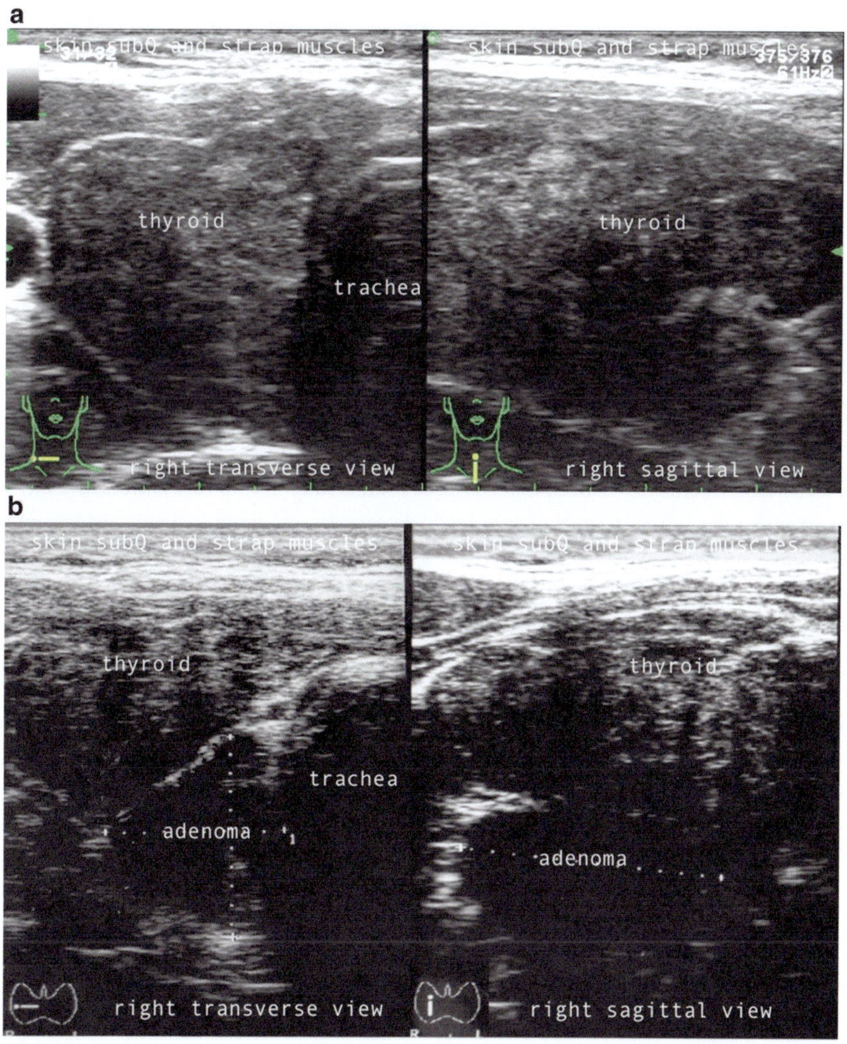

Fig. 34.4 Parathyroid adenoma identified on intraoperative ultrasound: (**a**) During ultrasound in the office setting, no parathyroid adenomas were identified in the neck. The subsequent nuclear medicine imaging (not shown) was also negative. (**b**) In the operating room, the patient received anesthetics and the neck was hyperextended. After gentle pressure with the transducer, a parathyroid adenoma was identified posterior to the right thyroid lobe

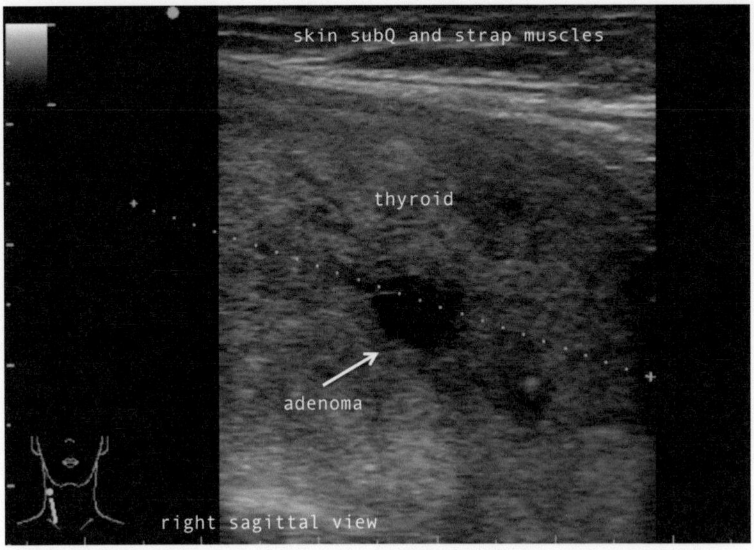

Fig. 34.5 Intrathyroidal parathyroid adenoma: During parathyroid exploration, the operative findings and intraoperative PTH levels indicated persistent disease. A hypoechoic lesion in the right thyroid lobe was identified during ultrasound. A right thyroid lobectomy was performed, which resulted in an appropriate decline of the intraoperative PTH level. Frozen section examination and final pathology confirmed intrathyroidal parathyroid adenoma

Cervical ultrasound is 55–69 % successful in identifying the offensive gland in patients with persistent or recurrent disease [7, 8]. If the patient's offending gland was identified on preoperative ultrasound, repeating the ultrasound in the operating room can facilitate targeted dissection in the scarred, reoperative field.

Similar to thyroid operations, IOUS can influence where to make the incision during parathyroid explorations. Surgeons who plan to perform a focal (single-gland) parathyroid exploration can use IOUS to guide placement of the incision [9]. Surgeons who plan to perform a comprehensive (four-gland) parathyroid exploration can use IOUS to make an incision that is centered over the thyroid or equidistant from the suspected location of all four parathyroid glands. For both operative approaches, ultrasound helps minimize the size of the incision.

34.4 Lymph Nodes

Preoperative lymph node mapping by ultrasound is recommended for all patients undergoing thyroidectomy for suspected malignant disease, especially to identify suspicious lateral neck lymph nodes [10]. Suspicious lateral neck lymph nodes should undergo preoperative biopsy, as the results will affect the extent of surgery (i.e., concurrent total thyroidectomy and lateral neck dissection). IOUS can enhance the completeness of lateral neck dissections by detecting additional nodes that were missed by visual inspection or palpation, specifically in levels II, IV, and V [11]. Additionally, suspicious central neck lymph nodes that were not seen in the office might now be identified on IOUS after the patient's neck is hyperextended. These nodes should then be addressed during thyroidectomy.

Ultrasonographic surveillance following thyroid cancer treatment is performed to identify non-palpable persistent or recurrent structural disease. If persistent/recurrent thyroid cancer is detected and large enough to be removed, repeating the ultrasound in the operating room greatly enhances the correct identification of the structural target within the scarred field [12]. Many series have described how IOUS (by itself or in combination with injections of methylene blue dye, charcoal, a localizing wire, or a radiotracer) facilitated successful resection of structural targets [13–16].

Intraoperative ultrasound is also helpful for incision planning in neck dissections. IOUS helps reveal the location and amount of disease burden, which can influence the location and size of the incision. In select cases, counter-incisions can made for high-level nodal disease (e.g., bulky level II nodes in a patient with a long neck) to minimize the size of the primary cervical incision.

34.5 Conclusions

IOUS provides many advantages in thyroid, parathyroid, and lymph nodes operations. A more complete ultrasound can be obtained when the patient's neck is optimally extended. IOUS facilitates incision planning, shapes intraoperative expectations, and improves operative success, especially in reoperations.

References

1. Jrearz R, Hart R, Jayaraman S. IOUS and surgical strategy in hepatic resection: what difference does it make? Can J Surg. 2015;58(5):318–22.
2. Mitchell J, Berber E, Siperstein A. Laparoscopic radiofrequency ablation of metastatic neuroendocrine tumors in the liver. In: Endocrine surgery: principles and practice. New York, NY: Springer; 2009.
3. Jaroszewski DE, Schlinkert RT, Thompson GB, Schlinkert DK. Laparoscopic localization and resection of insulinomas. Ann Surg. 2004;139(3):270–4.
4. Pautler SE, Choyke PL, Pavlovich CP, Daryanani K, Walther MM. IOUS aids in dissection during laparoscopic partial adrenalectomy. J Urol. 2002;168(4):1352–5.
5. Iacobone M, Citton M, Pagura G, Viel G, Nitti D. Increased and safer detection of nonrecurrent inferior laryngeal nerve after preoperative ultrasonography. Laryngoscope. 2015;125(7):1743–7.
6. Aliyev S, Agcaoglu O, Aksoy E, Birsen O, Milas M, Mitchell J, Siperstein A, Berber E. An analysis of whether surgeon-performed neck ultrasound can be used as the main localizing study in primary hyperparathyroidism. Surgery. 2014;156(5): 1127–31.
7. Parikh PPM, Farra JC, Allan BJ, Lew JI. Long-term effectiveness of localization studies and intraoperative parathormone monitoring in patients undergoing reoperative parathyroidectomy for persistent or recurrent hyperparathyroidism. Am J Surg. 2005;210(1):117–22.
8. Shin JJ, Milas M, Mitchell J, Berber E, Ross L, Siperstein A. Impact of localization studies and clinical scenario in patients with hyperparathyroidism being evaluated for reoperative neck surgery. Arch Surg. 2011;146(12):1397–403.
9. Soon PS, Delbridge LW, Sywak MS, Barraclough BM, Edhouse P, Sidhu SB. Surgeon performed ultrasound facilitates minimally invasive parathyroidectomy by the focused lateral mini-incision approach. World J Surg. 2008;32(5):766–71.
10. Haugen BR, Alexander EK, Bible KC, Doherty GM, Mandel SJ, Nikiforov YE, PAcini F, Randolph GW, Sawka AM, Schlumberger M, Schuff KG, Sherman SI, Sosa JA, Steward DL, Tuttle RM, Wartofsky L. American Thyroid Association management guidelines for adult patients with thyroid nodules and differentiated thyroid cancer. Thyroid. 2015;26:1.
11. Agcaoglu O, Aliyev S, Taskin HE, Aksoy E, Siperstein A, Berber E. The utility of IOUS in modified radical neck dissection: a pilot study. Surg Innov. 2014;21(2):166–9.
12. McCoy KL, Yim JH, Tublin ME, Burmeister LA, Ogilvie JB, McCarty SE. Same-day ultrasound guidance in reoperation for locally recurrent thyroid cancer. Surgery. 2007;142:965–72.
13. Harari A, Sippel RS, Goldstein R, Aziz S, Shen W, Gosnell J, Duh QY, Clark OH. Successful localization of recurrent thyroid cancer in reoperative neck surgery using ultrasound-guided methylene blue dye injection. J Am Coll Surg. 2012;215(4):555–61.
14. Chami L, Hartl D, Leboulleux S, Baudin E, Lumbroso J, Schlumberger M, Travagli JP. Preoperative localization of neck recurrences from thyroid cancer: charcoal tattooing under ultrasound guidance. Thyroid. 2015;25(3):341–6.
15. Triponez F, Poder L, Zarnegar R, Goldstein R, Roayie K, Feldstein V, Lee J, Kebebew E, Duh QY, Clark OH. Hook needle-guided excision of recurrent differentiated thyroid cancer in previously neck compartments: a safe technique for small, nonpalpable recurrent disease. J Clin Endocrinol Metab. 2006;91:4943–7.
16. Giles YS, Sarici IS, Tunca F, Sormaz IC, Salmashoglu A, Adalet I, Ozgur I, Tezelman S, Terzioglu T. The rate of operative success achieved with radioguided occult lesion localization and intraoperative ultrasonography in patients with recurrent papillary thyroid cancer. Surgery. 2014;156:1116–26.

Alcohol Ablation of Thyroid and Parathyroid Lesions and Lymph Nodes

35

Petros Tsamatropoulos and Andrea Frasoldati

35.1 Background/Introduction

Alcohol ablation is an image-guided, chemical ablation technique used to treat benign and malignant tumors [1–4]. Other terms for alcohol ablation are percutaneous ethanol injection (PEI) and ethanol ablation (EA), the latter being recommended by the Society of Interventional Radiology [5]. Cell dehydration and protein denaturation, resulting in coagulative necrosis and fibrotic changes, are the immediate toxic effect induced by instillation of ethanol into the target tissue. Furthermore, small vessel thrombosis due to endothelial cell necrosis severely impairs microcirculation with secondary ischemic damage [6]. At a histological level, hemorrhagic infarcts and reactive fibrosis are the most common changes reported after tissue exposure to ethanol [7, 8].

This chapter mainly focuses on EA application to treat thyroid cysts and nodules. The initial reports of ethanol injection into thyroid lesions dealt with sclerotherapy of thyroid cysts [9], and subsequently, this technique gained worldwide attention as an alternative tool to surgery and radioiodine in the treatment of "toxic" and "pre-toxic" nodules [10–13]. However, while the use of EA for autonomous functioning nodules (AFTNs) in the last 10–15 years has progressively declined, EA has established its position as first-line treatment for thyroid cysts [14, 15]. The role of EA in the treatment of other neck lesions, such as hyperfunctioning parathyroid glands, and metastatic lymph nodes, is also briefly addressed.

35.2 Alcohol Ablation of Thyroid Cystic Lesions

35.2.1 US-Guided Percutaneous Alcohol Injection: The Technique (See Also Video 35.1)

The patient is required to lie in a supine position, with a pillow under the shoulders to facilitate the hyperextension of the neck. A pair of glasses is useful to prevent any accidental contact of ethanol with the patient's eyes, while protection from external contamination is provided by the following simple, yet important, measures: (a) accurate disinfection of the neck skin; (b) placement of a sterile blanket over the patient's chest; (c) regular use of sterile devices (e.g., probe cover, ultrasound

Electronic supplementary material: The online version of this chapter (doi:10.1007/978-3-319-44100-9_35) contains supplementary material, which is available to authorized users. Videos can also be accessed at http://link.springer.com/chapter/10.1007/978-3-319-44100-9_35.

P. Tsamatropoulos, M.D. • A. Frasoldati, M.D. (✉)
Endocrine Unit, Arcispedale Santa Maria Nuova - Research Hospital (IRCCS) for Advanced Technologies and Clinical Pathways in Oncology, Viale Risorgimento, 80, Reggio Emilia 42123, Italy
e-mail: ptsamatropoulos@gmail.com; andrea.frasoldati@asmn.re.it

M. Milas et al. (eds.), *Advanced Thyroid and Parathyroid Ultrasound*, DOI 10.1007/978-3-319-44100-9_35

(US) gel and gloves). Local anesthesia is not routinely necessary. Nevertheless, it may be beneficial in selected cases to diminish local discomfort, especially when using larger (e.g., 16–18 gauge) needles. The EA procedure on thyroid cysts is performed on four stages: (a) needle insertion; (b) drainage of the fluid content of the cyst; (c) ethanol instillation into the cyst cavity; (d) needle extraction. The entire procedure, from needle insertion down to needle extraction, must be performed rigorously under US guidance (Fig. 35.1).

35.2.1.1 Needle Insertion

The needle may be either introduced through a guiding device connected to the US transducer (Fig. 35.1b), or alternatively, inserted free-hand

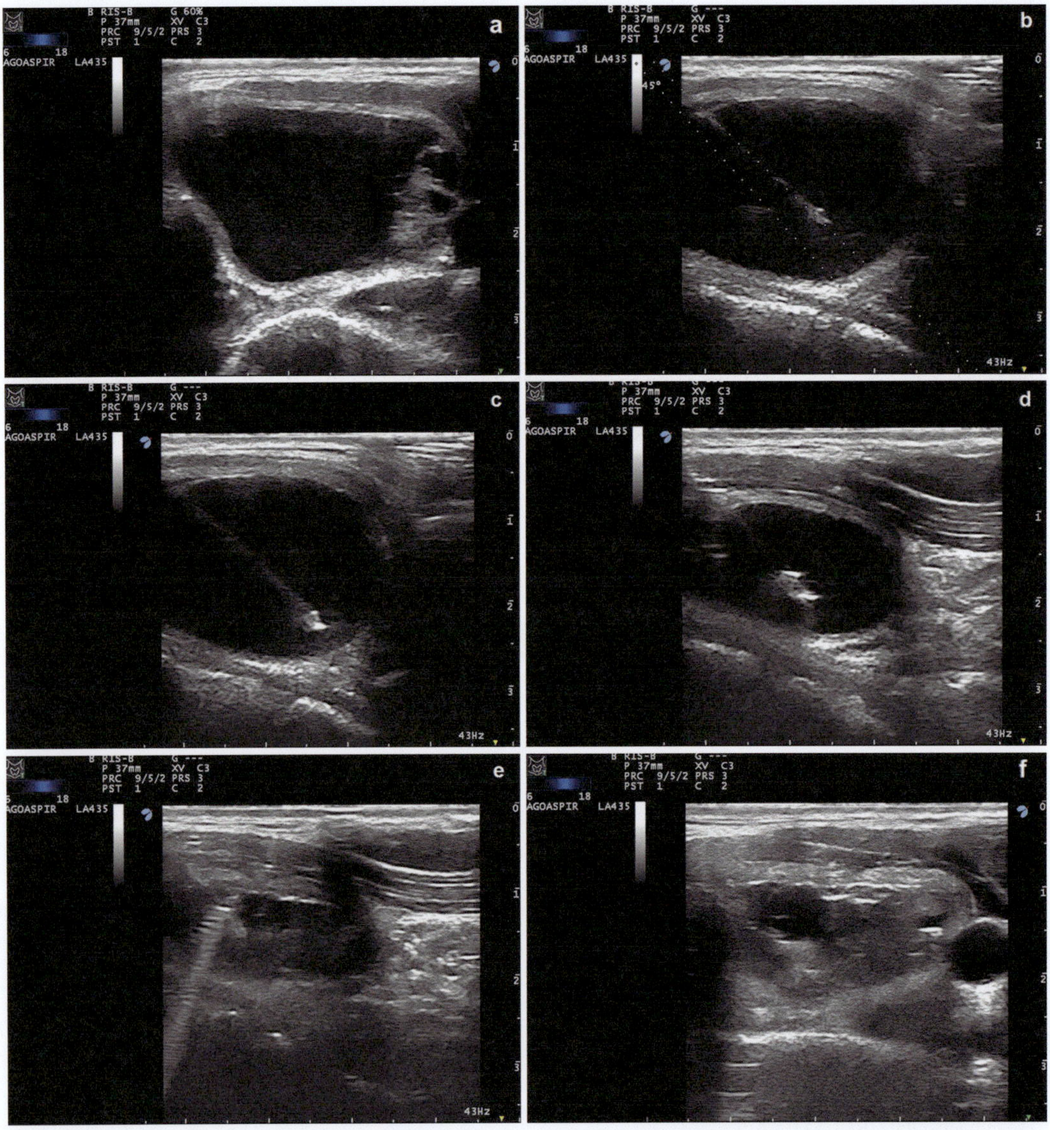

Fig. 35.1 US-guided ethanol ablation of a thyroid cyst. Basal US image of a left lobe thyroid cyst (B-mode, transverse view) (**a**). Needle insertion into the cyst using a needle track (**b**). Once the needle has been inserted, the needle track is removed from the screen image (**c**). Aspiration of fluid content of the cyst—the cyst shrinks—(**d**). Ethanol instillation—ethanol is visible as hyperechoic material—(**e**). The so called "mirror image" artifact of the needle can be observed. The thyroid cyst at the end of the procedure (**f**)

and cautiously directed into the lesion with continuous US imaging and probe adjustment to maintain the needle in the field of view (Fig. 35.1c). Neither approach is superior to the other in terms of results: however, the free-hand procedure is more widespread and offers the convenience of repositioning the needle along a wider range of spatial axes throughout the maneuver, a valuable option when treating large and complex cysts.

35.2.1.2 Drainage of the Fluid Content

After extraction of the needle stylet, a 20 ml syringe is connected to the needle for fluid drainage and collection. The use of two devices may quite effectively facilitate this phase: a syringe holder (e.g., the Cameco pistol) and a catheter (20–25 cm length) connecting the needle and the syringe. Both devices contribute to facilitating drainage of the fluid content, as well as the subsequent alcohol instillation; at the same time, the connecting tube prevents the transmission of abrupt traction and strain movements to the needle (Fig. 35.2). This is particularly relevant if we consider that the change of shape and size of the cyst during fluid drainage may result in needle tip mispositioning that requires correction by the operator. The aspiration of the cystic fluid should be slow, smooth and constant in order to minimize the risk of ex-vacuum hemorrhaging. Obviously, large cysts may require the use of more than 1–2 syringes. All the materials likely to be needed for each procedure should be readily available.

35.2.1.3 Ethanol Instillation

The 95 % sterile ethanol, usually contained in 10 ml syringes, is cautiously injected into the cyst. Other sclerosing agents that have been proposed for thyroid cysts are polydecanol [16], arginine hydrochloride [17], and sodium tetradecyl sulfate [18]; however none of these substances has proved to be superior to alcohol. During instillation, ethanol is usually visualized on US as a hyperechoic dense material that refills the anechoic empty chamber of the cyst. Since the needle may get occluded either during the fluid aspiration or the ethanol instillation phases, effective reaming may be achieved by repeatedly passing a stylet through the needle. In most instances, the volume of the ethanol injected corresponds to 50–70 % of the fluid volume drained from the cyst. However, the "right" ethanol amount should be chosen on individual basis, considering a number of factors: (a) the pattern of

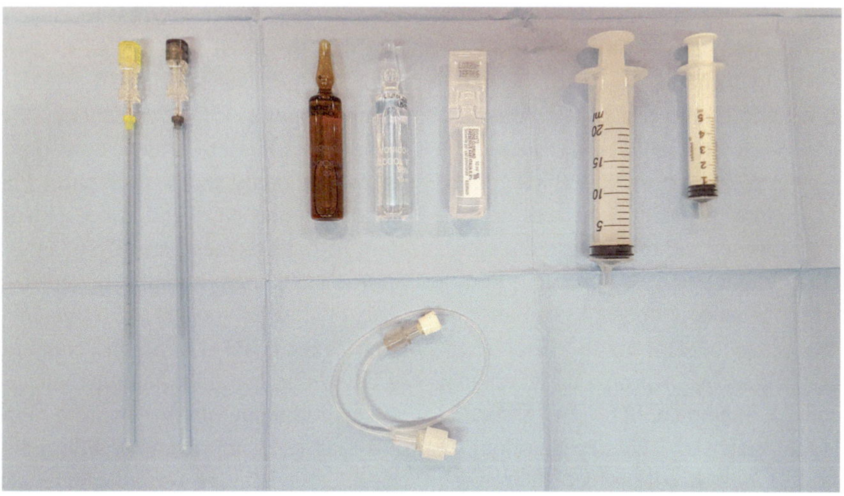

Fig. 35.2 Equipment for the ethanol ablation of a thyroid cyst (from the *left*): a 20- or a 22-gauge spinal needle with stylet; 2 % lidocaine for local anesthesia (seldom necessary); 95 % sterile alcohol; saline solution for washing the needle at the end of the procedure; a 20 mL syringe for alcohol injection; a 5 mL syringe for the administration of lidocaine in case of local anesthesia; a flexible extension tube (*bottom*) for connecting the hub of the needle to the tip of syringe

ethanol diffusion, (b) the degree of resistance applied to the tubing connection and the syringe, and (c) the subjective feedback from the patient. If the patient signals the sudden onset of intense pain or if there is resistance during ethanol injection, the administration of alcohol must be discontinued, and the position of the needle tip carefully checked.

After alcohol instillation, two alternative strategies have been used: (a) completely evacuate ethanol a short-time (3–10 min) after its instillation; (b) leave the cyst refilled with ethanol in order to prolong its sclerotic effect. Although the results obtained with these two modalities are similar [19] the latter strategy is probably preferred by most operators because is less cumbersome. Theoretically, the rationale for aspirating the ethanol-mixed fluid is to minimize the risk of ethanol leakage outside of the cyst into the surrounding tissue, an event that may lead to paraglandular fibrosis. Furthermore, there is a possible risk of post-surgical hypoparathyroidism and/or laryngeal nerve palsy in those patients previously submitted to PEI who are candidates for thyroid surgery [20].

35.2.1.4 Needle Extraction

At the end of the procedure, the needle is washed with saline solution to avoid minimal ethanol leakage to subcutaneous tissues and subsequent transient pain. Then, the needle is rapidly extracted. Firm compression and use of an ice pack for 5–10 min minimize bleeding. When the fluid is more viscous, the use of a larger bore needles (e.g., 18-gauge) should be considered for the drainage. For thyroid cysts with thick colloid material that cannot be easily aspirated, various authors have proposed modified EA techniques. The first strategy is a two-step approach: first, a small amount of ethanol is injected in an attempt to make the dense content more fluid. Then, 2–4 weeks later, a second aspiration with ethanol injection can be attempted [21, 22]. A second approach is the drainage of the dense colloid by means of a 16-gauge needle which is inserted into the nodule through a trans-isthmic approach and connected to a suction pump with a vacuum of 10–100 mmHg. If the content of the nodule cannot be aspirated, the 16-gauge needle is exchanged for an 8.5-French pigtail catheter. After more than 90 % of the viscous cystic content is aspirated, 99 % sterile ethanol is injected through the same needle or catheter. The amount of injected ethanol corresponds to 50 % of the aspirated fluid. After 10 min with the needle or catheter in place, the injected ethanol is removed completely [23]. This one-step EA method for viscous thyroid cysts is reported to produce volume reductions at 1 and 6 months of 78.4 % ± 14.4 % and 93.6 % ± 6.8 % respectively. Recently, a third option for the treatment of viscous cysts has been proposed utilizing a newly developed open-window needle that could efficiently aspirate dense gelatinous material from thyroid cysts [24].

35.2.2 Clinical Outcomes

A recently published Cochrane review concluded that, EA for cystic thyroid nodules results in a significant volume decrease, defined as a ≥50 % reduction, and improves pressure symptoms and cosmetic complaints with the only drawback of light pain after the procedure [25]. EA is considered the first-line treatment for thyroid cystic lesions [14, 15]. "Pure" thyroid cysts are exceedingly rare (<1 % of all thyroid nodules), and the majority of cystic thyroid lesions, about the 25–30 % of all thyroid nodules, correspond to mixed cystic solid lesions [26, 27] composed of an inhomogeneous fluid content of colloid, blood, and cell debris. Hemorrhagic cysts typically present as a suddenly visible neck lump which causes tenderness and pain, and is occasionally associated with hoarseness and dysphagia. Although these lesions may completely recede spontaneously or after fine-needle aspiration, they are quite likely to recur [28–31]. Studies comparing results of EA to simple fluid aspiration indicate that ethanol sclerotherapy offers a twofold higher chance of a long-term improvement with a 83 and 44 % of subjects achieving a significant reduction of the lesion volume after EA and aspiration alone, respectively [25, 32, 33]. Most studies report a low (<15–20 %) recurrence rate of thyroid cysts after ethanol sclerotherapy and recurrence rates of

3.4 % and 6.5 % at 5 years and 10 years, respectively [34, 35].

Interestingly, in spite of technical variations of the EA procedure, the results obtained across different studies report similar success rates, ranging from about 70 to 95 %, with a mean volume decrease between 65 and 90 % (Figs. 35.3 and 35.4) [32–37]. Resolution of local symptoms and cosmetic complains occurs in about 75–95 % of patients submitted to EA, although the quantification of symptom reduction is limited by the absence of standardized measurement tools. In a recent study, subjective symptoms were rated on a 10-cm visual analog scale [38]. Ethanol sclerotherapy was associated with a significant reduction of both symptom and cosmetic scores from 3.92 ± 1.54 to 0.39 ± 0.69 and from 3.31 ± 0.90 to 1.17 ± 0.56, respectively [38].

In another recently published series, a non-validated questionnaire including ten items related to goiter symptoms (visible enlargement, pressure in the neck, pain, difficulty in swallowing, shortness of breath and hoarseness, etc.) was created. Severity of each symptom was scored between 1 and 5 and a total score was calculated. EA reduced symptoms score from 22 ± 8 to 13 ± 5 ($p<0.05$) [39].

The efficacy of EA depends on a number of factors, e.g., the initial volume of the lesion, the amount of ethanol instilled, the proportion of the solid component of the mixed cystic solid lesion. The efficacy of EA in exceedingly large (e.g., >40–50 ml) cysts has long been debated [32, 40] but a negative prognostic role of a higher initial cystic volume on the final outcome has not yet been clearly demonstrated [20, 41, 42]. The type of the nodule structure is a more likely determinant of the final result. While EA is commonly used for treating “pure” cystic thyroid nodules (liquid component >90 %) as well as “mixed” nodules with a predominant (50–90 %) fluid component, the latter ones usually achieve a maximum

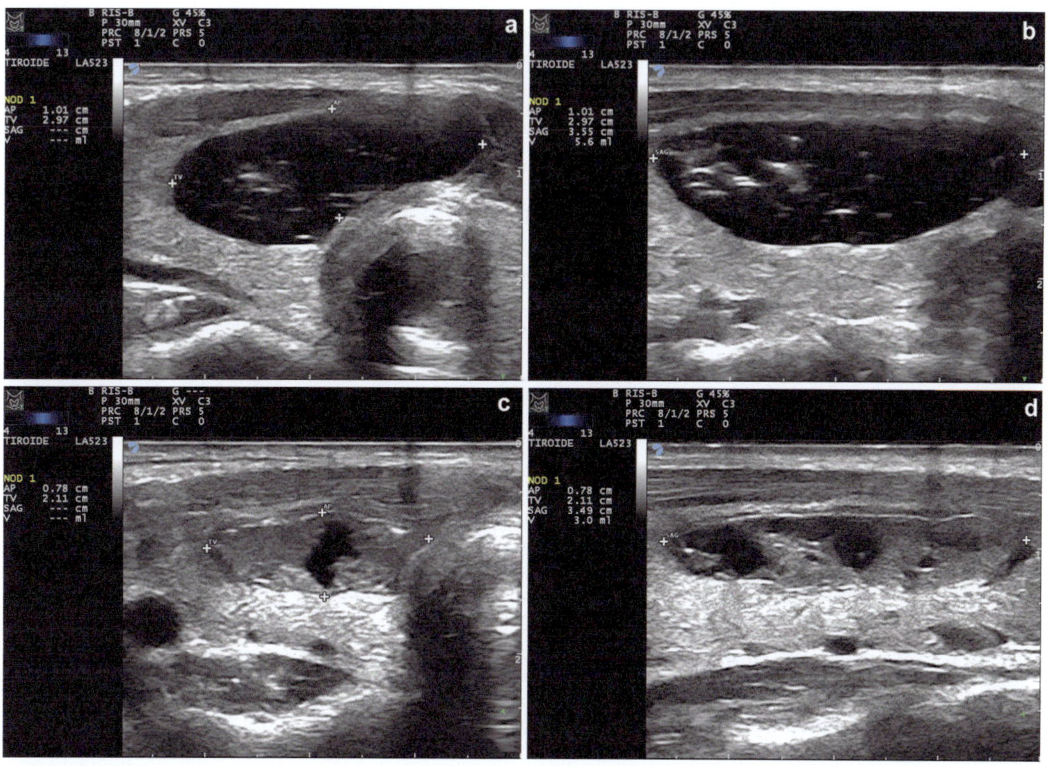

Fig. 35.3 A 6 mL right thyroid cyst before (**a** transverse view, **b** longitudinal view) and 2 weeks after (**c** transverse view, **d** longitudinal view) ethanol ablation. The thyroid cyst shrunk to 3 mL (50 % volume reduction)

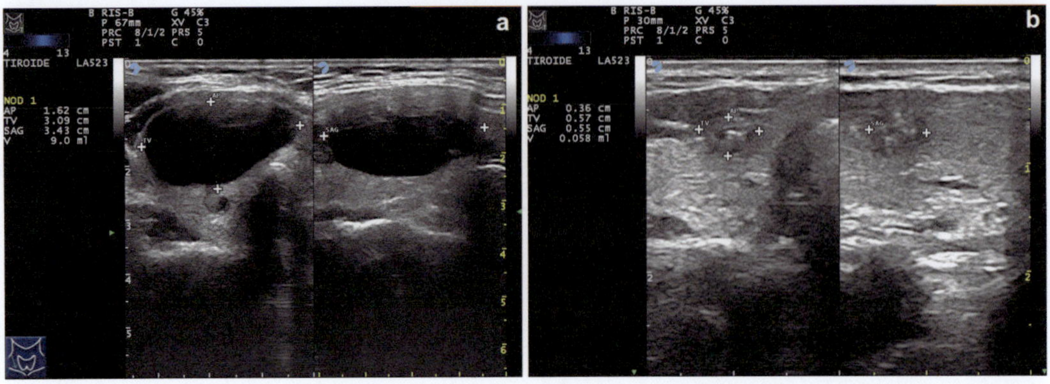

Fig. 35.4 Cystic thyroid nodule before (**a**) and 18 months after PEI (**b**). The thyroid cyst volume has been reduced from 9 to 0.06 mL (99.3 % volume reduction) with disappearance of patient's compressive and aesthetic problems

volume reduction of 60–65 %, less than the 90–95 % reduction achieved with "pure" cysts [43–48]. In "pure" cysts and in mixed nodules that are predominantly cystic, the final outcome is correlated to the volume of the fluid extracted, and to the amount of the instilled ethanol [20, 36]. Another, less predictable, obstacle to a successful PEI procedure is the finding of a viscous and dense cystic content [20, 36, 38]. A recent study based on 62 patients indicates that complete aspiration of the cystic content is the most important factor for achieving a successful EA in benign cystic thyroid nodules, as incomplete aspiration may significantly reduce the concentration of the injected ethanol [45]. Ethanol sclerotherapy has also been adapted, with encouraging results, to the treatment of thyroglossal duct cysts (TDC), a congenital neck abnormality deriving from the embryonic thyroglossal duct structures, located along the midline, between the hyoid bone and the thyroid gland [49–53].

35.2.3 Side Effects

EA of thyroid cystic lesions is a safe procedure and no relevant side effects are usually recorded [25]; nevertheless, because of the potential risk of recurrent laryngeal nerve (RLN) injury, vigilance with needle tip visualization is always required throughout the procedure. Ethanol injection into the cystic cavity is not likely to cause any major increase of pressure within the lesion and the integrity of the fibrous capsule surrounding the cyst should be fully preserved, thus preventing ethanol leakage into the perinodular tissues. As mentioned in the paragraph describing EA technique, the sudden pain during the phase of ethanol injection may signal improper alcohol diffusion outside the lesion. There are no reported differences in the risk profile of either complete aspiration of the ethanol-mixed fluid or leaving the ethanol within the lesion [19]. In one study, dysphonia, persistent nerve paralysis, and paranodular fibrosis were correlated to the use of larger ethanol doses while the occurrence of thyrotoxicosis and hyperpyrexia were unrelated to the amount of the instilled ethanol [54]. Most patients complain of a mild to moderate pain typically lasting a few minutes after the needle extraction. Pain, which can irradiate to the mandible angle or to the ear and rarely to the shoulder or to the back, may due to the contact of the needle tip with the subcutaneous tissues. Rinsing the needle with saline before its extraction may partially alleviate the discomfort but does not completely prevent it.

35.3 Alcohol Ablation of Thyroid Solid Nodules

35.3.1 Autonomously Functioning Thyroid Nodules

In the 1990s, several papers had enthusiastically proposed EA for the treatment of autonomously functioning thyroid nodules (AFTNs) as a reliable and cost-effective alternative to surgery and radioiodine [10, 55, 56]. An initial optimistic success rate of EA (about 90 %), defined as complete or partial restoration of normal thyroid function, was reported in over 400 patients with AFTNs in various studies from different institutions [10, 12, 13, 57, 58]. Improvement of thyroid functional data was associated with an impressive decrease (58.5–90 %) of the volume of the nodules [10, 12, 13, 57–59]. Patients presenting with pre-toxic nodules were far more likely to respond to ethanol sclerotherapy as compared to overtly hyperthyroid patients (83.4 % vs. 66.5 %) as shown by a multicentric Italian study [59]. Furthermore, better results were apparently obtained in smaller nodules although a variable range of cut-off volume values (15–40 ml) has been suggested by different authors [60–62]. Nodule composition is also a critical factor for EA outcome in AFTNs, with a >30 % fluid component associated with a long-term treatment success, unrelated to the degree of baseline thyroid dysfunction [35]. Importantly, although EA of cystic nodules is usually accomplished in 1–2 sessions, EA of AFTNs routinely requires a higher number of sessions.

Only a minority of the initial studies reported more than a 1-year follow-up. Subsequently, studies examining long-term effects of EA for AFTNs have demonstrated a 13–35 % recurrence rate for hyperthyroidism [63, 64]. This finding is not surprising because scintigraphic studies showed the persistence of autonomous function tissue in 30–50 % of cases performed ethanol sclerotherapy of AFTNs [65, 66].

The side effects of ethanol sclerotherapy for AFTNs also limit its use. RLN palsy has been reported in 0.7–3.9 % of patients, and although often transient, its complete resolution cannot be reliably predicted [58, 62, 64]. Other less common but serious adverse events reported after EA in AFTNs include hematomas, ipsilateral facial dysesthesia, jugular vein thrombosis, septic complications, worsening of thyrotoxicosis, and transient Horner's syndrome [67]. In addition, the later occurrence of Graves' disease in patients previously submitted to EA has been linked to possible induction of anti-thyroidal autoimmune response by the toxic action of ethanol in the thyroid tissue [68].

Controversy about long-term beneficial effects of EA, in conjunction with serious side effects induced by the leakage of alcohol outside the lesion, has resulted in the abandonment of EA as a treatment for AFTNs [14, 15, 25, 69, 70]. The role of EA is presently confined to selected cases not amenable to treatment by first-line therapies; for instance, a multimodal therapeutic approach combining EA and radioiodine administration has been proposed in selected cases of large AFTNs as an option to reduce the required amount of ^{131}I [65].

35.3.2 "Cold" Thyroid Nodules

Decreased nodule size has been reported after EA for benign nonfunctioning solid thyroid nodules [71, 72]. In a randomized, prospective study of 50 patients, EA achieved better results as compared to L-thyroxine (LT4) administration with a 47 % vs. 9 % mean volume reduction [72], while in a retrospective series on about 200 nodules a 75.1 % ± 12.3 (mean ± SD) volume reduction was reported [40]. The response of solid "cold" nodules, however, is less impressive than for cysts. Furthermore, repeated treatments are required with more frequent adverse effects [36, 54]. Thus, EA is not recommended for the treatment of solid cold thyroid nodules [14, 15, 25, 69, 70]. Today other more effective US-guided interventional techniques (e.g., laser thermal ablation and radiofrequency ablation) are available.

35.4 Alcohol Ablation in Other Neck Lesions

35.4.1 Parathyroid Lesions

EA of parathyroid (PT) lesions has been mainly applied in two clinical settings: treatment of non functional, large parathyroid cysts [73–75] and sclerotherapy of enlarged, hyperfunctioning PT glands in patients with chronic renal failure and tertiary hyperparathyroidism [76–79]. Cystic lesions of parathyroid origin may correspond either to a PT adenoma featuring a large fluid component or to nonfunctional “true” parathyroid cyst [80, 81]. A cystic PT adenoma is usually associated with primary hyperparathyroidism and sonographically demonstrates typically a solid, markedly vascularized portion in addition to a cystic area. Instead, non functional cysts have a “pure” fluid structure comprised of a watery, colorless fluid aspirate [73, 74, 81]. “True” PT cysts, which derive from embryological remnants [82, 83] are not as rare as once believed. Their incidence is underestimated because PT cysts are a rare cause of neck swelling, due to their usual deep location, posterior to the thyroid gland. Usually, PT cysts are incidentally detected during a neck US performed for various reasons, and they may be easily confused with a cystic lesion of thyroid origin [84, 85]. US-guided FNA with parathyroid hormone (PTH) assay in the aspiration fluid is useful for a correct diagnosis as well as recognition that an aspirate clear colorless fluid is almost pathognomonic for parathyroidal as opposed to thyroidal origin [3, 86, 87]. Similar to thyroid cysts, PT cysts frequently recur after FNA; therefore, ethanol and other sclerosing agents (e.g., tetracycline) are an effective alternative to surgery (Fig. 35.5) [73, 75–77, 88]. Although no major complications have been reported in published series, precaution should be taken to avoid ethanol leakage out of the cyst, because of close proximity to the laryngeal nerve in the tracheoesophageal groove. Severe tertiary hyperparathyroidism can be safely controlled using EA in patients with chronic renal failure [76–79, 89, 90]. Ethanol sclerotherapy of PT adenomas causing primary hyperparathyroidism should be restricted to patients at high-surgical risk [90, 91].

35.4.2 Alcohol Ablation of Metastatic Lymph Nodes

Ethanol sclerotherapy of metastatic lymph nodes from differentiated thyroid cancer was first performed as a palliative procedure at the Mayo Clinic in the 1990s [92, 93]. Based upon results from the first published series of 14 patients treated from 1993 to 2000, Lewis and colleagues concluded that EA was a valuable tool for patients who were not candidates for further surgical or radioiodine therapy, and that the procedure was safe, less invasive than reoperation and could be repeated without major problems [93]. The application of EA to thyroid cancer recurrences has gained popularity with papers from international centers reporting their experience [94–100]. EA of metastatic lymph nodes is no longer confined to the palliative setting but also is now regarded as potentially curative in patients with localized neck persistence of disease [98]. In a recent review article, an 87.5 % success rate was reported in 168 patients treated with EA for lymph node metastasis in different institutions with a very low (1.2 %) risk of complications [101]. Four published series of patients with papillary thyroid cancer [95–98] report a 16.5–66.0 % rate of complete regression of the treated lesions and a

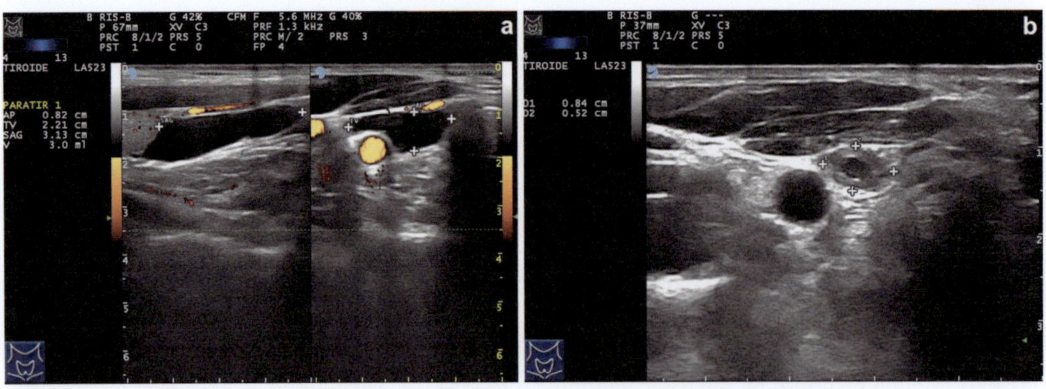

Fig. 35.5 A right, inferior, functional parathyroid cyst before (**a**) and after (**b**) ethanol ablation

remarkably low incidence of major complications. While EA of metastatic neck lymph nodes in the lateral neck compartments does not usually pose major concerns to the operators, apart from lesions strictly adjacent to large vessels, ethanol injections of lesions located in the central compartment may involve risk to the recurrent laryngeal nerves. The composition (solid vs. cystic) of the target lesion does not seem to influence the final outcome of the treatment. Furthermore, in the majority of patients treated by EA, subsequent progression of neck disease was not observed. Periodic measurement of serum thyroglobulin levels and US surveillance with color Doppler parameters are used to monitor the response to EA treatment. In conclusion, neck recurrences from thyroid cancer can profitably be treated by EA, after a careful risk-to-benefit balancing of the other therapeutic options. Future studies will help clarify advantages and limitations of ethanol sclerotherapy versus surgery and other interventional techniques in patients with neck recurrences from thyroid cancer [102–104].

References

1. Bean WJ. Renal cysts: treatment with alcohol. Radiology. 1981;138:329–31.
2. Livraghi T, Giorgio A, Marin G, Salmi A, de Sio I, Bolondi L, et al. Hepatocellular carcinoma and cirrhosis in 746 patients: long term results of percutaneous ethanol injection. Radiology. 1985;197:101–8.
3. Solbiati L, Giangrande A, De Pra L, Bellotti E, Cantù P, Ravetto C. Percutaneous ethanol injection of parathyroid tumors under US guidance: treatment for secondary hyperparathyroidism. Radiology. 1985;155:607–10.
4. Bean WJ, Rodan BA. Hepatic cysts: treatment with alcohol. AJR Am J Roentgenol. 1985;144:237–41.
5. Ahmed M, Solbiati L, Brace CL, Breen DJ, Callstrom MR, Charboneau JW, et al. International Working Group on Image-guided Tumor Ablation; Interventional Oncology Sans Frontières Expert Panel; Technology Assessment Committee of the Society of Interventional Radiology; Standard of Practice Committee of the Cardiovascular and Interventional Radiological Society of Europe. Image-guided tumor ablation: standardization of terminology and reporting criteria--a 10-year update. Radiology. 2014;273:241–60.
6. Lubiensky A, Simon M, Helmberger TK. Percutaneous alcohol instillation. In: Vogl TJ, Helmberger T, Mack MG, Reiser MF, editors. Percutaneous tumor ablation in medical radiology. New York, NY: Springer; 2008. p. 123–8.
7. Crescenzi A, Papini E, Pacella CM, Rinaldi R, Panunzi C, Petrucci L, et al. Morphological changes in a hyperfunctioning thyroid adenoma after percutaneous ethanol injection: histological, enzymatic and sub-microscopical alterations. J Endocrinol Invest. 1996;19:371–6.
8. Monzani F, Caraccio N, Basolo F, Iacconi P, LiVolsi V, Miccoli P. Surgical and pathological changes after percutaneous ethanol injection therapy of thyroid nodules. Thyroid. 2000;10:1087–92.
9. Rozman B, Bence-Zigman Z, Tomic-Brzac H, Skreb F, Pavlinovic Z, Simonovic I. Sclerosation of thyroid cysts by ethanol. Period Biol. 1989;91:1116–8.
10. Livraghi T, Paracchi A, Ferrari C, Bergonzi M, Garavaglia G, Raineri P, et al. Treatment of autonomous thyroid nodule with percutaneous ethanol injection: preliminary results. Radiology. 1990; 175:827–9.
11. Yasuda K, Ozaki O, Sugino K, Yamashita T, Toshima K, Ito K, et al. Treatment of cystic lesions of the thyroid by ethanol instillation. World J Surg. 1992;16:958–61.
12. Martino E, Murtas ML, Loviselli A, Piga M, Petrini L, Miccoli P, et al. Percutaneous intranodular ethanol injection for treatment of autonomously functioning thyroid nodules. Surgery. 1992;112:1161–5.
13. Papini E, Panunzi C, Pacella CM, Bizzarri G, Fabbrini R, Petrucci L, et al. Percutaneous ultrasound-guided ethanol injection: a new treatment of toxic autonomously functioning thyroid nodules? J Clin Endocrinol Metab. 1993;76:411–6.
14. Gharib H, Papini E, Paschke R, Duick DS, Valcavi R, et al. American Association of Clinical Endocrinologists, Associazione Medici Endocrinologi, and EuropeanThyroid Association Medical Guidelines for clinical practice for the diagnosis and management of thyroid nodules. Endocr Pract. 2010;16 Suppl 1:1–43.
15. Haugen BR, Alexander EK, Bible KC, Doherty G, Mandel SJ, Nikiforov YE, et al. 2015 American Thyroid Association Management Guidelines for adult patients with thyroid nodules and differentiated thyroid cancer. Thyroid. 2016;26:1.
16. Porenta M, Fettich JJ. Treatment of thyroid cysts by sclerosation. Radiobiol Radiother. 1985;26:249–54.
17. Zhao Y, Guan X, Liu Y, Liu S, Hussain A, Shi B. The efficacy of percutaneous AHI (arginine hydrochloride injection) for the treatment of recurrent thyroid cysts. Ann Endocrinol. 2015;76:281–5.
18. Kalra N, Ahuja CK, Dutta P, Rajwanshi A, Mittal BR, Bhansali A, et al. Comparison of sonographically guided percutaneous sodium tetradecyl sulfate injection with ethanol injection in the treatment of benign nonfunctioning thyroid nodules. J Vasc Interv Radiol. 2014;25:1218–24.
19. Kim DW, Rho MH, Kim HJ, Kwon JS, Sung YS, Lee SW. Percutaneous ethanol injection for benign

cystic thyroid nodules: is aspiration of ethanol-mixed fluid advantageous? AJNR Am J Neuroradiol. 2005;26:2122–7.
20. Cho YS, Lee HK, Ahn IM, Lim SM, Kim DH, Choi CG, et al. Sonographically guided ethanol sclerotherapy for benign thyroid cysts: results in 22 patients. AJR Am J Roentgenol. 2000;174:213–6.
21. Zingrillo M, Torlantano M, Ghiggi MR, D'Aloiso L, Nirchino V, Bisceglia M, et al. Percutaneous ethanol injection of large thyroid cystic nodules. Thyroid. 1996;6:403–8.
22. Zieleźnik W, Kawczyk-Krupka A, Peszel Barlik M, Cebula W, Sieroń A. Modified percutaneous ethanol injection in the treatment of viscous cystic thyroid nodules. Thyroid. 2005;15:683–7.
23. Sung JY, Baek JH, Kim YS, Jeong HJ, Kwak MS, Lee D, Moon W. One-step ethanol ablation viscous cystic thyroid nodules. AJR Am J Roentgenol. 2008;191:1730–3.
24. Lv G, Chen S, Li B, Chen X, Li S. Efficacy assessment of newly developed open-window intervention needles for the treatment of cystic thyroid nodules that cannot be aspirated. Thyroid. 2014;24:1012–7.
25. Bandeira-Echtler E, Bergerhoff K, Richter B. Levothyroxine or minimally invasive therapies for benign thyroid nodules. Cochrane Database Syst Rev. 2014; (6):CD004098.
26. de los Santos ET, Keyhani-Rofagha S, Cunningham JJ, Mazzaferri EL. Cystic thyroid nodules: the dilemma of malignant lesions. Arch Intern Med. 1990;150:422–7.
27. Sheppard MC, Franklyn JA. Management of the single thyroid nodule. Clin Endocrinol (Oxf). 1994;41:719–24.
28. Jensen F, Rasmussen SN. The treatment of thyroid cysts by ultrasonographically-guided fine needle aspiration. Acta Chir Scand. 1976;142:209–11.
29. Monzani F, Lippi F, Goletti O, Del Guerra P, Caraccio N, Lippolis PV, et al. Percutaneous aspiration and ethanol sclerotherapy for thyroid cysts. J Clin Endocrinol Metab. 1994;78:800–2.
30. Antonelli A, Campatelli A, Di Vito A, Alberti B, Baldi V, Salvioni G, et al. Comparison between ethanol sclerotherapy and emptying with injection of saline in treatment of thyroid cysts. Clin Investig. 1994;72:971–4.
31. Kim DW. Ultrasound-guided fine-needle aspiration of benign thyroid cysts or partially cystic thyroid nodules: a preliminary study for factors predicting successful collapse. Endocrine. 2014;45:67–72.
32. Bennedbaek FN, Hegedus L. Treatment of recurrent thyroid cysts with ethanol: a randomized double blind controlled trial. J Clin Endocrinol Metab. 2003;88:5773–7.
33. Valcavi R, Frasoldati A. Ultrasound-guided percutaneous ethanol injection therapy in thyroid cystic nodules. Endocr Pract. 2004;10:269–75.
34. Del Prete S, Caraglia M, Russo D, Vitale G, Giuberti G, Marra M, et al. Percutaneous ethanol injection efficacy in the treatment of large symptomatic thyroid cystic nodules: ten-year follow-up of a large series. Thyroid. 2002;12:815–21.
35. Guglielmi R, Pacella CM, Bianchini A, Bizzarri G, Rinaldi R, Graziano FM, et al. Percutaneous ethanol injection treatment in benign thyroid lesions: role and efficacy. Thyroid. 2004;14:125–31.
36. Kim JH, Lee HK, Lee JH, Ahn IM, Choi CG. Efficacy of sonographically guided percutaneous ethanol injection for treatment of thyroid cysts versus solid thyroid nodules. Am J Roentgenol. 2003;180:1623–726.
37. Verde G, Papini E, Pacella CM, Gallotti C, Delpiano S, Strada S, et al. Ultrasound guided percutaneous ethanol injection in the treatment of cystic thyroid nodules. Clin Endocrinol (Oxf). 1994;41:719–24.
38. Sung JY, Kim YS, Choi H, Lee JH, Baek JH. Optimum first-line treatment technique for benign cystic thyroid nodules: ethanol ablation or radiofrequency ablation? AJR Am J Roentgenol. 2011;196:W210–4.
39. Reverter JL, Alonso N, Avila M, Lucas A, Mauricio D, Puig-Domingo M. Evaluation of efficacy, safety, pain perception and health-related quality of life of percutaneous ethanol injection as first-line treatment in symptomatic thyroid cysts. BMC Endocr Disord. 2015;15:73.
40. Lee SJ, Ahn IM. Effectiveness of percutaneous ethanol injection therapy in benign nodular and cystic thyroid diseases: long-term follow-up experience. Endocr J. 2005;52:455–62.
41. Zingrillo M, Torlontano M, Chiarella R, Ghiggi MR, Nirchio V, Bisceglia M, et al. Percutaneous ethanol injection may be a definitive treatment for symptomatic thyroid cystic nodules not treatable by surgery: five-year follow-up study. Thyroid. 1999;9:763–7.
42. Kanotra SP, Lateef M, Kirmani O. Non-surgical management of benign thyroid cysts: use of ultrasound-guided ethanol ablation. Postgrad Med J. 2008;84:639–43.
43. Kim YJ, Baek JH, Ha EJ, Lim HK, Lee JH, Sung JY, et al. Cystic versus predominantly cystic thyroid nodules: efficacy of ethanol ablation and analysis of related factors. Eur Radiol. 2012;22:1573–8.
44. Kim DW, Rho MH, Park HJ, Kwag HJ. Ultrasonography-guided ethanol ablation of predominantly solid thyroid nodules: a preliminary study for factors that predict the outcome. Br J Radiol. 2012;85:930–6.
45. In HS, Kim DW, Choo HJ, Jung SJ, Kang T, Ryu JH. Ethanol ablation of benign thyroid cysts and predominantly cystic thyroid nodules: factors that predict outcome. Endocrine. 2014;46:107–13.
46. Suh CH, Baek JH, Ha EJ, Choi YJ, Lee JH, Kim JK, et al. Ethanol ablation of predominantly cystic thyroid nodules: evaluation of recurrence rate and factors related to recurrence. Clin Radiol. 2015;70:42–7.
47. Baek JH, Ha EJ, Choi YJ, Sung JY, Kim JK, Shong YK. Radiofrequency versus ethanol ablation for treating predominantly cystic thyroid nodules: a randomized clinical trial. Korean J Radiol. 2015;16:1332–40.

48. Kim DW. Usefulness of two-stage ethanol ablation in the treatment of benign predominantly cystic thyroid nodules. Endocr Pract. 2014;20:548–55.
49. Mondin V, Ferlito A, Muzzi E, Silver CE, Fagan JJ, Devaney KO, et al. Thyroglossal duct cyst: personal experience and literature review. Auris Nasus Larynx. 2008;35:11–25.
50. Clark OH. Parathyroid cysts. Am J Surg. 1978;35:395–402.
51. Fukumoto K, Kojima T, Tomonari H, Kontani K, Murai S, Tsujimoto F. Ethanol injection sclerotherapy for Baker's cysts, thyroglossal duct cysts, and branchial cleft cysts. Ann Plast Surg. 1994;33:615–9.
52. Baskin HJ. Percutaneous ethanol injection of thyroglossal duct cysts. Endocr Pract. 2006;12:355–7.
53. Kim SM, Baek JH, Kim YS, Sung JY, Lim HK, Choi H, et al. Efficacy and safety of ethanol ablation for thyroglossal duct cysts. AJNR Am J Neuroradiol. 2011;32:306–9.
54. Bennedbaek FN, Hegedüs L. Percutaneous ethanol injection therapy in benign solitary solid cold thyroid nodules: a randomized trial comparing one injection with three injections. Thyroid. 1999;9:225–33.
55. Goletti O, Monzani F, Caraccio N, Del Guerra P, Lippolis PV, Pucciarelli M, et al. Percutaneous ethanol injection treatment of autonomously functioning single thyroid nodules: optimization of treatment and short term outcome. World J Surg. 1992;16:784–9. discussion 789-90.
56. Monzani F, Goletti O, Caraccio N, Del Guerra P, Ferdeghini M, Pucci E, et al. Percutaneous ethanol injection treatment of autonomous thyroid adenoma: hormonal and clinical evaluation. Clin Endocrinol (Oxf). 1992;36:491–7.
57. Di Lelio A, Rivolta M, Casati M, Capra M. Treatment of autonomous thyroid nodules: value of percutaneous ethanol injection. Am J Roentgenol. 1995;164: 207–13.
58. Ferrari C, Reschini E, Paracchi A. Treatment of the autonomous thyroid nodule: a review. Eur J Endocrinol. 1996;135:383–90.
59. Lippi F, Ferrari C, Manetti L, Rago T, Santini F, Monzani F, et al. Treatment of solitary autonomous thyroid nodules by percutaneous etanol injection. Results of an Italian multicenter study. J Clin Endocrinol Metab. 1996;81:3261–4.
60. Monzani F, Caraccio N, Goletti O. Five year follow-up of percutaneous ethanol injection for the treatment of hyperfunctioning thyroid nodules: a study of 117 patients. Clin Endocrinol (Oxf). 1997;46:9–15.
61. Zingrillo M, Torlontano M, Ghiggi MR, Frusciante V, Varraso A, Liuzzi A, et al. Radioiodine and percutaneous ethanol injection in the treatment of large toxic thyroid nodule: a long-term study. Thyroid. 2000;10:985–9.
62. Del Prete S, Russo D, Caraglia M, Giuberti G, Marra M, Vitale G, et al. Percutaneous ethanol injection of autonomous thyroid nodules with a volume larger than 40 ml: three years of follow-up. Clin Radiol. 2001;56:895–901.
63. Tarantino L, Francica G, Sordelli I, Sperlongano P, Parmeggiani D, Ripa C, et al. Percutaneous ethanol injection of hyperfunctioning thyroid nodules: long-term follow-up in 125 patients. AJR Am J Roentgenol. 2008;190:800–8.
64. Yano Y, Sugino K, Akaishi J, Uruno T, Okuwa K, Shibuya H, et al. Treatment of autonomously functioning thyroid nodules at a single institution: radioiodine therapy, surgery, and ethanol injection therapy. Ann Nucl Med. 2011;25:749–54.
65. Zingrillo M, Modoni S, Conte M, Frusciante V, Trischitta V. Percutaneous ethanol injection plus radioiodine versus radioidine alone in the treatment of large toxic thyroid nodules. J Nucl Med. 2003;44:207–10.
66. Pacini F. Role of percutaneous ethanol injection in management of nodular lesions of the thyroid gland. J Nucl Med. 2003;44:211–2.
67. Pishdad GR, Pishdad P, Pishdad R. Horner's syndrome as a complication of percutaneous ethanol treatment of thyroid nodule. Thyroid. 2011;21:327–8.
68. Regalbuto C, Le Moli R, Muscia V, Russo M, Vigneri R, Pezzino V. Severe Graves' ophthalmopathy after percutaneous ethanol injection in a nontoxic thyroid nodule. Thyroid. 2012;22:210–3.
69. Papini E, Pacella CM, Hegedus L. Diagnosis of endocrine disease: thyroid ultrasound (US) and US-assisted procedures: from the shadows into an array of applications. Eur J Endocrinol. 2014;170: R133–46.
70. Papini E, Pacella CM, Misischi I, Guglielmi R, Bizzarri G, Døssing H, et al. The advent of ultrasound-guided ablation techniques in nodular thyroid disease: towards a patient-tailored approach. Best Pract Res Clin Endocrinol Metab. 2014;28:601–18.
71. Zingrillo M, Collura D, Ghiggi MR, Nirchio V, Trischitta V. Treatment of large cold benign thyroid nodules not eligible for surgery with percutaneous ethanol injection. J Clin Endocrinol Metab. 1998;83:3905–7.
72. Bennedbaek FN, Nielsen LK, Hegedus L. Effect of percutaneous ethanol injection therapy versus suppressive doses of L-thyroxine on benign solitary solid cold thyroid nodules: a randomized trial. J Clin Endocrinol Metab. 1998;83:830–5.
73. Sung JY, Baek JH, Kim KS, Lee D, Ha EJ, Lee JH. Symptomatic nonfunctioning parathyroid cysts: role of simple aspiration and ethanol ablation. Eur J Radiol. 2013;82:316–20.
74. Goomany A, Rafferty A, Smith I. An unusual neck mass: a case of a parathyroid cyst and review of the literature. Case Rep Surg. 2015;2015:243527.
75. Kim JH. Ultrasound-guided sclerotherapy for benign non-thyroid cystic mass in the neck. Ultrasonography. 2014;33:83–90.
76. Chen HH, Lin CJ, Wu CJ, Lai CT, Lin J, Cheng SP, et al. Chemical ablation of recurrent and persistent secondary hyperparathyroidism after subtotal parathyroidectomy. Ann Surg. 2011;253:786–90.

77. Douthat WG, Cardozo G, Garay G, Orozco S, Chiurchiu C, de la Fuente J, et al. Use of percutaneous ethanol injection therapy for recurrent secondary hyperparathyroidism after subtotal parathyroidectomy. Int J Nephrol. 2011;2011:246734.
78. Kitaoka M. Ultrasonographic diagnosis of parathyroid glands and percutaneous ethanol injection therapy. Nephrol Dial Transplant. 2003;18 Suppl 3:ii27–30.
79. Tanaka M, Itoh K, Matsushita K, Matsushita K, Fukagawa M. Efficacy of percutaneous ethanol injection therapy for secondary hyperparathyroidism in patients on hemodialysis as evaluated by parathyroid hormone levels according to K/DOQI guidelines. Ther Apher Dial. 2005;9:48–52.
80. Frasoldati A, Valcavi R. Challenges in neck ultrasonography: lymphadenopathy and parathyroid glands. Endocr Pract. 2004;10:261–8.
81. Sung JY. Parathyroid ultrasonography: the evolving role of the radiologist. Ultrasonography. 2015;34:268–74.
82. Clark OH, Okerlund MD, Cavalieri RR, Greenspan FS. Diagnosis and treatment of thyroid parathyroid and thyroglossal duct cysts. J Clin Endocrinol Metab. 1979;48:983–8.
83. Ippolito G, Palazzo FF, Sebag F, Sierra M, De Micco C, Henry JF. A single institution 25-year review of true parathyroid cysts. Langenbecks Arch Surg. 2006;391:13–8.
84. Prinz RA, Peters JR, Kane JM, Wood J. Needle aspiration of nonfunctioning parathyroid cysts. Am Surg. 1990;56:420–2.
85. Akel M, Salti I, Azar ST. Successful treatment of parathyroid cyst using ethanol sclerotherapy. Am J Med Sci. 1999;317:50–2.
86. Baskin HJ. New applications of thyroid and parathyroid ultrasound. Minerva Endocrinol. 2004;29:195–206.
87. Fukagawa M, Kitaoka M, Tominaga Y, Akizawa T, Kakuta T, Onoda N, et al. Guidelines for percutaneous ethanol injection therapy of the parathyroid glands in chronic dialysis patients. Nephrol Dial Transplant. 2003;18 Suppl 3:31–3.
88. Sanchez A, Carretto H. Treatment of nonfunctioning parathyroid cysts with tetracycline injection. Head Neck. 1993;15:263–5.
89. Koiwa F, Hasegawa T, Tanaka R, Kakuta T. Indication and efficacy of PEIT in the management of secondary hyperparathyroidism. NDT Plus. 2008;1 Suppl 3:14–7.
90. Cercueil JP, Jacob D, Verges B, Holtzmann P, Lerais JM, Krause D. Percutaneous ethanol injection into parathyroid adenomas: mid- and long-term results. Eur Radiol. 1998;8:1565–9.
91. Harman CR, Grant CS, Hay ID, Hurley DL, van Heerden JA, Thompson GB, et al. Indications, technique and efficacy of alcohol injection of enlarged parathyroid glands in patients with primary hyperparathyroidism. Surgery. 1998;124:1011–20.
92. Hay ID, Charboneau JW. The coming of age of ultrasound-guided percutaneous ethanol ablation of selected neck nodal metastases in well-differentiated thyroid carcinoma. J Clin Endocrinol Metab. 2011;96:2717–20.
93. Lewis BD, Hay ID, Charboneau JW, McIver B, Reading CC, Goellner JR. Percutaneous ethanol injection for treatment of cervical lymph node metastases in patients with papillary thyroid carcinoma. Am J Roentgenol. 2002;178:699–704.
94. Monchik JM, Donatini G, Iannuccilli J, Dupuy DE. Radiofrequency ablation and percutaneous ethanol injection treatment for recurrent local and distant well-differentiated thyroid carcinoma. Ann Surg. 2006;244:296–304.
95. Lim CY, Yun JS, Lee J, Nam KH, Chung WY, Park CS. Percutaneous ethanol injection therapy for locally recurrent papillary thyroid carcinoma. Thyroid. 2007;17:347–50.
96. Kim BM, Kim MJ, Kim EK, et al. Controlling recurrent papillary thyroid carcinoma in the neck by ultrasonography-guided percutaneous ethanol injection. Eur Radiol. 2008;18:835–42.
97. Sohn YM, Hong SW, Kim EK, Kim MJ, Moon HJ, Kim SJ, et al. Complete eradication of metastatic lymph node after percutaneous ethanol injection therapy: pathologic correlation. Thyroid. 2009;19:317–9.
98. Heilo A, Sigstad E, Fagerlid KH, Håskjold OI, Grøholt KK, Berner A, et al. Efficacy of ultrasound-guided percutaneous ethanol injection treatment in patients with a limited number of metastatic cervical lymph nodes from papillary thyroid carcinoma. J Clin Endocrinol Metab. 2011;96:2750–5.
99. Hay ID, Lee RA, Davidge-Pitts C, Reading CC, Charboneau JW. Long-term outcome of ultrasound-guided percutaneous ethanol ablation of selected "recurrent" neck nodal metastases in 25 patients with TNM stages III or IVA papillary thyroid carcinoma previously treated by surgery and 131I therapy. Surgery. 2013;154:1448–54. discussion 1454-5.
100. Vannucchi G, Covelli D, Perrino M, De Leo S, Fugazzola L. Ultrasound-guided percutaneous ethanol injection in papillary thyroid cancer metastatic lymph-nodes. Endocrine. 2014;47:648–51.
101. Fontenot TE, Deniwar A, Bhatia P, Al-Qurayshi Z, Randolph GW, Kandil E. Percutaneous ethanol injection vs reoperation for locally recurrent papillary thyroid cancer: a systematic review and pooled analysis. JAMA Otolaryngol Head Neck Surg. 2015;141:512–8.
102. Pacella CM, Papini E. Image-guided percutaneous ablation therapies for local recurrences of thyroid tumors. J Endocrinol Invest. 2013;36:61–70.
103. Yue W, Chen L, Wang S, Yu S. Locoregional control of recurrent papillary thyroid carcinoma by ultrasound-guided percutaneous microwave ablation: a prospective study. Int J Hyperthermia. 2015;3:403–8.
104. Lim HK, Baek JH, Lee JH, Kim WB, Kim TY, Shong YK, et al. Efficacy and safety of radiofrequency ablation for treating locoregional recurrence from papillary thyroid cancer. Eur Radiol. 2015;25:163–70.

36 HIFU and RFA Ablation for Thyroid and Parathyroid Disease

Petros Tsamatropoulos and Roberto Valcavi

36.1 Introduction

Interventional thyroidology encompasses minimally invasive ultrasound-guided techniques to treat diseases of the endocrine neck (i.e., diseases of thyroid and parathyroid glands). Radiofrequency ablation (RFA) and high-intensity focused ultrasound (HIFU) ablation are two of these techniques, used to destroy thyroid nodules and tumors using hyperthermia without surgical removal. Indications of RFA and HIFU ablation for the treatment of endocrine neck diseases include: symptomatic benign cold thyroid nodules, autonomously functioning thyroid nodules, and recurrent thyroid cancer. Both thermal techniques have also been used for the treatment of parathyroid adenomas, but with several drawbacks.

The advantages of in situ tumor ablation are reduced costs, the possibility of performing procedures on outpatients, and the possibility of treating patients who are poor candidates for surgery due to age or comorbidity. RFA and HIFU are performed by endocrinologists, interventional radiologists, and surgeons.

36.2 Radiofrequency Ablation

36.2.1 Principles

The aim of RFA is to induce thermal damage to the tissue through electromagnetic energy deposition. Passage of alternating high-frequency current, between 200 and 1200 kHz, through tissue causes agitation of ions, and consequently frictional heat [1]. In the monopolar mode, which is the one most commonly used in thyroid RFA, the patient is part of a closed-loop circuit that includes a radiofrequency generator, an electrode needle, and a large dispersive electrode (two grounding pads, one attached to each thigh) (Fig. 36.1). The discrepancy between the small surface area of the needle and the large area of the grounding pads causes the heat generated to be concentrated around the needle electrode inserted into target area. A typical RFA treatment produces temperatures of 90 °C, resulting in coagulative necrosis of the tissue,

Electronic supplementary material: The online version of this chapter (doi:10.1007/978-3-319-44100-9_36) contains supplementary material, which is available to authorized users. Videos can also be accessed at http://link.springer.com/chapter/10.1007/978-3-319-44100-9_36.

P. Tsamatropoulos, M.D. • R. Valcavi, M.D., F.A.C.E. (✉)
Endocrine Unit, Centro Palmer, Via Fratelli Cervi, 75/B, 42124 Reggio Emilia, Italy
e-mail: ptsamatropoulos@gmail.com; info@robertovalcavi.it

M. Milas et al. (eds.), *Advanced Thyroid and Parathyroid Ultrasound*,
DOI 10.1007/978-3-319-44100-9_36

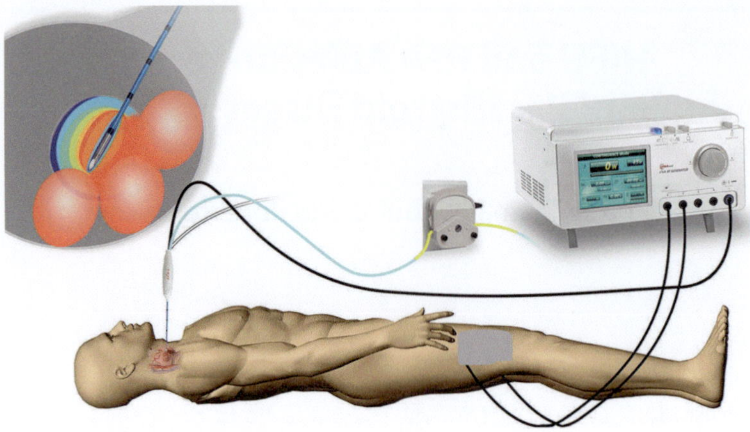

Fig. 36.1 Thyroid monopolar RFA system. The patient is part of a closed-loop circuit that includes a radiofrequency generator, an electrode needle for ablation, a pump for cooling the electrode needle, and a large dispersive electrode (ground pads). *Upper left*: multiple ellipsoid ablation areas around are obtained by moving the active tip of electrode needle (moving shot technique)

tissue desiccation, and consequent rise of impedance [2]. Small vessels are completely destroyed and larger vessels up to 0.3 cm in diameter are thrombosed. Internally cooled tip needles maintain temperatures around 90 °C in order to prevent tissue carbonization.

36.2.2 Devices

For monopolar thyroid RFA straight, internally cooled, short (7- or 10-cm), thin (18- or 19-gauge) electrode needles are currently used. The active tips of the electrode needles may have a different length (0.5–2.0 cm) according to the desired ablation area [3, 4]. Experience with bipolar radiofrequency electrode needles has not been reported for thyroid ablation. In the past other types of electrode needles (e.g., multi-tined expandable electrodes) had been used for thyroid RFA, but their use is no longer recommended [5–7].

36.2.3 Technique (See Video 36.1)

Thyroid RFA is performed as an outpatient procedure in an interventional suite. Patients should be fasting. The patient is placed on an operation bed in the supine position with hyperextended neck, and a venous catheter is inserted in a forearm vein. A multiparametric monitor is connected to the patient displaying a continuous single lead electrocardiogram, pulse oximetry, blood pressure, and respiratory rate. Conscious sedation is obtained with intravenous (i.v.) midazolam (2–5 mg) in fractionated boli in order to decrease the patient's anxiety, swallowing, cough, and movements. Local anesthesia with 2% ropivacaine pericapsular infiltration (2–5 mL) is performed under US assistance with thin (27-gauge) needles.

In the RFA monopolar technique, the patient is part of a closed-loop circuit: ground pads (dispersive electrodes) applied to both thighs are connected to a radiofrequency generator and the generator is connected to an electrode needle. These electrode needles are straight, internally cooled, 7-cm, 18-gauge and have active tips of usually 1.0 cm for most thyroid nodules.

The ablation is performed according to the "moving shot" technique: the nodule is divided into multiple conceptual areas and thereafter the nodule is ablated unit-by-unit by moving the electrode tip (Fig. 36.2) [1, 8–10]. The ablation starts from the deepest portion of the nodule with a transisthmic approach. The needle is inserted

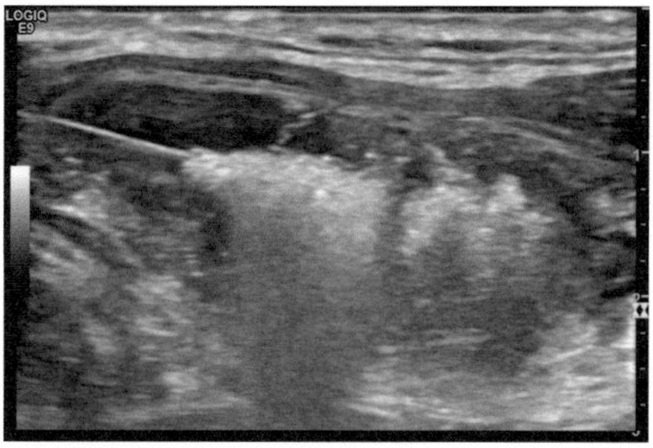

Fig. 36.2 The moving shot technique. According to the moving shot technique the electrode needle delivers energy and a hyperechoic area is seen along the track of the needle (sagittal view, B-mode)

transisthmically at the higher level according to patient anatomy. This insertion allows the repositioning of the needle as much as 60–90° with respect to the entry point in order to achieve ablation of more medially located tissue. This maneuver does not increase side effects, particularly vocal cord palsy, because while continuously tilting the probe, careful surveillance of the area medial to the needle is required to detect US signs of heating (gas microbubbles) when the needle is inserted close to the tracheoesophageal groove where the inferior laryngeal nerve runs (the so-called "danger triangle"). When a hyperechoic area appears and when impedance increases the tip is moved backward to an untreated more superficial area. The maneuver is repeated with repositioning the needle, until all areas are ablated (Fig. 36.3). Usually RF power starts with 30 W and 5-W upward adjustments are made up to 60 W. Higher RFA power is used in Korea [11]. The successful ablation of a unit is confirmed by the appearance of a hyperechoic area—due to microbubbles—and the abrupt increase of impedance (the so-called "break point") registered on the RF generator monitor.

To treat mixed nodules, the cystic fluid is first aspirated and then the ablation is performed. However, sometimes, bleeding occurs during cyst aspiration. To control the bleeding, 99 % ethanol can be injected into the evacuated cystic cavity [12]. The injected volume of ethanol corresponds to approximately 50 % of the aspirated fluid volume. Ethanol causes direct coagulative necrosis and local small vessel thrombosis, stopping the bleeding. After 2 min of ethanol retention, as much of the injected ethanol as possible is removed, and RFA may finally start.

Immediately after the RFA procedure, methylprednisolone 20 mg i.v. bolus may be administered in order to prevent pain. Patients are then brought to the recovery room and are kept under observation for 2 h. The day following the RFA procedure, patients can be started on oral methylprednisone taper of 16 mg daily for 5 days, 8 mg daily for 4 days, and 4 mg daily for 3 days. Oral proton pump inhibitors are administered for 12 days [10].

36.2.4 Indications

RFA can be used to treat [3, 4]:

- Nonfunctioning, benign, solid or predominantly solid, thyroid nodules in patients presenting with local symptoms or cosmetic complaints when surgery is contraindicated or declined.
- Autonomously functioning thyroid nodules (AFTNs) causing problems related to thyrotoxicosis when surgery or radioiodine are contraindicated or declined.
- Recurrent thyroid cancers located in the thyroid bed as well as metastatic lymph nodes when surgery is contraindicated and radioiodine is ineffective.

RFA is not recommended for the treatment of primary thyroid cancers because there is no evidence of its efficacy for malignancy. Similarly it is not recommended for treatment of nodules with follicular neoplasm cytology since, about 15–30 % of cases labelled as follicular neoplasm prove to be malignant [13].

Finally, there is very limited experience of treating primary hyperparathyroidism [14, 15] and secondary hyperparathyroidism [16] with RFA, and thus no recommendation can be made.

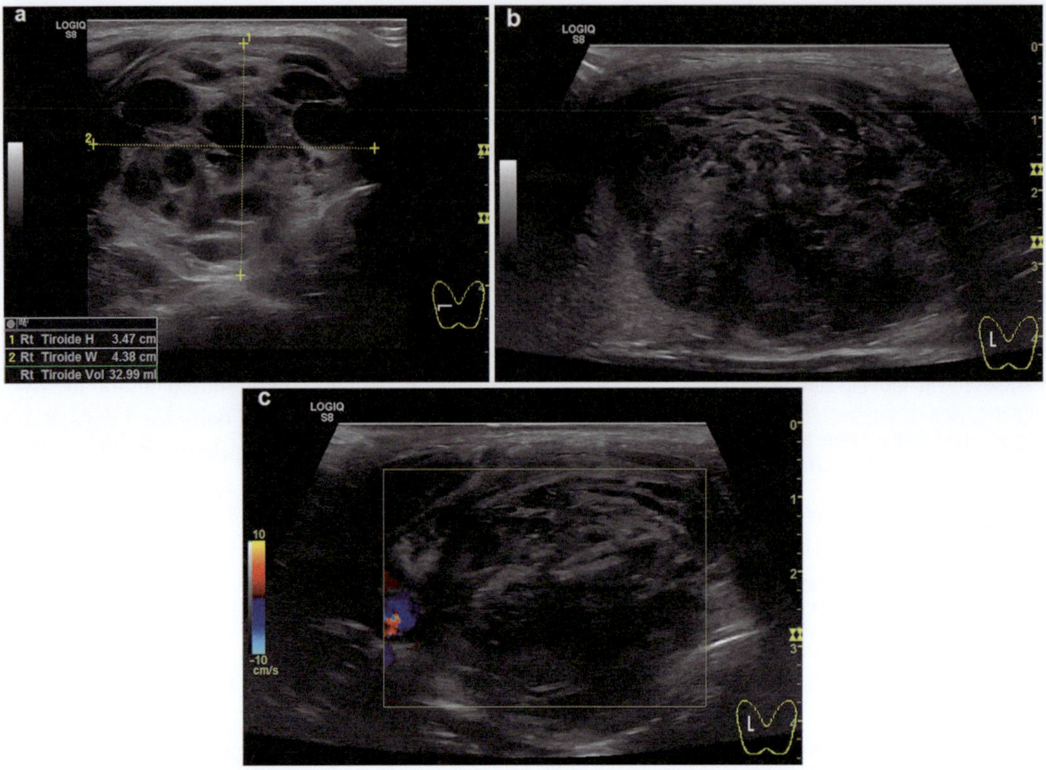

Fig. 36.3 A large (33 mL) spongiform thyroid nodule before RFA (**a**) and immediately after the procedure in B-mode (**b**) and with color Doppler (**c**). After RFA the nodule is unstructured and not vascularized. The color spot of (**c**) (*lower left*) is the common carotid artery

36.2.5 Clinical Results in Benign Cold Thyroid Nodules

At present, the most important indication for RFA in the thyroid gland is to reduce the volume of benign cold thyroid nodules in patients with local pressure symptoms or cosmetic complaints. Benignity of thyroid nodules is usually confirmed by at least two separate fine needle aspiration (FNA) biopsies. The first study suggesting the use of RFA to treat symptomatic thyroid nodules was published in 2006 [17]. Since then, many studies have confirmed the efficacy and safety of treating benign thyroid nodules with RFA. Recently, two systematic reviews with meta-analyses have confirmed that RFA is effective in both reducing the volume of thyroid nodules and improving the related compressive symptoms and aesthetic problems, without causing thyroid dysfunction or serious complications [18, 19]. Moreover, RFA of symptomatic thyroid nodules improves patients' health-related quality of life [10]. Some authors have found that the efficacy of thyroid RFA is similar to that of thyroid surgery [20, 21].

The reduction in thyroid nodule volume after RFA ranges from 50 to 90 % [22–28]. The heterogeneity of results among studies can be explained by a number of factors: (a) different types of electrodes used; (b) a single treatment versus repeated RFA sessions; (c) different initial volume of treated nodules; (d) different composition (solid, cystic, or mixed) of the target nodules. Nodule volume reduction is gradual and final results are achieved approximately 1 year after RFA or even more in case of large lesions (Fig. 36.4). The goal of thyroid RFA is to perform the procedure only once. Additional ablation can

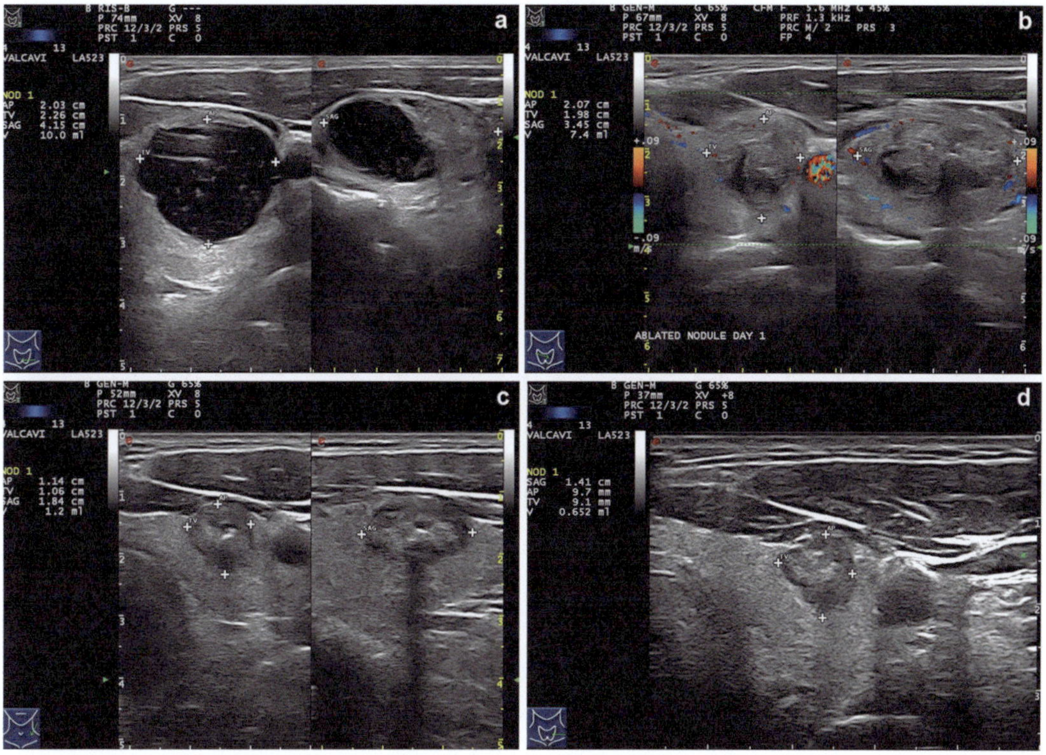

Fig. 36.4 US follow-up images of a mixed thyroid nodule treated with RFA. The nodule had a volume of 10 ml (**a**). Before RFA application the fluid component was drained. The day after RFA there was no fluid component and the nodule measured 7.4 ml (**b**). After 6 months the nodule measured 1.2 ml (**c**). After 1 year the nodule had shrunk to 0.65 ml (**d**). The ablated nodule shrinks over time and becomes inhomogeneous and hypoechoic

be performed if results are partial or in case of thyroid nodule regrowth [29–31]. In a 4-year follow-up study thyroid nodule regrowth was recorded in only 5.6 % of the patients (7/126) [31]. Importantly, RFA does not affect eventual subsequent thyroid surgery [32].

RFA does not alter the thyroid function [10]. This is also true for extended thyroid tissue thermal ablation. Indeed, in patients with previous lobectomy, RFA does not affect blood thyroid hormone levels [33]. Similarly, the thyroid function of patients treated with RFA for bilateral benign nodules is also preserved [34]. We need to keep in mind that an ablated thyroid nodule becomes hypoechoic, inhomogeneous, and avascular on color Doppler ultrasonography [35]. Therefore, it is important not to confound a treated thyroid nodule with a thyroid cancer.

Ethanol ablation (EA) is the first-line treatment for benign, symptomatic, cystic (cystic portion >90 %) or predominantly cystic (cystic portion less than 90 % and greater than 50 %) thyroid nodules [36–38]. Notwithstanding, RFA is also effective in treating cystic or predominantly cystic thyroid nodules, but is more expensive than EA and requires more sessions [39–41]. Despite the effectiveness of EA, some patients may have unsatisfactory results, mostly because of the solid component of the nodule which does not respond to alcohol. In this case, RFA has been used successfully to solve persistent clinical problems after an EA session [42, 43].

36.2.6 Clinical Results in Benign Autonomous Functioning Thyroid Nodules

The first case report of the successful treatment of an autonomous functioning thyroid nodule (AFTN) was published in 2008 [44]. Subsequently, additional reports demonstrate that RFA is effective in patients with AFTNs since it reduces the nodule volume and controls hyperthyroidism [6, 8, 45]. RFA ablation of AFTNs requires a complete ablation, as untreated peripheral areas tend to regrow, causing relapse of hyperthyroidism. It has been shown that for the treatment of AFTNs more than one RFA session may be necessary. However, there are no studies comparing RFA to radioiodine for the treatment of AFTNs.

36.2.7 Clinical Results in Recurrent Thyroid Cancer

Occasionally well-differentiated thyroid cancer (DTC) may recur, mainly in the thyroid bed or in lymph nodes [46]. In this case, surgical removal is recommended, sometimes followed by radioiodine [38]. However, repeated neck dissection is difficult due to distortion of normal tissue planes by scar tissue formation, and such operations are associated with a higher rate of complications such as recurrent laryngeal nerve injury, hypoparathyroidism, and skin scar formation [47]. In 2001, RFA was proposed as a treatment for regional recurrence from DTC [48]. Subsequently, other studies have also confirmed the efficacy of RFA for treating thyroid cancer recurrences to cause volume reduction or complete disappearance of tumor in some cases, decrease of serum thyroglobulin concentrations, and improvement of clinical symptoms if present. The RFA technique used for the treatment of DTC recurrences is similar to that used for benign thyroid nodules, but has additional precautions. First, the lesion has to be confirmed to be malignant by US-guided FNA biopsy and FNA thyroglobulin measurement. Second, since these lesions are usually small, use of electrode needles with a shorter active tip (i.e., 0.5 or 0.7 cm) is generally more appropriate. RFA starts with low power (5 W) and the power is gradually increased until a hyperechoic area forms. Thermal damage to nerves, especially recurrent laryngeal nerve and vagus nerve, during RFA treatment is of more concern than damage to blood vessels, as blood flow within the vessels dissipates the heat (the so-called heat sink effect). On the other hand, there is the possibility that the heat sink effect might reduce RFA efficacy if treating lesions close to a large vessel (common carotid artery or internal jugular vein) because of the cooling effect of blood flow. In order to avoid thermal injury of neck nerves during RFA, sterile water or 5 % dextrose solution can be injected with a 23-gauge needle between the expected location of these vital structures and the tumor (hydrodissection technique). Thus, a protective barrier displaces the target from critical structures (not only nerves, but also trachea and esophagus). Saline solution is not recommended for hydrodissection in RFA because it conducts electricity. During hydrodissection technique, if a continuous infusion of fluid is deemed necessary, the tip of the hydrodissection needle should be placed at least 1 cm away from the tip of the RF applicator. Another strategy that prevents thermal injury is the use of the electrode needle as a lever to increase the distance between tumor and critical structures. Using this technique, tumor is pulled away from vital structures by tilting the electrode needle during ablation under continuous US guidance [49–56].

36.2.8 Complications of Thyroid Radiofrequency Ablation

Various complications may occur during thyroid RFA. A large multicenter Korean study reported an overall complication rate of 3.3 % associated with the RFA treatment of benign thyroid nodules [57]. In order to minimize complications, it is important to have a thorough knowledge of sonographic anatomy of the neck [58].

Intraoperative pain is usually well controlled by means of local anesthesia with ropivacaine and conscious sedation with midazolam [10]. Notwithstanding, in case of intense pain, local or radiating to the jaw, teeth, chest, or back, the RF generator is turned off. Subsequently, the electrode needle is repositioned in a more central area of the nodule and the ablation can proceed. Intranodular bleeding during needle insertion may occur and is seen as a rapidly expanding hypo/anechoic signal within nodular tissue. It can be stopped by swift needle-electrode insertion and heat administration. Intranodular bleeding does not prevent ablation procedure. Thyroid pericapsular bleeding is seen as a hypoechoic layer surrounding the thyroid. Pericapsular hematomas can be controlled by compression of the neck for a few minutes. Neck bruising may follow a few days later, and it disappears in about 3–4 weeks. A rarely reported complication is vasovagal reaction which presents with bradycardia, hypotension, vomiting and defecation. If this reaction is observed, the bed is tilted in Trendelenburg position and maneuvers are temporarily interrupted until spontaneous recovery, which occurs in a few minutes. Vasovagal syncope is due to vagus nerve stimulation as the nodule may displace the common carotid artery and the internal jugular vein. For this reason, knowledge of cervical vagus nerve localization is of paramount importance in thyroid RFA [59]. Cough during thermal ablation is due to trachea stimulation and the tip of the needle should be pulled back.

Nodule rupture presents with sudden neck bulging and pain during the early follow-up period (2–4 weeks) [60]. The rupture might occur due to volume expansion because of intranodular bleeding. An initial conservative treatment with compression is recommended. Another cause for tumor rupture may be liquefaction which occurs typically 2–4 weeks after RFA procedure. However, in case of deterioration of symptoms, drainage or excision may be required. Infection or abscess formation is rare, since the skin is sterilized with povidone–iodine solution. Skin burns have been reported at the electrode needle puncture site. Application of an ice bag during ablation or injection of fluid between the nodule and skin may prevent skin burns. Voice change is a serious complication of thyroid RFA which is due to thermal injury of the recurrent laryngeal nerve. This phenomenon may be prevented by undertreating the area near the danger triangle (i.e., the tracheoesophageal groove which contains the recurrent laryngeal nerve). Finally, RFA may cause the new appearance of thyroid antibodies (anti-thyroglobulin, anti-thyroid peroxidase, or anti-thyrotropin receptor antibodies), but no subsequent clinical consequences (hypothyroidism or hyperthyroidism) have been reported.

36.2.9 Comparison Between RFA and Other Nonsurgical Techniques for Benign Thyroid Nodules

There are no head-to-head comparisons between RFA and other US-guided nonsurgical techniques for the treatment of benign thyroid nodules. However, a recent systematic review including traditional pooling and Bayesian network meta-analysis found that RFA is superior to laser ablation in reducing benign solid thyroid nodule volume, despite the smaller number of treatment sessions without major side effects [61]. It is clear that interventional thyroidology, and especially RFA, is playing an increasing role in the management of thyroid nodule pathology [62].

36.3 High-Intensity Focus Ultrasound

36.3.1 Device and Technique

High intensity focused ultrasound (HIFU) ablation is an extracorporeal thermal treatment that is used in the endocrine neck diseases for treating benign thyroid nodules (cold or hot) and parathyroid adenomas or hyperplastic parathyroids since 2010. High intensity ultrasound beam, as opposed to the low energy field used for ultrasound imaging, when absorbed by tissue, creates a rise in temperatures (approximately 80–95 °C) with subsequent nodular coagulation and cavitation. The ultrasound beam

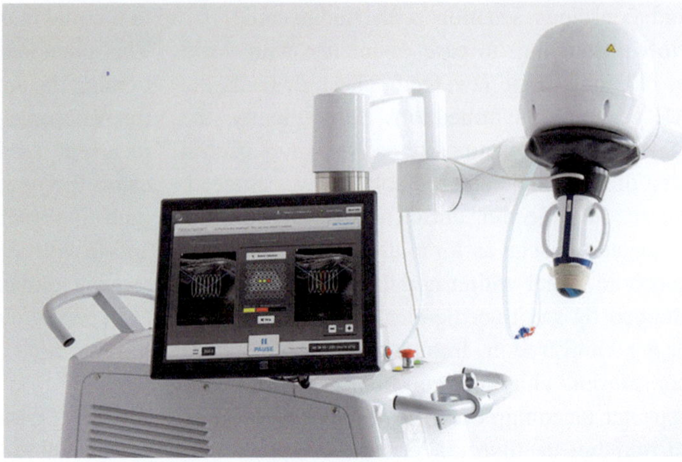

Fig. 36.5 The EchoPulse HIFU device is composed of an electronic mobile unit with energy generator, a robotic articulated arm with a visualization and treatment unit (VTU), and a touch-screen monitor for ablation planning and follow-up

is focused, and for this reason the tissue thermal injury is confined only to a well delimited area, minimizing the effects on surrounding structures. At the present time, the only available system for HIFU treatment of thyroid and parathyroid lesions is the EchoPulse (Theraclion, Paris, France). The EchoPulse device is composed of a mobile electronic unit with energy generator, a robotic articulated arm with a visualization and treatment unit (VTU) and a touch-screen monitor for ablation planning and follow-up (Fig. 36.5). The VTU contains both the ultrasound imaging transducer (7.5 MHz) and the HIFU transducer (3 MHz) for delivering the energy to the target (Fig. 36.6). A cooling circuit specific for the device lowers the temperature between consecutive pulses. The HIFU pulse produces an ablation area of 9 mm in length and a 2-mm diameter. After manually drawing the area to treat on the touch screen monitor, multiple pulses are automatically delivered to carry out the ablation. The safe margins of the treated area are 3 mm from trachea, 2 mm from carotid artery, and 5 mm from skin. The maximum treatable depth from the skin surface is 28 mm. The procedure is usually performed under conscious sedation and seldom local anesthesia is required.

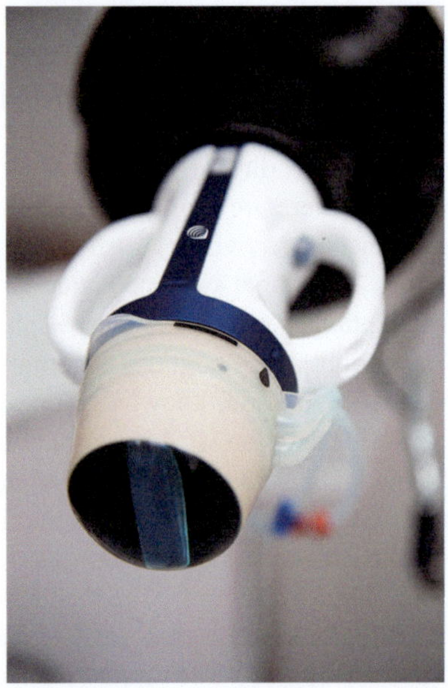

Fig. 36.6 The VTU contains both the ultrasound imaging transducer (7.5 MHz) and the HIFU transducer (3 MHz) for delivering the energy to the target. A cooling circuit specific for the device turns down temperature among consecutive pulses

36.4 Clinical Results

Initial HIFU experimental studies on animal thyroid ablation were published in 2004 [63] and 2009 [64]. The first case report of a successful

HIFU ablation of a human AFTN was published on 2010 [65]. Since then, a few studies of a relatively limited number of patients have assessed the HIFU treatment efficacy and safety profile for the ablation of cold and hot thyroid nodules [66–71] and of parathyroid lesions linked to primary and secondary hyperparathyroidism [72–75]. The results of these studies are encouraging, but the HIFU procedure still carries some limiting factors. The procedure is time consuming. The patient has to remain still during the entire ablation time since if he or she moves, the treatment planning has to be restarted from the beginning. In addition more treatments are necessary to treat large lesions and deep lesions cannot be ablated since the maximum treatable depth is only 28 mm from the skin. If there are skin scars or moles between the probe and the skin, HIFU ablation is not possible. Larger studies are needed to integrate HIFU ablation of neck diseases into clinical practice.

References

1. Baek JH, Lee JH, Valcavi R, Pacella CM, Rhim H, Na DG. Thermal ablation for benign thyroid nodules: radiofrequency and laser. Korean J Radiol. 2011;12(5):525–40.
2. Ha EJ, Baek JH, Lee JH. The efficacy and complications of radiofrequency ablation of thyroid nodules. Curr Opin Endocrinol Diabetes Obes. 2011;18(5):310–4.
3. Na DG, Lee JH, Jung SL, Kim JH, Sung JY, Shin JH, et al. Korean Society of Thyroid Radiology (KSThR); Korean Society of Radiology Radiofrequency ablation of benign thyroid nodules and recurrent thyroid cancers: consensus statement and recommendations. Korean J Radiol. 2012;13(2):117–25.
4. Garberoglio R, Aliberti C, Appetecchia M, Attard M, Boccuzzi G, Boraso F, et al. Radiofrequency ablation for thyroid nodules: which indications? The first Italian opinion statement. J Ultrasound. 2015;18(4):423–30.
5. Spiezia S, Garberoglio R, Di Somma C, Deandrea M, Basso E, Limone PP, et al. Efficacy and safety of radiofrequency thermal ablation in the treatment of thyroid nodules with pressure symptoms in elderly patients. J Am Geriatr Soc. 2007;55(9):1478–9.
6. Deandrea M, Limone P, Basso E, Mormile A, Ragazzoni F, Gamarra E, et al. US-guided percutaneous radiofrequency thermal ablation for the treatment of solid benign hyperfunctioning or compressive thyroid nodules. Ultrasound Med Biol. 2008;34(5):784–91.
7. Spiezia S, Garberoglio R, Milone F, Ramundo V, Caiazzo C, Assanti AP, et al. Thyroid nodules and related symptoms are stably controlled two years after radiofrequency thermal ablation. Thyroid. 2009;19(3):219–25.
8. Baek JH, Moon WJ, Kim YS, Lee JH, Lee D. Radiofrequency ablation for the treatment of autonomously functioning thyroid nodules. World J Surg. 2009;33(9):1971–7.
9. Shin JH, Baek JH, Ha EJ, Lee JH. Radiofrequency ablation of thyroid nodules: basic principles and clinical application. Int J Endocrinol. 2012;2012:919650.
10. Valcavi R, Tsamatropoulos P. Health-related quality of life after percutaneous radiofrequency ablation of cold, solid, benign thyroid nodules: a 2-year follow-up study in 40 patients. Endocr Pract. 2015;21(8):887–96.
11. Deandrea M, Sung JY, Limone P, Mormile A, Garino F, Ragazzoni F, et al. Efficacy and safety of radiofrequency ablation versus observation for nonfunctioning benign thyroid nodules: a randomized controlled international collaborative trial. Thyroid. 2015;25(8):890–6.
12. Yoon HM, Baek JH, Lee JH, Ha EJ, Kim JK, Yoon JH, et al. Combination therapy consisting of ethanol and radiofrequency ablation for predominantly cystic thyroid nodules. AJNR Am J Neuroradiol. 2014;35(3):582–6.
13. Cibas ES, Ali SZ. NCI Thyroid FNA State of the Science Conference. the Bethesda system for reporting thyroid cytopathology. Am J Clin Pathol. 2009;132(5):658–65.
14. Kim HS, Choi BH, Park JR, Hahm JR, Jung JH, Kim SK, et al. Delayed surgery for parathyroid adenoma misdiagnosed as a thyroid nodule and treated with radiofrequency ablation. Endocrinol Metab (Seoul). 2013;28(3):231–5.
15. Xu SY, Wang Y, Xie Q, Wu HY. Percutaneous sonography guided radiofrequency ablation in the management of parathyroid adenoma. Singapore Med J. 2013;54(7):e137–40.
16. Carrafiello G, Laganà D, Mangini M, Dionigi G, Rovera F, Carcano G, et al. Treatment of secondary hyperparathyroidism with ultrasonographically guided percutaneous radiofrequency thermoablation. Surg Laparosc Endosc Percutan Tech. 2006;16(2):112–6.
17. Kim YS, Rhim H, Tae K, Park DW, Kim ST. Radiofrequency ablation of benign cold thyroid nodules: initial clinical experience. Thyroid. 2006;16(4):361–7.
18. Fuller CW, Nguyen SA, Lohia S, Gillespie MB. Radiofrequency ablation for treatment of benign thyroid nodules: systematic review. Laryngoscope. 2014;124(1):346–53.

19. Bandeira-Echtler E, Bergerhoff K, Richter B. Levothyroxine or minimally invasive therapies for benign thyroid nodules. Cochrane Database Syst Rev. 2014;(6):CD004098.
20. Bernardi S, Dobrinja C, Fabris B, Bazzocchi G, Sabato N, Ulcigrai V, et al. Radiofrequency ablation compared to surgery for the treatment of benign thyroid nodules. Int J Endocrinol. 2014;2014:934595.
21. Che Y, Jin S, Shi C, Wang L, Zhang X, Li Y, Baek JH. Treatment of benign thyroid nodules: comparison of surgery with radiofrequency ablation. AJNR Am J Neuroradiol. 2015;36(7):1321–5.
22. Baek JH, Kim YS, Lee D, Huh JY, Lee JH. Benign predominantly solid thyroid nodules: prospective study of efficacy of sonographically guided radiofrequency ablation versus control condition. AJR Am J Roentgenol. 2010;194(4):1137–42.
23. Faggiano A, Ramundo V, Assanti AP, Fonderico F, Macchia PE, Misso C, et al. Thyroid nodules treated with percutaneous radiofrequency thermal ablation: a comparative study. J Clin Endocrinol Metab. 2012;97(12):4439–45.
24. Wong KP, Lang BH. Use of radiofrequency ablation in benign thyroid nodules: a literature review and updates. Int J Endocrinol. 2013;2013:428363.
25. Turtulici G, Orlandi D, Corazza A, Sartoris R, Derchi LE, Silvestri E, et al. Percutaneous radiofrequency ablation of benign thyroid nodules assisted by a virtual needle tracking system. Ultrasound Med Biol. 2014;40(7):1447–52.
26. Cesareo R, Pasqualini V, Simeoni C, Sacchi M, Saralli E, Campagna G, et al. Prospective study of effectiveness of ultrasound-guided radiofrequency ablation versus control group in patients affected by benign thyroid nodules. J Clin Endocrinol Metab. 2015;100(2):460–6.
27. Ugurlu MU, Uprak K, Akpinar IN, Attaallah W, Yegen C, Gulluoglu BM. Radiofrequency ablation of benign symptomatic thyroid nodules: prospective safety and efficacy study. World J Surg. 2015;39(4):961–8.
28. De Bernardi IC, Floridi C, Muollo A, Giacchero R, Dionigi GL, Reginelli A, et al. Vascular and interventional radiology radiofrequency ablation of benign thyroid nodules and recurrent thyroid cancers: literature review. Radiol Med. 2014;119(7):512–20.
29. Jeong WK, Baek JH, Rhim H, Kim YS, Kwak MS, Jeong HJ, et al. Radiofrequency ablation of benign thyroid nodules: safety and imaging follow-up in 236 patients. Eur Radiol. 2008;18(6):1244–50.
30. Huh JY, Baek JH, Choi H, Kim JK, Lee JH. Symptomatic benign thyroid nodules: efficacy of additional radiofrequency ablation treatment session-Prospective randomized study. Radiology. 2012;263(3):909–16.
31. Lim HK, Lee JH, Ha EJ, Sung JY, Kim JK, Baek JH. Radiofrequency ablation of benign non-functioning thyroid nodules: 4-year follow-up results for 111 patients. Eur Radiol. 2013;23(4):1044–9.
32. Dobrinja C, Bernardi S, Fabris B, Eramo R, Makovac P, Bazzocchi G, et al. Surgical and pathological changes after radiofrequency ablation of thyroid nodules. Int J Endocrinol. 2015;2015:576576.
33. Ha EJ, Baek JH, Lee JH, Sung JY, Lee D, Kim JK, et al. Radiofrequency ablation of benign thyroid nodules does not affect thyroid function in patients with previous lobectomy. Thyroid. 2013;23(3): 289–93.
34. Ji Hong M, Baek JH, Choi YJ, Lee JH, Lim HK, Shong YK, et al. Radiofrequency ablation is a thyroid function-preserving treatment for patients with bilateral benign thyroid nodules. J Vasc Interv Radiol. 2015;26(1):55–61.
35. Andrioli M, Valcavi R. The peculiar ultrasonographic and elastographic features of thyroid nodules after treatment with laser or radiofrequency: similarities and differences. Endocrine. 2014;47(3):967–8.
36. Valcavi R, Frasoldati A. Ultrasound-guided percutaneous ethanol injection therapy in thyroid cystic nodules. Endocr Pract. 2004;10(3):269–75.
37. Gharib H, Papini E, Paschke R, Duick DS, Valcavi R, Hegedüs L, et al. AACE/AME/ETA Task Force on Thyroid Nodules. American Association of Clinical Endocrinologists, Associazione Medici Endocrinologi, and European Thyroid Association Medical Guidelines for clinical practice for the diagnosis and management of thyroid nodules. Endocr Pract. 2010;16 Suppl 1:1–43.
38. Haugen BR, Alexander EK, Bible KC, Doherty G, Mandel SJ, Nikiforov YE, et al. 2015 American Thyroid Association Management Guidelines for adult patients with thyroid nodules and differentiated thyroid cancer. Thyroid. 2016;26:1.
39. Sung JY, Kim YS, Choi H, Lee JH, Baek JH. Optimum first-line treatment technique for benign cystic thyroid nodules: ethanol ablation or radiofrequency ablation? AJR Am J Roentgenol. 2011;196(2):W210–4.
40. Sung JY, Baek JH, Kim KS, Lee D, Yoo H, Kim JK, Park SH. Single-session treatment of benign cystic thyroid nodules with ethanol versus radiofrequency ablation: a prospective randomized study. Radiology. 2013;269(1):293–300.
41. Baek JH, Ha EJ, Choi YJ, Sung JY, Kim JK, Shong YK. Radiofrequency versus ethanol ablation for treating predominantly cystic thyroid nodules: a randomized clinical trial. Korean J Radiol. 2015;16(6):1332–40.
42. Lee JH, Kim YS, Lee D, Choi H, Yoo H, Baek JH. Radiofrequency ablation (RFA) of benign thyroid nodules in patients with incompletely resolved clinical problems after ethanol ablation (EA). World J Surg. 2010;34(7):1488–93.
43. Jang SW, Baek JH, Kim JK, Sung JY, Choi H, Lim HK, et al. How to manage the patients with unsatisfactory results after ethanol ablation for thyroid nodules: role of radiofrequency ablation. Eur J Radiol. 2012;81(5):905–10.

44. Baek JH, Jeong HJ, Kim YS, Kwak MS, Lee D. Radiofrequency ablation for an autonomously functioning thyroid nodule. Thyroid. 2008;18(6):675–6.
45. Sung JY, Baek JH, Jung SL, Kim JH, Kim KS, Lee D, et al. Radiofrequency ablation for autonomously functioning thyroid nodules: a multicenter study. Thyroid. 2015;25(1):112–7.
46. Durante C, Montesano T, Torlontano M, Attard M, Monzani F, Tumino S, et al. Papillary thyroid cancer: time course of recurrences during post surgery surveillance. Clin Endocrinol Metab. 2013;98(2):636–42.
47. Samaan NA, Schultz PN, Hickey RC, Goepfert H, Haynie TP, Johnston DA, et al. The results of various modalities of treatment of well differentiated thyroid carcinomas: a retrospective review of 1599 patients. J Clin Endocrinol Metab. 1992;75(3):714–20.
48. Dupuy DE, Monchik JM, Decrea C, Pisharodi L. Radiofrequency ablation of regional recurrence from well-differentiated thyroid malignancy. Surgery. 2001;130(6):971–7.
49. Monchik JM, Donatini G, Iannuccilli J, Dupuy DE. Radiofrequency ablation and percutaneous ethanol injection treatment for recurrent local and distant well-differentiated thyroid carcinoma. Ann Surg. 2006;244(2):296–304.
50. Baek JH, Kim YS, Sung JY, Choi H, Lee JH. Locoregional control of metastatic well-differentiated thyroid cancer by ultrasound-guided radiofrequency ablation. AJR Am J Roentgenol. 2011;197(2):W331–6.
51. Park KW, Shin JH, Han BK, Ko EY, Chung JH. Inoperable symptomatic recurrent thyroid cancers: preliminary result of radiofrequency ablation. Ann Surg Oncol. 2011;18(9):2564–8.
52. Shin JE, Baek JH, Lee JH. Radiofrequency and ethanol ablation for the treatment of recurrent thyroid cancers: current status and challenges. Curr Opin Oncol. 2013;25(1):14–9.
53. Lee SJ, Jung SL, Kim BS, Ahn KJ, Choi HS, Lim DJ, et al. Radiofrequency ablation to treat loco-regional recurrence of well-differentiated thyroid carcinoma. Korean J Radiol. 2014;15(6):817–26.
54. Wang L, Ge M, Xu D, Chen L, Qian C, Shi K, et al. Ultrasonography-guided percutaneous radiofrequency ablation for cervical lymph node metastasis from thyroid carcinoma. J Cancer Res Ther. 2014;10(Suppl):C144–9.
55. Lim HK, Baek JH, Lee JH, Kim WB, Kim TY, Shong YK, et al. Efficacy and safety of radiofrequency ablation for treating locoregional recurrence from papillary thyroid cancer. Eur Radiol. 2015;25(1):163–70.
56. Kim JH, Yoo WS, Park YJ, Park DJ, Yun TJ, Choi SH, et al. Efficacy and safety of radiofrequency ablation for treatment of locally recurrent thyroid cancers smaller than 2 cm. Radiology. 2015;276(3):909–18.
57. Baek JH, Lee JH, Sung JY, Bae JI, Kim KT, Sim J, et al. Korean Society of Thyroid Radiology. Complications encountered in the treatment of benign thyroid nodules with US-guided radiofrequency ablation: a multicenter study. Radiology. 2012;262(1):335–42.
58. Ha EJ, Baek JH, Lee JH. Ultrasonography-based thyroidal and perithyroidal anatomy and its clinical significance. Korean J Radiol. 2015;16(4):749–66.
59. Ha EJ, Baek JH, Lee JH, Kim JK, Shong YK. Clinical significance of vagus nerve variation in radiofrequency ablation of thyroid nodules. Eur Radiol. 2011;21(10):2151–7.
60. Shin JH, Jung SL, Baek JH, Kim JH. Rupture of benign thyroid tumors after radio-frequency ablation. AJNR Am J Neuroradiol. 2011;32(11):2165–9.
61. Ha EJ, Baek JH, Kim KW, Pyo J, Lee JH, Baek SH, et al. Comparative efficacy of radiofrequency and laser ablation for the treatment of benign thyroid nodules: systematic review including traditional pooling and Bayesian network meta-analysis. J Clin Endocrinol Metab. 2015;100(5):1903–11.
62. Lupo MA. Radiofrequency ablation for benign thyroid nodules - a look towards the future of interventional thyroidology. Endocr Pract. 2015;21(8):972–4.
63. Esnault O, Franc B, Monteil JP, Chapelon JY. High-intensity focused ultrasound for localized thyroid-tissue ablation: preliminary experimental animal study. Thyroid. 2004;14(12):1072–6.
64. Esnault O, Franc B, Chapelon YJ. Localized ablation of thyroid tissue by high-intensity focused ultrasound: improvement of noninvasive tissue necrosis methods. Thyroid. 2009;19(10):1085–91.
65. Esnault O, Rouxel A, Le Nestour E, Gheron G, Leenhardt L. Minimally invasive ablation of a toxic thyroid nodule by high-intensity focused ultrasound. AJNR Am J Neuroradiol. 2010;31(10):1967–8.
66. Esnault O, Franc B, Ménégaux F, Rouxel A, De Kerviler E, Bourrier P, et al. High-intensity focused ultrasound ablation of thyroid nodules: first human feasibility study. Thyroid. 2011;21(9):965–73.
67. Korkusuz H, Fehre N, Sennert M, Happel C, Grünwald F. Early assessment of high-intensity focused ultrasound treatment of benign thyroid nodules by scintigraphic means. J Ther Ultrasound. 2014;2:18.
68. Korkusuz H, Sennert M, Fehre N, Happel C, Grünwald F. Local thyroid tissue ablation by high-intensity focused ultrasound: effects on thyroid function and first human feasibility study with hot and cold thyroid nodules. Int J Hyperthermia. 2014;30(7):480–5.
69. Korkusuz H, Fehre N, Sennert M, Happel C, Grünwald F. Volume reduction of benign thyroid nodules 3 months after a single treatment with high-intensity focused ultrasound (HIFU). J Ther Ultrasound. 2015;3:4.
70. Korkusuz H, Sennert M, Fehre N, Happel C, Grünwald F. Localized thyroid tissue ablation by high intensity focused ultrasound: volume reduction, effects on thyroid function and immune response. Röfo. 2015;187(11):1011–5.
71. Kovatcheva RD, Vlahov JD, Stoinov JI, Zaletel K. Benign solid thyroid nodules: US-guided

high-intensity focused ultrasound ablation-initial clinical outcomes. Radiology. 2015;276(2):597–605.
72. Kovatcheva RD, Vlahov JD, Shinkov AD, Borissova AM, Hwang JH, Arnaud F, et al. High-intensity focused ultrasound to treat primary hyperparathyroidism: a feasibility study in four patients. AJR Am J Roentgenol. 2010;195(4):830–5.
73. Kovatcheva RD, Vlahov JD, Stoinov JI, Kirilov GG, Krivoshiev SG, Arnaud F, et al. High-intensity focussed ultrasound (HIFU) treatment in uraemic secondary hyperparathyroidism. Nephrol Dial Transplant. 2012;27(1):76–80.
74. Kovatcheva R, Vlahov J, Stoinov J, Lacoste F, Ortuno C, Zaletel K. US-guided high-intensity focused ultrasound as a promising non-invasive method for treatment of primary hyperparathyroidism. Eur Radiol. 2014;24(9):2052–8.
75. Ambrosini CE, Cianferotti L, Picone A, Torregrossa L, Segnini G, Frustaci G, Cetani F, Basolo F, Marcocci C, Miccoli P. High-intensity focused ultrasound as an alternative to the surgical approach in primary hyperparathyroidism: a preliminary experience. J Endocrinol Invest. 2011;34(9):655–9.

37 Ultrasound-Guided Laser Ablation

Claudio Maurizio Pacella and Enrico Papini

37.1 Introduction

The use of laser energy was first proposed in 1983 for the treatment of tumors [1] and later, in the 1990s for the nonsurgical management of benign symptomatic thyroid nodules [2–4]. Ultrasound-guided percutaneous laser ablation is now an evaluated and accepted minimally invasive procedure in several thyroid referral centers for the treatment of selected patients with thyroid lesions.

37.2 Why Ultrasound-Guided Laser Ablation for Thyroid Nodules?

Thyroid nodules are a clinical finding frequently encountered in clinical practice. Solid or cystic thyroid lesions are revealed by ultrasound (US) evaluation in 20–70 % of the general population [5–11], with a prevalence that is now similar to that formerly described at post-mortem assessment [12]. Most of these lesions are clinically insignificant because they are benign, small and unchanging over time [13]. A minority of them, from 15 to 20 %, progressively increase in size and some may induce pressure symptoms, concern and, finally, surgical consultation as no useful medical treatment can be presently offered [14, 15]. However, the expenses related to thyroid surgery, the risk of surgical complications, and the consequences on the quality of life should be carefully considered when this widespread clinical problem is approached [16, 17]. Patients' quality of life may be adversely influenced by the permanent requirement of thyroid hormone and/or calcium substitution therapy, and by cervical cosmetic damage [17]. Due to these reasons, nonsurgical image-guided ablation techniques have been extensively investigated over the last two decades and are now increasingly used for the management of symptomatic benign thyroid nodules [18].

Electronic supplementary material: The online version of this chapter (doi:10.1007/978-3-319-44100-9_37) contains supplementary material, which is available to authorized users. Videos can also be accessed at http://link.springer.com/chapter/10.1007/978-3-319-44100-9_37.

C.M. Pacella, M.D. (✉)
Department of Diagnostic Imaging and Interventional Radiology, Regina Apostolorum Hospital, Via San Francesco, 50, Albano Laziale, Rome 00041, Italy
e-mail: claudiomauriziopacella@gmail.com

E. Papini
Department of Endocrinology and Metabolism, Regina Apostolorum Hospital, Albano Laziale, Rome, Italy
e-mail: papinie@gmail.com

M. Milas et al. (eds.), *Advanced Thyroid and Parathyroid Ultrasound*,
DOI 10.1007/978-3-319-44100-9_37

37.3 Minimally Invasive Techniques

Minimally invasive image-guided percutaneous techniques are used for the treatment of selected focal malignancies in various organs [19]. Numerous studies over the last two decades have defined the basic principles of ablative therapies and research is currently focused on new devices especially suited for energy delivery to specific tumors [20]. Various modalities for minimally invasive treatment, directed at the ablation of the target lesion with the smallest damage to the surrounding tissues, and without necessity of general anesthesia are currently available. Among them, thermal ablation procedures appear as the most thoroughly evaluated, widely used and easiest to master. Either US or computed tomography (CT) or magnetic resonance imaging (MRI) may be employed to guide the proper placement of applicators and to monitor the progression of the coagulation zone during ablation [20].

37.4 Basic Principles

Laser light ("light amplification by stimulated emission of radiation") is coherent and monochromatic may be carefully focused and allows the transmission of a considerable quantity of energy at long distance. Laser light may be transmitted from the source to the target tissue through an "optical fiber," which consists of a silica-based core with a surrounding cladding also made of silica or a hard polymer material. These flexible optical fibers are 400–600 μm in diameter and convey laser light to the tip of the fiber optic, which is directly inserted into the tissue to be treated. So laser light is a fast-delivered, precise, and relatively tissue-insensitive energy [20–22]. When laser light interacts with biological tissues, scattering and absorption occur, followed by thermal injury [21].

A variety of laser sources and wavelengths are available and different types of fibers, modified tips, and applicators can be used. Nd:YAG lasers, operating at 1064 nm, seem most suited for procedures in deep-seated organs because of their superior penetration and absorption properties in perfused soft tissues. Currently, the majority of laser procedures use either Nd:YAG or diode lasers ($\lambda = 800–980$ nm) operating in the range of 2–40 W.

Thermal ablation destroys the tissues by increasing their temperature so as to induce irreversible cellular damage. Complete destruction by thermal ablation requires that the entire target lesion, ideally including an additional 0.5–1.0-cm safety margin (ablative margin) of normal surrounding parenchyma, is subjected to cytotoxic temperatures: "The extent of coagulation zone induced in a lesion is equal to the energy deposited, modified by local tissue interactions, minus the heat lost before inducing thermal damage"[23]. However, achievement of an elevated mean temperature within the lesion, may not result in a complete destruction of a tumor due to some heterogeneity of heating throughout the different areas of the volume subjected to the procedure.

With a temperature increase to approximately 40 °C, cellular homeostasis is usually not affected. When the temperature level arrives at 42–45 °C (hyperthermia), the cells become susceptible to damage induced by various agents (e.g., irradiation or chemotherapy) [24]. At these temperatures, however, cell function and tumor growth may endure even after a protracted exposure [23, 25–28]. Irreversible cellular damage occurs only when cells are heated to 46 °C for 60 min, and the injury takes place with increasing rapidity as the temperature level rises [29, 30]. When temperature is increased to between 60 and 100 °C, there is a fast coagulation of the proteins that permanently injuries cytosolic and mitochondrial enzymes and nucleic acid proteins. As this damage causes cellular death over the course of several days [26, 31–38] an early (24 h) post-treatment percutaneous biopsy will provide an adequate assessment of the ablation. Critical temperature at the edge of the coagulative zone has been shown to range from 30 to 77 °C for normal tissue and from 41 to 64 °C for neoplastic tissues [39–41], with relevant variation of the thermal dose required to induce cell death in different tissues [39]. On the basis of an experimental study [30] that demonstrated tissue coagulation after tissue heating to approximately 50 °C for less than 5 min, these parameters are used as the standard surrogate endpoint for thermal ablation therapies in current clinical paradigms. Finally, temperatures over 105–110 °C induce tissue carbonization and vaporization. These changes may hamper a complete ablation because of an insulating effect on energy diffusion in radiofrequency (RF) or LA-based systems [30, 42–45]. In microwave systems, on the other hand, high-grade temperatures do not interfere with the deposition of energy, although microwave energy is inherently more difficult to distribute than laser or RF energy.

37.5 Technique and Devices

Treatment algorithms and laser equipment differs among centers. The laser source is either a continuous diode laser of varying power and wavelength [46–59] or a continuous wave Nd:YAG laser with optical fibers and applicators of different gauge [60–69]. Operators may insert the applicator(s) in the appropriate area of the targeted lesion and terminate the procedure when the area of echogenicity (identifiable by "white spots" caused by evaporation), generated by energy delivery, is stationary in size [49, 54–59]. The energy may be also delivered continuously while retracting the applicators [47, 70]. The most frequently used laser is continuous wave Nd:YAG 1064 nm with an output power of 3–5 W and flat-tipped quartz fibers of 300 μm. Energy is directed towards the tissue using a 21 G needle [61]. LA sessions may be performed either under US guidance (US-g) or assistance using a commercially available US system equipped with a high-frequency linear transducer (7.5–15 MHz).

The patient is placed on an operating table in the supine position with hyperextended neck. The majority of operators perform the treatment after local anesthesia, both at the entry site and on the thyroid capsule, and under conscious sedation. Under US-guidance, the introducer needles are inserted into the target thyroid nodule along its longest axis. Treatments are preferentially performed with a fixed-power protocol (usually 3 W) while the illumination time changes case by case. Each illumination time ranges from a minimum of 400 s to a maximum of 600 s to deliver a total energy from 1200 to 1800 J per fiber. The use of thin (<1 mm in diameter) needles, positioned on planes as parallel as possible to the horizontal plane of the nodule, permits the safe positioning of one or more needles depending on the size, shape, and location of the nodule. The applicators, when multiple, must be inserted one at a time, spaced least 0.8 cm apart and next to each other on the same plane. Placement on the same plane allows simultaneous monitoring in real time (see Video 37.1 included). The tip of the optical fiber should be positioned at a safety distance of 10–15 mm from the critical structures of the neck, such as the epiaortic vessels and the trachea, and this safety criterion should be carefully checked by means of biplanar ultrasound imaging. Depending on the size of the nodule, from one to three consecutive illuminations are performed with a "pullback" technique during the same treatment session. A reliable assessment of the actual extent of the ablated area is obtained a few hours after treatment, when the hyperechoic spots due to gas microbubbles within the tissue are disappeared, with the intravenous injection of a second-generation ultrasound contrast medium (SonoVue, Bracco, Italy). The area of coagulative necrosis achieves its maximum extension 72 h after treatment [71] because the cellular injury and the microvascular occlusion of the vessels that supply the tissue progress during the days following the procedure.

37.6 Indications for Laser Treatment

Laser treatment for nodule volume reduction should be considered if all the following conditions are met: (a) evidence at ultrasound examination of a single nodule or of a dominant lesion clearly detectable in a multinodular goiter; (b) hypo- ("cold") or iso- ("warm") active appearance at radioisotope thyroid scintiscan; (c) serum TSH and thyroid hormones within normal range; (d) two benign cytological diagnoses (class II of the Bethesda classification system) [72] obtained by ultrasound guided fine-needle aspiration performed within the last 6 months; (e) presence of either local pressure symptoms or cosmetic concern.

For an optimal treatment, nodules to be ablated should be solid or nearly completely solid, with a <20 % cystic component. Solid lesions with a large fluid component should be evaluated case by case by the operator, who may aspirate the fluid component immediately before the laser treatment of the remaining solid parenchyma [59] or may perform the procedure after a few weeks, following the liquid drainage and the percutaneous ethanol injection of the cystic component.

Anticoagulant or antiplatelet therapy should be stopped for 72 h prior to the procedure. Routine coagulation tests, including prothrombin time, partial thromboplastin time, and complete blood cell count, should be anyway performed before the procedure. We also recommend that patients should undergo a pre procedure direct laryngoscopy.

The risk of overlooking a thyroid malignancy should be carefully assessed. Subjects with a family history of thyroid cancer and those who have undergone previous neck radiation therapy for any reason should have a careful sonographic examination to identify high suspicion thyroid nodules. The presence of suspicious US findings is a partial contraindication to laser ablation even in case of benign cytological findings. Finally, the patient should be informed that regular US follow-up is recommended even after a successful minimally invasive treatment and the disappearance of local symptoms.

37.7 Clinical Results

37.7.1 Hypo- or Iso-functioning Thyroid Nodules

After a series of preliminary in vivo studies on animal models [33] and ex-vivo tests on resected thyroid glands [4], the initial feasibility study in humans on the use of image-guided percutaneous thermal ablation for the treatment of thyroid nodules was published in 2000 [4]. Since then, numerous case reports [48, 55], non-randomized series [47, 49, 54, 60, 61, 65, 66], and randomized cohort studies [57, 63, 64, 67] have validated on the clinical use of US-guided laser ablation. Even though the treatment plan and the equipment differ in the various centers, this large body of data has established the clinical effectiveness and substantial safety of laser thermal ablation for thyroid lesions. The range of reported volume reductions ranges from 43 to 84 % [64, 68] at 1 year (Table 37.1), while follow-up studies at three [66] and 5 years [58] report a persistent mean nodule volume decrease of 48 % and 51 %, respectively. A recent multicenter prospective randomized trial, performed with a single ablation session and fixed treatment parameters, demonstrated nodule volume reduction ranging from 49 to 60 % 36 months after a single LA session [67]. Of note, only 9 % of these patients showed an initial regrowth after 3 years after treatment [66]. Moreover, the majority of LA-treated patients reported a significant and persistent improvement in their local pressure symptoms or discomfort using a visual-analogue questionnaire [57, 58, 64, 67].

Finally, in 2015, an externally monitored multicenter retrospective study of 1531 patients confirmed both the efficacy and the safety in clinical practice of the multiple thin needle ablation technique [2, 3] for the nonsurgical management of benign symptomatic thyroid nodules. Because this population included those who both received multiple treatments for large nodules and had complex lesions, the results demonstrated an up to 80 % decrease of thyroid nodules.

The histopathologic changes on the basis of nodule shrinkage in humans are the same as in experimental models [4]. Cytological and histological samples obtained in 15 cold thyroid nodules 12 months after multiple LA procedures demonstrated coagulative necrosis, degenerative changes, and signs of inflammatory reaction in the ablated areas [73]. No malignant change has been reported even in nodules resected 24 months after laser ablation [53].

Table 37.1 Clinical outcomes of patients with symptomatic benign thyroid cold nodules treated with laser ablation (major series)

	Pts/Nodules		US pattern	Baseline Vol		Energy load	Number of		Volume reduction
Author	no.	RCT	solid-cystic[a]	mL (mean)	Laser source	Joules/mL (mean)	sessions (mean)	FU month	% (mean)
Dossing et al.	16		solid	10.0	820 diode	761 (median)	1	6	46
Spiezia et al.	5		solid	11.1	Nd:YAG	2.2	12	61	
Pacella et al.	8		solid	22.7	Nd:YAG	788	4.1	6	63
Papini et al.	20		solid	24.1	Nd:YAG	300	2.2	6	64
Dossing et al.	15 vs 15	yes	solid	8.2	820 diode	224 (median)	1	6	44 (median)
Dossing et al.	10		cystic-solid	9.6	820 diode	254 (median)	1	12	57
Amabile et al.	23		solid	15.0	980 diode	33	1.2	3	36
Dossing et al.	15 vs 15[b]	yes	solid	10.1/10.7	820 diode	262 vs 412	1	6	45 vs 58 (median)
Gambelunghe et al.	13 vs 13	yes	solid	8.2	Nd:YAG	1900 (median)	1	30 weeks	44
Cakir et al.	12/15		solid	11.9	810 diode	2726	1.5	12	82
Papini et al.	21 vs 21 vs 20[c]	yes	solid	11.7/13.6/12.1	Nd:YAG	1221	1	12	>40
Valcavi et al.	119		solid	24.8	Nd:YAG	1	12	56	
Valcavi et al.	122[d]		solid	23.1	Nd:YAG	484 (median)	1	36	48
Dossing et al.	78	yes	solid	8.2	820 diode	242 (median)	1	67	51 (median)
Amabile et al.	51[e]		solid	53.5	980 diode	391	3.2 cycle	12	81
Gambelunghe et al.	20/20[f]		solid	15/14	Nd:YAG	71/579 (median)	1	36	+11/57
Gambelunghe et al.	50/50[l]		solid	21/21	Nd:YAG	502/499	1	6	55/56 (median)
Papini et al.	101/99	yes	solid	12	Nd:YAG	—	1	36	57
Achille et al.	45		solid	24	Nd:YAG	—	1	12	84
Pacella et al.	1531/1534		solid	27	Nd:YAG	—	1.2	12	72

Pts = Patients

[a]Uniformly solid or predominantly solid with not more than 20 % fluid component

[b]One laser session vs three laser sessions

[c]Pts treated with laser energy vs patients treated with L-T4 or no treated

[d]The energy was delivered continuously while retracting the applicators in a single session

[e]The energy was delivered continuously while extracting the needle in multiple sessions

[f]Retrospective comparison between a group treated with low amount of energy and one treated with a high amount of energy

[l]Retrospective comparison between patients treated with local anesthetic and patients treated without local anesthetic

37.7.2 Hyper-Functioning Thyroid Nodules

Reports evaluating the efficacy of LA for therapy of hyperthyroidism due to hyperfunctioning nodules have less consistent results. A few small series of hyper-functioning thyroid nodules treated with laser ablation report normalization of thyroid function and the resolution of the previously hyperfunctioning area at post-treatment radioisotope scan [50, 55, 60]. Others demonstrated that LA was not invariably effective, and that multiple LA sessions were required to normalize TSH levels [48, 61, 74]. Finally, a randomized trial on 30 solitary hot nodules with extraglandular suppression, treated either with a single LA session or one radioiodine dose, demonstrated that LA and ^{131}I therapy had a similar effect on nodule volume reduction. However in contrast to ^{131}I, LA was less likely to results in a normal serum TSH (only 50 % of patients) [75]. Overall, these results demonstrate the effectiveness of LA when treating small, solitary and mildly hyperfunctioning nodules [65, 74]. In toxic nodular goiters or large autonomously functioning thyroid nodules, LA therapy results are more inconsistent and the normalization of thyroid function usually requires repeated treatment sessions [48] (Table 37.2). A recent pilot study [76] compared outcomes in patients large toxic nodules treated with LA followed by ^{131}I with those treated by ^{131}I only, and demonstrated that combined treatment induced a more rapid and substantial improvement in local and systemic symptoms compared to ^{131}I only. In addition, for three patients, no ^{131}I treatment was needed after LA. This approach seems a possible alternative to thyroidectomy in patients who refuse surgery.

37.7.3 Cystic Lesions

In a recent report, 44 subjects with predominantly cystic thyroid nodules were randomly assigned to aspiration alone or to fluid drainage immediately followed by laser ablation [59]. At 6 month follow-up, both clinically significant volume decrease and improvement of local symptoms were observed in 15 of 22 (68 %) of cases in the thermal ablation group compared to only 4 of 22 (18 %) cases in the fluid drainage group. Laser ablation significant decreased the solid component of the cystic lesion (from 1.8 to 1.0 mL), while in the drainage alone group, the solid part was not reduced. No side effects were reported and thyroid function was maintained.

Even if the outcomes of laser ablation for cystic nodules are favorable, percutaneous ethanol injection still remains the first-line minimally invasive treatment for predominantly cystic lesions due to its low cost, safety, and easiness [77]. Laser ablation should be considered only for the management of complex lesions with a relevant solid component because it will both prevent fluid recurrence and reduce of the solid part of the nodule.

37.8 Complications and Side Effects

Laser ablation is a fairly well tolerated procedure. Mild to moderate cervical pain, minor neck swelling and a low-grade fever may occur after treatment and commonly last 1 or 2 days. These side effects may be controlled with the oral administration of acetaminophen.

Minor complications are infrequent and include persistent cervical pain that radiates to the ear, lower jaw or chest that does not dissipate after the laser ablation procedure. Pain subsides spontaneously but may last up to 24 h is done [61, 62]. Subcapsular hematoma and skin burns are extremely rare [52, 69]. Severe neck swelling due to subcutaneous edema, and cystic transformation have been occasionally reported [66]. The occurrence of transitory hyperthyroidism or late hypothyroidism is rare in patients with normal thyroid function [66].

Clinically significant damage or fibrosis have not been reported in the tissues contiguous to the area of treatment in subjects who subsequently underwent thyroidectomy because of unrelated problems [53, 73]. A single case of damage to the trachea wall was caused by the erroneous placing of the optical fiber by an inexperienced operator and required a surgical repair after 1 month [78].

Table 37.2 Clinical outcomes of patients with symptomatic benign hot thyroid nodules treated with laser ablation (major series)

Author	Nodules	RCT	US pattern	Baseline Vol	Laser source	Total Energy load or	Number of sessions	FU	Volume Reduction	TSH changes	Hormones changes
		No.		mL (mean)		Joules/mL (mean)	(mean)	moth	% (mean)	(%)*	(%)*
Dossing et al.	1		solid	8.2	820 diode	1950	1	9	40	N^a	N^a
Spiezia et al.	7		solid	3.2	Nd:YAG		1	12	74	N^b	7/7 (100)
Pacella et al.	16		solid	7.9	Nd:YAG	816 (J/mL)	2.7	6	62	5/16 (31) 5/16 (31)	
Gambelunghe et al.	13		solid	8.2	Nd:YAG	1900 (J/mL)	1	30 weeks	44	13/13 (100)	13/13 (100)
Barbaro et al.	18		solid	21.1	Nd:YAG		3	12	59	N^c	
Dossing et al.	14 vs 15	yes**	solid	10.6/11.2	820 diode	217 (J/mL)	1	6	44/47	7/14–15/15 (50–100)	
Valcavi et al.	1		solid	2.5	Nd:YAG		1	—	95	N^d	N^d
Rotondi et al.	1		solid	55.0	980 diode		4	10	91	N^e	N^e
Amabile et al.	26		solid	55.3	980 diode	379 (J/mL)	3.2 cycle	12	82	23/26 (88)	—

No. = nodules numbers; * = Improvement rate (%); N^a = Normalization of serum TSH and peripheral hormones within 2 months who remained normal during additional 9 months; N^b = Normalization: no recurrence of hyperthyroidism up to 12 months.; N^c = Normalization: after a time ranging from 3 to 6 weeks to 2–3 months all patients with single AFTN ($n = 8$) and 5 pts (50 %) of 10 with multinodular goiter had improvement of serum levels of FT3 and FT4 and a complete normalization of TSH that remained unaltered during follow-up; ** = RCT comparing a single radioiodine dose and a single laser therapy (see text); N^d = Complete normalization of TSH and peripheral hormones; N^e = 6 month after LA normalization of TSH and thyroid hormones that remained so throughout a 30-month follow-up

In a series of 122 patients treated by operators in the initial part of their learning curve, recurrent nerve damage was reported in 1.6 % of patients [66]. On the other hand, a recent study carried out by four centers demonstrated a very low risk of major complications if treatment is performed by adequately trained operators [67]. Only one case (<1 %) of vocal cord paresis that spontaneously resolved within 1 month, was reported while the use of analgesics was required in about 5 % of cases [67]. The very low incidence (0.5 %) of minor and major complications has been reported in a recent multicenter retrospective study on 1534 thyroid nodules treated with the same procedure [69]. The risk of vocal cord paresis was extremely low and occurred during the training period of operators and with treatment of nodules in close proximity to the trachea wall.

As a general rule, the occurrence of pain during the laser treatment is a useful warning symptom that may prevent the risk of procedural complications and the procedure should be halted to check and reposition the fiber tip within the target lesion [61, 68, 69, 74, 79].

37.9 Costs

The price of a state-of-the art ultrasound equipment with a built-in laser source is about $120,000, while a separate diode or Nd-YAG laser source is much less expensive (about $15–20,000). The expense for a complete kit including the fiberoptics and other required disposables is about $400 for a single treatment. The cost of local anesthetic, dressings, and antiseptics must be included. Treatments, which require about 30 min, may be performed as either an outpatient or day hospitalization by an operator and a sonographer.

37.10 Conclusions for Clinical Practice

Percutaneous laser ablation is indicated for the treatment of solid, or predominantly solid, nonfunctioning cytologically benign thyroid nodules that progressively enlarge and become symptomatic or cause cosmetic concern. Laser-induced nodule volume reduction usually persists over several years and may be repeated in case of late regrowth without risk of cosmetic damage or loss of thyroid function.

If the procedure is properly performed with experienced operators, the risk of periprocedural complications is low.

Laser ablation may be used for the treatment of small hyperfunctioning thyroid nodules that do not cause suppression of the perinodular thyroid tissue. In these pre-toxic nodules, especially in young patients, normalization of serum TSH is attained without radiation exposure or risk of late hypothyroidism. In large hyperfunctioning nodules, laser ablation may not be cost-effective compared with 131-I treatment. Before treatment, efficacy, complications and side-effects of traditional management options should be discussed with the patient and compared with those of LA. Specifically, the possibility of late regrowth and the need of follow-up after thermal ablation should be clearly stated.

Percutaneous ethanol injection remains the treatment of choice for relapsing large-volume cystic nodules due to its excellent clinical results, absence of permanent complications and nearly negligible cost.

References

1. Bown SG. Phototherapy in tumors. World J Surg. 1983;7(6):700–9.
2. Pacella CM, Papini E, Fabbrini R, Bizzarri G, Anelli V, Guglielmi R, et al. Ultrasound-guided percutaneous interstitial laser ablation of thyroid nodules. Feasibility study. In: European Congress Radiology (abstract).
3. Pacella CM, Papini E, Bizzarri G, Anelli V, Crescenzi A, Pacella S. Ultrasound-guided (US) percutaneous interstitial laser photo-coagulation of thyroid tissue. Feasibility study. In: RSNA, editor. 84th Scientific Assembly and Annual Meeting Chicago, November 29–December 4, 1998 (abstract).
4. Pacella CM, Bizzarri G, Guglielmi R, Anelli V, Bianchini A, Crescenzi A, et al. Thyroid tissue: US-guided percutaneous interstitial laser ablation-a feasibility study. Radiology. 2000;217(3):673–7.
5. Carroll BA. Asymptomatic thyroid nodules: incidental sonographic detection. AJR Am J Roentgenol. 1982;138(3):499–501.

6. Harach HR, Franssila KO, Wasenius VM. Occult papillary carcinoma of the thyroid. A "normal" finding in Finland. A systematic autopsy study. Cancer. 1985;56(3):531–8.
7. Tan GH, Gharib H. Thyroid incidentalomas: management approaches to nonpalpable nodules discovered incidentally on thyroid imaging. Ann Intern Med. 1997;126(3):226–31.
8. Wiest PW, Hartshorne MF, Inskip PD, Crooks LA, Vela BS, Telepak RJ, et al. Thyroid palpation versus high-resolution thyroid ultrasonography in the detection of nodules. J Ultrasound Med. 1998;17(8):487–96.
9. Brander AE, Viikinkoski VP, Nickels JI, Kivisaari LM. Importance of thyroid abnormalities detected at US screening: a 5-year follow-up. Radiology. 2000;215(3):801–6.
10. Frates MC, Benson CB, Charboneau JW, Cibas ES, Clark OH, Coleman BG, et al. Management of thyroid nodules detected at US: Society of Radiologists in Ultrasound consensus conference statement. Radiology. 2005;237(3):794–800.
11. Gharib H, Papini E. Thyroid nodules: clinical importance, assessment, and treatment. Endocrinol Metab Clin North Am. 2007;36(3):707–35. vi.
12. Mortensen JD, Woolner LB, Bennett WA. Gross and microscopic findings in clinically normal thyroid glands. J Clin Endocrinol Metab. 1955;15(10):1270–80.
13. Durante C, Costante G, Lucisano G, Bruno R, Meringolo D, Paciaroni A, et al. The natural history of benign thyroid nodules. JAMA. 2015;313(9):926–35.
14. Cooper DS, Doherty GM, Haugen BR, Kloos RT, Lee SL, Mandel SJ, et al. Revised American Thyroid Association management guidelines for patients with thyroid nodules and differentiated thyroid cancer. Thyroid. 2009;19(11):1167–214.
15. Gharib H, Papini E, Paschke R, Duick DS, Valcavi R, Hegedus L, et al. American Association of Clinical Endocrinologists, Associazione Medici Endocrinologi, and European Thyroid Association medical guidelines for clinical practice for the diagnosis and management of thyroid nodules: executive summary of recommendations. J Endocrinol Invest. 2010;33(5 Suppl):51–6.
16. Bergenfelz A, Jansson S, Kristoffersson A, Martensson H, Reihner E, Wallin G, et al. Complications to thyroid surgery: results as reported in a database from a multicenter audit comprising 3,660 patients. Langenbecks Arch Surg. 2008;393(5):667–73.
17. Watt T, Hegedus L, Groenvold M, Bjorner JB, Rasmussen AK, Bonnema SJ, et al. Validity and reliability of the novel thyroid-specific quality of life questionnaire, ThyPRO. Eur J Endocrinol. 2010;162(1):161–7.
18. Gharib H, Hegedus L, Pacella CM, Baek JH, Papini E. Clinical review: nonsurgical, image-guided, minimally invasive therapy for thyroid nodules. J Clin Endocrinol Metab. 2013;98(10):3949–57.
19. Gazelle GS, Goldberg SN, Solbiati L, Livraghi T. Tumor ablation with radio-frequency energy. Radiology. 2000;217(3):633–46.
20. Ahmed M, Brace CL, Lee Jr FT, Goldberg SN. Principles of and advances in percutaneous ablation. Radiology. 2011;258(2):351–69.
21. Stafford RJ, Fuentes D, Elliott AA, Weinberg JS, Ahrar K. Laser-induced thermal therapy for tumor ablation. Crit Rev Biomed Eng. 2010;38(1):79–100.
22. Ahrar K, Gowda A, Javadi S, Borne A, Fox M, McNichols R, et al. Preclinical assessment of a 980-nm diode laser ablation system in a large animal tumor model. J Vasc Interv Radiol. 2010;21(4):555–61.
23. Goldberg SN, Gazelle GS, Mueller PR. Thermal ablation therapy for focal malignancy: a unified approach to underlying principles, techniques, and diagnostic imaging guidance. AJR Am J Roentgenol. 2000;174(2):323–31.
24. Solazzo S, Mertyna P, Peddi H, Ahmed M, Horkan C, Goldberg SN. RF ablation with adjuvant therapy: comparison of external beam radiation and liposomal doxorubicin on ablation efficacy in an animal tumor model. Int J Hyperthermia. 2008;24(7):560–7.
25. Christophi C, Winkworth A, Muralihdaran V, Evans P. The treatment of malignancy by hyperthermia. Surg Oncol. 1998;7(1-2):83–90.
26. Thomsen S. Pathologic analysis of photothermal and photomechanical effects of laser-tissue interactions. Photochem Photobiol. 1991;53(6):825–35.
27. Trembley H, Ryan T, Strohbehn J. Interstitial hyperthermia: physics, biology, and clinical aspects. Hyperthermia and oncology. Utrecht: VSP; 1992. p. 11–98.
28. Jacques SL. Laser-tissue interactions. Photochemical, photothermal, and photomechanical. Surg Clin North Am. 1992;72(3):531–58.
29. Larson TR, Bostwick DG, Corica A. Temperature-correlated histopathologic changes following microwave thermoablation of obstructive tissue in patients with benign prostatic hyperplasia. Urology. 1996;47(4):463–9.
30. Goldberg SN, Gazelle GS, Halpern EF, Rittman WJ, Mueller PR, Rosenthal DI. Radiofrequency tissue ablation: importance of local temperature along the electrode tip exposure in determining lesion shape and size. Acad Radiol. 1996;3(3):212–8.
31. Zervas NT, Kuwayama A. Pathological characteristics of experimental thermal lesions. Comparison of induction heating and radiofrequency electrocoagulation. J Neurosurg. 1972;37(4):418–22.
32. Matthewson K, Coleridge-Smith P, O'Sullivan JP, Northfield TC, Bown SG. Biological effects of intrahepatic neodymium:yttrium-aluminum-garnet laser photocoagulation in rats. Gastroenterology. 1987;93(3):550–7.
33. Pacella CM, Rossi Z, Bizzarri G, Papini E, Marinozzi V, Paliotta D, et al. Ultrasound-guided percutaneous laser ablation of liver tissue in a rabbit model. Eur Radiol. 1993;3:26–32.

34. Muller G, Roggan A. Laser-induced interstitial thermotherapy. Bellingham, WA: SPIE-The International Society for Optical Engineering; 1995.
35. Heisterkamp J, van Hillegersberg R, IJzermans JN. Critical temperature and heating time for coagulation damage: implications for interstitial laser coagulation (ILC) of tumors. Lasers Surg Med. 1999;25(3):257–62.
36. Goldberg SN, Gazelle GS, Compton CC, Mueller PR, Tanabe KK. Treatment of intrahepatic malignancy with radiofrequency ablation: radiologic-pathologic correlation. Cancer. 2000;88(11):2452–63.
37. Nikfarjam M, Muralidharan V, Christophi C. Mechanisms of focal heat destruction of liver tumors. J Surg Res. 2005;127(2):208–23.
38. Nikfarjam M, Malcontenti-Wilson C, Christophi C. Focal hyperthermia produces progressive tumor necrosis independent of the initial thermal effects. J Gastrointest Surg. 2005;9(3):410–7.
39. Mertyna P, Hines-Peralta A, Liu ZJ, Halpern E, Goldberg W, Goldberg SN. Radiofrequency ablation: variability in heat sensitivity in tumors and tissues. J Vasc Interv Radiol. 2007;18(5):647–54.
40. Mertyna P, Dewhirst MW, Halpern E, Goldberg W, Goldberg SN. Radiofrequency ablation: the effect of distance and baseline temperature on thermal dose required for coagulation. Int J Hyperthermia. 2008;24(7):550–9.
41. Mertyna P, Goldberg W, Yang W, Goldberg SN. Thermal ablation a comparison of thermal dose required for radiofrequency-, microwave-, and laser-induced coagulation in an ex vivo bovine liver model. Acad Radiol. 2009;16(12):1539–48.
42. Dachman A, Smith M, Burris J, VanDeMerwe W. Interstitial laser ablation in experimental models and in clinical use. Semin Interv Radiol. 1993;10:101–12.
43. McGahan JP, Browning PD, Brock JM, Tesluk H. Hepatic ablation using radiofrequency electrocautery. Invest Radiol. 1990;25(3):267–70.
44. Nolsoe CP, Torp-Pedersen S, Burcharth F, Horn T, Pedersen S, Christensen NE, et al. Interstitial hyperthermia of colorectal liver metastases with a US-guided Nd-YAG laser with a diffuser tip: a pilot clinical study. Radiology. 1993;187(2):333–7.
45. McGahan JP, Dodd GDI. Radiofrequency ablation of the liver: current status. AJR Am J Roentgenol. 2001;176:3–16.
46. Amabile G, Rotondi M, De Chiara G, Silvestri A, Di Filippo B, Bellastella A, et al. Low-energy interstitial laser photocoagulation for treatment of nonfunctioning thyroid nodules: therapeutic outcome in relation to pretreatment and treatment parameters. Thyroid. 2006;16(8):749–55.
47. Amabile G, Rotondi M, Pirali B, Dionisio R, Agozzino L, Lanza M, et al. Interstitial laser photocoagulation for benign thyroid nodules: time to treat large nodules. Lasers Surg Med. 2011;43(8):797–803.
48. Rotondi M, Amabile G, Leporati P, Di Filippo B, Chiovato L. Repeated laser thermal ablation of a large functioning thyroid nodule restores euthyroidism and ameliorates constrictive symptoms. J Clin Endocrinol Metab. 2009;94(2):382–3.
49. Cakir B, Topaloglu O, Gul K, Agac T, Aydin C, Dirikoc A, et al. Effects of percutaneous laser ablation treatment in benign solitary thyroid nodules on nodule volume, thyroglobulin and anti-thyroglobulin levels, and cytopathology of nodule in 1 yr follow-up. J Endocrinol Invest. 2006;29(10):876–84.
50. Cakir B, Gul K, Ugras S, Ersoy R, Topaloglu O, Agac T, et al. Percutaneous laser ablation of an autonomous thyroid nodule: effects on nodule size and histopathology of the nodule 2 years after the procedure. Thyroid. 2008;18(7):803–5.
51. Cakir B, Topaloglu O, Gul K, Agac T, Aydin C, Dirikoc A, et al. Ultrasound-guided percutaneous laser ablation treatment in inoperable aggressive course anaplastic thyroid carcinoma: the introduction of a novel alternative palliative therapy--second experience in the literature. J Endocrinol Invest. 2007;30(7):624–5.
52. Cakir B, Gul K, Ersoy R, Topaloglu O, Korukluoglu B. Subcapsular hematoma complication during percutaneous laser ablation to a hypoactive benign solitary thyroid nodule. Thyroid. 2008;18(8):917–8.
53. Cakir B, Ugras NS, Gul K, Ersoy R, Korukluoglu B. Initial report of the results of percutaneous laser ablation of benign cold thyroid nodules: evaluation of histopathological changes after 2 years. Endocr Pathol. 2009;20(3):170–6.
54. Dossing H, Bennedbaek FN, Karstrup S, Hegedus L. Benign solitary solid cold thyroid nodules: US-guided interstitial laser photocoagulation--initial experience. Radiology. 2002;225(1):53–7.
55. Dossing H, Bennedbaek FN, Hegedus L. Ultrasound-guided interstitial laser photocoagulation of an autonomous thyroid nodule: the introduction of a novel alternative. Thyroid. 2003;13(9):885–8.
56. Dossing H, Bennedbaek FN, Hegedus L. Effect of ultrasound-guided interstitial laser photocoagulation on benign solitary solid cold thyroid nodules: one versus three treatments. Thyroid. 2006;16(8):763–8.
57. Dossing H, Bennedbaek FN, Hegedus L. Effect of ultrasound-guided interstitial laser photocoagulation on benign solitary solid cold thyroid nodules—a randomised study. Eur J Endocrinol. 2005;152(3):341–5.
58. Dossing H, Bennedbaek FN, Hegedus L. Long-term outcome following interstitial laser photocoagulation of benign cold thyroid nodules. Eur J Endocrinol. 2011;165(1):123–8.
59. Dossing H, Bennedbaek FN, Hegedus L. Interstitial laser photocoagulation (ILP) of benign cystic thyroid nodules--a prospective randomized trial. J Clin Endocrinol Metab. 2013;98(7):E1213–7.
60. Spiezia S, Vitale G, Di Somma C, Pio Assanti A, Ciccarelli A, Lombardi G, et al. Ultrasound-guided laser thermal ablation in the treatment of autonomous hyperfunctioning thyroid nodules and compressive nontoxic nodular goiter. Thyroid. 2003;13(10):941–7.

61. Pacella CM, Bizzarri G, Spiezia S, Bianchini A, Guglielmi R, Crescenzi A, et al. Thyroid tissue: US-guided percutaneous laser thermal ablation. Radiology. 2004;232(1):272–80.
62. Papini E, Guglielmi R, Bizzarri G, Pacella CM. Ultrasound-guided laser thermal ablation for treatment of benign thyroid nodules. Endocr Pract. 2004;10(3):276–83.
63. Gambelunghe G, Fatone C, Ranchelli A, Fanelli C, Lucidi P, Cavaliere A, et al. A randomized controlled trial to evaluate the efficacy of ultrasound-guided laser photocoagulation for treatment of benign thyroid nodules. J Endocrinol Invest. 2006;29(9):RC23–6.
64. Papini E, Guglielmi R, Bizzarri G, Graziano F, Bianchini A, Brufani C, et al. Treatment of benign cold thyroid nodules: a randomized clinical trial of percutaneous laser ablation versus levothyroxine therapy or follow-up. Thyroid. 2007;17(3):229–35.
65. Valcavi R, Bertani A, Pesenti M, Al Jandali Rifa'Y LR, Frasoldati A, Formisano D, et al. Laser and radiofrequency ablation procedures. In: Baskin HJ, Duick DS, Levine RA, editors. Thyroid ultrasound and ultrasound guided FNA biopsy. 2nd ed. New York, NY: Springer; 2008. p. 191–218.
66. Valcavi R, Riganti F, Bertani A, Formisano D, Pacella CM. Percutaneous laser ablation of cold benign thyroid nodules: a 3-year follow-up study in 122 patients. Thyroid. 2010;20(11):1253–61.
67. Papini E, Rago T, Gambelunghe G, Valcavi R, Bizzarri G, Vitti P, et al. Long-term efficacy of ultrasound-guided laser ablation for benign solid thyroid nodules. Results of a three-year multicenter prospective randomized trial. J Clin Endocrinol Metab. 2014;99(10):3653–9.
68. Achille G, Zizzi S, Di Stasio E, Grammatica A, Grammatica L. Ultrasound-guided percutaneous laser ablation in treating symptomatic solid benign thyroid nodules: our experience in 45 patients. Head Neck. 2016;38:677.
69. Pacella CM, Mauri G, Achille G, Barbaro D, Bizzarri G, De Feo P, et al. Outcomes and risk factors for complications of laser ablation for thyroid nodules: a multicenter study on 1531 patients. J Clin Endocrinol Metab. 2015;100(10):3903–10.
70. Valcavi R, Piana S, Bortolan GS, Lai R, Barbieri V, Negro R. Ultrasound-guided percutaneous laser ablation of papillary thyroid microcarcinoma: a feasibility study on three cases with pathological and immunohistochemical evaluation. Thyroid. 2013;23(12):1578–82.
71. Nikfarjam M, Muralidharan V, Malcontenti-Wilson C, Christophi C. Progressive microvascular injury in liver and colorectal liver metastases following laser induced focal hyperthermia therapy. Lasers Surg Med. 2005;37(1):64–73.
72. Bongiovanni M, Spitale A, Faquin WC, Mazzucchelli L, Baloch ZW. The Bethesda System for reporting thyroid cytopathology: a meta-analysis. Acta Cytol. 2012;56(4):333–9.
73. Piana S, Riganti F, Froio E, Andrioli M, Pacella CM, Valcavi R. Pathological findings of thyroid nodules after percutaneous laser ablation: a series of 22 cases with cyto-histological correlation. Endocr Pathol. 2012;23(2):94–100.
74. Barbaro D, Orsini P, Lapi P, Pasquini C, Tuco A, Righini A, et al. Percutaneous laser ablation in the treatment of toxic and pretoxic nodular goiter. Endocr Pract. 2007;13(1):30–6.
75. Dossing H, Bennedbaek FN, Bonnema SJ, Grupe P, Hegedus L. Randomized prospective study comparing a single radioiodine dose and a single laser therapy session in autonomously functioning thyroid nodules. Eur J Endocrinol. 2007;157(1):95–100.
76. Chianelli M, Bizzarri G, Todino V, Misischi I, Bianchini A, Graziano F, et al. Laser ablation and 131-iodine: a 24-month pilot study of combined treatment for large toxic nodular goitre. J Clin Endocrinol Metab. 2014;99:e1283.
77. Guglielmi R, Pacella CM, Bianchini A, Bizzarri G, Rinaldi R, Graziano FM, et al. Percutaneous ethanol injection treatment in benign thyroid lesions: role and efficacy. Thyroid. 2004;14(2):125–31.
78. Di Rienzo G, Surrente C, Lopez C, Quercia R. Tracheal laceration after laser ablation of nodular goitre. Interact Cardiovasc Thorac Surg. 2010;14(1):115–6.
79. Gambelunghe G, Bini V, Monacelli M, Avenia N, D'Ajello M, Colella R, et al. The administration of anesthetic in the thyroid pericapsular region increases the possibility of side effects during percutaneous laser photocoagulation of thyroid nodules. Lasers Surg Med. 2013;45(1):34–7.

Part VIII

Ultrasound in Advanced and Novel Applications

38 Ultrasound for Surgeons: What I Learned from Lifetime Practice

Allan E. Siperstein

38.1 Introduction

Surgeon-performed ultrasound is a necessary tool in the evaluation of patients with thyroid and parathyroid disease. On a daily basis, I am able to demonstrate to my residents and fellows key decisions that hinged upon the ultrasound evaluation performed by the surgeon that were not apparent by review of images or reports. For a surgical practice, both the indications for surgery as well as the extent of the surgical procedure are driven by the findings on ultrasound evaluation. This benefit is apparent when applied in the clinic as well as in the operating room setting. In addition to the ability to identify structural lesions, fine needle aspiration under ultrasound guidance is an invaluable adjunct for clinical decision-making.

38.2 Adaptation of Ultrasound into Surgical Practice

Prior to the 1990s, ultrasonography was almost exclusively the purview of the radiologist. With the development of higher quality ultrasound machines and, in particular, ultrasound probes for use in the operating room, it became apparent that intraoperative ultrasonography had areas of particular clinical advantage. One key area is in the identification of liver tumors in patients undergoing hepatic surgery. Intraoperative ultrasound was able to identify tumors that were not apparent on preoperative CT scan imaging and thus had a direct effect on intraoperative decision-making. In addition, it was realized that ultrasound could be used repeatedly during the procedure to identify the relationship between the tumor and the surrounding vasculature and thus guide the resection. Early papers also demonstrated the advantage of intraoperative ultrasound in identifying pancreatic islet tumors.

In my surgical training, I was exposed to two studies that drove home the value of ultrasound technology. First was a study that used intraoperative ultrasound at the completion of a carotid endarterectomy devote to assess the anatomy, in particular intimal flaps as well is to study the flow dynamics. It became apparent that a repair that appeared perfect from visual examination of the external vessel wall did not necessarily correlate with an adequate restoration of internal flow. The second study was the use of transabdominal ultrasound to diagnose patients with suspected acute appendicitis. This was an era where history, laboratory studies and importantly physical examination was the key to determining whether surgical exploration was warranted. This preceded routine CT scan and the use of diagnostic laparoscopy.

A.E. Siperstein, M.D. (✉)
Endocrine Surgery Department, Cleveland Clinic, 9500 Euclid Ave. F-20, Cleveland, OH 44195, USA
e-mail: SIPERSA@ccf.org

M. Milas et al. (eds.), *Advanced Thyroid and Parathyroid Ultrasound*,
DOI 10.1007/978-3-319-44100-9_38

Having made the decision to operate, it was initially frustrating as part of this study to have to call the radiology resident to perform an abdominal ultrasound while waiting to take the patient to the operating room. In observing these studies being performed, I became aware of the advantages of this preoperative evaluation. Obviously imaging a clearly inflamed appendix, typically with an appendicolith, clearly established the diagnosis. It was also apparent that ultrasound was a dynamic study as the point of maximal tenderness could be reproduced with graded compression of the transducer. The conduct of the operation was also facilitated by knowing in advance the anatomic relationship of the appendix to the cecum and surrounding structures.

Although the organ systems may be different, these principles apply equally well to the management of patients with thyroid and parathyroid disease. What is not apparent on physical examination becomes clearly defined when viewed sonographically. Diagnoses can be confirmed with a high degree of accuracy and operative strategy is thus directly affected.

In the 1990s, incorporation of ultrasound into surgical practice was challenging. At the local level, there was opposition to non-radiologists performing "radiologic" studies. Pathways for training were also challenging. Despite these obstacles, there was a group that recognized that surgeon-performed ultrasound held particular value for patient care. This was despite the fact that in this era, there was no financial incentive for the surgeon. Other countries, in particular Germany had recognized the value of surgical sonography and had incorporated it into resident training and clinical care. In 1992, in collaboration with German colleagues, I was able to establish an early course in surgical sonography. This included office ultrasound evaluation of the thyroid and parathyroid, as well as techniques for ultrasound guided fine needle aspiration. Surgeons were able to learn these skills quickly. Having an intimate knowledge of the three dimensional anatomy, correlating this to the two-dimensional grayscale ultrasound image was intuitive. In fact when performing an ultrasound study, I imagine the three dimensional color structures that live beneath the skin.

38.3 Overall Philosophy of Surgeon-Performed Ultrasound

The value of ultrasound in an endocrine surgical practice is the identification of structural disease, appropriate diagnosis to determine whether surgical intervention is warranted, determination of the appropriate extent of surgery. It has been repeatedly stated, with great truth, that ultrasound is an extension of the physical exam. In the office setting, physical examination skills are enhanced by performing a subsequent ultrasound evaluation. When sonographic lesions are not appreciated on initial physical examination, it reinforces the more subtle examination skills such as head position, intensity of palpation, and swallowing to appreciate more subtle lesions.

The value of a real-time ultrasound examination cannot be over emphasized. Almost all patients coming to the office with thyroid disease and many with parathyroid disease have had prior ultrasound imaging. Review of the printed reports alone, in many cases, would not have led to appropriate clinical decision-making. In addition, even review of the static images typically yields far less diagnostic information than preforming the evaluation yourself.

I feel the reasons for this are multifactorial. Typically, the sonographer performing the initial evaluation is hindered by having a very limited clinical history. As a surgeon, I have assembled the history of the patient's condition, reviewed medications and laboratory studies, as well as the prior imaging. After performing a physical examination, the ultrasound is then performed in a much richer clinical context. The ultrasound is therefore performed in a more strategic fashion to determine the best clinical course of action. Specific examples as they pertain to thyroid, parathyroid, and fine needle aspiration are discussed below.

An additional limitation in reviewing prior ultrasound reports and images is lack of completeness of the exam. Thyroid nodules may lack a description of key characteristics such as calcification or blood flow. Typical spongiform nodules may be described only as complex. Even when suspicious thyroid nodules are identified, nodal surveys are often not done. Many centers lack familiarity with the subtleties of parathyroid localization. What is important, particularly for thyroid evaluation, is that lesions have been identified and documented to require further evaluation.

38.4 Know How to Use Your Equipment

Modern ultrasound machines perform complex computerized digital image processing to produce the images we see on the screen. Although many standard functions are quite similar from manufacturer to manufacturer, there are many subtleties available to enhance the quality of the images. We tend to rely quite heavily on preprogrammed settings that are suitable for most routine studies. Although laborious to read through the supplied instruction manuals, I have found it helpful, particularly in more unusual clinical situations. A patient technician who will take the time to demonstrate some of the more subtle features of the equipment is also valuable.

There is an initial tendency to prefer images with greater contrast. Many important structures are best appreciated with a more subtle grayscale. With larger goiters, it is useful to decrease the ultrasound frequency to achieve a deeper depth of penetration. The size of larger lesions are often challenging to measure. Most machines allow for 2B mode images to be placed side-by-side such that the lesion spans both images. Angulation of the transducer, often helped with the use of a curved array probe, may allow the long axis of a nodule to fit on a single screen, making this distance easier to measure. Many linear array probes may allow for a "trapezoidal" view such that with a subtle compromise in resolution a wider field of view is obtained. Understanding these settings to optimize color flow Doppler imaging is also essential. To evaluate color flow signal within a thyroid nodule is important to understand how to obtain highly sensitive settings on a particular model of ultrasound machine. Most machines also have a "power flow" mode where increased sensitivity is obtained with the loss of flow direction information (see Figs. 38.1 and 38.2).

38.5 Optimizing the Use of Ultrasound in the Office

The vast majority of patients presenting to a surgical practice have had prior ultrasound evaluations. Findings on that study often prompted the surgical consultation. It is essential to review those prior reports and images so as to fully understand the issues to address at that consultation as well as to better hone in on what needs to be evaluated during that office ultrasound.

- The patient with Hashimoto's thyroiditis may be referred due to suspicion of multiple thyroid nodules. The prior imaging may demonstrate the measurement of multiple small lesions within the thyroid gland. Upon your ultrasound evaluation, you appreciate that on the real-time examination these findings reflect the heterogeneity within the thyroid parenchyma rather than true nodules, often called pseudonodules.
- In patients with multinodular goiter, the size of purported nodules may have increased over a short period of time. Careful comparison of prior images to the real-time examination may reveal that different nodules were reported from one examination to another or, as is often the case, two adjacent nodules may be subsequently reported as one much larger nodule. Reported increase in size of the thyroid also needs to be carefully evaluated.
- A patient with the length of a thyroid lobe reported as 5 cm on one examination may subsequently be reported as having increased to 6.5 cm. This may simply reflect, as the thyroid parenchyma gradually tapers out at its superior and inferior most aspect, that the placement of the measurement calipers may vary significantly. For this reason, the overall width and depth of a thyroid lobe are much more reliably followed on serial examination (Fig. 38.3).
- The patient referred with a worrisome thyroid nodule due to multiple "fine calcifications" many in fact be a typical benign spongiform nodule with inspissated colloid within the cystic areas mimicking calcifications. An understanding of these discrepancies will allow for an appropriate clinical decision to be made.

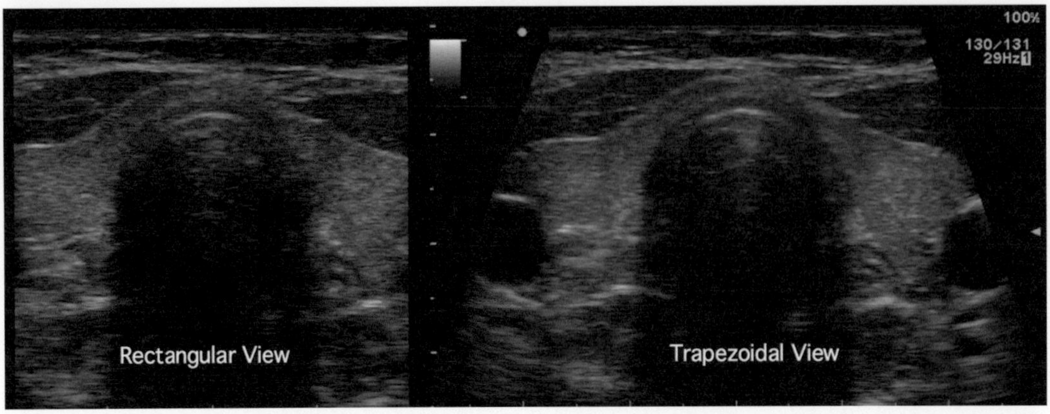

Fig. 38.1 Understanding how to use the variety of features on a modern ultrasound machine will optimize imaging ability. A rectangular image is unable to fully encompass the width of the thyroid, whereas using the trapezoidal imaging feature of the same probe allows the entire gland to be seen

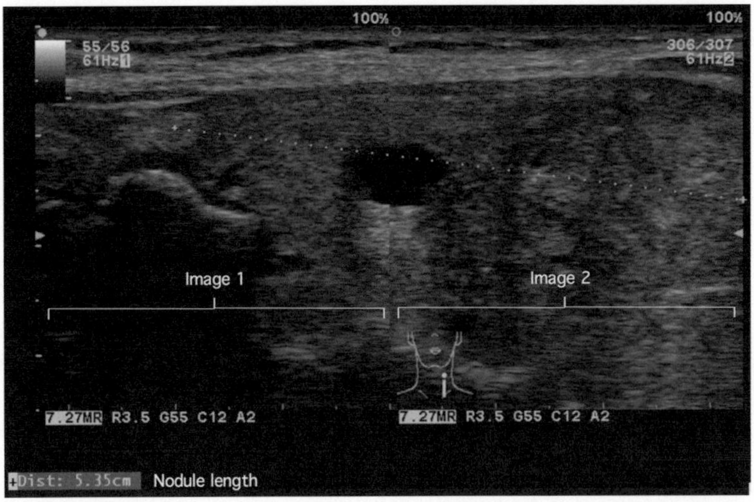

Fig. 38.2 The measurement of a large lesion may not be possible if it exceeds the width of the ultrasound probe. By "fusing" two images side-by-side, the length may be accurately measured

Patients typically come into the office very concerned that there have been untoward changes in their thyroid and are typically told that they need biopsy and/or surgery. I find it quite useful at the completion of the ultrasound examination to show the patient their findings in real time on the ultrasound screen. This provides better reassurance, typically, that intervention is not required at this point and gives them an understanding as to any discrepancy between prior imaging and the current evaluation. To reassure these patients that important findings have not been overlooked, I will typically see them back for a follow-up evaluation. To this end, it is extremely useful to have the ability to capture images into the hospitals electronic medical record. This is key for image comparison both on a follow-up office visit and in the operating room.

The technique and conduct of the ultrasound evaluation is key for extracting the maximal amount of information from the examination and arriving at the proper clinical decision. Although aware of prior examination and imaging findings, it is important to keep an open and unprejudiced

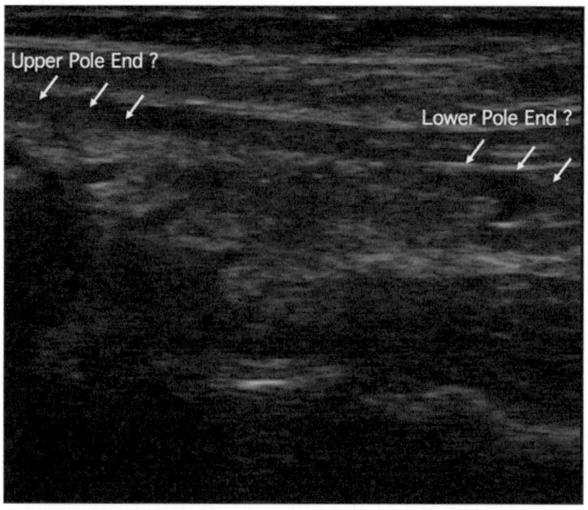

Fig. 38.3 Although the longest dimension of a thyroid lobe, the exact length may not be easily appreciated given tapering of the thyroid parenchyma. This results in potential variability on serial studies that may be misinterpreted as a true increase in size

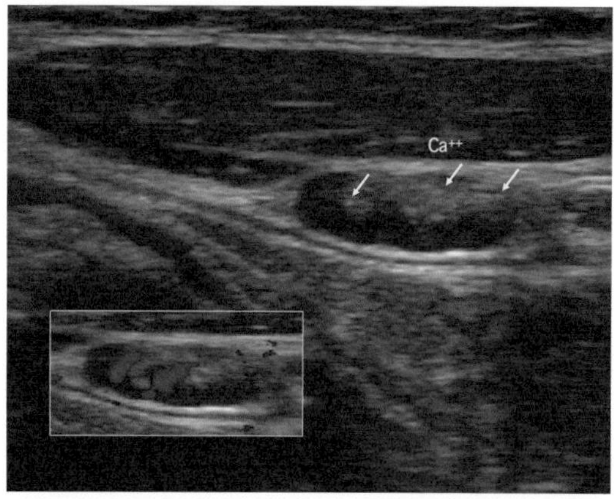

Fig. 38.4 Pathologic lymph nodes with partial tumor replacement will show more subtle features such as subcapsular areas of microcalcification with corresponding increase in color flow Doppler signal

frame of mind while conducting the examination. Prior documentation of a benign thyroid nodule by FNA should not dissuade careful examination of the contralateral lobe nor of lymph nodes demonstrating worrisome sonographic features. Parathyroid adenomas may occasionally be identified in patients without prior suspicion of primary hyperparathyroidism.

In performing a thyroid ultrasound, it is important to conduct the examination in a standard fashion as well as to perform image capture and annotation systematically. There is no absolute right or wrong way to form this study, but establishing a routine will guarantee that a thorough examination has been performed and that essential elements are not omitted due to attention being focused on a major finding. It is also essential to understand that although we may use the term "thyroid" ultrasound, what this means in the surgeon's office is a comprehensive neck ultrasound. Although our initial attention may be directed at a thyroid nodule that prompted surgical consultation, careful evaluation must be performed of the contralateral lobe, potential cervical adenopathy or other unexpected anatomic findings that may be key to directing needle aspiration or indication for surgery.

I prefer to start with a transverse view centered over the thyroid isthmus. This gives me a "lay of the land" in terms of the overall thyroid appearance as well as determining whether the trachea remains in the midline. By determining the shift from the midpoint of the transducer centered over the trachea to the sternal notch, quantitative measurement of tracheal deviation is included in the ultrasound report.

I then perform transverse imaging of one lobe with care to examine all of the central neck compartment tissue from well above to well below the limits of the thyroid parenchyma itself. This includes attention to any central neck lymph nodes. I then perform longitudinal imaging of the same region. Any thyroidal or extra thyroidal abnormalities are then assessed with color flow Doppler (Fig. 38.4).

As is typically done, axial measurement of nodule length is done on longitudinal imaging with width and depth done on transverse imaging. Capturing these images on a side-by-side view so that all three measurements are displayed in a single image is particularly helpful to avoid confusion with subsequent imaging, especially if multiple nodules are being measured.

I find it useful to document nodule characteristics in a systematic, essentially templated, fashion. Also useful are dynamic assessments of a nodule. With graded compression of the ultrasound probe, deformability of a nodule can hint at whether it is more firm or softer in texture. Also useful is to have the patient swallow while imaging a nodule longitudinally. Lack of motion of the nodule distinct from the overlying strap muscles or from the posterior tissues may predict gross extra-thyroidal extension.

After assessing the contralateral lobe in an identical manner, careful examination of the midline structures is then performed. Although typically covered while assessing each lobe, particular attention is paid at this point to subtle lesions within the thyroid isthmus. Key points to focus attention to at this time are anterior tracheal nodes, prominent pyramidal lobes or even unexpected thyroglossal duct cysts. An assessment of vocal cord function can also be made in most patients. I still assess any patient with voice changes, high-risk lesions or reoperative cases with direct laryngoscopy.

Careful examination is then done both transversely and longitudinally for any lateral neck lymph nodes. This evaluation will reimage any notes in the central neck as well. More prominent nodes are typically encountered just beneath the salivary glands. These may have been reported as "concerning" on a prior ultrasound study. If they are of a benign sono-morphology, and in particular bilateral and symmetric, needle biopsy is rarely warranted. The classic pathologic lymph node completely replaced with tumor is easily spotted: typically round, lacking a hyperechoic stripe, often with micro calcifications and increased color flow doppler signal. Attention must be paid to the node with partial tumor replacement. These findings are more subtle, often with a cluster of micro calcifications at the periphery of a somewhat more prominent node that otherwise has benign sonographic features.

Almost subconsciously, I assess the presence of a carotid subclavian junction on the right side. Although arch abnormalities are uncommon, this finding would predict the presence of a nonrecurrent laryngeal nerve on the right side.

For patients who have undergone surgery for thyroid cancer, a key component of oncologic surveillance is periodic neck ultrasound, in particular to assess abnormal lymph nodes, the most common site of recurrence. The algorithm for performing the study is the same as when the thyroid is in place. Examination of the central neck compartment may be less sensitive at the carotid arteries with shadowing from their edges obscuring a key area of interest. This is helped by graded compression of the transducer with the intention of displacing the carotid laterally. In addition, the anterior tracheal area requires special attention as it is a common sight of recurrence; however, the quality of the image may be impaired by being so close to the transducer. When first learning to perform this examination, trainees often focus their attention on the obvious structures such as the carotid artery and jugular vein. What must be taught is to retrain your focus to those soft tissues, which bear the lymph nodes, surrounding the obvious structures.

Parathyroid localization is also an important component of a surgical practice. This examination should be comprehensive to include the thyroid and lateral neck nodes as well. It is very common to identify previously unsuspected thyroid pathology that may directly impact the extent of any planned operation. I find that the most common indication for an unplanned thyroid fine needle aspiration is in a patient being evaluated for primary hyperparathyroidism.

As with any ultrasound examination, a systematic approach is important. As with the thyroid, I perform transverse and longitudinal imaging on each side of the neck. Attention is initially placed on the typical anatomic locations for parathyroid glands. Following this, the ectopic sites are evaluated. For lower glands, it is important to assess the areas of the cervical thymus inferior to the lower poles of the thyroid. Proper neck hyperextension and angulation of the transducer are employed to image as much of the upper mediastinum as possible. The upper parathyroid glands very commonly are found in a descended location along the tracheal esophageal groove. Compression with the transducer is an important component of this examination. It allows displacement of the esophagus that commonly reveals glands hidden behind this organ. It may not be immediately apparent whether a suspected structure is in fact a parathyroid located beyond the margins of the thyroid versus a nodule at the periphery of the thyroid. With compression of the transducer, the structure may be seen to move separately from the thyroid, particularly in the transverse orientation, thus confirming that it is a parathyroid.

Although the typical hypoechoic parathyroid with a hyperechoic rim and teardrop configuration is easily recognized, parathyroid appearance may be variable. Hyperplastic glands may appear more heterogeneous given their multinodular makeup. Parathyroids may also have cystic areas or even areas of calcification. Being aware of this variable appearance will improve localization accuracy. Some very large glands are missed as they spanned the entire width of the transducer and are not recognized as a distinct structure.

38.6 Optimizing Fine Needle Aspiration Results

The ability to perform accurate fine needle aspirations is a key diagnostic tool for the endocrine surgeon. As a commitment to providing quality patient care, the practitioner should monitor their rate of inadequate aspirations. If higher than desired, additional training or proctoring should be undertaken.

Variable techniques have been described performing the aspiration. Training and personal preference will establish the best technique for an individual provider. I prefer to perform my diagnostic examination standing to the patient's right, but perform the fine needle aspiration standing to the patient's left. This allows my right hand holding the syringe and my left hand holding the transducer to be in the same field of view as the ultrasound screen. I find this to be a more natural ergonomic positioning. Although diagnostic examinations are performed with a linear transducer, I perform almost all aspirations with a small footprint curved array probe. I find that this provides increased degrees of freedom of movement of the probe, particularly useful when aspirating lesions in the central neck. There is also a shorter length of tissue that the needle must traverse before coming into view on the ultrasound screen.

Discussions of needle diameter and aspiration technique and number of needle passes constitute a complex area. I find it to be the most emotionally charged and dogmatic area with near religious conviction to a given technique. Given this variability, it may imply that, in the end, there is little difference in outcome, with operator dependency, the key variable. Regardless of technique, it is essential to clearly identify the tip of the needle within the target lesion. It is important to collaborate with the cytologist to provide smears and/or suspensions so as to get an optimal reading.

The indications to perform a fine needle aspiration on a given thyroid lesion based on sonographic criteria have been detailed in other chapters. A key determination of whether to perform an aspiration hinges on whether it will alter the treatment course for the patient. A given lesion, in and of itself, may meet criteria for aspiration; however, the patient's clinical context would make performing an aspiration of no value in clinical decision making. In a patient with a bilateral nodular goiter and no worrisome adenopathy, where total thyroidectomy is the planned procedure, fine needle aspiration will not affect the clinical course. At the time of surgery, attention is paid to enlarge nodes and these should be sampled, if identified. The same procedure would be followed whether the aspiration were benign or malignant. The only exception would be for those groups who choose to perform routine prophylactic central neck dissection in malignant cases. Similarly, patients with a history of external beam radiation treatment and multiple thyroid nodules typically need total thyroidectomy given the high rate of malignancy and thus do not require fine needle aspiration.

In addition to cytology, measurement of thyroglobulin, calcitonin, or parathyroid hormone in the appropriate clinical setting provides very useful adjunctive information. I routinely send all aspirated lymph nodes for thyroglobulin measurements. Any structure aspirated in a patient with known medullary cancer is sent for calcitonin. In patients with primary hyperparathyroidism,

I routinely send any suspected thyroid nodules for parathyroid hormone measurement. I have had many intrathyroidal masses return with high PTH values and a sonographic appearance atypical for a parathyroid gland. Armed with this information preoperatively is key to avoiding what otherwise would be a prolonged parathyroid exploration. Any aspiration of a suspected parathyroid should be sent for PTH as the cytology on the cells mimics a thyroid follicular neoplasm.

38.7 Use of Ultrasound in the Operating Room

Prior to thyroid or parathyroid surgery, I routinely ultrasound the patient when they are asleep in the operating room and properly positioned. For patients with thyroid disease, this confirms the presence and features of the index lesions. Additional unsuspected pathology may be identified such as lymph nodes that will have a direct impact on the extent of the planned procedure. For patients with parathyroid disease, the greater degree of compression that may be applied can identify previously unsuspected glands. Knowing the exact anatomic relation between the localized parathyroid and the surrounding structures facilitates its removal. Knowing that a gland is located just inferior to lower pole of the thyroid versus tucked just posterior to the lower pole, directs the surgeon to the abnormal gland with minimal dissection. I often refer to this as an "ultrasound guided parathyroidectomy." The ultrasound is also useful at judging the optimal level at which to place the surgical incision, particularly in obese patients when the thyroid may not be palpable.

There is also an important educational benefit for trainees. Is entirely non-threatening for the trainee to perform the examination and to have the instructor give direction or take over movement of the probe with a patient being asleep. It clearly reinforces ultrasound findings to image the lesion preoperatively then to directly observe the pathology several minutes later.

In certain complex situations, there is a value to performing true intraoperative ultrasonography with the probe placed within the surgical wound. Particularly in reoperative situations with extensive neck scarring, the location of a nodal recurrence in the central neck or enlarged parathyroid may not be apparent at initial exploration. Bringing the ultrasound probe, covered by a sterile see-through bag, into the wound allows clear identification of the pathology and therefore a more focused dissection.

38.8 Conclusion

Ultrasound is an indispensable tool in the practice of an endocrine surgeon. With equipment costs decreasing, availability of excellent training courses, and limited resistance by radiologists of surgeons performing these procedures, barriers to incorporating this into a surgical practice are limited. That said, there is a time commitment and learning curve. Once adopted, however, the value of surgeon-performed ultrasound becomes apparent in improving diagnostic accuracy and appropriate clinical decision-making.

39 Ultrasound for Otolaryngologists and Head and Neck Surgeons: What I Learned from Lifetime Practice

Robert A. Sofferman and Merry E. Sebelik

39.1 Pro

39.1.1 Convenience and Efficiency of Patient Care

Imagine the patient who must travel 3–4 h from a small town for an appointment for a suspected thyroid mass. Appropriate imaging and up-to-date cytology are not possible near or within the local community. The receiving physician at our tertiary medical center would perform a standard examination and the patient scheduled for a return visit to radiology for ultrasound. Often, the radiologist will ask the patient to come back yet again for an ultrasound-guided biopsy.

After the cytology is confirmed, a fourth visit to the head and neck surgeon would be required to round out the preoperative program.

Consider the same patient circumstances but availability of office-based ultrasound at the initial visit. Upon receipt of referral with a thyroid mass, the scheduler sets several elements in motion for the initial visit. A complete history and physical are performed along with a complete diagnostic ultrasound of the thyroid and head and neck. An FNA with cytology is accomplished with or without an on-site cytotechnologist. If lymphoma is suspected, an aspirate can be placed in special media at the outset. With thyroid masses, all elements of thyroid surgery are discussed with the patient including risks and complications and consents are signed. The cytology results are reported to the patient and referring physician by telephone in the ensuing week as well as any unexpected changes in surgical management. This scenario is followed with every routine thyroid patient and reduces the patient inconvenience from 4 visits to 1. For head and neck tumor (non-thyroid) patients, the efficiency of obtaining imaging and tissue biopsy at the first visit can translate into reduced time to staging and initiation of treatment. Head and neck cancer patients face many challenges in obtaining multidisciplinary consultations, and point-of-care ultrasound has greatly improved the way I “package” the patient prior to treatment planning.

39.1.2 Comprehensive Attention to Relevant Details

The surgeon who performs his/her own ultrasound has the opportunity to look at more areas and details than that by a radiography technician.

R.A. Sofferman, M.D., F.A.C.S.
Professor Emeritus and Chairman, Division of Otolaryngology-HNS, University of Vermont Medical Center, Burlington, VT, USA

M.E. Sebelik, M.D., F.A.C.S. (✉)
Department of Otolaryngology, Head & Neck Surgery, Veterans Affairs Medical Center-Atlanta, Emory University School of Medicine, 550 Peachtree St NE, Suite 1135, Atlanta, GA 30308, USA
e-mail: msebeli@emory.edu

M. Milas et al. (eds.), *Advanced Thyroid and Parathyroid Ultrasound*,
DOI 10.1007/978-3-319-44100-9_39

Static images described by someone else with a different set of views and annotation are often difficult to interpret. Ideally, appropriate cine loops are the best way to recall important dynamic information and not every radiology study includes them.

39.1.3 Use in Operating Room

Frequently, the study needs to be repeated pre or even intraoperatively and the same surgeon will be better equipped to do the repeat study rather than expecting another radiologist to offer efficiency and an accurate assessment. Pre-incision, surgeon-performed ultrasound has become the ultimate "time-out", confirming the correct side, correct patient, correct procedure, and ensuring that no additional pathology has developed in the interim.

39.1.4 Continuity of Care

Follow-up of a mass for change in dimension and/or character is ideally accomplished by the same examiner on the same machine. Surgeon-performed ultrasound eliminates the errors in communication that occur when the imaging study is performed off-site and by non-treating sonographers. It also engages the patient in a direct conversation with the treating physician about the implications of any change in findings.

39.1.5 Comfort with Use of Invasive Procedures

Occasionally, a core biopsy is preferable to an FNA with cytology. The surgeon experienced with obtaining core samples is best suited to make this decision. In fact, it is frequently obtained at the time of initial visit to the office, increasing efficiency of treatment. Some lesions which are reasonable candidates for core under ultrasound guidance are anaplastic thyroid carcinoma, Reidel's struma, and neck and large thyroid lymphoma.

39.1.6 Low-Resource Settings

Head and neck pathology often requires imaging studies to best make diagnosis and management decisions. However, in many parts of the world, there is a paucity of imaging equipment and radiologists, as well as surgeons. Portable ultrasound brings imaging capabilities to patients who otherwise would not have access to such care. Patients with head and neck tumors who live in rural, remote, or low-resource settings can enjoy the benefits of immediate imaging and tissue procurement, with a much smaller investment in infrastructure and personnel than a traditional radiology department requires. The World Health Organization recognized the unique value of ultrasound imaging in basic health care, and published its first manual of ultrasound technique in 1995. Surgeon-performed ultrasound closes the loop between diagnosis and treatment without requiring a radiologist and/or technician.

39.2 Con

39.2.1 Ongoing Education Needs

Head and neck ultrasound requires a continual self-education and hands-on experience. The individual who is not committed to properly developing the examining skills, proper reporting language, and interpretation of images will do a disservice to patients.

39.2.2 Time Challenges

For the first few months, this will add time to the outpatient visit. The surgeon must adjust the schedule accordingly with the expectation that over time the frustration associated with this prolongation will diminish substantially and the study can be accelerated to an acceptable level.

39.3 Conclusions

This is an overview of the relevance of ultrasound to the arsenal of the head and neck surgeon. Generally, surgeons enjoy applied anatomy; ultrasound offers the consummate opportunity to examine structures in real time. Arguments have been rendered concerning potential conflict with referring endocrinologists and radiologists who perform other imaging studies on rush request. The surgeon wants to retain their friendship and lines of referral. It is helpful to discuss mutual interests with the endocrinologist, emphasizing that a full screening and mapping of lymph nodes is critical to the design of the procedure as well as defining long term follow-up issues. Patients who have previously been studied with ultrasound in the radiology department should nevertheless have the study repeated by the surgeon. Of course, if the study is available in a PACS system with cine loops this step can be omitted. Regardless, no charge should be submitted by the surgeon. The relationship with radiology will depend to some degree on expertise. Learning their preferred construction of a report and specific terminology will give the surgeon credibility. Providing a DVD or PACS image of interesting images for the radiology teaching file will be appreciated and will demonstrate that a spirit of collegiality can exist.

R.S. Lastly, after my surgical career terminated I have continued to enjoy the care and management of endocrine surgery of the head and neck through ultrasound. It has allowed me to perform appropriate imaging, perform biopsies, and follow patients. And it really is fun. I have been part of the National Ultrasound Faculty of the American College of Surgeons since 2001 and Chairman of the Thyroid and Parathyroid Module for 10 years ending in 2013. We have sponsored introductory courses at the American College of Surgeons (ACS) Congress and American Association-Head and Neck Surgery (AAO-HNS) and numerous exported courses to universities, resort, and hotel courses. These are all designed to teach the didactic elements of ultrasound to include hands-on skills. This is just the beginning as it does not guarantee any degree of quality. Accreditation of expertise from an independent agency is now available and I predict under mandate in the future as insurance carriers and government agencies will insist on parameters of ability. The American Institute of Ultrasound in Medicine (AIUM) in conjunction with the AAO-HNS has been able to develop the opportunity for surgeons, residents, and radiologists to submit cases to a Review Board. The AIUM website with head and neck concentration is clear and the only means of obtaining Accreditation at the present. Managing this process has become my current primary medical activity. Hopefully, individuals who complete the ACS courses and continue performing ultrasound will want to pursue Accreditation for the reasons outlined above.

M.S. As I incorporated point-of-care ultrasound into my head and neck surgery practice, I found that ultrasound became the "stethoscope" for my fingers in examining my patients. The longer I have had a machine in my office, the more applications I find. It has invigorated my practice and career tremendously: my patients welcome the convenience and enhanced information, my students and trainees enthusiastically embrace ultrasound practice, and I've taken point-of-care head and neck ultrasound around the globe to bring imaging capabilities into remote settings. The network of surgeon sonographers is growing rapidly, thanks to the vision and leadership of Dr. Sofferman and other pioneers in the field.

40 Ultrasound for Endocrinologists: What I Learned from Lifetime Practice

Susan J. Mandel

Reflections on ultrasound imaging of the thyroid and the neck over more than two decades of use as an endocrinologist trigger both exhilaration and humility, which are persistently coupled as I continue to practice of the art of imaging. Throughout my career, I have been fortunate to partner with and learn from skilled and dedicated colleagues from multiple specialties to provide optimal care for my patients.

40.1 Exhilaration

40.1.1 What You Can See

Anatomy is awesome. There is the thrill of visualizing the intricacies and three-dimensional relationships of the neck structures which may particularly resonate with those physicians in disciplines where these spatial relationships have not been encountered since first year medical school anatomy. Ultrasound (US) demonstrates transverse processes of the cervical vertebrae, vagal nerves, the esophagus, great vessels and smaller ones, the vocal cords, salivary glands, the thymus, the origin of the superior thyroidal artery from the carotid and the inferior thyroidal artery the traverses the great vessels to originate from the thyrocervical trunk. And US allows unforeseen detection of nonthyroid pathology—sarcoidosis based upon lymph node appearance, Sjogren's because of heterogeneity of the salivary glands, thyroglossal duct cysts, lymphomas, and other malignancies associated with metastatic cervical adenopathy.

Sonographic imaging of the thyroid enhances our understanding of pathophysiology. We can diagnose autoimmune thyroid disease based upon parenchymal heterogeneity and detect thyroid nodules that we otherwise cannot palpate, measuring a few millimeters to over 3 cm. The compendium of literature informs us about the association of a nodule's malignancy risk with its sonographic appearance. For patients undergoing thyroid surgery, imaging of cervical lymph nodes can optimize the surgical procedure by detecting nonpalpable metastatic disease.

As an educator, sonographic imaging complements physical diagnosis. US delineates the anterior contour of the thyroid gland, making evident what should be detected on a physical examination. An irregular thyroid contour as found in Hashimoto's thyroiditis translates to the firm gritty sensation felt on exam. And US makes it clear that the 2 cm nodule thought to be palpable by another clinician is clearly not because there is no forward displacement of the anterior

S.J. Mandel, M.D., M.P.H. (✉)
Division of Endocrinology, Diabetes and Metabolism, Perelman School of Medicine, University of Pennsylvania, Philadelphia, PA 19104, USA
e-mail: Susan.Mandel@uphs.upenn.edu

M. Milas et al. (eds.), *Advanced Thyroid and Parathyroid Ultrasound*,
DOI 10.1007/978-3-319-44100-9_40

surface of the thyroid. Conversely, US confirms that the 8 mm isthmus nodule located only 6 mm below the skin surface should be evident on a physical examination.

40.1.2 What You Can Do

Ultrasound guided fine-needle aspiration biopsies (US FNA) of thyroid nodules and lymph nodes. Using ultrasound guidance, it is technically possible for a skilled operator to target lesions as small as 5 mm, although we now know this is generally not clinically indicated (see below). Ultrasound facilitates accurate targeting of posterior nodules or those located lower or deeper in the neck as well as the solid areas of cystic nodules, otherwise inaccessible for palpation FNA. Furthermore, by taking advantage of the sector imaging properties of a lower frequency curvilinear versus a linear probe, it is possible to target suspicious lymph nodules located posterior to the great vessels in the inferior lateral neck.

40.1.3 Whom You Can Work With

Ultrasound imaging and FNA of thyroid and neck structures transcend specialties, endocrinology, radiology, cytology, head and neck surgery and endocrine surgery, with opportunities for multidisciplinary collaboration, research, patient care, and education—all of which have resulted in cross discipline collegiality and friendships. In fact, the concept of this textbook originated at an ultrasound course 4 years ago, where Mira Milas, Jill Langer, and I were faculty. We reflected upon how the synergy of our disciplines broadened our understanding of imaging, physiology and pathophysiology and how this could benefit learners of US. Both the Endocrine Society and American Thyroid Association US courses for continuing medical education (CME) include surgeons, endocrinologists, cytologists, and radiologists from the United States and from abroad. Furthermore, as US workshops have become increasing refined to become more effective learning venues, opportunities for international education have increased.

There are two collaborative endeavors that have most contributed to my professional satisfaction as an endocrinologist. The first is the multidisciplinary Thyroid Nodule Clinic at my own institution. Here, I work with Jill Langer, our Ultrasound section chief, Zubair Baloch, a cytologist known for his thyroid expertise, and their colleagues to optimize efficient and quality care for patients with thyroid nodules. A patient undergoes a diagnostic ultrasound exam, followed by US-guided fine needle aspiration (FNA) when clinically indicated, with onsite cytology examination and discussion of preliminary cytology results. The synergistic learning over the last two decades has enhanced all of our careers. The second is my partnership with the endocrine faculty at Chris Hani Baragwanath Hospital in Soweto, South Africa to initiate a multidisciplinary thyroid nodule clinic that started in 2014. This clinic has directly impacted quality of care, decreasing the time from diagnosis of thyroid cancer to surgery from 3 months to as little as 2 weeks.

40.2 Humility—So Much Still to Learn

40.2.1 What You See May Not Be What It Is

Studies investigating interobserver reproducibility for identification of both individual features and composite sonographic patterns report that at most, agreement just reaches the lower limit of what is considered as good. Some of the variability has been attributed to operator experience or US equipment. Working with high end radiology machines, and with years of experience, daily I confront challenges in classification of what are even considered basic features, such as composition and echogenicity. The same nodule may appear isoechoic on one static image and hypoechoic on another and this may be influenced by probe angle or adjacent structures on that view. In addition, high frequency linear probes are generally used for diagnostic imaging and we have observed that a nodule that images as uniformly solid may appear to have a more mixed cystic solid composition with a lower frequency curvilinear or sector probe, subsequently abrogating the recommendation for FNA. The classifications of borders that are not smooth as infiltrative or microlobulated versus just poorly defined, and the classifications of bright reflectors as either more (microcalcifications) or less worrisome, are frequent grey areas in image interpretation. And this all directly affects patient care by impacting FNA decision making.

40.2.2 Not Everything You See Merits a Needle

I began my career as a thyroidologist in the era of palpation FNA, with the pervasive mantra of aspiration of all nodules over 1 cm. So in the 1990s, I recommended US FNA for all such sonographically detected nodules—so many FNAs. I would aspirate up to four nodules in a single patient. In fact, the first version of the ATA Guidelines for management of thyroid nodules, published only 10 years ago, recommended FNA for all supracentimetric nodules [1]. The first refinement to my FNA practice was the incorporation of risk stratification using sonographic features, which then determined variable size cutoffs for FNA. But still many nodules were submitted to FNA because our mission objective remained cancer detection.

Now, we recognize that the almost exponential rise in thyroid cancer incidence over the last decade epitomizes the concept of cancer overdiagnosis [2]. This trend is strongly correlated with increased use of imaging pervasive in medicine that leads to incidental detection of nodules, with subsequent FNA. The cancers we are currently diagnosing are significantly smaller than 15 years ago and many are low risk or indolent [3, 4]. Therefore, confronted with the burgeoning number of detected thyroid nodules, FNA should be reserved for nodules with the potential to be clinically more aggressive cancers, and surveillance is appropriate for smaller sonographically suspicious nodules 1 cm or less, confined to the thyroid, without metastatic adenopathy. Furthermore, given the very low cancer risk of <3 % associated with certain sonographic patterns such as spongiform, FNA can be deferred even for large nodules. Therefore, at this stage of my career, I adhere to a more holistic approach to FNA decision making, where knowing more may actually mean doing less. And this model is currently promoted internationally by leading practitioners of sonography, be they radiologists, endocrinologists or surgeons, as we strive to maximize benefit to patients, while minimizing harm.

References

1. Cooper DS, Doherty GM, Haugen BR, Kloos RT, Lee SL, Mandel SJ, et al. Management guidelines for patients with thyroid nodules and differentiated thyroid cancer. Thyroid. 2006;16(2):109–42.
2. Welch HG, Black WC. Overdiagnosis in cancer. J Natl Cancer Inst. 2010;102(9):605–13.
3. Ahn HS, Kim HJ, Welch HG. Korea's thyroid-cancer "epidemic"--screening and overdiagnosis. N Engl J Med. 2014;371(19):1765–7.
4. Davies L, Welch HG. Current thyroid cancer trends in the United States. JAMA Otolaryngol Head Neck Surg. 2014;140(4):317–22.

41 Ultrasound for Radiologists: What I Learned from Lifetime Practice

Jill E. Langer

The rapid expansion of technology has caused most radiology practices to focus on the so-called "high-tech" diagnostic radiology exams, such as magnetic resonance imaging (MRI), computed tomography (CT), and positron emission tomography (PET). There is likely a subconscious bias among most radiologists (and perhaps non-radiologists), that these complex and expensive exams with hundreds, and sometimes over a thousand images, displayed from multiple imaging planes with the aid of advanced reconstruction platforms, must always be superior for diagnosis as compared to the low-tech radiology exams. As a subspecialist radiologist in diagnostic and interventional sonography for the last 25 years, I can proclaim with pride that for imaging of the thyroid and cervical nodes, sonography completely outperforms all other exams. The superficial location of the majority of the structures in the neck affords an unhindered view with the ultrasound probe and the spatial resolution of sonography surpasses that of MR and CT, uniquely allowing the detection of subtle and critically important findings such as microcalcifications and infiltrative margins within thyroid nodules and tiny cystic regions in cervical nodes. The real time nature of sonography allows for dynamic assessment which can be useful for diagnosis but more importantly provides the safest and most efficient guidance for biopsies and other interventions in the neck. Sonography is unquestionably the most essential imaging tool for the care of patients with thyroid (and in many cases, parathyroid) disease. I must admit that it is a sort of a moral victory that my dedication to and passion for the practice of sonography is affirmed by the superiority of sonography in this clinical context.

The practice of sonography is incredibly appealing to me because the field ranges broadly across nearly all aspects of health care. This challenges me to be knowledgeable and current about so many different medical and surgical subspecialties in order to provide meaningful interpretation of the images, as well as being skillful in the performance of the exam and biopsy procedures. More importantly, the practice of sonography offers the ability to provide direct patient care. The sonography exam and the performance of an ultrasound-guided procedure are among the most intimate patient care experiences in the practice of radiology both from the patient perspective and (in my practice) from the physician perspective. It is a hands-on encounter with an opportunity for the radiologists to truly care for a patient,

J.E. Langer, M.D. (✉)
Department of Radiology, The Perelman School of Medicine at the University of Pennsylvania, 3400 Spruce Street, Philadelphia, PA 19104, USA
e-mail: jill.langer@uphs.upenn.edu

M. Milas et al. (eds.), *Advanced Thyroid and Parathyroid Ultrasound*,
DOI 10.1007/978-3-319-44100-9_41

by listening to them, examining them and having dialogue about the findings, an experience quite similar to a typical physician office visit.

41.1 The Art of Sonography

Technologic advances in the last several years have allowed for the development of good quality, portable and inexpensive sonographic instruments that can be used in the office setting and in the operating room. This availability has motivated a variety of subspecialties that care for patients with thyroid and parathyroid abnormalities to encourage physicians and other care providers to learn to become adept at examining the neck with ultrasound and incorporate sonography as a routine part of their practice.

It is wonderful to witness the ever expanding role of sonography in the care of patients. The challenge is that, unlike CT and MR, the sonographic exam is not an automated process; it is an exam that needs to be created by the sonologist (noting that term sonologist refers to the person operating the ultrasound equipment without distinction by medical background or training) by using skillful manipulation of the probe and sonographic controls. The sonologist must pay incredible attention to small details while adhering to imaging protocols to be thorough, but must also be prepared appropriately to expand the exam to assure that they have fully investigated the entire neck when abnormalities are noted. Therefore, it remains essential that all sonologists recognize that, in order to provide optimal patient care, the exam needs to be both expertly performed *and* expertly interpreted. It is incumbent upon the sonologist to maintain a healthy respect for the challenges that the performance of high quality sonography presents and an appreciation that the recognition of incredible subtleties will dramatically alter the diagnosis. In the radiology practice model, the ultrasound lab is responsible for performing a complete and comprehensive diagnostic exam of the neck whereas in the non-radiology practice model it is acceptable to use sonography in a more limited capacity or so-called point-of care sonography. In most radiology practices in the USA, the images are typically acquired by ultrasound technologists (sonographers), who are highly trained medical professionals who need to be certified and work within an institution accredited to perform sonography. It is the responsibility of the sonographers to take a brief patient history, to perform the real time exam, and capture the required images as stipulated by practice guidelines. The thoroughness with which the neck is interrogated, the number of captured images and the diagnostic quality of the captured images will vary greatly depending on the skill and experience of the sonographer. I have worked with a number of outstanding technologists who are not only extremely skilled at the technical aspect of their craft but who are dedicated and caring professionals. They have strived to become educated about both the imaging findings and the clinical presentations of the disease processes of their patients in an effort to provide optimal patient care. Their diagnostic excellence has indeed been essential in the care of many patients seen in our ultrasound lab and I am incredibly indebted to all of them. There are too many technologists that I would like to publically recognize to list all by name, but I would like to give special recognition to a few. Caren Levine, RDMS, assumed the role as our first lead technologist in our multidisciplinary thyroid clinic. Caren is the consummate perfectionist in her scanning, consistently providing images of the highest quality and often capturing the most subtle abnormalities that I am sure would go undetected under another's watch. Her expertise and compassionate care have made her the most sought after technologist for our returning patients, many of whom will only schedule their appointment with the knowledge that Caren will be there to perform their scan. Christopher Iyoob, RDMS (our ultrasound supervisor) and Bonnie Brake, RDMS, RVT (our lead technologist for interventional ultrasound) have provided the leadership and mentorship necessary to make sure all of our technologists meet our lab's high expectations for diagnostic quality.

41.2 The Role of the Radiologist

The role of the radiologist is to (a) provide medical and technical guidance to the sonographers, (b) assure that the lab is adhering to practice guidelines in the performance of the sonographic exams and the maintenance standards of its equipment, (c) accurately interpret the images, and (d) generate a radiology report that describes the pertinent findings, and when appropriate, provide recommendations for further testing or follow-up evaluation. Certainly the interpretation of the images and the generation of the report require the most expertise on the part of the radiologist. Similar to the expected variances of diagnostic expertise in all medical disciplines, the diagnostic skill of the physicians interpreting ultrasound exams will vary, and an interpretation, even among the most skilled, may be compromised by technically limited or incomplete imaging. Certainly my diagnostic skills and knowledge base have evolved over the course of my training and throughout my career. I am fortunate to practice in an outstanding academic institution where I have had the benefit of working with and learning from some of the most gifted and knowledgeable physicians in the fields of Endocrinology, Head and Neck Surgery, Oncologic Surgery, Anatomic Pathology and Cytopathology over my career at the University of Pennsylvania. A major turning point in our institution's quest for clinical and research excellence in the care of patients with thyroid disease was the recruitment of Susan Mandel, MD, MPH in 1998. Under her guidance and leadership as an endocrinologist specializing in thyroid disease, an open line of communication and a culture of mutual respect were established with our radiology department as well as with all clinicians caring for her patients. Our institution and more importantly, the patients for whom we all provide care, have greatly benefited from this respectful spirit of clinical collaboration. These colleagues have made me a better diagnostician by respectfully discussing what pertinent information the radiologist needs to provide to them to optimize the care of *our* patients. In fact, it has been our (Mira Milas, Susan Mandel, and myself) collective experience to recognize that when the pathologist, radiologist, endocrinologist, and surgeon, all communicate their findings, clinical impressions, and diagnostic dilemmas to each other, this exchange translates into optimal patient care. This was the inspiration and motivation for writing this book, to share expertise among all subspecialties caring for these patients.

In just the last decade, the leading national and international organizations of thyroidologists have dramatically changed their recommendations for the management of thyroid nodules from a lesion size approach to one which is nearly entirely based on the sonographic appearance of the nodule, especially in the most common scenario of detection of nodules in patients without risk factors for thyroid cancer. Sonographic assessment has become the single most important determinant in the management of the thyroid nodules and in determining the extent of thyroid surgery, which makes accurate assessment and reporting of sonographic findings essential. I caution those who trivialize the interpretation of the thyroid or parathyroid ultrasound exam as simplistic. The technologists and physicians in our lab find the nuances of sonographic assessment of the thyroid, parathyroid glands, and lymph nodes in the neck among our most challenging work. After reviewing the images acquired by our sonologists, it is at the discretion of the interpreting physicians as to whether additional imaging is necessary or if the exam is considered complete. Among all of the varied, highly complex exams we perform, it is far and away the neck exam that requires the most physician involvement prior to discharging the patient from our lab. Our physicians are diligent about scanning patients themselves to be sure they can properly characterize the type of echoic foci in a thyroid nodule as suspicious or nonsuspicious and that a hidden, hyperplastic parathyroid gland can be coaxed into view by having the patient swallow or changing to a lower frequency probe and severely angling into the upper mediastinum. I realize that an academic practice affords me the luxury of being on-site to trouble shoot and work dynamically with our excellent sonographers. In other practices, the radiologist may be off-site during the acquisition of the exam, such that it is paramount that the radiologist and the sonographers work together to understand the nuances and diagnostic pitfalls of the neck ultrasound exam and develop imaging protocols that help to improve diagnostic accuracy. The most effective radiologist is one who not only has a keen eye for detecting abnormalities, but one who understands their relevance and what necessary information needs to be conveyed in the report.

41.3 Radiologist as Gate Keeper

Over the last few years, there has been much appropriate discussion about the necessity or lack of necessity to biopsy all detected thyroid nodules. The remarkable sensitivity of sonography, and to a lesser extent CT and MR, leads to the identification of thyroid nodules in many adults, and in older individuals, thyroid nodules will be seen in the majority of those examined by imaging, especially by sonography. A majority of these nodules are detected by the radiologist outside of the context of clinical evaluation for known or suspected thyroid cancer and are therefore termed incidental thyroid nodules (ITNs). Fortunately, only a very small minority of incidentally detected nodules will show obvious imaging signs of malignant or aggressive behavior at the time of detection. For the vast majority of nonsuspicious appearing ITNs, medical decision making as to the need for further evaluation and the specifics of that evaluation will need to be addressed. What is the radiologist's role in the decision making and medical management of these ITNs?

The majority of the ITNs are noted in patients referred for imaging exams by non-thyroidologists. These clinicians therefore are looking for guidance from the radiologist about how to manage the incidental finding. It is common to see incidentally detected lesions in almost all organs among patients undergoing diagnostic evaluation by CT, MR and sonography. Referring clinicians rely on the radiologists to perform a careful assessment of imaging features of the incidentally detected lesion and based on evidence-based guidelines, provide a management recommendation for the need or lack of need of follow-up in the radiology report. Similar to thyroid nodules, the vast majority of these incidentally detected lesions are also benign and therefore follow-up imaging is not recommended in many instances. It is not the expectation that this approach will detect all malignant lesions but that unnecessary additional testing and, in some instances, surgery can be avoided in the majority of patients due to a very low probability of malignancy among the entire patient group. The recent American Thyroid Association (ATA) guidelines have embraced this strategy by recommending against follow-up of nodules under 10 mm with a very low suspicion sonographic appearance in low-risk patients [1]. Certainly it is possible that not 100 % of these nodules are benign but the risk of malignancy is deemed exceedingly low such that it is not practical to perform surveillance sonography on a huge number of patients to detect very few cancers. I believe that this is an appropriate and medically responsible strategy, and one that can be extrapolated to the incidental detection of small nodules on CT or MR in adult low risk patients. The impetus to abandon nodule size of 10 mm or greater as the sole indication for biopsy, and instead place a greater emphasis on the analysis of sonographic appearance of ITNs in medical decision making was brought forth by The Society of Radiologists in Ultrasound (SRU) at a consensus conference in 2004 and published in 2005 [2]. At first, this concept was met with resistance by some, concerned that malignant thyroid nodules over 10 mm would go undetected, but now this is the cornerstone of all nodule evaluation algorithms. The concept of imaging-based risk stratification of thyroid nodules and the need to less aggressively pursue evaluation of nonsuspicious appearing nodules is fully now supported by the non-radiology community. The ATA has recently adopted a more conservative approach in the management of very low suspicion pattern nodules over 20 mm, now allowing for sonographic surveillance rather than recommending biopsy in all patients. This more closely aligns with the recommendations of the SRU for low risk adults as well. Certainly, any clinician may elect to pursue a different management plan for any incidental or nonincidental finding than that recommended by the radiologist, based on risk factors potentially not known at the time of the radiology report, abnormal physical exam or laboratory findings, or personal preference of the physician. The future likely holds an expanding role of sonography in medical decision making about thyroid nodules. As we accumulate more knowledge about the natural history of benign (or presumed benign) thyroid nodules of larger size, our concepts regarding for the need for biopsy or sonographic follow-up to exclude malignancy from nodules that have a very low suspicion pattern may also change.

Overall, I am proud and enthusiastic about the central role that sonography has come to play in the sphere of thyroid and parathyroid disease. Sonography is an incredibly patient-friendly imaging tool that can provide remarkably high-resolution images. It is wonderful to see so many clinicians from so many varied disciplines not only acknowledge but ardently support the use of sonography in the care of patients.

References

1. Haugen BR, Alexander EK, Bible KC, Doherty GM, Mandel SJ, Nikiforov YE, et al. 2015 American Thyroid Association Management Guidelines for adult patients with thyroid nodules and differentiated thyroid cancer: the American Thyroid Association Guidelines Task Force on thyroid nodules and differentiated thyroid cancer. Thyroid. 2016;26(1):1–133.
2. Frates MC, Benson CB, Charboneau JW, Cibas ES, Clark OH, Coleman BG, Cronan JJ, Doubilet PM, Evans DB, Goellner JR, Hay ID, Hertzberg BS, Intenzo CM, Jeffrey RB, Langer JE, Larsen PR, Mandel SJ, Middleton WD, Reading CC, Sherman SI, Tessler FN, Society of Radiologists in Ultrasound. Management of thyroid nodules detected at US: Society of Radiologists in Ultrasound consensus conference statement. Radiology. 2005;237(3):794–800.

Ultrasound for Primary Care Practitioners and Emergency Medicine Physicians

42

Renee K. Dversdal and Teresa Wu

42.1 "Top 10" Favorite Ultrasound Pearls

1. Most thyroid glands should be evaluated using a high frequency, linear array transducer.
2. In the acute care setting, it is helpful to place the patient in a supine position with a pillow under the patient's shoulders to help extend the patient's neck.
3. Begin the scan by orienting the transducer so that the indicator marker is pointing towards the patient's right side.
4. Do not mistake the longus colli muscles or esophagus for nodules.
5. Do not mistake the four hypoechoic parathyroid glands for cysts or masses.
6. Nodules seen in only one plane are likely "pseudonodules."
7. Pay close attention to microcalcifications, or punctate echogenic foci seen within the thyroid gland. Microcalcifications are very specific for thyroid malignancy.
8. While many handheld and basic point-of-care ultrasound machines do not have time-gain compensation, in some, users can selectively change near and far-field gain.
9. In morbidly obese patients, it may be necessary to use a low-frequency curvilinear probe to penetrate deep enough to appreciate the entire thyroid gland and surrounding structures.
10. Know your machine: while many basic point-of-care machines will not have as many knobs and buttons for fine adjustments, there are usually several "soft key" or "auto" options to optimize images.

42.2 "Top 10" Lexicon Terms

1. *Acoustic shadowing*: When the ultrasound beam hits a strong reflector (like calcium), the reflective surface can block the beam from reaching deeper structures. Structures distal to the reflector will not be imaged, and

Electronic supplementary material: The online version of this chapter (doi:10.1007/978-3-319-44100-9_42) contains supplementary material, which is available to authorized users. Videos can also be accessed at http://link.springer.com/chapter/10.1007/978-3-319-44100-9_42.

R.K. Dversdal, M.D.
Division of Hospital Medicine, Department of Medicine, Oregon Health & Science University, 3181 SW Sam Jackson Park Rd, OP30, Portland, OR 97239, USA
e-mail: dversdar@ohsu.edu

T. Wu, M.D. (✉)
Center for Simulation & Innovation, University of Arizona, College of Medicine-Phoenix, 435 N. 5th Street, B420, Phoenix, AZ 85004, USA

Department of Emergency Medicine, Banner - University Medical Center Phoenix, 1111 E. McDowell Road, Phoenix, AZ 85006, USA
e-mail: teresawumd@gmail.com

M. Milas et al. (eds.), *Advanced Thyroid and Parathyroid Ultrasound*,
DOI 10.1007/978-3-319-44100-9_42

a dark, acoustic shadow is seen farfield to the reflective material.

2. *Comet-tail artifact*: Echogenic focus with reverberation artifact.
3. Eggshell calcification: Hyperechoic, bright white enhancement of the peripheral rim of a nodule or mass typically secondary to calcium deposition.
4. *Hypoechogenic areas* (*HEAs*): Term specifically describing hypoechoic regions in the thyroid associated with subacute thyroiditis.
5. *Irregular*: A thyroid nodule that is not ovoid, round or taller-than-wide.
6. *Macrocalcifications*: Hyperechoic calcifications large enough to cause posterior acoustic shadowing.
7. *Microcalcifications*: Punctate hyperechoic calcifications that are too small to cause posterior acoustic shadowing.
8. *Edge-artifact*: Thin acoustic shadows may appear behind the edges of cystic structures. Sound waves that bounce off a cystic wall or a curved surface at a tangential angle are scattered and refracted, leading to energy loss and formation of an edge shadow.
9. *Reverberation*: When sound waves bounce back and forth between two layers before traveling back to the transducer. This is interpreted by the probe as a prolonged travel time so an additional reverberated image is produced in the adjacent, deeper tissue layer.
10. *Taller-than-wide*: When the anteroposterior diameter of a nodule is longer than its transverse diameter in either the transverse or longitudinal plane.

42.3 Background

Over the past decade, there has been a dramatic increase in the number of health care providers learning how to incorporate point-of-care ultrasound (POCUS) into their clinical practices. Multiple medical specialties have integrated clinician-performed sonography into the assessment, evaluation, and management of patients at the bedside. As the number of bedside ultrasound applications continues to grow, specialties such as surgery, pediatrics, internal medicine, family practice, and emergency medicine are now beginning to develop policies and procedures on how to obtain, interpret, and integrate point-of-care thyroid ultrasonography into patient care pathways.

The integration of point-of-care thyroid sonography is still a relatively novel application in both the primary care and acute care settings. As such, it is important to recognize that early adopters of point-of-care thyroid ultrasound will have varying amounts of experience and expertise. Over the past few years, there has been a concerted movement to introduce point-of-care ultrasound education into both medical school curricula and post-graduate residency and fellowship training. Recent reports suggest that several medical schools are now graduating physicians with 4 years of integrated ultrasound experience [1, 2], while in 2012 over 62 % of curricula at responding medical schools contained at least some ultrasound component, with 78 % of schools agreeing that ultrasound should be a part of the undergraduate medical curriculum [3]. At the Graduate Medical Education level, Emergency Medicine and Pulmonary Critical Medicine now have ultrasound-related ACGME program requirements, and accrediting bodies such as American College of Emergency Physicians have published guidelines on required ultrasound training via Residency-based or Practice-based pathways. In the USA, several Internal Medicine residency programs have also published data on introducing ultrasound curricula [4, 5]; however, in 2012 only 25 % of programs had formal ultrasound curricula [6]. Because point-of-care thyroid ultrasound is still quite novel, the clinicians currently performing bedside thyroid scans may have varying image acquisition and interpretation skills based on their experiences and training.

It is important to note that most point-of-care ultrasound is performed using simple, compact, and portable ultrasound machines that have different settings frequently encountered on machines used in sonography suites and thyroid clinics (Fig. 42.1 (GE V-Scan, Wauwatosa, WI, USA), and Fig. 42.2a (SonoSite M-turbo), Fig. 42.2b (SonoSite X-porte), and Fig. 42.2c (SonoSite EDGE) (SonoSite, Bothell, WA)). Many of these portable ultrasound machines have

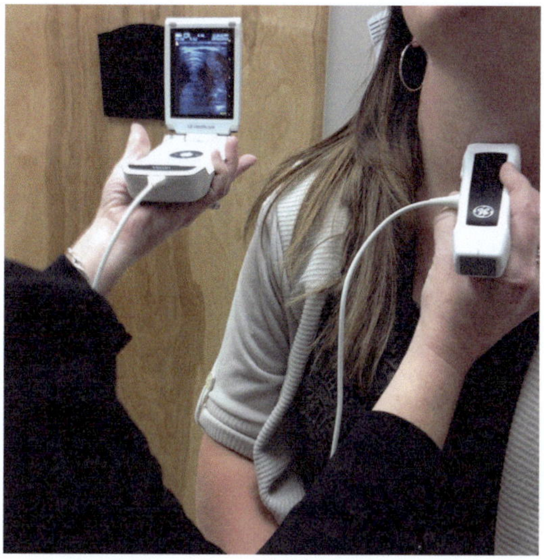

Fig. 42.1 A dual-probe handheld ultrasound unit is used in the linear, nonvascular setting to visualize a young woman's thyroid in a primary care clinic. GE V-Scan used with permission of GE Healthcare, Wauwatosa, WI, USA

automatically set focal zones and lack time gain compensation (TGC), which makes image acquisition easier for the novice, but can also impair ultimate image quality. Most point-of-care scans of the thyroid gland and surrounding structures are performed in B-mode, using basic standard settings. Color Doppler and power Doppler can be applied to help evaluate surrounding vasculature and to determine if there is increased blood flow to the target organ.

Point-of-care ultrasound of the thyroid is typically utilized to answer a specific set of questions at the bedside. Most practitioners who are performing POCUS of the thyroid have imposed time constraints that prohibit the acquisition and interpretation of a comprehensive thyroid ultrasound that is typically obtained in radiology or thyroid centers. When focused, point-of-care thyroid ultrasounds are being performed at the bedside, the clinician is usually interested in answering the following questions:

1. Does the patient have an enlarged thyroid gland?
2. Does the patient have a focal or discrete thyroid mass?
3. Does the patient's ultrasound demonstrate findings suggestive of thyroiditis?
4. Does the patient have a goiter?

Clinicians who are performing these point-of-care ultrasound examinations of the thyroid have been trained to obtain useful sonographic information at the bedside that can be used to help tailor future treatment, management, and follow-up options for the patient.

42.4 Technique

As with other point-of-care ultrasound examinations, clinicians in the primary care and acute care settings are performing focused, goal-directed imaging of the target structures. During a point-of-care ultrasound of the thyroid, the patient is placed in a supine position with the neck in slight hyperextension. Using a high-frequency linear transducer, the clinician will typically start by obtaining an image of the trachea in the midline and note the right and left thyroid lobes adjacent to the thyroid. An image of the thyroid isthmus is typically recorded in this transverse plane. It is important to confirm that the orientation is in the conventional position: for transverse views (the patient's right side is displayed on the left of the monitor as physician faces monitor); for longitudinal views, the superior thyroid pole is on monitor left. This is easiest to do with finger pressing one edge of the probe's flat footprint to detect where the motion displays on the monitor; alternately the marker facing the patient's right side can be helpful but this varies with machines and can change when machine settings are changed. The clinician will then scan through each thyroid lobe and the isthmus in both the longitudinal and transverse planes. During the scan, the clinician will sweep entirely through both glands and adjust the depth to ensure adequate imaging of posterior and far field structures.

Some clinicians practice a basic "eyeball" or global evaluation of the thyroid echotexture and size and will recommend referral for comprehen-

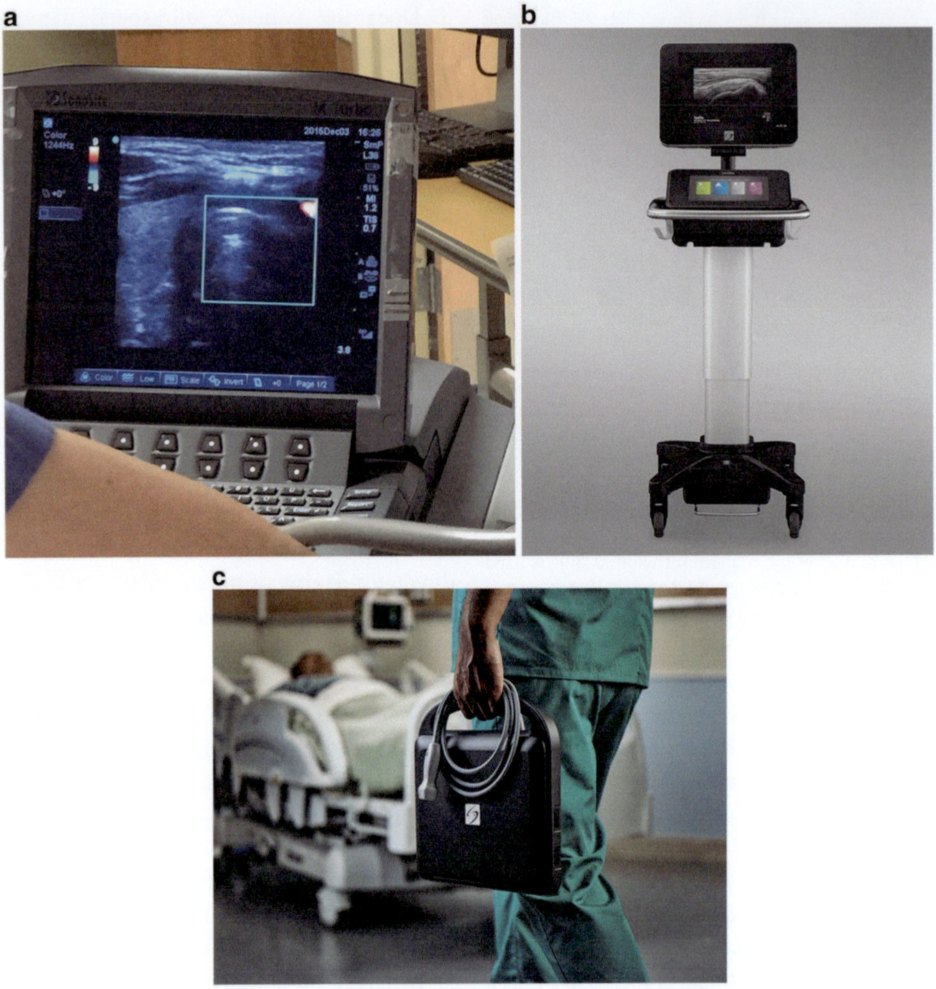

Fig. 42.2 A basic point-of-care ultrasound machine is used by an Emergency Medicine resident to practice thyroid ultrasound during ultrasound rounds. (**a**) SonoSite M-turbo; (**b**) X-porte; and (**c**) EDGE. Used with permission of SonoSite, Bothell, WA, USA

sive imaging if any obvious abnormalities are noted. Others will perform a more comprehensive and detailed ultrasound evaluation of the thyroid gland at the bedside. Clinicians performing point-of-care ultrasound evaluations of the thyroid as a regular part of their practice will often seek to obtain transverse images of the superior, mid, and inferior portions of the right and left thyroid lobes. In addition, images will be recorded of the medial, mid, and lateral portions of both lobes in a longitudinal fashion. The size of each thyroid lobe is generally recorded in three dimensions: anteroposterior, transverse, and longitudinal, and color or power Doppler examination can also be used to supplement grayscale evaluation of any focal or diffuse abnormalities noted. It is often useful to extend the scan to include the soft tissue above the isthmus (e.g., to evaluate a possible pyramidal lobe congenital abnormalities such as a thyroglossal duct cyst, or if any superior palpable abnormality is noted.)

It is important to obtain both still images and to record short video clips for archiving, documentation and billing purposes. These still images and video clips should include standardized images of the entire thyroid gland in both longitudinal and transverse planes, and also recordings of any abnormalities noted in the gland and surrounding structures. Current research is underway to delineate which abnormal sonographic findings are likely non-pathologic (i.e., nodules <1 cm with no findings associated with malignancy), in comparison to those that require urgent or expedited follow up with comprehensive thyroid imaging with dedicated specialists.

42.5 Thyroid Ultrasound in the Non-acute Care Setting

The thyroid examination is a classic component of the complete physical examination, and despite profound technological advancements and innumerable changes in medicine, it is still deemed important enough to be listed as #1 on the Stanford Medicine 25 [7]. However, when compared with postmortem thyroid weight and sonographically determined thyroid volume, palpation has been shown to be highly inaccurate for estimating thyroid size [8]. In surveys of medical students, interns, residents, and attending internists detecting a thyroid nodule had one of the lowest self-confidence scores of 15 key physical examination skills, along with one of the highest perceived utility scores [9].

Below are some cases encountered in the clinical setting where a portable thyroid ultrasound can be useful in the patient's assessment and management.

42.5.1 Case 1: Why Is Her Heart Racing?

While on a medical service trip in extremely rural Haiti a 32-year-old woman presents with a chief complaint of heart racing. The only available diagnostic tools are your stethoscope and your portable ultrasound.

On examination her heart rate is about 110 beats per minute, she has an enlarged, smooth thyroid, and a very soft bruit. The rest of her exam is unremarkable. With handheld ultrasound you confirm thyromegaly (Fig. 42.3, Video 42.1). To further assess her tachycardia you perform focused cardiac ultrasound to rule out congenital or acquired heart disease, and assessed volume status via inferior vena cava ultrasound. These studies are unremarkable.

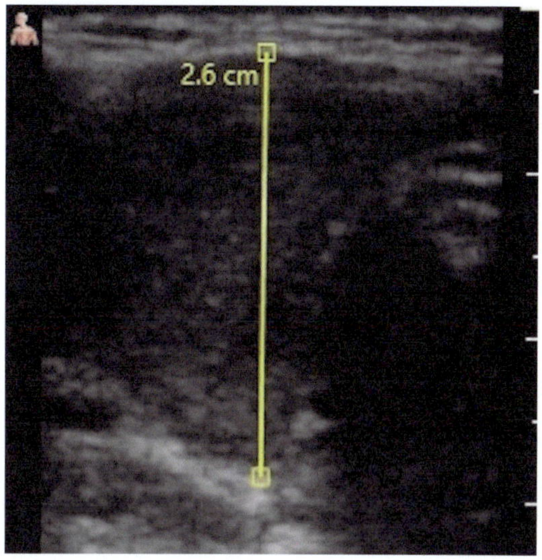

Fig. 42.3 An enlarged right lobe of the thyroid as captured on a handheld ultrasound unit. This measures 2.6 cm in depth as demonstrated by the yellow annotation

Your clinical diagnosis is Graves' disease; however, with no other diagnostic or treatment capabilities you are only able to advise travel to the nearest clinic which is 2h away, and some money, as they only perform basic testing and will likely have to refer her onward via ferry to Port-au-Prince, which you know she cannot afford.

Thyroid ultrasonography for goiter prevalence assessment in developing countries has been shown to be feasible [10], and has been used to assess iodine deficiency via World Health Organization recommended surveillance methods in rural/mountain areas as well [11]. This case demonstrates the utility of point-of-care ultrasound in resource-limited settings for detecting thyroid pathology in addition to simple screening/prevalence assessment purposes.

42.5.2 Case 2: Does She Have a Thyroid Nodule?

A healthy 24-year-old medical student presents to your primary care clinic after learning the thyroid examination in her Endocrine clinical skills lab. She has been more anxious lately, always "runs hot," and has self-diagnosed Irritable Bowel Syndrome, but thinks her bowel movements have been more loose lately. She is concerned she found a thyroid nodule on herself, though her clinical skills teacher on further examination did not appreciate this. However, she asserts that she does have some symptoms of hyperthyroidism, and worries she could have a "hot" nodule that her clinical skills teacher could not palpate.

You are up to date on clinical recommendations and well aware that the American Thyroid Association (ATA) recommends formal thyroid sonography for all patients with known or suspected nodules, while at the same time acknowledging that high-resolution thyroid ultrasound is able to detect thyroid nodule in 19–67 % of individuals [12]. You recall your own erroneous self-diagnosis of hypothyroidism in the setting of fatigue from studying long hours and being persistently cold (while in Boston for the winter!). You ask yourself "Am I ***really*** going to order a formal ultrasound for a ***suspected*** thyroid nodule that the most respected clinician at the university could not palpate?" Thankfully, the answer is no, as you have been attending ultrasound training sessions for years and incorporated point-of-care ultrasound in your practice for reasons just like this, along with a plethora of other clinical indications. You are actually one of the proponents for point of care ultrasound incorporation into the medical school curriculum.

Her traditional physical examination is completely normal, as is her thyroid ultrasound (Fig. 42.4), which you are able to demonstrate to her as you perform. Seeing the normal thyroid parenchyma seems to appease her, however she still convinces you to get thyroid function tests, just in case.

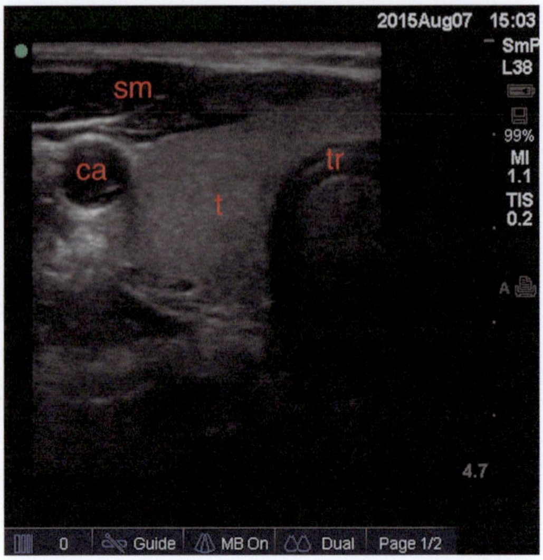

Fig. 42.4 In this transverse view of a normal R thyroid lobe the isoechoic (*grey*) thyroid tissue (t) is seen below the strap muscles (sm) and between the carotid artery (ca) and trachea (tr)

42.5.3 Case 3: What Is the Etiology of His Throat Pain?

A 55-year-old man with a history of hypertension, stage III chronic kidney disease, and well-controlled type-2 diabetes mellitus on insulin presents to your Urgent Care clinic with progressive anterior neck pain. He notes a mild cold last week, followed by muscle aches, alternating chills with hot flashes (no thermometer at home), fatigue and this neck pain that has progressed to the point that it hurts when he swallows or turns his head too far. Acetaminophen has helped a bit, but he is still very uncomfortable and worries he might have strep throat again, although he does note that this pain, while as severe, is different in nature than his past strep infection.

On exam his vital signs are notable for a temperature of 100 °C Fahrenheit, and heart rate of 110 bpm. His posterior oropharynx is completely unremarkable, and he has an exquisitely tender, enlarged thyroid. Your suspicion is for subacute thyroiditis and you are considering prednisone given his kidney disease barring use of nonsteroidal anti-inflammatory agents (NSAID) and pain severity; however, with diabetes you are reticent to start corticosteroids without additional confirmation of disease. You order thyroid function tests, but know that they get sent out to the hospital lab and will not be back for a few days.

You recall that thyroid ultrasound can also be helpful in subacute thyroiditis in addition to nodules and hyperthyroid states, so you grab the machine usually used for musculoskeletal purposes, knowing you are looking for enlargement (confirmed on physical examination) and more importantly, hypoechogenic areas (HEA) [13, 14]. On ultrasound examination you find multiple bilateral HEAs with normal-appearing thyroid parenchyma interspersed, and reduced flow on color Doppler (Fig. 42.5, Video 42.2).

With point of care ultrasound findings supporting your clinical impression you proceed with prednisone treatment more confidently, in addition to increasing his morning insulin NPH dose and setting up primary care follow-up in 1 week.

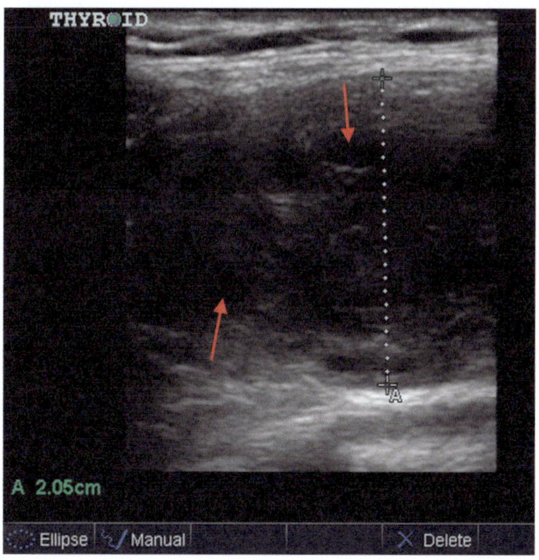

Fig. 42.5 In this longitudinal view of a diffusely abnormal thyroid one can appreciate an increased depth of 2.05 cm along with poorly defined hypoechogenic areas (two are highlighted with *arrows*)

42.6 Thyroid Ultrasound in the Acute or Emergent Setting

Disorders of the thyroid may be difficult to diagnose in the acute care or emergency setting. Patients may not know that they have an underlying thyroid disorder, and signs and symptoms of hyper or hypothyroidism can often manifest in varying manners. A thyroid ultrasound can be performed quickly at the bedside where valuable information can be obtained without exposing the patient to any radiation or delay in their diagnosis and treatment. Many urgent care centers and emergency departments have portable ultrasound machines that the practitioner will use during the initial assessment of patients presenting with a potential thyroid disorder. Acute care clinicians are being trained to evaluate the thyroid for size, presence of focal or discrete masses, increased vascular flow, and global appearance of the thyroid tissue on bedside ultrasound.

42.6.1 Case 4: Fever, Palpitations, and Diaphoresis

A 50-year-old female presents to the emergency department with a chief complaint of fever, palpitations and diaphoresis. Over the past few weeks, she has been feeling more "jittery" and she has recently developed some nausea, vomiting, and diarrhea. She is unemployed and has not been able to see a physician for "quite some time." She denies any past medical history and is not taking any medications.

She presents to the emergency department, tachycardic, hypertensive, febrile, and vomiting. Her initial physical exam is otherwise notable for a slender woman of stated age, with who appears in moderate distress from her symptoms. During her initial assessment, the team is concerned about a potential infection and risk for sepsis. A peripheral intravenous line is placed, blood tests are drawn for analysis, and a chest X-ray and electrocardiogram are obtained. As part of the

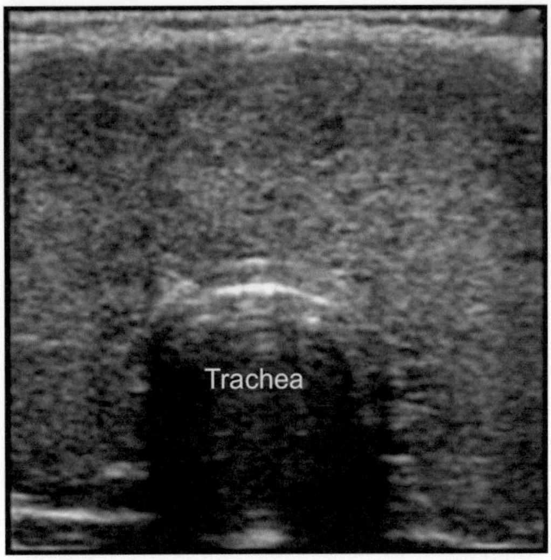

Fig. 42.6 In this longitudinal view, you can see a diffusely enlarged thyroid gland surrounding the normal trachea

patient's emergency department evaluation, a bedside, point-of-care ultrasound evaluation is performed to evaluate the patient's heart, lungs, and thyroid.

The patient is noted to have a small pericardial effusion, mild pulmonary edema with bilateral pleural effusions, and an enlarged thyroid gland with increased heterogeneity and Doppler flow on bedside ultrasound (Fig. 42.6). Based on her findings, a thyroid stimulating hormone (TSH) and Free T4 are added onto the initial blood tests, and aggressive supportive measures are started. The patient receives IV beta-blockade, glucocorticoids, potassium iodide, and methimazole or propylthiouracil (PTU). The diagnosis of thyrotoxicosis is made in the acute care setting and the patient's treatment is expedited based on the point-of-care ultrasound findings.

42.7 Conclusion

As technology progresses and becomes more readily available at the bedside, an increasing number of health care practitioners will begin to incorporate thyroid ultrasound into the assessment, treatment, and management of their patients. It will be important to define the types of thyroid and parathyroid abnormalities that may be optimal for evaluation in the primary and acute care settings, and to determine the appropriate follow-up and subsequent imaging required for these findings. The incorporation of thyroid ultrasonography into the initial assessment and management of patients at the bedside can provide invaluable information, and its use and integration has the potential to improve time to diagnosis and treatment for patients in multiple health care settings.

References

1. Hoppmann RA, Rao VV, Poston MB, Howe DB, Hunt PS, Fowler SD, et al. An integrated ultrasound curriculum (iUSC) for medical students: 4-year experience. Crit Ultrasound J. 2011;3(1):1–12. Available from: http://www.pubmedcentral.nih.gov/articlerender.fcgi?artid=3064888&tool=pmcentrez&rendertype=abstract.
2. Bahner DP, Adkins EJ, Hughes D, Barrie M, Boulger CT, Royall NA. Integrated medical school ultrasound: development of an ultrasound vertical curriculum. Crit Ultrasound J. 2013;5(1):6. Available from: http://www.pubmedcentral.nih.gov/articlerender.fcgi?artid=3701608&tool=pmcentrez&rendertype=abstract.
3. Bahner DP, Goldman E, Way D, Royall NA, Liu YT. The state of ultrasound education in U.S. medical schools: results of a national survey. Acad Med. 2014;89(12):1681–6. Available from: http://www.ncbi.nlm.nih.gov/pubmed/25099238.
4. Keddis MT, Cullen MW, Reed DA, Halvorsen AJ, McDonald FS, Takahashi PY, et al. Effectiveness of an ultrasound training module for internal medicine residents. BMC Med Educ. 2011;11:75. Available from: http://www.pubmedcentral.nih.gov/articlerender.fcgi?artid=3196730&tool=pmcentrez&rendertype=abstract.
5. Schnobrich DJ, Olson APJ, Broccard A, Duran-Nelson A. Feasibility and acceptability of a structured curriculum in teaching procedural and basic diagnostic ultrasound skills to internal medicine residents. J Grad Med Educ. 2013;5(3):493–7. Available from: http://www.pubmedcentral.nih.gov/articlerender.fcgi?artid=3771182&tool=pmcentrez&rendertype=abstract.
6. Schnobrich DJ, Gladding S, Olson APJ, Duran-Nelson A. Point-of-care ultrasound in internal medicine: a national survey of educational leadership. J Grad Med Educ. 2013;5(3):498–502. Available from: http://www.pubmedcentral.nih.gov/articlerender.fcgi?artid=3771183&tool=pmcentrez&rendertype=abstract.
7. Verghese AM. Stanford Medicine 25. Available from: http://stanfordmedicine25.stanford.edu/the25/thyro.

8. Langer P. Normal thyroid size versus goiter—postmortem thyroid weight and ultrasonographic volumetry versus physical examination. Endocrinol Exp. 1989;23(2):67–76. Available from: http://www.ncbi.nlm.nih.gov/pubmed/2673744.
9. Wu EH, Fagan MJ, Reinert SE, Diaz JA. Self-confidence in and perceived utility of the physical examination: a comparison of medical students, residents, and faculty internists. J Gen Intern Med. 2007;22(12):1725–30. Available from: http://www.pubmedcentral.nih.gov/articlerender.fcgi?artid=2219827&tool=pmcentrez&rendertype=abstract.
10. Amoah AGB, Asibey-Berko E, Ayettey OM, Addo F, Agyepong E, Lartey A, et al. Feasibility of thyroid ultrasonography in field studies in a developing country, Ghana. Afr J Med Med Sci. 2004;33(2):161–4. Available from: http://www.ncbi.nlm.nih.gov/pubmed/15565936.
11. Saggiorato E, Arecco F, Mussa A, Sacerdote C, Rossetto R, Origlia C, et al. Goiter prevalence and urinary iodine status in urban and rural/mountain areas of Piedmont region. J Endocrinol Invest. 2006;29(1):67–73. Available from: http://www.ncbi.nlm.nih.gov/pubmed/16553036.
12. Haugen BR, Alexander EK, Bible KC, Doherty GM, Mandel SJ, Nikiforov YE, Pacini F, Randolph GW, Sawka AM, Schlumberger M, Schuff KG, Sherman SI, Sosa JA, Steward DL, Tuttle RM, Wartofsky L. 2015 American Thyroid Association Management Guidelines for adult patients with thyroid nodules and differentiated thyroid cancer: the American Thyroid Association Guidelines Task Force on thyroid nodules and differentiated thyroid cancer. Thyroid. 2016;26(1):1–133. doi:10.1089/thy.2015.0020.
13. Park SY, Kim E-K, Kim MJ, Kim BM, Oh KK, Hong SW, et al. Ultrasonographic characteristics of subacute granulomatous thyroiditis. Korean J Radiol. 2015;7(4):229–34. Available from: http://www.pubmedcentral.nih.gov/articlerender.fcgi?artid=2667608&tool=pmcentrez&rendertype=abstract.
14. Nishihara E, Amino N, Ohye H, Ota H, Ito M, Kubota S, et al. Extent of hypoechogenic area in the thyroid is related with thyroid dysfunction after subacute thyroiditis. J Endocrinol Invest. 2009;32(1):33–6. Available from: http://www.ncbi.nlm.nih.gov/pubmed/19337012.

Ultrasound as a Component of Medical School Curriculum/Simulation Training

43

Emily Watters and Amy Sisley

43.1 Introduction

The use of ultrasound (US) in the practice of clinical medicine has expanded rapidly in the past two decades, and now encompasses multiple clinical specialties. This is in part due to the portability of newer US machines and a significant increase in image quality even in the smaller US machines, which has encouraged clinicians to adopt point of care (POC) US [1]. Currently, US comprises almost 25 % of all imaging in the world [2]. US imaging is now an integral part of specialties ranging from anesthesia to trauma surgery to sports medicine. In consequence, there is a growing demand for undergraduate medical education to include teaching and training in US. Early exposure to this modality will facilitate skills in image acquisition and interpretation likely to be necessary in residency and beyond.

43.2 Ultrasound in Undergraduate Medical Education

In addition to preparing medical students for mastering US skills during residency, early training in US has been shown to enhance students' mastery of anatomy and physical diagnosis skills [3, 4].

43.3 Gross Anatomy

US training was first incorporated into the undergraduate medical curriculum at Hannover Medical School, Hannover, Germany in 1996 [3]. US was used in conjunction with the gross anatomy course to better understand and visualize organ systems. The course combined cadaver dissections, radiology sessions, and clinical cases. In addition, the students practiced US on live models (volunteer students); each student would have a turn performing a series of US examinations of the abdomen, with instructors correcting their form. Students reported that their skills in ultrasound improved with just a 2 h

E. Watters, M.D., M.P.H. (✉)
Phoenix Integrated Surgery Residency, University of Arizona College of Medicine Phoenix, Banner – University Medical Center Phoenix,
925 E. McDowell Road, Second Floor, Phoenix, AZ 85006, USA
e-mail: watters.e@gmail.com

A. Sisley, M.D. (✉)
University of Arizona College of Medicine Phoenix, Banner – University Medical Center Phoenix,
Phoenix, AZ, USA
e-mail: Amy.Sisley@bannerhealth.com

M. Milas et al. (eds.), *Advanced Thyroid and Parathyroid Ultrasound*,
DOI 10.1007/978-3-319-44100-9_43

course. Importantly, they also reported enhanced understanding of abdominal anatomy with the addition of the US module.

Ultrasound provides a unique window on human anatomy. Many undergraduate medical schools have found that teaching US is incorporated smoothly with their gross anatomy course. A variety of methods are being used to accomplish this goal such as practicing US on live models and reviewing sonographic images. One school found it useful to teach US using a live model while in the anatomy lab so students would have a better understanding of the anatomy before they were to dissect on the cadaver [5]. When US was used in combination with anatomy courses, 98 % of students were able to correctly identify vascular anatomy on sonographic images [4].

43.4 Physical Diagnosis

As basic physical examination skills are taught during medical school, US should be as well since it is proving itself to be a useful adjunct to the physical exam.

Wayne State University (WSU) in Detroit, MI, incorporated US training into their first and second year curriculum in physical diagnosis (PD) [4]. The first year curriculum emphasized basic image acquisition skills in abdominal, cardiovascular, musculoskeletal, and genitourinary systems as well as basic US physics and knobology. In the second year, both cardiovascular and abdominal ultrasounds were incorporated into the PD course using standardized patients. Significant improvements in image recognition were documented. In addition, 89 % of the students felt that US is a valuable tool.

Interestingly, multiple studies have shown that medical students using US are better at diagnosing certain conditions than seasoned physicians who are only using their physical exam skills. Students trained in US were able to better identify cardiac abnormalities with the US than cardiologists were able to with just their bedside physical exam skills [6]. Students were also able to use US to diagnose hepatomegaly more accurately than internists who only used their physical exam skills [7]. US, of course, is not intended to replace the physical examination, but rather to enhance it, much as the stethoscope has done. By incorporating US with the physical exam, accuracy is improved and diagnostic capabilities are increased. Hence it seems a wise investment to teach medical students how to use US so that they have attained some degree of proficiency prior to entering residency training.

43.5 Ultrasound Guided Procedures

One of the key advantages of US is that it is both diagnostic and therapeutic. Many basic procedures such as central line placement, thoracentesis, paracentesis, abscess drainage, and biopsy are routinely performed using US guidance. When trained in medical school, students are more confident in using US for procedures than students who did not learn US in medical school [1]. Students introduced to US in the first year of medical school were also more likely to want to continue their use of US throughout their practice [8].

43.6 Ultrasound Curriculum for Undergraduate Medical Education

The incorporation of US into medical school curricula has taken several different forms. These include a vertical (or longitudinal) curriculum in which US education starts in the first year and continues throughout all 4 years, in only select years, as an elective, or in a seminar format. The most popular approach is the vertical integration of the US curriculum [9].

In the vertical approach, the curriculum is divided into preclinical and clinical years. During the preclinical years, students are taught about the physics behind US, how to use the probes, and normal anatomy as seen on US. Many programs incorporate US into the gross anatomy course as well. In the first 2 years, students' skills can be assessed with standardized patients during an objective structured clinical examination (OSCE).

In the clinical years, US is used to identify abnormal anatomy and pathological conditions. Ultrasound is also used in teaching students how to perform procedures such as central lines, thoracentesis, and liver biopsy. Students are taught US skills specific to their clinical rotation such as identifying hypertrophic pyloric stenosis on pediatrics and gallstone on a general surgery rotation. As US is invaluable in many of the specialties, students are exposed to US during multiple rotations throughout third and fourth year. It is important to know the common pathology seen in different specialties such as hypertrophic pyloric stenosis in pediatrics or gallstones in a general surgery rotation. Recognition of the pros and cons of using US and applying it in the correct situation is also a goal of the clinical years. These are the basic premises of the vertical curriculum although variations exist between the different schools.

In the USA, one of the first medical schools to use a formalized 4 year US curriculum was the University of South Carolina (USC) in 2006. The curriculum is divided into preclinical and clinical applications. The preclinical US is focused on image acquisition related to anatomy, physiology and pathology. The clinical applications are focused on using US as part of clinical decision making in various case scenarios [10]. US proficiency is tested by an OSCE. The curriculum is highly rated by students: over 90 % felt that the integration of US in the preclinical curriculum was a valuable addition and improved their understanding of the basic sciences [11]. Subsequently, several other medical schools have implemented a fully integrated 4 year US curriculum similar to that of USC.

WSU began giving first year students a portable US device in 2006 [12]. The majority of students found the US sessions to be effective teaching tools. Students continued to use US throughout all 4 years. Thyroid ultrasound is part of the curriculum at USC, with training modules and a library of cine-clips; even the main page display of their website features an ultrasound probe positioned to image the thyroid in longitudinal mode (http://ultrasoundinstitute.med.sc.edu/UIlearning.asp; www searched June 6, 2016).

Ohio State University uses a vertical approach with the first 2 years focused on basic science and using the US machine [13]. The last 2 years are focused on the indications for US and interpreting images.

University of California Irvine has also integrated a 4 year US curriculum with special features such as podcasts, iPAD centric curriculum, and hands-on skills lab. Instructors at UC Irvine have also experimented with teaching US in remote locations via the internet with live feedback from instructors [14].

Rather than use an integrated vertical curriculum, some medical schools have opted to focus on US education in certain years such as the University of Chicago and the Mayo clinic who teach students in their fourth year how to perform echocardiography. Some programs do a 3 day course (Thomas Jefferson) and the National US Curriculum has developed a 3 day course outline. US can also be taught as a fourth year elective [15].

To encourage US education, some schools have started an intercollegiate competition to help students learn US [10]. This competition gives students time to practice using US then allows students to compete against students from other schools in categories such as identifying anatomy and measuring structures. In a different creative way to expose students to US, schools have started US interest groups and are also teaching US via internet based modules [16]. A formal professional society with annual meetings (World Congress on Ultrasound in Medical Education) serves to advance these themes of ultrasound training and networking between institutions who have or hope to develop ultrasound curricula (http://www.wcume.org/).

43.7 The Future of Ultrasound Training in Undergraduate and Graduate Medical Education

Currently, there is no standardized curriculum for US in medical education or even milestones for teaching US in undergraduate medical education. For this reason, US is being taught (or not taught) in many different ways. A national survey of allopathic medical schools showed that of the curriculum administrators who responded, 62 % stated US was part of their school's curriculum [17]. A survey of incoming interns at the University of Birmingham, in 2012 and 2013, showed one-fourth of survey participants had never performed a bedside US scan [13].

At the University of Arizona College of Medicine Phoenix, US education is incorporated as part of the simulation center and is taught both individually and in small group sessions (Figs. 43.1, 43.2, and 43.3). Education in ultrasound is provided to both medical students and residents. Several faculty members at the University of Arizona—Phoenix are also members of their respective professional society leadership panels on clinician-performed ultrasound, especially in surgery and emergency medicine. Therefore, the curriculum for residents and medical students who rotate on these services is rich in clinical ultrasound exposures in real-time settings. A separate simulation center for skills training is present both at the hospital campus (Banner-University Medical Center Phoenix) and the medical school campus.

In the national survey of curriculum administrators, the most common reasons for not implementing US were time in the curriculum and money. US machines are not inexpensive, with even the smaller, basic machines costing 20,000–55,000. Also as medical schools pressured pressure are pressured to cut down the amount of hours spent in the classroom, it seems a daunting task to add more material to an already overloaded curriculum. Just as curriculum administrators are having a hard time finding

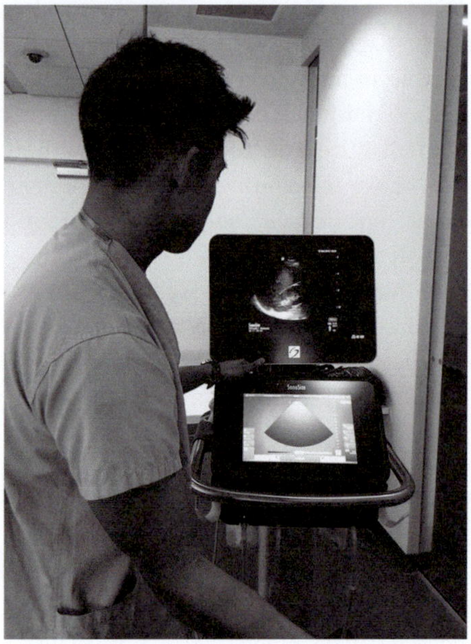

Fig. 43.1 Early exposure to ultrasound techniques improves understanding of both anatomy and pathophysiology. These ultrasound skills can also be readily transferred to clinical practice during the latter part of medical training and throughout a medical career

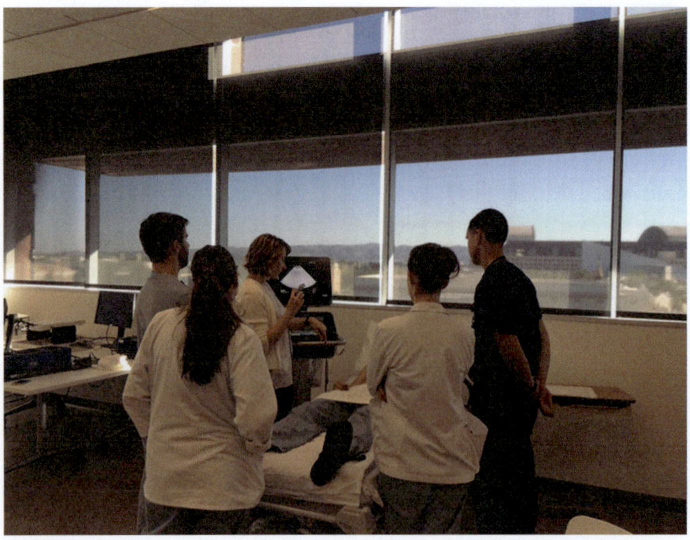

Fig. 43.2 Faculty member practicing ultrasound with third year medical students at the University of Arizona College of Medicine, Phoenix. These students are about to begin their clinical rotations

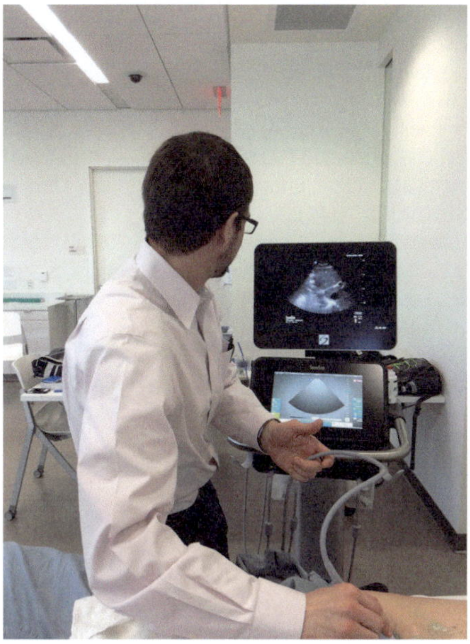

Fig. 43.3 Medical students practicing the Focused Assessment with Sonography in Trauma (FAST) examination on each other prior to their trauma surgery rotation at the University of Arizona College of Medicine, Phoenix

time in the curriculum to teach US, students also report that time is a barrier in learning US [8].

A well-run US program requires faculty fully committed to US and teaching. It also requires a significant commitment on the part of the administration as the US machines and servers for image archives are costly to purchase and maintain [8].

However, it is necessary for students to be exposed to US early since the abilities of the US user correlates positively with the number of scans performed [14]. US skills must also be frequently practiced and reinforced, or they diminish significantly [18].

43.8 Conclusion

Ultrasound is an increasingly important imaging modality which has become an integral part of many clinical specialties. It functions as a screening, diagnostic, and procedural tool. As the technology continues to advance and US becomes ever more accessible, the demand for US proficiency will continue to increase. US training should begin in medical school so that students can better understand and learn anatomy, can have supervised practice of US use, increase student satisfaction in learning anatomy, and improve physical exam skills. Significantly, early exposure and development of US skills ensures that students are familiar with the basic components of US by the time they reach residency and, during residency, this enhances the potential to incorporate US in subsequent professional careers.

References

1. Lane N, Lahham S, Joseph L, Bahner DP, Fox JC. Ultrasound in medical education: listening to the echoes of the past to shape a vision for the future. Eur J Trauma Emerg Surg. 2015;41(5):461–7.
2. McLachlan JC, Bligh J, Bradley P, Searle J. Teaching anatomy without cadavers. Med Educ. 2004;38(4):418–24.
3. Teichgräber UK, Meyer JM, Poulsen Nautrup C, von Rautenfeld DB. Ultrasound anatomy: a practical teaching system in human gross anatomy. Med Educ. 1996;30(4):296–8.
4. Afonso N, Amponsah D, Yang J, Mendez J, Bridge P, Hays G, et al. Adding new tools to the black bag—introduction of ultrasound into the physical diagnosis course. J Gen Intern Med. 2010;25(11):1248–52.
5. Swamy M, Searle RF. Anatomy teaching with portable ultrasound to medical students. BMC Med Educ. 2012;12:99.
6. Kobal SL, Trento L, Baharami S, Tolstrup K, Naqvi TZ, Cercek B, Neuman Y, et al. Comparison of effectiveness of hand-carried ultrasound to bedside cardiovascular physical examination. Am J Cardiol. 2005;96(7):1002–6.
7. Mouratev G, Howe D, Hoppmann R, Poston MB, Reid R, Varnadoe J, et al. Teaching medical students ultrasound to measure liver size: comparison with experienced clinicians using physical examination alone. Teach Learn Med. 2013;25(1):84–8.
8. Brown B, Adhikari S, Marx J, Lander L, Todd GL. Introduction of ultrasound into gross anatomy curriculum: perceptions of medical students. J Emerg Med. 2012;43(6):1098–102.
9. Gogalniceanu P, Sheena Y, Kashef E, Purkayastha S, Darzi A, Paraskeva P. Is basic emergency ultrasound training feasible as part of standard undergraduate medical education? J Surg Educ. 2010;67(3):152–6.
10. Cook T, Hunt P, Hoppman R. Emergency medicine leads the way for training medical students in clinician-based ultrasound: a radical paradigm shift in patient imaging. Acad Emerg Med. 2007;14(6):558–61.

11. Hoppmann RA, Fletcher S. An integrated ultrasound curriculum (iUSC) for medical students: 4-year experience. Crit Ultrasound J. 2011;3(1):1–12.
12. Rao S, van Holsbeeck L, Musial JL, Parker A, Bouffard JA, Bridge P, et al. A pilot study of comprehensive ultrasound education at the Wayne State University School of Medicine: a pioneer year review. J Ultrasound Med. 2008;27(5):745–9.
13. Bahner DP, Adkins EJ, Hughes D, Barrie M, Boulger CT, Royall NA. Integrated medical school ultrasound: development of an ultrasound vertical curriculum. Crit Ultrasound J. 2013;5(1):6.
14. Winn S, McKeown P, Lotfipour S, Maguire GA, Youm JH, Wiechmann W, et al. Remote, synchronous, hands-on ultrasound education. Telemed J E Health. 2015;21(7):593–7.
15. Baltarowich OH, Di Salvo DN, Scoutt LM, Brown DL, Cox CW, DiPietro MA, et al. National ultrasound curriculum for medical students. Ultrasound Q. 2014;30(1):13–9.
16. Bahner DP, Jasne A, Boore S, Mueller A, Cortez E. The ultrasound challenge: a novel approach to medical student ultrasound education. J Ultrasound Med. 2012;31(12):2013–6.
17. Bahner DP, Goldman E, Way D, Royall NA, Liu YT. The state of ultrasound education in US medical schools: results of a national survey. Acad Med. 2014;89(12):1681–6.
18. Gracias VH, Frankel HL, Gupta R, Malcynski J, Gandhi R, Collazzo L, et al. Defining the learning curve for the Focused Abdominal Sonogram for Trauma (FAST) examination: implications for credentialing. Am Surg. 2001;67(4):364–8.

Part IX

Resources, Tools, and Tips for the Sonographer

44 The Ultrasound Lexicon: Common Terminology for Thyroid and Parathyroid Sonography

Mira Milas

44.1 Pattern Recognition and Risk Stratification

The modern approach to ultrasound image interpretation that seeks to arrive at a global, holistic assessment of the thyroid diagnosis and relevant risks of thyroid malignancy based on multiple coordinated features of a thyroid abnormality, such as a thyroid nodule [1].

44.2 Knobology

The science of knowing control buttons on the ultrasound instrument console that adjust the function and settings of ultrasound applications [2].

44.3 Delphian Lymph Node

A lymph node located in the pre-cricoid area above the thyroid isthmus. The eponym relates to the expectation that an abnormal or enlarged lymph node in this area may predict the presence of thyroid cancer; hence, the reference is to foretelling of the future as did the Oracle of Delphi from ancient Greek mythology. Enlarged lymph nodes in this area may also be benign and seen in Hashimoto's thyroiditis [3].

44.4 Tubercle of Zuckerkandl

This is a knuckle of thyroid tissue projecting from the deep border of a thyroid lobe, typically at the posterior midpoint. It represents an embryologic remnant of the lateral cervical migration of thyroid cells, which later fail to involute and disappear. Thus, the Tubercle of Zuckerkandl is similar to the pyramidal lobe, an embryologic remnant of midline migration. The tubercle sometimes gives the impression that a "cleft" (hyperechoic bright line) separates it from the main thyroid lobe. Thus, it may be misinterpreted as a nodule and unnecessarily biopsied. It can range in size from a small round tissue fragment to 2–3 cm oval structure. Surgically, the Tubercle of Zuckerkandl can be a marker of the nearby trajectory of the recurrent laryngeal nerve.

Electronic supplementary material: The online version of this chapter (doi:10.1007/978-3-319-44100-9_44) contains supplementary material, which is available to authorized users. Videos can also be accessed at http://link.springer.com/chapter/10.1007/978-3-319-44100-9_44.

M. Milas, M.D., F.A.C.S. (✉)
Department of Surgery and the Endocrinology & Metabolism Institute, University of Arizona College of Medicine - Phoenix, Banner - University Medical Center Phoenix, 1441 North 12th Street 2nd floor, Phoenix, AZ 85006, USA
e-mail: Mira.Milas@bannerhealth.com

M. Milas et al. (eds.), *Advanced Thyroid and Parathyroid Ultrasound*,
DOI 10.1007/978-3-319-44100-9_44

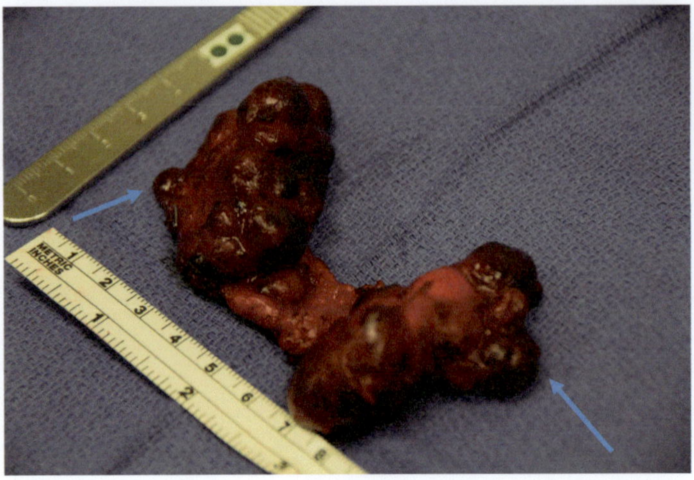

Fig. 44.1 Tubercle of Zuckerkandl: surgical specimen with *arrows* pointing to bilateral tubercles

Please see Videos 44.1, 44.2, and 44.3, and surgical thyroidectomy specimen photo (Fig. 44.1) [4].

44.5 White Knight

A hyperechoic ("white") nodule in Hashimoto's thyroiditis thought to represent regenerative benign tissue nodule appearing within the inflammation of the thyroid. This entity is discussed also in Chap. 16 (Lupo) and described in detail in the following two publications. Please see Video 44.4 [5, 6].

44.6 Starry Starry Night

A dense collection of microcalcifications that appear to "sparkle" like stars in the nighttime sky. This is a sonographic sign that is highly suspicious for thyroid cancer. The microcalcifications represent psammoma bodies, which in turn are involuted and necrotic papillae of papillary thyroid cancer. Please see Video 44.5 [7].

44.7 Comet Tail Artifact

A reverberation of sound waves caused by inspissated colloid and a marker of a benign process. This sonographic sign is often misinterpreted as microcalcifications. A key feature to recognize is that colloid fragments precipitate in cystic structures. In contrast, microcalcifications associated with thyroid cancer occur in solid nodules. Please see Videos 44.6 and 44.7 [8–10].

44.8 Giraffe Pattern

A sonographic pattern seen with Hashimoto's thyroiditis and described by Bonavita and colleagues as a "giraffe" pattern similar to the two-tone coloring of a giraffe (see cartoon example). The ultrasound appearance is described as globular, block-like, or plate-like areas of hyperechogenicity surrounded by linear thin areas of hypoechogenicity [5] (Fig. 44.2a–d).

44.9 Three Circle Sign

This lexicon terminology was first reported in the textbook, *Diseases of the Parathyroid Glands*, published by Springer in 2012. It describes the arrangement of circular cross-sections of the internal jugular vein (IJ), common carotid artery (CA), and the enlarged parathyroid gland when viewed by ultrasound in a transverse orientation. Figure 44.3 illustrates this orientation. The unique aspects of the "three circle sign" include the following: the uniform hypoechoic echogenicity of

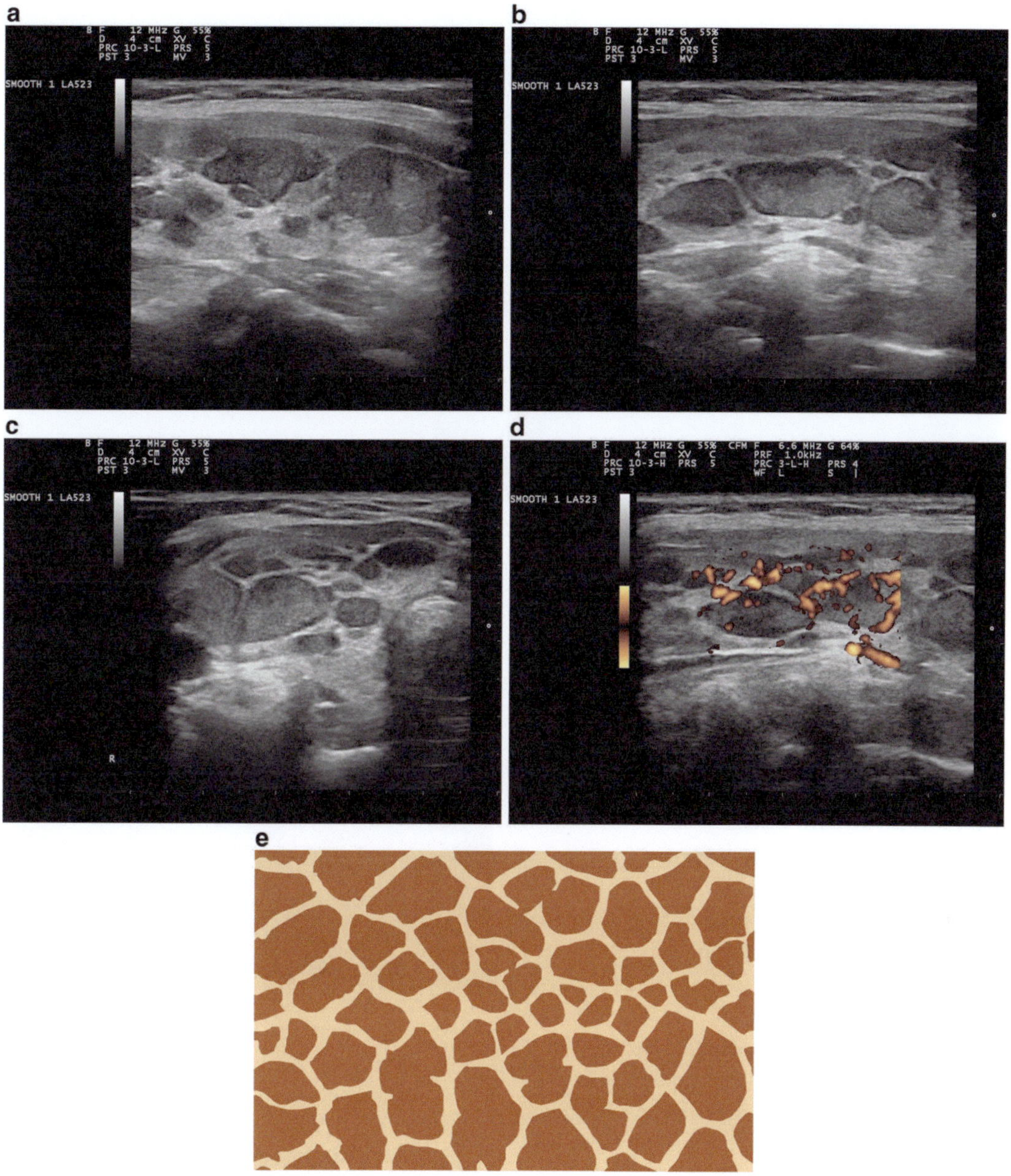

Fig. 44.2 (**a**–**d**). Giraffe pattern. Images are courtesy of the personal image collection of Dr. John S. Abele, Sacramento, California. (**e**) Giraffe skin pattern

all three structures (a thyroid nodule may not exhibit this) and the absence of a rim of normal thyroid tissue between the endocrine gland and the carotid artery (a thyroid nodule will typically be within the gland parenchyma and the abnormal parathyroid gland is almost always extracapsular to the thyroid). The arrangement can be observed with both superior and inferior enlarged parathyroid glands. Video 44.8 demonstrates in color Doppler mode a very small caliber IJ at the left of the screen, the CA in the center of the video and the hypoechoic enlarged parathyroid gland at the

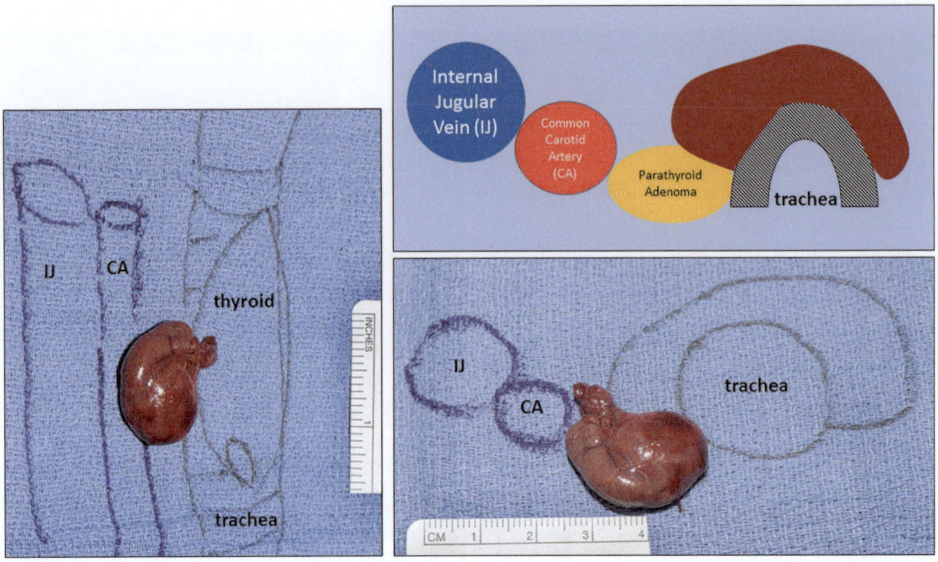

Fig. 44.3 Three circle sign

right of the screen. Video 44.9 illustrates all three round structures, with a valve seen fluttering within the IJ at the left of the screen [11].

44.10 Pseudonodules and Cobblestones

The presence of thyroiditis can distort the thyroid architecture into globular arrangements that may appear to be discreet nodules but are really a conglomerate of round shapes of varying sizes that reflect inflammation and compartmentalization of tissue. These round areas, especially if they represent the pattern of the entire thyroid gland, should not be viewed as discreet nodules and should not undergo biopsy. Please see Figs. 44.4 and 44.5, and Videos 44.10, 44.11, 44.12, and 44.13 [12, 13]

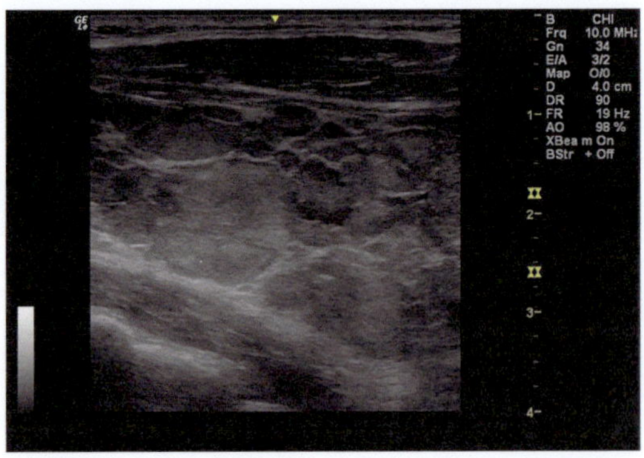

Fig. 44.4 Pseudonodules, longitudinal

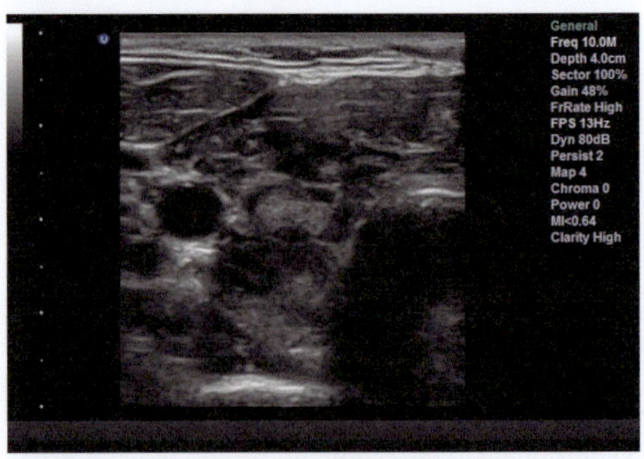

Fig. 44.5 Pseudonodules, transverse

44.11 Spongiform/Honeycomb Nodule

The appearance of a thyroid nodule when at least 50 % of its composition is cystic, including a pattern with small cystic structures that mimics the scattering of holes in a sponge or a honeycomb

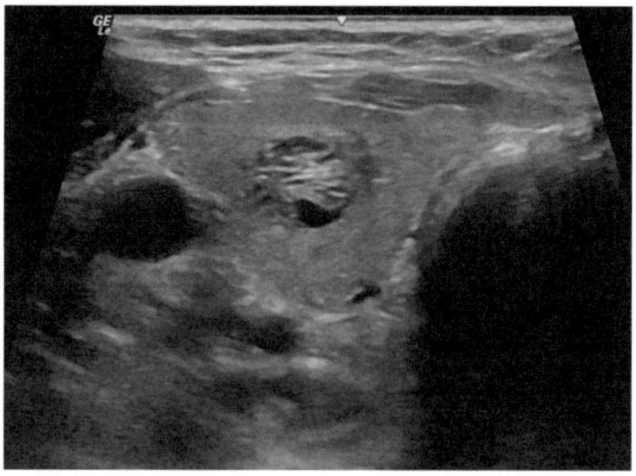

Fig. 44.6 Spongiform

panel. This feature is described in detail in Chap. 10 (Langer). It is highly associated with a benign pathology with minimal risk of thyroid cancer. Please see Fig. 44.6 and Video 44.14 [5].

References

1. ATA. Revised American Thyroid Association management guidelines for patients with thyroid nodules and differentiated thyroid cancer: the American Thyroid Association (ATA) Guidelines Taskforce on thyroid nodules and differentiated thyroid cancer. Thyroid. 2015;19:1167–214.
2. Enriquez JL, Wu TS. An introduction to ultrasound equipment and knobology. Crit Care Clin. 2014;30(1):25–45.
3. Iyer NG, Kumar A, Nixon IJ, Patel SG, Ganly I, Tuttle RM, Shah JP, Shaha AR. Incidence and significance of Delphian node metastasis in papillary thyroid cancer. Ann Surg. 2011;253(5):988–91.
4. Lee TC, Selvarajan SK, Curtin H, Mukundan S. Zuckerkandl tubercle of the thyroid: a common imaging finding that may mimic pathology. AJNR Am J Neuroradiol. 2012;33(6):1134–8.
5. Bonavita JA, Mayo J, Babb J, et al. Pattern recognition of benign nodules at ultrasound of the thyroid: which nodules can be left alone? AJR. 2009;193:207–13.
6. Virmani V, Hammond I. Sonographic patterns of benign thyroid nodules: verification at our institution. AJR Am J Roentgenol. 2011;196(4):891–5.
7. Bongiovanni M, Mazzucchelli L, Martin V, Crippa S, Bolli M, Suriano S, Giovanella L. Images in endocrine pathology: a starry-sky in the thyroid. Endocr Pathol. 2012;23(1):79–81.
8. Ahuja A, Chick W, King W, Metreweli C. Clinical significance of the comet-tail artifact in thyroid ultrasound. J Clin Ultrasound. 1996;24(3):129–33.
9. Beland MD, Kwon L, Delellis RA, Cronan JJ, Grant EG. Nonshadowing echogenic foci in thyroid nodules: are certain appearances enough to avoid thyroid biopsy? J Ultrasound Med. 2011;30(6):753–60.
10. Malhi H, Beland MD, Cen SY, Allgood E, Daley K, Martin SE, Cronan JJ, Grant EG. Echogenic foci in thyroid nodules: significance of posterior acoustic artifacts. AJR Am J Roentgenol. 2014;203(6):1310–6.
11. Milas Z, Milas M. The use of ultrasonography in the management of parathyroid disease, Chapter 18. In: Licata AA, Lerma EV, editors. Diseases of the parathyroid glands. New York, NY: Springer; 2012. p. 323–41.
12. Jung SJ, Kim DW. Ultrasonographic and cytopathological features of an inflammatorypseudonodule in the thyroid gland. Diagn Cytopathol. 2016. doi: 10.1002/dc.23516
13. Yildirim D, Gurses B, Gurpinar B, Ekci B, Colakoglu B, Kaur A. Nodule or pseudonodule? Differentiation in Hashimoto's thyroiditis with sonoelastography. J Int Med Res. 2011;39(6):2360–9.

Educational Resources for Training in Thyroid and Parathyroid Ultrasound

45

Barbra S. Miller

45.1 Introduction to the History of Ultrasound and Ultrasound Training

Since the proposal of the Theory of Sound in 1877 and subsequent discovery of the Piezoelectric Effect in 1880, the potential for imaging using US was born. The first diagnostic application of US was reportedly in 1942 by Karl Dussik from Vienna, Austria, using amplitude (A) mode for diagnosis of brain tumors. US was first used in a therapeutic manner in the late 1940s as a destructive treatment. Later on, with advances in computers, the development of brightness (B) mode US imaging was pioneered by Douglass Howry and Joseph Holmes at University of Colorado. With this technique, the development of a gray-scale display improved image quality and the ability to interpret images. Resolution, along with overall image quality and decreasing size of US machines continues to improve. In 1951, the technology was first used to describe the acoustic characteristics of breast tumors. During the 1960s research into breast ultrasound began in Australia, and in 1966 the first ultrasonic breast scanner in the world was installed at Royal North Shore Hospital in Sydney under endocrine surgeon Tom Reeve's clinical supervision. It was a bistable machine capable of imaging in linear, sector, and compound scanning modes. The combination of gray scale imaging and focused array techniques enabled gray scale ultrasonography to be applied to all soft tissue lesions. The Australian Society for Ultrasound in Medicine was established in 1970, another world first. In 1974, the breast scanner was then modified and applied to the thyroid, parathyroid, and testis. The increasing experience of this group with the clinical application of small parts US led to the 1978 sentinel publication on small parts US of breast, testicle, thyroid, and parathyroid. Two thyroid and parathyroid publications [3, 4] were among the first in the world to utilize the technology and set the scene for the use of US in endocrine practice for decades to follow. Hereafter, dissemination of the technique through various educational opportunities was imparted and has grown exponentially.

45.1.1 Expansion of Ultrasound Use Outside the Radiology Department into Specialty Practices

In the past 30 years, US has become an increasingly important tool employed by clinicians as an extension of the physical examination.

B.S. Miller, M.D., F.A.C.S. (✉)
Division of Endocrine Surgery, Section of General Surgery, University of Michigan, Ann Arbor, MI, USA
e-mail: barbram@med.umich.edu

M. Milas et al. (eds.), *Advanced Thyroid and Parathyroid Ultrasound*, DOI 10.1007/978-3-319-44100-9_45

These clinicians range from entry level ancillary care providers to physicians. Along with an increase in types of users and settings in which US technology is employed, there has been an expansion of diagnostic, therapeutic, and surveillance applications for US to endocrine disorders including thyroid, parathyroid, and cervical US.

Various avenues for training and dissemination of techniques for performing and interpreting thyroid and parathyroid US have evolved over time. Non-physician sonographers working in radiology based settings are classically trained in image acquisition. Many radiologists do not perform their own ultrasound exams and instead interpret images acquired by sonographers. Important and many times subtle findings may be less likely appreciated or common findings misinterpreted using this workflow, especially if key clinical information about the disease process is not available, communicated or familiar to the radiologist. A lack of understanding of current diagnostic and treatment algorithms, provided by professional endocrine societies, can limit the clinical utility of information relayed to the managing physician. This in turn may lead to the need to repeat examinations searching for additional findings or clarification of reported findings. Clinicians of varying levels of expertise in many specialties, such as trauma, breast disease, emergency medicine, obstetrics and gynecology in addition to endocrinology have similarly identified the great utility of US technology and apply it outside the radiology suite. As an example, in the 1990s surgeons and emergency medicine physicians began to perform Focused Assessment with Sonography for Trauma (FAST) exams for trauma patients and noted equivalent sensitivity in identifying fluid within the peritoneal cavity [5–8]. The ability of trauma and emergency medicine physicians to perform FAST exams in sequence with the primary and secondary physical examinations in the trauma bay decreased the time to definitive treatment and need to involve additional personnel. Other specialties have noted similar advantages of performing bedside or in-office US exams.

45.2 Current Resources for Ultrasound Education and Training

A trained sonographer must be able to repeatedly and accurately acquire and interpret high quality images. A thorough understanding of US physics, methods for image optimization, knowledge of artifacts that may lead to a critical change in image interpretation, and bio-effects of US which may affect patient safety as well as any complications that may result from procedures performed under US guidance is required and must be emphasized in any training course. The format for US education and training varies widely. Many basic US concepts can be taught as didactic lectures in various settings (classroom, Internet-based modules, live versus taped, remote video feed). Following this, proctored practical sessions are key to transfer knowledge gained and instruct students on simultaneously incorporating information learned from multiple lectures. Techniques for generating and optimizing an image are refined as much as possible in a given short period of time. Ideally, additional practice is pursued by the student after completing the course as competence requires practice, especially with regard to image interpretation and invasive procedures. Additional study may include self-study and practice using phantom models for image acquisition, fine needle aspiration of thyroid nodules, as well as supervision from an experienced sonographer during initial exams while the learner is on the learning curve [9].

45.2.1 Available Training Courses from Professional Societies

With the rapid expansion of US imaging technology to a wide variety of clinical specialties, numerous training opportunities exist in formal and informal settings, with and without certification. Some courses are offered through practice specific societies [American Association of Clinical Endocrinologists (AACE), American College of Surgeons

(ACS), The Endocrine Society (ENDO), American Head and Neck Society (ANHS)] while others are more informal. Sisley has emphasized the importance of using the objective structured clinical examination (OSCE) in pre-course and post-course settings. OSCE can be used not only in evaluating the effectiveness of a course but also in assessing physician competency in performance and interpretation of the US exam [10].

45.2.2 Ultrasound Training During Medical School, Residency, Fellowship, Clinical Practice

Opportunities for incorporation of US technology into the medical curriculum exist at earlier stages than ever before. Some medical schools incorporate US education into anatomy courses offered during the first and second years with additional training when students partake in third and fourth year clinical rotations [11–22]. While a good number of programs across many specialties also incorporate US training into residency and fellowship training, this is often informal with little didactic coursework or supervised practical sessions. Training as part of graduate medical education may range from incidental clinical contact to a single didactic lecture up to progressive vertical multi-year curricula depending on the training program. Most commonly, one resident teaches another, and appropriate education may not occur. In some situations, incorrect methods and interpretation are perpetuated. Some clinicians opt to pursue training in new techniques after they begin their clinical practice. Most attend societal based courses; however, some receive instruction from a partner in their practice. It is currently unknown what the difference in competency is between those who have had formal versus informal US training, and this issue is further expanded to US training while in clinical practice [23].

45.2.3 Remote Distance Learning Opportunities

For those unable to travel to more formal courses due to financial hardship, distance, length of the course, or other reasons, unique opportunities for remote learning are available. Transducer simulators can be purchased to use in conjunction with online courses (Ex. SonoSim®). Simple didactic courses with the completion of formal or informal on-line materials may also be pursued for additional training. Live videoconferences may also be remotely attended.

45.2.4 Learning Curve

Literature from various sources has described the attempts to define a learning curve for transition to independence regarding performance and interpretation of US exams. Studies of learners in emergency department settings suggest the need to perform 50–75 exams to reach minimum standards for image acquisition, although this varied with the type of exam being performed, from as little as 18 exams for soft tissue and up to 90 exams for structures of the right upper quadrant of the abdomen [24]. Some have suggested there is little to no learning curve for some types of US examinations. One group suggests the learning curve for some types of exams can be accomplished on a virtual reality simulator alone [25, 26]. The learning curve has neither been formally described for thyroid and parathyroid ultrasound nor for US-guided needle biopsy.

45.2.5 Adjuncts for Training

In addition to standard didactic materials such as books and articles, additional educational materials are available. These include on-line resources and training courses, manufactured phantom models (Ex. Blue Phantom™), and homemade gelatin or animal-based models [27, 28]. More complex training models and mannequins are also available. Cost ranges from pennies to thousands of dollars.

45.3 Certification and Accreditation

45.3.1 What Does Certification Mean?

While participants of a program may receive a certification, in many instances it is solely a certification of attendance or medical education credits. Some certifications, such as those offered by the American College of Surgeons require students to successfully pass a written test and practical exam, but this does not equate to proficiency in a clinical setting. The student is expected to pursue additional practice and obtain feedback from those who are proficient at their home institution. The quality and accuracy with which examinations are performed and interpreted after training has not been well studied, nor has the time or number of examinations performed to be considered proficient or an expert. The AACE Endocrine Certification in Neck Ultrasound (ECNU) program requires successful completion of a comprehensive certification examination as well as completion of the validation of competency process which requires submission of 15 exams performed and reports generated for review, although long-term performance issues and quality control are left to the clinician. ECNU, currently the most involved level of certification available to nonradiologists performing thyroid and parathyroid US in the USA, is addressed in detail in an earlier chapter of this textbook. Certification again does not necessarily equal proficiency. While most organizations recommend some sort of assessment of proficiency, the means to do this long-term and document continued proficiency is lacking. It is the individual clinician's responsibility to assess outcomes and correct if necessary.

45.3.2 The Role of AIUM in and Beyond Radiology Based Practices

The AIUM is a recognized group that provides opinions regarding training in the application of ultrasound to various clinical areas by organ system or body area. Current recommendations for physicians who perform, interpret, and evaluate head and neck US examinations are the following:

1. Completion of an Accreditation Council for Graduate Medical Education (ACGME)-approved radiology residency program, fellowship, or postgraduate training within the previous 36 months that included structured training in diagnostic head and neck ultrasound under the supervision of a qualified physician(s), during which the trainees had evidence of being involved with the performance, evaluation, interpretation, and reporting of at least 150 diagnostic head and neck ultrasound examinations; and the physicians must be board certified or board eligible.
2. Completion of an approved radiology residency and/or fellowship program that did not include structured training in diagnostic head and neck ultrasound or completion of a residency and/or fellowship program that involved such training more than 36 months ago and must have documented: supervision and/or performance, interpretation, and reporting of at least 150 diagnostic head and neck ultrasound examinations in the previous 36 months; and 12 *AMA PRA Category 1 Credits*™ dedicated to diagnostic head and neck ultrasound within the previous 36 months.
3. Completion of an ACGME-approved residency in otolaryngology or general surgery within the previous 36 months with structured didactic training in diagnostic head and neck ultrasound and evidence of being involved with the performance, evaluation, interpretation, and reporting of at least 150

diagnostic head and neck ultrasound examinations under the supervision of a qualified physician(s); and the physicians must be board certified or eligible by the American Board of Otolaryngology or the American Board of Surgery.

4. Completion of an approved residency in otolaryngology or general surgery more than 36 months ago; and the physicians must be board certified or eligible by the American Board of Otolaryngology or the American Board of Surgery and provide documentation of the following: successful completion of the American College of Surgeons Postgraduate Course in Head and Neck Ultrasound; a passing grade on the American College of Surgeons Basic Pretest and Posttest for Head and Neck Ultrasound; and evidence of being involved with the performance, evaluation, interpretation, and reporting of at least 150 diagnostic head and neck ultrasound examinations under the supervision of a qualified physician(s) within the previous 36 months.
5. All physicians performing diagnostic head and neck ultrasound examinations must be involved in the performance and/or interpretation and reporting of a minimum of 50 ultrasound examinations of the head and neck per year to maintain competence. All physicians performing diagnostic head and neck ultrasound examinations are required to obtain a minimum of 12 *AMA PRA Category 1 Credits*™ in head and neck ultrasound every 3 years.

While AIUM is often referenced as an authoritative body, it is unclear where the recommendation for 150 exams comes from or from where the CME recommendations originate. These requirements have decreased from 300 examinations and 100 h of category 1 CME dedicated to diagnostic US in the area of practice. Specialties beyond radiology aside from general surgery and otolaryngology are not recognized in these guidelines; however, AIUM does recognize the ECNU certification of medical endocrinologists offered by the American Association of Clinical Endocrinologists and surgeons are eligible for ECNU. Other societies (AAEP, SAGES, ASBS) have developed their own specialty specific certification and practice guidelines for performance and interpretation of US as they relate to these specialty fields (emergency medicine, laparoscopic and gastrointestinal surgeons, and breast surgeons, respectively).

45.3.3 Variations in Performance of Diagnostic Ultrasound and Reporting Practices Based on Clinical Specialty

What constitutes adequate training in thyroid and parathyroid US will be different for different specialties as information needed from assessment of one organ or region of the body may vary between specialties depending on the utility of that information as it pertains to the clinical issue. Various measurements or views obtained as required by one set of guidelines may have no bearing on the clinical care of the patient. Lack of assessment of various areas not required by certain groups or guidelines may lead to important missed findings and information. For example, thyroid and parathyroid surgeons often examine specific areas of the neck for findings that will impact the decision for and extent of surgery. These are not areas routinely evaluated by other specialists as that particular information does not impact their care of the patient. In a single patient, multiple US exams may need to be performed by multiple clinicians of differing backgrounds to gain information needed for the overall care of the patient. Inter-observer variation in acquisition and interpretation of US images also impacts patient care.

45.3.4 Safe Incorporation of New Ultrasound Techniques into Practice

New techniques utilizing US technology in some way naturally emerge over time. This has been the case with US guided fine needle aspiration, percutaneous US guided ethanol injection and

Table 45.1 Educational resources for thyroid and parathyroid ultrasound[a]

ACS	American College of Surgeons https://www.facs.org/clincon2016
AACE	American Association of Clinical Endocrinologists https://www.aace.com/
ECNU	Endocrine Certification in Neck Ultrasound https://www.aace.com/ecnu
ENDO	The Endocrine Society https://www.aace.com/ecnu
AAES	American Association of Endocrine Surgeons https://www.endocrinesurgery.org/meeting/meeting.html
AHNS	American Head and Neck Society http://www.ahns.info/
AIUM	American Institute of Ultrasound in Medicine http://www.aium.org/
WCUME	World Congress on Ultrasound in Medical Education http://www.wcume.org/
TCCC	Thyroid Cancer Care Collaborative https://www.thyroidccc.org/
Ultrasound manufacturer websites	
SonoSim	Ultrasound Simulation Systems http://sonosim.com/
Blue Phantom	Ultrasound Training Models https://www.bluephantom.com/
Collected Med/ECHO	Ultrasound Interactive Interpretation https://collectedmed.com/
Ultrasound Institute	Ultrasound Education http://ultrasoundinstitute.med.sc.edu/

[a]Accessed via www on June 14th 2016

ablation of various targets (nodules, lymph nodes, etc.), US guided radiofrequency ablation, and US examination of the vocal cords [29–31]. One must be cautious in their exuberance for and acceptance of any new technique. Rigorous testing must ensure at least equivalence in outcome and safety compared to the existing gold standard method. Opinions from multiple practitioners across multiple specialties must be sought to understand the true impact and relevance of a new procedure or technique.

45.4 Summary

US is no longer an emerging technology. It is a routinely employed diagnostic and therapeutic modality necessary for the optimal care of patients with thyroid and parathyroid disorders. Educational opportunities to gain fundamental and advanced skills in thyroid, parathyroid, and cervical US are abundant (Table 45.1). The ultimate goal of the training, rigorousness of training, didactic work included, existence and means of post-course assessment as well as ongoing maintenance of skills should be examined carefully to ensure optimal training of the student. US education should be incorporated into training programs at the earliest level possible as it has become a natural extension of the physical examination and is applicable to nearly every area of the body. It should be recognized that the extent of examination and need for information provided by US imaging will vary by clinician specialty.

References

1. Baskin HJ. Thyroid ultrasound-just do it. Thyroid. 2004;14(2):91–2.
2. Bumpous JM, Randolph GW. The expanding utility of office-based ultrasound for the head and neck surgeon. Otolaryngol Clin North Am. 2010;43(6):1203–8.
3. Crocker EF, Jellins J. Grey scale ultrasonic examination of the thyroid gland. Med J Aust. 1978;9:244.
4. Crocker ED, Bautovich GJ, Jellins J. Gray-scale echographic visualisation of parathyroid adenoma. Radiology. 1978;126:233–4.
5. Rozycki GS, Ochsner MG, Jaffin JH, et al. Prospective evaluation of surgeons' use of ultrasound in the evaluation of trauma patients. J Trauma. 1993;34:516–27.
6. Shackford SR, Rogers FB, Osler TM, et al. Focused abdominal sonogram for trauma: the learning curve of nonradiologist clinicians in detecting hemoperitoneum. J Trauma. 1999;46:553–62.
7. Scalea TM, Rodriguez A, Chiu WC, FAST Consensus Conference Committee, et al. Focused Assessment with Sonography for Trauma (FAST): results from an International Consensus Conference. J Trauma. 1999;46:466–72.
8. Rozycki GS, Shackford SR. Ultrasound, what every trauma surgeon should know. J Trauma. 1996;40:1–4.

9. Nagarkatti SS, Mekel M, Sofferman RA, Parangi S. Overcoming obstacles to setting up office-based ultrasound for evaluation of thyroid and parathyroid diseases. Laryngoscope. 2011;121(3):548–54.
10. Sisley AC, Johnson SB, Erickson W, Fortune JB. Use of an Objective Structured Clinical Examination (OSCE) for the assessment of physician performance in the ultrasound evaluation of trauma. J Trauma. 1999;47(4):627–31.
11. Bahner DP, Goldman E, Way D, Royall NA, Liu YT. The State of Ultrasound Education in U.S. Medical Schools: results of a National Survey. Acad Med. 2014;89:1681–6.
12. Accreditation Council for Graduate Medical Education. ACGME Program Requirements for Graduate Medical Education in Emergency Medicine. Effective July 1, 2013. http://www.acgme.org/acgmeweb/Portals/0/PFAssets/2013-PR-FAQ-PIF/110_emergency_medicine_07012013.pdf. Accessed May 23, 2014.
13. Accreditation Council for Graduate Medical Education. ACGME Program Requirements for Graduate Medical Education in Internal Medicine. Effective July 1, 2013. http://www.acgme.org/acgmeweb/Portals/0/PFAssets/2013-PR-FAQ-PIF/140_internal_medicine_07012013.pdf. Accessed May 23, 2014.
14. Accreditation Council for Graduate Medical Education. ACGME Program Requirements for Graduate Medical Education in Diagnostic Radiology. Effective July 1, 2013. https://www.acgme.org/acgmeweb/Portals/0/PFAssets/2013-PR-FAQ-PIF/420_diagnostic_radiology_07012013.pdf. Accessed May 23, 2014.
15. Accreditation Council for Graduate Medical Education. ACGME Program Requirements for Graduate Medical Education in Obstetrics and Gynecology. Effective January 1, 2008. https://www.acgme.org/acgmeweb/Portals/0/PFAssets/ProgramRequirements/220obstetricsandgynecology01012008.pdf. Accessed May 23, 2014.
16. Hoppmann RA, Rao VV, Poston MB, et al. An integrated ultrasound curriculum (iUSC) for medical students: 4-year experience. Crit Ultrasound J. 2011;3:1–12.
17. Rao S, van Holsbeeck L, Musial JL, et al. A pilot study of comprehensive ultrasound education at the Wayne State University School of Medicine: a pioneer year review. J Ultrasound Med. 2008;27:745–9.
18. Tshibwabwa ET, Groves HM, Levine MA. Teaching musculoskeletal ultrasound in the undergraduate medical curriculum. Med Educ. 2007;41:517–8.
19. Angtuaco TL, Hopkins RH, DuBose TJ, Bursac Z, Angtuaco MJ, Ferris EJ. Sonographic physical diagnosis 101: teaching senior medical students basic ultrasound scanning skills using a compact ultrasound system. Ultrasound Q. 2007;23:157–60.
20. Afonso N, Amponsah D, Yang J, et al. Adding new tools to the black bag: introduction of ultrasound into the physical diagnosis course. J Gen Intern Med. 2010;25:1248–52.
21. Hoppmann R, Cook T, Hunt P, et al. Ultrasound in medical education: a vertical curriculum at the University of South Carolina School of Medicine. J S C Med Assoc. 2006;102:330–4.
22. Bahner DP, Adkins EJ, Hughes D, Barrie M, Boulger CT, Royall NA. Integrated medical school ultrasound: development of an ultrasound vertical curriculum. Crit Ultrasound J. 2013;5:1–9.
23. Miller BS, Gauger PG, Broome JT, Burney RE, Doherty GM. An international perspective on ultrasound training and use for thyroid and parathyroid disease. World J Surg. 2010;34(6):1157–63.
24. Blehar DJ, Barton B, Gaspari RJ. Learning curves in emergency ultrasound education. Acad Emerg Med. 2015;22(5):574–82. doi:10.1111/acem.12653.
25. Madsen ME, Konge L, Nørgaard LN, Tabor A, Ringsted C, Klemmensen AK, Ottesen B, Tolsgaard MG. Assessment of performance measures and learning curves for use of a virtual-reality ultrasound simulator in transvaginal ultrasound examination. Ultrasound Obstet Gynecol. 2014;44(6):693–9.
26. Tolsgaard MG, Ringsted C, Dreisler E, Nørgaard LN, Petersen JH, Madsen ME, Freiesleben NL, Sørensen JL, Tabor A. Sustained effect of simulation-based ultrasound training on clinical performance: a randomized trial. Ultrasound Obstet Gynecol. 2015;46(3):312–8.
27. Richardson C, Bernard S, Dinh VA. A cost-effective, gelatin-based phantom model for learning ultrasound-guided fine-needle aspiration procedures of the head and neck. J Ultrasound Med. 2015; 34(8):1479–84.
28. Bude RO, Adler RS. An easily made, low-cost, tissue-like ultrasound phantom material. J Clin Ultrasound. 1995;23(4):271–3.
29. Baskin HJ. New applications of thyroid and parathyroid ultrasound. Minerva Endocrinol. 2004;29(4):195–206.
30. Miller BS. Perspective: laryngoscopy of vocal cords avoided with ultrasound. ACS Surg News. 2015; 11(7):17. http://www.acssurgerynews.com/viewdf.html?file=fileadmin/content_pdf/sn/past_issues/SURG_JUL2015_LowRes.
31. Parangi S. Translaryngeal vocal cord ultrasound: ready for prime time. Surgery. 2015;159:67. doi:10.1016/j.surg.2015.10.014. pii: S0039-6060(15)00841-7.

Index

M. Milas et al. (eds.), *Advanced Thyroid and Parathyroid Ultrasound*,
DOI 10.1007/978-3-319-44100-9

V

W

MIX
Papier aus verantwortungsvollen Quellen
Paper from responsible sources
FSC® C105338

If you have any concerns about our products,
you can contact us on
ProductSafety@springernature.com

In case Publisher is established outside the EU,
the EU authorized representative is:
Springer Nature Customer Service Center GmbH
Europaplatz 3, 69115 Heidelberg, Germany

Printed by Libri Plureos GmbH
in Hamburg, Germany